HOSPITAL
PHARMACY

HOSPITAL PHARMACY

William E. Hassan, Jr., Ph.D., LL.B., FACA, FACHA

Vice President and General Counsel
Brigham and Women's Hospital, Inc.
A teaching hospital of the Harvard Medical School.

Chairman
Board of Trustees
Massachusetts College of Pharmacy and Allied Health
Sciences

Formerly:

Pharmacist-in-Chief
Peter Bent Brigham Hospital

Adjunct Professor of Hospital Pharmacy
Massachusetts College of Pharmacy

Fifth Edition

Lea & Febiger

Philadelphia   1986

Lea & Febiger
600 Washington Square
Philadelphia, PA 19106-4198
U.S.A.
(215) 922-1330

First Edition, 1965

Second Edition, 1967
  Reprinted September, 1968

Third Edition, 1973
  Reprinted February, 1977

Fourth Edition, 1981

Fifth Edition, 1986

Library of Congress Cataloging-in-Publication Data

Hassan, William E.
  Hospital pharmacy.

  Includes bibliographies and index.
  1. Hospital pharmacies. I. Title. [DNLM:
1. Pharmacy Service, Hospital. WX 179 H353h]
RA975.5.P5H3   1986   362.1′782   85-16027
ISBN 0-8121-1014-5

Printed in the United States of America

Print number   3   2   1

PREFACE

Since the publication of the first edition of *Hospital Pharmacy* in 1965, the institutional practice of pharmacy has made great progress. Professional hospital and clinical pharmacists now practice in hospitals, extended care facilities, nursing homes, neighborhood health centers and satellite clinics. Within these environments, pharmacists contribute to the triad of *patient care, teaching* and *research* through clinical programs involving the taking of patient drug histories, maintaining patient drug profiles and providing surveillance for drug interactions. Also, of great importance are programs in unit dose dispensing, preparation of hyperalimentation fluids, drug abuse education, drug utilization review, the development of systems for the control of drugs, poison control centers and post-marketing surveillance of prescription drugs.

Notwithstanding the above cited developments within the profession, the original purposes and scope of the book as well as my philosophy relative to the methodology of presentation have not changed. Thus, new material has been added and no longer pertinent subjects have been deleted. Hopefully, the end result is a useful text which permits the teacher the opportunity to provide the student with academically cogent supplementary data via classroom lectures, yet provides the practitioner guidance in the development of a pharmaceutical service to meet the needs of the particular institution served.

Thanks and appreciation are hereby extended to all of my friends, colleagues and organizations who have offered their counsel and suggestions for the improvement of the book. All material quoted from the American Society of Hospital Pharmacists, Joint Commission on Accreditation of Hospitals and National Association of Boards of Pharmacy is copyrighted and used with their permission.

Boston, Massachusetts WILLIAM E. HASSAN, JR.

CONTENTS

1

Introduction

The specialty of hospital pharmacy has been defined as follows:[1]

... the department or service in a hospital which is under the direction of a professionally competent, legally qualified pharmacist, and from which all medications are supplied to the nursing units and other services, where special prescriptions are filled for patients in the hospital, where prescriptions are filled for ambulatory patients and out-patients, where pharmaceuticals are manufactured in bulk, where narcotic and other prescribed drugs are dispensed, where biologicals are stored and dispensed, where injectable preparations should be prepared and sterilized, and where professional supplies are often stocked and dispensed.

Although the above definition may have been applicable at the time that it was written, the modern practice of hospital pharmacy involves much more. The computerization of the pharmacy department makes it possible for the staff to participate in patient education programs, poison control center activities, preparation of patient drug use profiles, parenteral nutrition program participation, cooperating in the teaching and research programs of the hospital, communicating new product information to nursing service and other hospital personnel and dispensing radiopharmaceuticals.

With such a broad definition of purpose, one might wonder about the origin of this branch of the profession of pharmacy. According to Urdang,[2] the hospital pharmacist was the first recognized representative of the pharmaceutical profession. He states that hospital pharmacists were employed in the hospitals which were a part of many early monasteries. Many of the descriptions of these old hospitals include a description of the "apothecary shop" and its garden for the cultivation of medicinal herbs.

From this ancient period, hospital pharmacy passes into the early American era, 1752 to be exact, when Pennsylvania Hospital, the first in North America was opened, with Jonathan Roberts as its hospital pharmacist. Since this historic date, two hundred and twenty-nine years have passed, and a number of outstanding persons associated with the hospital pharmacy have received professional recognition and the accolade of pharmaceutical historians.

The greatest strides in the profession were made in the early 1940s.

It was during this period that the American Society of Hospital Pharmacists was formed, August 21, 1942. Besides the formation of a distinct professional society, the other major contributing factors were the publishing of the Society's official organ, the *American Journal of Hospital Pharmacy,* the formation of affiliated chapters at the state level, the acceptance of the Society as a member of the United States Pharmacopoeial Convention, the establishment of minimum standards for pharmacies in hospitals, the institution of internships and training programs in connection with accredited colleges of pharmacy, and the institutes and continuing education programs which the Society has cosponsored with its affiliates and other hospital organizations. These are only a few of the many advances made by this hitherto unheard-of body of pharmacists. It is no wonder that those who have watched this remarkable progress during the past 3 decades foresee an even brighter and more successful future.

Today, the prognosticators of the past can take pride in their prediction of the progress to be made in the practice of hospital pharmacy. Clearly, the definition cited in the opening paragraph of this chapter is deficient in that it does not encompass the newer areas of institutional pharmacy practice. Of necessity, it must include the responsibility for unit dose, hyperalimentation, intravenous additive, and educational and clinical pharmacy programs. In certain locales, it could even involve participation in scientific and administrative research endeavors. By the same token, such activities as bulk manufacturing and dispensing of professional supplies should properly be de-emphasized.

In 1982 there were 6983 hospitals registered by the American Hospital Association. Community hospitals numbered approximately 5800 and large hospitals (those with 400 or more beds) numbered 605. Hospitals in 1982 handled 36,379,000 admissions, performed 19,539,639 surgical operations, delivered 3,514,457 babies and treated 248,124,000 ambulatory patients. The average daily census was 762,000 patients and the average length of stay was 7.6 days. Community hospital expenditures totaled $104.9 billion in 1982. Payroll represented 48.3% of community hospital expenditures for more than $8.8 billion.

Average inpatient revenue per inpatient day was $392.11 in U.S. community hospitals in 1982. Revenue per inpatient day showd a strong correlation to hospital size. As community hospitals increased in size, so did the inpatient revenue, ranging from $270.66 per day for hospitals with fewer than 25 beds to $451.79 per day for those with 500 beds or more. Total revenue for outpatient care in community hospitals was $16.7 billion in 1982.

Many modern hospital administrators, after surveying this tremendous purchase and use of drugs, have suddenly realized that only trained pharmaceutical personnel are capable of storing, handling, pricing, and dispensing these products. As a result, many hospitals have retained the services of a pharmacist either on a full-time or part-time basis.

The presence of adequate pharmaceutical personnel in many hospitals has benefited both patient and staff members, for hospital manufacture of various pharmaceutical products as well as parenteral solutions has reduced the cost of medication. In addition, it enables the members of the staff to prescribe mixtures which require compounding skill. Also, hospital pharmacists have become involved in the preparation of hyperalimentation products, dialysis fluids, intravenous additive programs, unit dose packaging and unit dose dispensing. Without the knowledge possessed by a trained pharmacist, these preparations could not be properly or safely prepared in the hospital.

Whereas in the past, pharmacists acted as pharmacologic advisor to the physician concerning the pharmacology, toxicology, and posology of the new classes of drugs, today this clinical role has expanded to the point where it is a specialty unto itself. These clinical pharmacists are involved in the preparation of patient drug profiles, recording patient drug history, advising physicians of possible drug-drug interactions and drug effects on clinical laboratory test results.

Because of their special training, hospital pharmacists are now serving on the faculties of many of the hospital schools of nursing, teaching courses in pharmaceutical mathematics and pharmacology. This particular duty helps immeasurably to strengthen the professional bond between these two allied health professions.

In addition, the hospital pharmacists of today's hospitals serve on such vital committees as the Pharmacy and Therapeutics Committee, the Safety Committee, Committee on Standardization, the Antibiotics Committee, the Committee on Environmental Sepsis, the Policy Committee of the Administrative Staff, Research Committee, Planning Committee, Loss Control Risk Management Committee and the Ambulatory Care Committee.

These paragraphs have briefly summed up the past and present of hospital pharmacy. Consideration must now be given to its future.

The American Hospital Association has registered 6,983 hospitals. Of these, about 1,000 hospitals are more than 200-bed capacity, whereas the remainder of them have 100 or fewer beds. It is in the hospitals of no more than 100 beds that the greatest challenge for providing adequate pharmaceutical services exists. Statistics show that less than 70% of all hospitals possess a pharmacy.

With these figures in mind, it would seem that the profession of hospital pharmacy must now satisfy a newly recognized need, that of placing a hospital pharmacist in every hospital throughout the country. This is necessary since the hospital pharmacist, in his new role, is a vital link in the chain of health professions dedicated to the care of hospitalized patients.

Another advantage to the hospital resulting from the specialized training of the hospital pharmacist manifests itself in the smaller hospital. In these institutions, the individual serving as a hospital pharmacist may also serve as an assistant to the administrator, purchasing agent, supervisor of the central sterile supply room and in some instances as a laboratory technician. By combining his duties, a hospital pharmacist is within the financial reach of every hospital, irrespective of size.

Archambault,[4] in a study on the manpower needs of hospital pharmacists, arrived at the conclusion that there is an annual need for more than 400 hospital pharmacists.

Competition for the services of qualified hospital and clinical pharmacists by hospitals is best evidenced by a perusal of some of the listings in hospital journals. It will be noted that many positions are available and range from staff pharmacist to Chief Pharmacist. Salaries range from $30,000 to $60,000 or more depending upon the size and location of the hospital. Some of the inducements offered include 4 weeks' vacation with pay, liberal sick leave, meals free while on duty, 100% hospital paid health policy for the pharmacist and his/her family, hospitalization, pension plan, and 9 to 11 paid holidays. The work week ranged from a low of 35 hours to a high of 44 hours with the majority of institutions adhering to the standard 40 hours.

Dr. Charles Letourneau,[5] a consultant in a hospital administration and Editorial Director of the Journal, *Hospital Management,* wrote—

". . . the function of the hospital pharmacist is vital not only to the professional care of the patient but to the management of the hospital as well. The management function of the hospital pharmacist is a relatively recent concept which is rapidly achieving recognition in the hospital field. Hospital administration is the coordination of men, money and materials to provide facilities to assist a physician to treat his patient. The pharmacist participates in hospital administration in addition to his professional obligations."

Should the profession meet the challenge of the future, the opportunities and resources of institutional pharmacy practice would be greatly increased. With this increase, it is inevitable that new young blood with administrative and clinical qualifications must be attracted to the profession in sufficient quantity to make this a profession with a notable past, a noble and invigorating present, and a brilliant future.

The following ASHP *Statement of Goals for Institutional Pharmacy* was developed by the ASHP Council on Professional Affairs, approved by the ASHP Board of Directors on March 20, 1980 and by the ASHP House of Delegates on April 21, 1980.

ASHP STATEMENT OF GOALS FOR INSTITUTIONAL PHARMACY

Just as any organization must have long-range goals toward which its daily activities are directed, so must a profession, its members, and their representative societies. This document, intended to be a basic statement of purpose for the American Society of Hospital Pharmacists and its membership, has been prepared with this in mind.

The American Society of Hospital Pharmacists, in its Constitution and Bylaws, sets forth the following objectives:

1. To provide the benefits of a qualified hospital pharmacist to patients and health care institutions, to the allied health professions, and to the profession of pharmacy.
2. To assist in providing an adequate supply of such qualified hospital pharmacists.
3. To assure a high quality of professional practice through the establishment and maintenance of standards of professional ethics, education, and attainments and through the promotion of economic welfare.
4. To promote research in hospital pharmacy practices and in the pharmaceutical sciences in general.
5. To disseminate pharmaceutical knowledge by providing for interchange of information among hospital pharmacists and with members of allied specialties and professions.

More broadly, the Society's primary purpose is the advancement of rational, patient-oriented drug therapy in hospitals and other organized health care settings.[a]

To the preceding can be added the following objectives:

1. To expand and strengthen institutional pharmacists' abilities to: (a) effectively manage an organized pharmaceutical service; (b) develop and provide clinical services[b]; (c) conduct and participate in clinical and pharmaceutical research; (d) conduct and participate in educational programs for health practitioners, students, and the public.
2. To increase the knowledge and understanding of contemporary institutional pharmacy practice by the public, government, pharmaceutical industry, and other health care professionals.
3. To promote compensation and benefits commensurate with pharmacists' responsibilities and contributions to patient care.
4. To help provide an adequate supply of qualified supportive personnel for institutional pharmacy services.
5. To help ensure that health care reimbursement and payment systems do not inhibit the implementation of innovative pharmaceutical services or adversely reflect on institutional pharmacy practice.

---

[a]Directions for the American Society of Hospital Pharmacists in organized health care delivery. *Am J Hosp Pharm.* 1975; 32:702–3.

[b]ASHP statement on clinical functions in institutional pharmacy practice. *Am J Hosp Pharm.* 1978; 35:813.

6. To assist in the development and advancement of the pharmacy profession.

The foregoing serves as a collective statement of goals of the Society and its constituency. Transforming these goals into realities will require the dedicated efforts of all institutional pharmacists, both as individuals and as members of the Society.

Minimum Standards

The original *Minimum Standard for Pharmacies in Hospitals* was developed and adopted by the American College of Surgeons in 1935. A revised version was adopted by the American Society of Hospital Pharmacists in 1950 and such was approved by the American Pharmaceutical Association. Later, a *"Guide to Application"* for each of the six sections of the *Minimum Standard* was appended as supplementary material. This *"Guide to Application"* was developed by the American Society of Hospital Pharmacists without approval from other organizations. Thus, there is an important differentiation which must be recognized between the two documents—the former is an official document, whereas the latter is supplementary information.

Because the new practitioner and the student may not have available to them the journals carrying the *ASHP Guidelines Minimum Standard for Pharmacies in Institutions,* they are hereinafter reproduced in detail.[7]

ASHP GUIDELINES: MINIMUM STANDARD FOR PHARMACIES IN INSTITUTIONS[a]

Am J Hosp Pharm. 1985; 42:372–5

Pharmaceutical services[b] in institutions have numerous components, the most prominent being (1) the procurement, distribution, and control of all pharmaceuticals used within the facility, (2) the evaluation and dissemination of comprehensive information about drugs and their use to the institution's staff and patients, and (3) the monitoring, evaluation, and assurance of the quality of drug use. These functions are carried out in cooperation with other institutional departments and programs.

---

[a]Approved by the ASPH Board of Directors, November 14–15, 1984. Revised by the ASHP Council on Clinical Affairs. Supersedes the previous version, which was approved on August 1, 1977.

[b]The terms "pharmaceutical services" and "pharmacy" as used in this document are synonymous. The term "pharmacist" is used in the collective sense, referring to the pharmacy staff.

The primary function of this document is to serve as a guide for the development and provision of pharmaceutical services in institutions. It will also be useful in evaluating the scope and quality of these services. It does not, however, provide detailed instructions for operating a pharmacy—other Society publications serve this function.

Standard I: Administration

The pharmaceutical service shall[a] be directed by a professionally competent, legally qualified pharmacist. He or she must be on the same level within the institution's administrative structure as directors of other clinical services. The director of pharmaceutical services[b] is responsible for (1) setting the long- and short-range goals of the pharmacy based on developments and trends in health care and institutional pharmacy practice and the specific needs of the institution, (2) developing a plan and schedule for achieving these goals, (3) supervising the implementation of the plan and the day-to-day activities associated with it, and (4) determining if the goals and schedule are being met and instituting corrective actions where necessary.

The director of pharmaceutical services, in carrying out these tasks, shall employ an adequate number of completent and qualified personnel.

- The director of pharmaceutical services must be thoroughly knowledgeable about hospital pharmacy practice and management. He or she should have completed a pharmacy residency program accredited by the American Society of Hospital Pharmacists.
- Sufficient supportive personnel (technical, clerical, secretarial) shall be available in order to minimize the use of pharmacists in nonjudgmental tasks. Appropriate supervisory controls[c] for supportive personnel must be maintained.
- The director of pharmaceutical services shall assure that work schedules, procedures, and assignments use pharmacy personnel and resources in the most efficient manner possible.
- All personnel must possess the education and training needed for their responsibilities. Competence of all staff must be maintained through relevant continuing-education programs and activities.
- Personnel must be selected and assigned solely on the basis of job-related qualifications and performance. The employment and discharge of pharmacy personnel shall be the responsibility of the director of pharmaceutical services. There should be an established procedure, based on

---

[a]The terms "shall" and "must" are used to indicate a mandatory statement. The term "should" reflects the commonly accepted or recommended method; it permits the use of equally effective alternatives.

[b]The title "director of pharmaceutical services" or a similar title is preferred over "chief pharmacist" or "consultant pharmacist."

[c]Any system of control which assures the quality of the outcome of the work performed by supportive personnel is deemed to be "appropriate."

predetermined objectives, for orienting new personnel to the pharmacy and their respective positions. Procedures for the routine evaluation of pharmacy personnel performance shall be established.

- Lines of authority and areas of responsibility within the pharmacy shall be clearly defined. Written position descriptions for all categories of pharmacy personnel must be prepared and revised as necessary.
- An operations manual governing all pharmacy functions should be prepared. It should be continually revised to reflect changes in procedures, organization, etc. All pharmacy personnel should be familiar with the contents of the manual.
- Policies and procedures for managing drug expenditures should be established. They should include such methods as controlled formularies, competitive bid and group purchasing, drug-use review programs, and cost-effective clinical services.
- The director of pharmaceutical services should prepare periodic reports to the institution's administration containing qualitative and quantitative information on the pharmacy's activities for the period plus the current position of the pharmacy with respect to its long- and short-range plans. These reports require that a system for routinely monitoring pharmacy workload and expenses be established. The system should provide for the determination and analysis of the amounts and costs of drugs and services furnished to specific patients and/or patient categories.
- There shall be an ongoing, systematic program for assuring the quality of pharmaceutical services. This program should be integrated with the institution's organized quality assurance program.
- Hospitals provide services to patients 24 hours a day. Pharmaceutical services are an integral part of the total care provided by the hospital, and the services of a pharmacist should, therefore, be available at all times. Where around-the-clock operation of the pharmacy is not feasible, a pharmacist must be available on an "on-call" basis. The use of night cabinets and drug dispensing by nonpharmacists should be minimized and eliminated wherever possible.
- Some small facilities may not require, or be able to obtain, the services of a full-time pharmacist. However, it should be noted that the concepts, principles, and recommendations contained in this standard apply to *all* hospitals, regardless of size or type. Thus, the part-time director of pharmaceutical services has the same basic obligations and responsibilities as his or her full-time counterpart in the larger institution.
- The relevant standards and guidelines of the American Society of Hospital Pharmacists and the Joint Commission on Accreditation of Hospitals must be adhered to regardless of the particular financial and organizational arrangements by which pharmaceutical services are provided to the facility and its patients.

Standard II: Facilities

There shall be adequate space, equipment, and supplies for the professional and administrative functions of the pharmacy.

- The pharmacy shall be located in an area (or areas) that facilitate(s) the provision of services to patients. It must be integrated with the facility's communication and transportation systems.

- Space and equipment, in an amount and type to provide secure, environmentally controlled storage of drugs, shall be available.
- There shall be designated space and equipment suitable for the preparation of sterile products and other drug compounding and packaging operations.
- The pharmacy should have a private area for pharmacist-patient consultations. The director of pharmaceutical services should also have a private office or area.
- Current drug information resources must be available. These should include appropriate pharmacy and medical journals and texts and drug literature search and retrieval resources.

Standard III: Drug Distribution and Control

The pharmacy shall be responsible for the procurement, distribution, and control of *all* drugs used within the institution. This responsibility extends to drugs and related services provided to ambulatory patients. Policies and procedures governing these functions shall be developed by the pharmacist with input from other involved hospital staff (e.g., nurses) and committees (pharmacy and therapeutics committee, patient-care committee, etc.). In doing so, it is essential that the pharmacist routinely be present in all patient-care areas, establish rapport with the personnel, and become familiar with and contribute to medical and nursing procedures relating to drugs.

- The pharmacist shall maintain an up-to-date formulary of drug products approved for use in the institution. While the items to be included in the formulary are selected by the pharmacy and therapeutics committee (or its equivalent), it is the pharmacist's responsibility to establish specifications for these drug products and to select their source of supply. In doing so, it is advisable that written specifications for multisource items be prepared and used in the acquisition process.
- Policies and procedures controlling the use of investigational drugs (if used in the institution) shall be developed and followed. The pharmacy shall be responsible for storing, packaging, labeling, distributing, and maintaining inventory records of investigational drugs. It should also be responsible (in cooperation with the principal investigator) for providing information about these drugs.
- There shall be a procedure for providing drugs and pharmaceutical services in the event of a disaster.
- Written policies governing the activities of medical sales representatives within the hospital shall be prepared and approved by the pharmacy and therapeutics committee. Sales representatives should receive a copy of these policies and their activities should be controlled. The use of drug samples within the institution should be eliminated to the extent possible. However, if the use of drug samples is permitted, they must be controlled and distributed only through the pharmacy.
- The pharmacist must review the physician's original order, or a direct copy thereof, prior to dispensing any drug (except for emergency use). There shall be no transcribing of medication orders by nursing or clerical staffs (except for their own records). Hospitalwide and pharmacy stand-

alone computer systems must be secure against unauthorized entry. All systems must provide for review and verification of the physician's original order before the drug is dispensed.

- A medication profile for all inpatients and all (or selected) outpatients shall be maintained and used.
- The pharmacist must institute the control procedures needed to ensure that patients receive the correct drugs at the proper times. In accomplishing this, it is necessary that all drugs used in the institution (including i.v. fluids) be distributed by the pharmacy. All drugs must be packaged, labeled, and distributed in a manner that meets applicable professional standards and legal requirements. An accountability system for controlled substances that meets all applicable governmental requirements must be maintained.
- In the interest of patient safety, all drugs dispensed by the pharmacist for administration to patients should be in single unit packages and, to the extent possible, in ready-to-administer form. The need for nurses to manipulate drugs (i.e., withdraw doses from multidose containers, label containers, etc.) prior to their administration should be minimized; thus, the unit dose system of preparing and distributing drugs should be used.
- Pharmacy personel shall prepare all sterile products (e.g., chemotherapy injections, continuous and intermittent i.v. preparations, irrigation solutions), except in emergencies.
- The pharmacist, in cooperation with hospital staff, must establish policies and procedures for handling drugs that are putative occupational hazards. The procedures should maintain the integrity of the drug and protect hospital personnel.
- Floor stocks of drugs must be kept as small as possible and limited to drugs for emergency use and routinely used "safe" items, such as mouthwash and antiseptic solutions. All drug storage areas within the hospital must be routinely inspected to ensure that no outdated or unusable items are present, that all stock items are properly labeled and stored, etc.[a]
- There shall be a system for removing from use any drugs subjected to a product recall.
- When feasible, the pharmacist should prepare those drug formulations, strenths, dosage forms, and packages that are not available commercially but which are useful in the care of patients. Adequate quality assurance procedures shall be developed for these operations.
- A written stop-order policy or other system shall be established to ensure that drug orders are not inappropriately continued.
- Policies and procedures shall be established for the identification and use of medications brought into the institution by patients.

Standard IV: Drug Information

The pharmacy is responsible for providing the institution's staff and patients with accurate, comprehensive information about drugs and their use and shall serve as its center for drug information.

- The pharmacist (in cooperation with the organization's librarian, if any)

---

[a]Examples of nursing unit inspection forms are available upon request from the American Society of Hospital Pharmacists.

is responsible for maintaining up-to-date drug information resources (both in the pharmacy and at patient-care areas) and using them effectively. The pharmacist, in addition to supplying specific drug information, must be able to furnish objective evaluations of the drug literature and to provide informed opinion on drug-related matters.

- The pharmacist must keep the institution's staff well informed about the drugs used in the institution and their various dosage forms and packagings. This is accomplished through newsletters, seminars, displays, etc., developed by the pharmacy. No drug shall be administerd unless the medical and nursing personnel have received adequate information about, and are familiar with, its therapeutic use, adverse effects, and dosage.
- The pharmacist must help ensure that all patients are given adequate information about the drugs they receive. This is particularly important for ambulatory, home care, and discharge patients. These patient education activities shall be coordinated with the nursing and medical staffs and patient education department (if any).

Standard V: Assuring Rational Drug Therapy

An important aspect of pharmaceutical services is that of maximizing rational drug use. In this regard, the pharmacist, in concert with the medical staff, must develop policies and procedures for assuring the quality of drug therapy.

- Sufficient patient information must be collected, maintained, and reviewed by the pharmacist to ensure meaningful and effective participation in patient care. This requires that a medication profile be maintained for all inpatients and for those ambulatory patients routinely receiving care at the hospital. A pharmacist-conducted medication history from patients may be useful in this regard.
- All physicians' medication orders (except in emergency situations) must be reviewed for appropriateness by the pharmacist prior to the dispensing of the first dose. Any questions regarding the order must be resolved with the prescriber at this time and a written notation of these discussions made in the chart or copy of the physician's order. The nursing staff must be informed of any changes made in the order.
- The pharmacist, in cooperation with the pharmacy and therapeutics committee, shall develop a mechanism for the reporting and review (by the committee or other appropriate medical staff group) of adverse drug reactions.
- Appropriate clinical information about patients must be available and accessible to the pharmacist for use in his or her daily practice activities.
- The pharmacist must review each patient's drug regimen on a concurrent basis and directly communicate any suggested changes to the prescriber.
- A formalized drug-use program, developed and conducted jointly with the medical staff, shall be initiated and integrated with the overall hospital patient-care evaluation program. This program should include, but not be limited to, the use of antibiotics and other anti-infective agents.
- The pharmacist must actively participate in developing and maintaining the hospital formulary. This is particularly important in small hospitals lacking the services of various medical specialists.

- The pharmacist shall be a member of the pharmacy and therapeutics, infection control, patient-care, use review, and other committees where input concerning the use of drugs is required.

Standard VI: Research

The pharmacist should conduct, participate in, and support medical and pharmaceutical research appropriate to the goals, objectives, and resources of the pharmacy and the institution.

- The pharmacist should maintain adequate information on all investigational drug studies and similar research projects involving drugs in which the facility's patients are participants.
- The pharmacist should be represented on the institution's Institutional Review Board.
- The pharmacist shall ensure that policies and procedures for the safe and proper use of investigational drugs are established and followed.

Supplemental References

The American Society of Hospital Pharmacists (4630 Montgomery Avenue, Bethesda, MD 20814) has numerous publications which elaborate on many of the concepts embodied in this Standard. They are described in the Society's publications catalog, available upon request.

ABILITIES REQUIRED OF HOSPITAL PHARMACISTS

The American Society of Hospital Pharmacists and the American Association of Colleges of Pharmacy, recognizing the specialty of hospital pharmacy and the fact that qualified practitioners must be specially educated, have developed and approved *ASHP Guidelines on the Competencies Required in Institutional Pharmacy Practice.*

For the convenience of the practitioner and student, the *Statement* is hereinafter reproduced.[8]

ASHP GUIDELINES ON THE COMPETENCIES REQUIRED IN INSTITUTIONAL PHARMACY PRACTICE[a]

Preface

The practice of pharmacy in health care institutions continues to undergo evolutionary and even radical changes. It has changed to a personal health service charged with assuring pharmaceutic and therapeutic appropriateness of all its functions in the care of patients. Professional, societal, governmental and economic factors will continue to force further changes and the pharmacist practicing in an institution must be ready not only to adapt to these changes but to take the lead in introducing them. In all cases, the basis for the institutional pharmacist's contribution to health care is a thorough knowledge of drugs and their actions. To bring this expertise to bear in the most effective manner, the institutional pharmacist must interact and cooperate closely with all other health professionals practicing in the institution and he must assist the patient and the patient's family to cope with the problems of illness.

It is recognized that a large and diverse body of expertise is required in the operation of a pharmacy department. No one pharmacist may possess or have opportunity to demonstrate this breadth of expertise. For a variety of reasons, some institutions offer greater opportunity than others for the pharmacist to use his unique skills. All institutional pharmacists should, however, develop minimal competencies in each area and be capable of becoming expert in any one or several of them. This requires more than casual acquaintance with a broad area of knowledge and emphasizes the need for a sound professional education grounded on a firm base of physical, biological and social sciences.

This statement addresses itself to the various competencies which must be demonstrated collectively by the professional staff of an institutional pharmacy department. The statement recognizes not only the need for but the responsibility of a department to make pharmaceutical services available to both inpatients and ambulatory patients as well as to promote the rational use of drugs by health professionals and the public. The department must participate in all programs and functions of the institution where pharmaceutical expertise is needed. The professional staff of the pharmacy department must have the ability to carry out collectively the following service functions.

I. Effective Administration and Management of a Pharmacy Department in an Institution

The successful delivery of any pharmacy service offered will be based on expert management and administrative procedures. The director of pharmacy services or personnel specializing in departmental administration must be familiar with the health care system in general and the specific function of the institution in particular so that the pharmacy's goals can be achieved in cooperation with all other departments in the institution and with other programs that insure continuity of care for the patient.

Broad areas of administrative and management responsibilities include planning and integrating professional services, budgeting, inventory control, cost review, cost effectiveness, audit, maintenance of records and preparation of reports. As a basis for this responsibility, pharmacy personnel must be thoroughly familiar with the organization of a hospital, with staff and line relationships and with appropriate lines of communication.

Pharmacy activities must be coordinated with medical, nursing and other services and with the administrative elements of the hospital. Pharmacy administrative personnel must be able to prepare suitable written communications to the hospital staff concerning pertinent pharmacy matters.

The director of pharmacy services, or his designee, is responsible for the justification and accountability of all pharmaceutical services in terms of patient care and the expenditure of funds. He must be able to analyze and interpret prescribing trends and the economic impact of new drug developments, which for budgeting purposes are translated to his forecast of future drug expenditures. He must maintain an adequate system of stock and inventory control. He must have the ability to control operational costs without compromising services.

The director of pharmacy services is responsible for records on all pharmacy operations which may be legally or administratively required. The data collected should be translated into periodic or special reports. These may include, but usually are not limited to, data on prescriptions dispensed, controlled drugs dispensed, drug purchases, inspections and improvements in operations. The use of automated data processing systems may allow more effective and efficient handling of pharmacy records and data. A basic knowledge and understanding of the applications of such systems to pharmacy operations is important to the department.

II. Assimilation and Provision of Comprehensive Information on Drugs and Their Actions

Fundamental to the pharmacist's contribution to health care is his knowledge of drugs and their actions. The pharmacy department is the primary source of information concerning drugs. The pharmacy must maintain the appropriate information sources and develop mechanisms for evaluating information and transmitting it to the institution's professional staff and to patients.

The pharmacist must have the ability to use his basic science knowledge and his knowledge of the effects of drugs on biological systems in assessing such determinants of drug action as absorption, distribution, metabolism and excretion of a drug; drug interactions with other drugs, foods or diagnostic agents; effects of a disease state on the drug's action; and miscellaneous patient and drug variables. Thus, the pharmacist practicing in an institution must be knowledgeable in chemistry, pharmacology, toxicology, pathophysiology, pharmaceutics, therapeutics, and patient care techniques, and he should have some background in the social sciences.

III. Development and Conduct of a Product Formulation and Packaging Program

Frequently, the institutional pharmacist must respond to the need for special dosage forms and formulations not available commercially. Not infrequently, this also involves a knowledge of appropriate packaging. An adequate understanding of the principles involved in the formulation and preparation of pharmaceutical dosage forms is needed. This involves the concepts of biopharmaceutics, bioavailability, pharmacokinetics, pharmaceutics, stability, physicochemical, kinetics, microbiology, quality assurance and techniques of medication administration. In some instances, as in the case of intravenous admixtures and total parenteral nutrition, the pharmacist must also be familiar with patient variables such as electrolyte and fluid balance, and such factors as personal hygiene, environmental control and equipment performance. Similar concepts hold true in radiopharmacy. Furthermore, the pharmacist must be able to evaluate the economic factors involved, including the cost of labor, raw materials, space, equipment depreciation and other items of fixed overhead.

IV. Conduct of and Participation in Research

The institutional pharmacist must be prepared to participate in clinical research originated by the medical staff and to conduct pharmaceutical research or initiate research himself. In doing so, he may act as the principal or coprincipal investigator or he may use the resources of the department to support a particular research study. The pharmacist must be able to establish a data base, either for the drugs being used or the patients participating in the study. Equally important, he must have the ability to collect appropriate data, interpret them, apply the conclusions drawn from the data and transmit the results in an adequate manner.

An educational background with appropriate orientation and training in research methodology, including criteria for and structure of a research report, is mandatory.

V. Development and Conduct of Patient-oriented Services

Pharmacy, as practiced in health care institutions, is developing a wide spectrum of clinical services which have become part of overall pharmaceutical service but may not be directly associated with drug distribution. Fundamental to these clinical services is the pharmacist's knowledge of drugs, diseases and patient and drug variables, and his ability to interact closely on a personal basis with other health professionals. Academic training in such areas as toxicology, pathophysiology and therapeutics, as well as extensive clinical experience, provide the background for a pharmacist to function in this clinical role.

These services include (1) drug information, which encompasses the collection, organization, retrieval, interpretation and evaluation of the applicable literature and the ability to present the excerpted data in an appropriate fashion; (2) collection of the pharmacy patient data base; (3) patient education; (4) the monitoring (either subjectively or objectively) and auditing of therapeutic regimens; (5) drug use review; (6) the monitoring of specific adverse drug reactions to decrease their incidence; and (7) other similar functions designed to improve patient care by optimizing drug use. Further, clinical functions may extend to the pharmacist's role in primary care as well as in the management of chronic care patients.

VI. Conduct of and Participation in Educational Activities

A wide range of educational activities is performed routinely in the institution and involves all health practitioners and students of the various health professions. The director of pharmacy services, or his designee, is responsible for coordinating the department's contribution to these educational activities. Further, he is responsible for training new personnel and for carrying on a continuous educational program for pharmacists and pharmacy supportive personnel. In institutions having a pharmacy residency program, the pharmacist must develop a well planned and coordinated program so that the residency is a meaningful educational experience in the development of future practitioners. In institutions offering a pharmacy residency program in conjunction with an academic program, the pharmacist must have a thorough understanding of his own program and the course material and objectives of the academic phase to assist in coordinating one with the other.

VII. Development and Conduct of a Quality Assurance Program for Pharmaceutical Services

A major responsibility of the department must be the assurance of the quality of its services and of products dispensed, coupled with a control program for the distribution of drugs throughout the institution.

The pharmacist must conduct service audits, either by process or outcome, or both, to assure the quality of patient care services rendered and to assure the appropriate patient benefit of all pharmaceutical services offered.

RESEARCH IN HOSPITAL PHARMACY

It has been stated that for hospital pharmacy to continue its advancement as a contributing member of the health professions, it must encourage its practitioners towards greater participation in research.

To achieve this objective the American Society of Hospital Pharmacists issued the following guidelines.[9]*

The promotion of scientific research in institutional pharmacy and in pharmaceutical problems in general is an objective of the American Society of Hospital Pharmacists, as stated in its Constitution and Bylaws. In keeping with this objective, institutional pharmacists should, therefore, have the ability to conduct and participate in research.[1]

There are differing views about the proper function of scientific research. Some feel that the purpose of research is to improve things, while others say that the proper function of research is to establish general laws regarding the behavior of events or objects which may be used to predict. All of these functions are apropos institutional pharmacy research activities. The institutional pharmacist should, to the extent possible, participate in clinical research with other health care disciplines, in pharmaceutical sciences research, and in operations research in pharmaceutical services and systems.

The Nature of Scientific Research

Scientific research is the systematic, controlled, empirical and critical investigation of hypothetical propositions about the presumed relations among natural phenomena.[2]

It is a method of acquiring knowledge based on the faith that there are real things whose characteristics are entirely independent of our opinions about them, and that objective propositions can be stated about them and subject to empirical tests.

There are two broad views of science: the *static* and the *dynamic*.[1] The static view, held by most students and laymen, is that science is an activity that contributes systematized information to the world. The scientist's job is to

---

*Approved by the ASHP Board of Directors, November 15, 1977.

This document replaces the ASHP Guidelines for Scientific Research in Hospital Pharmacy and the ASHP Statement on Research in Hospital Pharmacy.

discover new facts and to add them to the already existing body of information. Science is even conceived to be a body of fact. The emphasis is on the present state of knowledge and adding to it.

The dynamic view regards science more as an activity—what scientists do. The present state of knowledge is considered to be important, but mainly because it is a base for further scientific theory and research. This has been called the heuristic view (meaning serving to discover or reveal). The heuristic view in science emphasizes theory and interconnected conceptual schemata that are fruitful for further research. It is an emphasis upon discovery. The heuristic view stresses problem-solving rather than facts and bodies of information, and distinguishes scientific research from engineering and technology.

Although research is problem-solving, not all problem-solving is research. The difference that distinguishes research is a primary concern for theory, rather than just the immediate answer to one specific problem at one place at one time.

The basic aim of scientific research is theory.[4] A theory is defined as a set of interrelated constructs (concepts), definitions and propositions that presents a systematic view of phenomena by specifing relations among variables, for the purpose of explaining and predicting phenomena. Theory sets out the relationship between variables and explains phenomena by stating what variables are related and how the variables are related.

Theories are general explanations of natural events. Their value lies in their generality, because they can be applied widely and to many people in many places.

Realistically, much that has been identified as research in institutional pharmacy, although often quite valuable, is more accurately described as problem-solving through the use of research methods. The subject matter of such activity has included the development of new pharmaceutical dosage forms, the identification of unknown drugs in poisoning cases, the development of new drug tests and assays, exploratory studies of various aspects of the pharmacist's work role, attitudinal studies of acceptance of innovations, and descriptive studies of drug prescribing, drug use and adverse drug reactions. Many (but not all) of these research "studies" would probably be better identified by such terms as methods improvement studies, product development, demonstration projects with built-in evaluation, etc.

Scientific research in general can be divided by using many different classification schemes, for example:

1. Experimental/nonexperimental
2. Exploratory/descriptive/predictive
3. Whether or not stimulus-variables are under control of the experimenter.

Special Types of Research

Two special types of research are historical research and methodological research.

Historical research is the critical investigation of events, developments and experiences of the past, the careful weighing of evidence, the validating of sources of information on the past and the interpretation of the weighed evidence. The historical investigator collects data, evaluates the data for validity and interprets the data. The historical method, or historiography, differs from scientific research only in its focus upon the past and the peculiarly difficult interpretative tasks imposed by the elusive nature of its subject matter.

Methodological research is the controlled investigation of the theoretical and applied aspects of measurement and ways of attaining and analyzing data. Areas of investigation include the theoretical and practical problems of identifying and measuring variables, including reliability and validity. The application of mathematics (e.g., statistics and predictive equations) may be investigated. Methods of data collection and analysis may be studied.

Scope of Research

Pharmacy is based on the theories of the medical, pharmaceutical and social sciences. Therefore, every pharmacist has an obligation to support the advancement of these sciences through research in order that they may continue to grow. History has shown that the results of such research by practitioners can make a vital contribution to the improvement of patient care, and the support of such research has become one of the fundamental objectives of most health care facilities. It is, therefore, logical and in accord with the fundamental purposes of these facilities that they provide their pharmacists with at least a modest level of resources to control research. Institutions such as university teaching hospitals with a primary emphasis upon research objectives may be expected to provide more elaborate research facilities than other health care facilities.

The amount and quality of the education and training in research possessed by most institutional pharmacists are important, if temporary, limitations in the advance of research in institutional pharmacy. Those pharmacists who do have adequate preparation may, by reason of their training of interests, or both, wish to make their research contribution in any of the several sciences basic to pharmacy practice—pharmacology, pharmacognosy, the social sciences, etc. As research in these fields will require greatly differing needs for facilities and equipment, it is difficult to provide a general recommendation for institutional pharmacy research facilities.

No limit should be placed on the scope of scientific research to be undertaken by the institutional pharmacist. Free and unhindered inquiry is the basic tenet given to all research workers in keeping with skills and facilities available for research. The primary areas for research by institutional pharmacists are those areas in which pharmacists possess a body of knowledge which is uniquely theirs. A research problem involving the delivery of pharmaceutical services would be an example of such an area.

The Scientific Approach

Problem—Obstacle—Idea.[5] The scientist experiences an obstacle to understanding, or curiosity as to why something is as it is. His first step is to get the idea out in the open and express it in some reasonably manageable form. He states the problem, even if ill-defined and tentative.

Hypothesis. The scientist looks back on experience for possible solutions—his own experience, the literature and contacts with other scientists. He formulates an hypothesis, a tentative proposition about the relation between two or more variables. He says, "If such and such occurs, then so and so results."

Reasoning—Deduction. The scientist deduces the consequences of the hypothesis he has formulated. He may find that the deductions formulated as a consequence of his hypothesis cause him to arrive at a new problem quite different from the one with which he started. On the other hand, his deductions may lead him to believe that the problem cannot be solved with existing technical tools. Such reasoning can help lead to wider, more basic, and more significant problems, as well as provide operational (i.e., testable) implications of the original hypothesis.

Observation—Test—Experiment. If the problem has been well stated, the hypotheses adequately formulated and the implications of the hypotheses carefully deduced, this next step is almost automatic for the competent investigator. To test an hypothesis is to test the relation expressed by the hypothesis, that is, the relation between the variables. All testing is for one purpose: putting the problem relation to an empirical test.

It is not the hypotheses that are tested, but the deduced implications of the hypotheses. On the basis of the research evidence, the hypothesis is either accepted or rejected.

Criteria for a Research Report

Area of the Study. The area selected leads meaningfully to some more encompassing concept or theory.

The hypothesis concerns specific problems which are capable of being solved.

The boundaries of the study are limited to practical proportions without being overly simplified to the point of being out of context to the overall problem.

Variables and terms used to identify variables are operationally defined.

Hypotheses are identified clearly and simply.

Evidence is given as to the relationship of this research to the work of others in this area.

Design of the Study. Procedures and methods used are clearly described in order to permit reproducibility. Where interview schedules or questionnaires are used, such items are included with the study report.

The overall plan of this design permits drawing a valid conclusion. Groups used for inferences are equated as to variables, or the inequalities among the groups are compensated for. The design eliminates the possibility of confusing the results or manipulating the desired variable and the results of other variables.

Assumptions underlying the study are given explicit recognition.

The plan of design permits collection of sufficient information to make reliable inferences.

The design allows equal opportunity for evidence that would prove and evidence that would disprove the hypotheses.

The methods of drawing the sample and the universe from which it was drawn are stated clearly.

The representativeness of the population studied to the population to which the reslts are generalized is substantiated.

Consideration is given to the permanency of the results of the study.

Quantitative or qualitative measurements are appropriate for and applicable to the type of data collected.

Statistical treatment is appropriate to the type of data collected, the population and the sample involved.

The statistical results are interpreted correctly.

Evidence is given of the degree of probablility that the statistical results could have been chance variations or errors of measurement.

Conclusion of the Study. All conclusions are justified by the procedures used and the data obtained.

Conclusions *supported* by the data are clearly differentiated from conclusions *suggested* by the data.

The limitations imposed by underlying assumptions are readily admitted when drawing conclusions.

Personal opinions and impressions of the research worker are included only if they are identified as such.

Structure of a Research Report

The structure of a research report is relatively simple and is almost the same as the structure of the research itself: the problem, the methodology and the results. The general outline is as follows:

1. Problem
    a. Theory, hypotheses, definitions
    b. Previous research: the literature
2. Methodology—data collection
    a. Sample and sampling method
    b. How hypotheses were tested, experimental procedures, instrumentation
    c. Measurement of variables
    d. Methods of analysis, statistics
    e. Pretesting and pilot studies
3. Results, interpretation and conclusions

The statement of the general problem sets the general stage for the reader and is usually in question form. A good practice is to state the broader, general problem and then to state the hypotheses, both general and specific. All the important variables should be defined, both in general and in operational terms, giving a justification for the definitions used.

The two reasons for discussing the general and research literature related to the problem are (1) to explain the theoretical rationale of the problem and (2) to tell the reader what research has and has not been carried out on the problem and show that this particular investigation has not been conducted before.

The methodology-data collection section of the report should meticulously describe what was done so as to enable another investigator to reproduce the research, reanalyze the data and arrive at unambiguous conclusions as to the adequacy of the methods and data collection. This criterion may be difficult to meet in a published article in view of the lack of journal space; nevertheless, it remains valid, and such material should be made available in unpublished form to other researchers on request. This section should tell what samples were used, how they were selected and why they were selected. An account of the measurement of the variables of the study must be included.

An account of the data analysis methods used is sometimes included in the methodology section and sometimes in the analysis/interpretations section; in either case, the analysis methods must be outlined and justified. Where pilot studies and pretesting are used, they must be described; however, if the purpose of the pilot study was solely to try out instruments or the methodology on a small scale, little may be said.

Before writing the results and interpretations and conclusions, the author should reduce the data to condensed form, usually tables. The limitations and weaknesses of the study should be discussed. In writing this section, the question, "Do the data support the hypotheses?" must be foremost in mind, and everything written should be geared to letting the data bear on the problem and the hypotheses.

Facilities for Scientific Research

Facilities for scientific research in the institutional pharmacy should be appropriate for the type of research conducted. It is a mistake to identify the research function solely with the analytical chemistry function of the pharmacy, although the analytical equipment and facilities may be used for research. The single piece of equipment most commonly needed for research of all types is an electronic calculator.

Research Staff

Pharmacists conducting scientific research must have an adequate educational background in research methodology and in the preparation of research reports.

Summary

For institutional pharmacy to continue to be successful it must be able to adapt to an ever-increasing rate of change. The best type of scientific thinking will be required to attempt to understand these changes and to keep the profession relevant.[a]

SCOPE OF HOSPITAL PHARMACY RESEARCH

The hospital pharmacist who possesses adequate education and training can conduct a protracted investigation in the various scientific disciplines which comprise the profession of pharmacy. In addition, the hospital pharmacist may become involved in research pertaining to packaging, distribution, manufacture and storage of pharmaceutical preparations. There exists also the opportunity to develop new dosage forms, improve existing ones and to develop new and more accurate methods for analyzing the final product.

Some writers even suggest that the hospital pharmacist and/or the clinical pharmacist become involved, along with other members of the hospital's clinical research team, in studies on the absorption, distribution and excretion of drugs and their metabolites. The feeling being that these pharmacists possess the analytical chemical knowledge to make a worthy contribution in this type of applied research.

By the same token, many hospital pharmacists are capable of conducting a studious inquiry into problems of pharmaceutical adminis-

---

[a](References to ASHP Guidelines for Scientific Research in Institutional Pharmacy) Anon: Statement on the competencies required in institutional pharmacy practice, Am. J. Hosp. Pharm., *37*:917, (Sep.) 1975. Kerlinger, F.: Foundations of behavioral research, New York, Holt, Rinehart and Winston, Inc., 1964, p. 13. Conant, J.: Science and common sense, New Haven, Yale University Press, 1951, p. 23–27. Braithwaite, R.: Scientific explanation, Cambridge, Cambridge University Press, 1955, p. 1. Dewey, J.: How we think, Boston, Heath, 1933, p. 106–117, as adapted to the scientific framework by Kerlinger, op cit, p. 13–15.

tration, quality control, professional practice, and the sociological aspects of patient care as they relate to the practice of hospital pharmacy.

PHARMACEUTICAL SERVICES IN ACCREDITED HOSPITALS

The Joint Commission on Accreditation of Hospitals was incorporated in 1952 through a joint effort of the primary associations of North American medicine and hospitals for the purpose of encouraging the voluntary attainment of uniformly high standards of institutional medical care. The founding sponsors of the Joint Commission on Accreditation of Hospitals were the American College of Surgeons, the American College of Physicians, the American Hospital Association, the American Medical Association and the Canadian Medical Association. On December 15, 1979 the board of commissioners took the "unprecedented" action of expanding the commission by granting board membership and one voting seat to the American Dental Association. It was the first time that the board has been enlarged since the commission's inception in 1951.

JCAH STANDARDS FOR PHARMACEUTICAL SERVICES

The purpose of the Joint Commission on Accreditation of Hospital (JCAH) are:

1. to establish standards for the operation of hospitals and other health-related facilities and services;
2. to conduct survey and accreditation programs that will encourage members of the health professions, hospitals, and other health-related facilities and services voluntarily:
   a. to promote high quality of care in all aspects in order to give patients the optimum benefits that medical science has to offer,
   b. to apply certain basic principles of physical plant safety and maintenance, and of organization and administration of function for efficient care of the patient, and
   c. to maintain the essential services in the facilities through coordinated effort of the organized staffs and the governing bodies of the facilities;
3. to recognize compliance with standards by issuance of certificates of accreditation;
4. to conduct programs of education and research and publish the results thereof, which will further the other purposes of the corporation, and to accept grants, gifts, bequests, and devices in support of the purposes of the corporation; and
5. to assume such other responsibilities and to conduct such other

activities as are compatible with the operation of such standard-setting, survey and accreditation programs.

In 1965, Public Law 89-97 (Medicare) was enacted. Reference to JCAH in this law represented the confidence of Congress in the ability of the private health care sector to voluntarily assess the quality of care being provided. Written into the Medicare Act was the provision that hospitals participating in that program were to maintain the level of patient care that has come to be recognized as the norm. The standards of JCAH are specifically referred to in the law, and the Conditions of Participation for Hospitals, subsequently promulgated and published by the Social Security Administration, reflected the 1965 standards of JCAH.

One result of the 1965 Medicare legislation was that hospitals accredited by JCAH were "deemed" to be in compliance with most of the federal Medicare Conditions of Participation for Hospitals and, thus, deemed to meet eligibility requirements for participation in Medicare. (The 1972 Amendments to the Social Security Act, Public Law 92-603, provide for "validation" surveys of JCAH-accredited hospitals. This means that, while JCAH-accredited hospitals continue to be deemed to meet eligibility requirements for participation in Medicare, the Secretary of the Department of Health and Human Services is authorized to validate JCAH findings, either on a selective sample basis or on the basis of substantial complaint.)

Recognizing that most of the nation's hospitals are eager to achieve a level higher than a required minimum, the Board of Commissioners, in August 1966, voted to review, reevaluate, and rewrite the accreditation standards to encourage hospitals to strive for excellence in the provision of patient care. Consequently, the standards underwent extensive revision, resulting in the 1970 edition, called, for the first time, the Accreditation Manual for Hospitals. Since then, the Accreditation Manual for Hospitals has undergone continuous review and revision to keep abreast of the state of the act.[10]

Accordingly, the following pharmaceutical service standards and their interpretations are published verbatim from the *Accreditation Manual for Hospitals 1985*.[10]

PRINCIPLE

The hospital shall maintain a pharmaceutical department/service that is conducted in accordance with accepted ethical and professional practices and all legal requirements.

Standard I

The pharmaceutical department/service shall be directed by a professionally competent and legally qualified pharmacist. It shall be staffed by a sufficient number of competent personnel, in keeping with the size and scope of services of the hospital.

The pharmaceutical department/service shall be directed by a competent pharmacist who is appropriately licensed and who is responsible to the chief executive officer of the hospital or his designee. The director should either be a graduate of a college of pharmacy accredited by the American Council on Pharmaceutical Education and be oriented and knowledgeable in the specialized functions of hospital pharmacies, or have completed a hospital pharmacy residency program accredited by the American Society of Hospital Pharmacists. Consideration may be given to graduates of foreign colleges of pharmacy who are appropriately licensed and otherwise qualified to perform the responsibilities of the job. The director may be employed full-time or part-time.

The pharmaceutical services provided shall be sufficient to meet the needs of the patients as determined by the medical staff. It is recommended that a pharmacist be available at all times. Whether this is on an on duty, on call, or consultative basis should be determined by the pharmacy work load.

When the hospital pharmaceutical department/service in decentralized, a licensed pharmacist, responsible to the director of the pharmaceutical department/service, shall supervise each satellite pharmacy or separate organizational element involved with the preparation and dispensing of drugs and with the provision of drug information and other pharmaceutical services.

The director of the pharmaceutical department/service should be assisted by additional qualified pharmacists and pharmacy supportive personnel commensurate with the scope of services provided. Nonpharmacist personnel shall work under the direct supervision of a licensed pharmacist and in such a relationship that the supervising pharmacist is fully aware of all activities involved in the preparation and dispensing of medications, including the maintenance of appropriate records. The duties and responsibilities of nonpharmacist personnel must be consistent with their training and experience, and they shall not be assigned duties that by law or regulation must be performed only by a licensed pharmacist. Clerical and stenographic assistance should be provided as needed to assist with records, reports, and correspondence.

The organizational structure of the pharmaceutical department/service will vary with the size and complexity of the hospital and the scope of services provided. The pharmacy shall be licensed as required.

If the hospital does not have an organized pharmacy, pharmaceutical services shall be obtained from another hospital having such services or from a community pharmacy. Prepackaged drugs then shall be stored in, and distributed from, the hospital drug storage area, under the supervision of the director of the pharmaceutical department/service. Prepackaged drugs obtained from pharmacies outside the hospital shall be identified and labeled so that recalls can be effected as necessary and the proper controls established. There shall be an approved written procedure for obtaining drugs from another hospital or community pharmacy on a routine basis and in emergencies.

Standard II

Space, equipment, and supplies shall be provided for the professional and administrative functions of the pharmaceutical department/service as required, to promote patient safety through the proper storage, preparation, dispensing, and administration of drugs.

Hospitals with an organized pharmaceutical department/service shall have the necessary space, equipment, and supplies for the storage, preparation (compounding, packaging, labeling), and dispensing of parenteral products and radio-pharmaceuticals.

Drug storage and preparation areas within the pharmacy and throughout the hospital must be under the supervision of the director of the pharmaceutical department/service or his pharmacist-designee. Drugs must be stored under proper conditions of sanitation, temperature, light, moisture, ventilation, segregation, and security. Properly controlled drug preparation areas should be designated, and locked storage areas or locked medication carts provided, for each nursing unit as required. Drug preparation areas should be well-lighted and should be located where personnel preparing drugs for dispensing or administration will not be interrupted. The directors of the pharmaceutical department/service or his qualified designee must conduct at least monthly inspections of all nursing care units or other areas of the hospital where medications are dispensed, administered, or stored.

A record of all such monthly inspections shall be maintained to verify the following:

Antiseptics, other drugs for external use, and disinfectants are stored separately from internal and injectable medications.

Drugs requiring special conditions for storage to assure stability are properly stored. For example, biologicals and other thermolabile medications shall be stored in a separate compartment within a refrigerator that is capable of maintaining the necessary temperature. All drugs must be stored in accordance with current established standards (United States Pharmacopeia). Drugs not listed in the official compendia must be stored so that their integrity, stability, and effectiveness are maintained.

Outdated or otherwise unusable drugs have been identified and their distribution and administration prevented. The director of the pharmaceutical department/service, with the approval of the chief executive officer, shall designate one or more areas for the authorized storage of such drugs prior to their proper disposition.

Distribution and administration of controlled drugs are adequately documented by the pharmacy, nursing service, and other involved services or personnel, and are in accordance with federal and state law.

Any investigational drugs in use are properly stored, distributed, and controlled.

Emergency drugs, as approved by the medical staff, are in adequate and proper supply within the pharmacy and in designated hospital areas. The pharmacist should be responsible for both the contents of emergency medication carts, kits, and so forth, and for the inspection procedure to be used.

The metric weight system is in use for all medications. Metric-apothecaries' weight and measure conversion charts should be available to those professional individuals who may require them.

There should be a suitable area for the manipulation of parenteral medications. When laminar airflow hoods are used, quality control requirements shall include cleaning of the equipment used on each shift, microbiological monitoring as required by the infection control committee, and periodic checks for operational efficiency at least every 12 months by a qualified inspector. Appropriate records shall be maintained.

Materials and equipment necessary for the administration of the pharmaceutical department/service should be provided. Effective messenger and delivery service, when appropriate, should be provided for the pharmacy.

Up-to-date pharmaceutical reference materials shall be provided in order to furnish the pharmaceutical, medical, and nursing staffs with adequate information concerning drugs. These should include official pharmaceutical compendia and periodicals, as well as current editions of text and reference books covering the following: theoretical and practical pharmacy; general, organic, pharmaceutical, and biological chemistry; toxicology; pharmacology; therapeutics; bacteriology; sterilization and disinfection; compatibility and drug interaction references; and other related matters important to good pharmaceutical practice in its relation to patient care. Authoritative, current antidote information and the telephone number of the regional poison control information center should be readily available in the pharmacy for emergency reference. Current federal and state drug law information should be readily available to the pharmaceutical department/service.

Standard III

The scope of the pharmaceutical department/service shall be consistent with the medication needs of the patients as determined by the medical staff.

All drugs, chemicals, and biologicals shall meet national standards of quality or shall be clearly and accurately labeled as to contents, and such information shall be disclosed to the medical staff. All drugs should be obtained and used in accordance with written policies and procedures that have been approved by the medical staff. Such policies and procedures should relate to the selection, the distribution, and the safe and effective use of drugs in the hospital, and should be established by the combined effort of the director of the pharmaceutical department/service, the medical staff, the nursing service, and the administration.

Within this framework, the director of the pharmaceutical department/service should be responsible for at least the following:

Maintaining an adequate drug supply.

Establishing specifications for the procurement of all approved drugs, and those chemicals and biologicals related to the practice of pharmacy.

Preparing and dispensing drugs and chemicals.

Preparing, sterilizing, and labeling parenteral medications and solutions that are manufactured in the hospital. There shall be an associated quality control program to monitor personnel qualifications, training and performance, and equipment and facilities. The end product should be examined on a sampling basis, as determined by the director of the pharmaceutical department/service, to assure that it meets with the required specifications. Appropriate records shall be maintained. The compounding and admixture of large volume parenterals should ordinarily be the responsibility of a qualified pharmacist. Individuals who prepare or administer large volume parenterals should have special training to do so. When any part of the above functions (preparing, sterilizing, and labeling parenteral medications and solutions) is performed within the hospital but not under direct pharmacy supervision, the director of the pharmaceutical department/service shall be responsible for providing written guidelines and for approving the procedure to assure that all pharmaceutical requirements are met. In the interest of safety of preparation and administration, and effective nutritional content, overall direction shall be provided by a qualified physician when total parenteral nutrition products (hyperalimentation) are required.

Participating in the initial orientation and subsequent in-service education, including the provision of appropriate incompatibility information, of all personnel involved in the preparation or administration of sterile parenteral medications and solutions.

Any in-hospital manufacturing of pharmaceuticals, with proper control procedures.

Maintaining and keeping available the medical staff-approved stock of antidotes and other emergency drugs, both in the pharmacy and in patient care areas. Authoritative, current antidote information, as well as the phone number of the regional poison control information center, should also be readily available in areas outside the pharmacy where these drugs are stored.

Filling and labeling all drug containers issued to the departments/services from which medications are to be administered.

Maintaining records of the transactions of the pharmacy as required by federal, state, and local laws, and as necessary to maintain adequate control and accountability of all drugs. This should include a system of controls and records for the requisitioning and dispensing of pharmaceutical supplies to nursing care units and to other departments/services of the hospital.

Assuring the monitoring and evaluation, with medical staff input, of the quality and appropriateness of patient services provided by the pharmaceutical department/service.

Participating in the development and subsequent updating of a hospital formulary or drug list. The medical staff, through its pharmacy and therapeutics function, shall determine the hospital formulary to be used. When properly annotated, a formulary developed outside the hospital will suffice if it is maintained as a current document and if it has been approved by the medical staff. Any hospital formulary or drug list should be readily available to the professional staff who use it, and the staff should be kept informed of any changes. The formulary or drug list should also include the availability of non-legend medications. The existence of a formulary does not preclude the use of unlisted drugs, and there should be a written policy and procedure for their procurement.

Requiring and documenting the participation of pharmacy personnel in relevant education programs, including orientation of new employees, as well as in-service and outside continuing education programs. Frequency of programs and participation shall be related to the scope of the pharmaceutical services offered and shall be established with the approval of the chief executive officer.

Participating in those aspects of the overall hospital quality assurance program that relate to drug utilization and effectiveness. This may include determining usage patterns for each drug according to clinical department/service or individual prescribers, and assisting in the setting of drug use criteria. Refer also to the Quality Assurance section of the *JCAH Manual.*

Participating in all meetings of the pharmacy and therapeutics committee and implementing the decisions of that committee throughout the hospital.

Communicating new product information to nursing service and other hospital personnel, as required.

Performing an annual review of all pharmaceutical policies and procedures for the purpose of establishing their consistency with current practices within the hospital.

Maintaining confidentiality of patient/medical staff information.

Maintaining a means of identifying the signature of all practitioners authorized to use the pharmaceutical services for ambulatory care patient prescriptions, as well as a listing of their Drug Enforcement Administration numbers.

Cooperating in the teaching and research programs of the hospital.

Within the limits of available resources, the pharmaceutical department/service should provide drug monitoring services in keeping with each patient's needs. These may include, but are not necessarily limited to, the following:

The maintenance of a medication record of drug profile for each patient, which is based on available drug history and current therapy and includes the name, age, and weight of the patient, the current diagnosis(es), the current drug therapy, any drug allergies or sensitivities, and other pertinent information relating to the patient's drug regimen. This information should be available to the responsible practitioners at all times.

A review of the patient's drug regimen for any potential interactions, interferences, or incompatibilities, prior to dispensing drugs to the patient. Such irregularities must be resolved promptly with the prescribing practitioner, and, when appropriate, with notification of the nursing service and administration.

The instruction of the patient or of the appropriate nursing department/service personnel who advise the patient, verbally or in writing, on the importance and correct use of medication to be taken following discharge, in the interest of assuring safe and correct self-administration, when such instruction is requested by the responsible practitioner or as provided by written medical staff policy.

The director of the pharmaceutical department/service and staff pharmacists should be invited to participate on a regular basis in the education of medical staff and nursing service personnel in regard to drugs and biologicals in use in the hospital. This may include information on drug incompatibilities and sensitivities, on the monitoring of end-points for initial signs of toxicity or optimum drug effect, and on new drugs. Individuals who have responsibility for drug storage or administration should be instructed in the recognition of signs of drug deterioration. Greatest benefit occurs when qualified pharmaceutical department/service staffing permits the establishment of a drug information center in the hospital, which is available at all times to professional staff members.

Standard IV

Written policies and procedures that pertain to the intrahospital drug distribution system shall be developed by the director of the pharmaceutical department/service in concert with the medical staff and, as appropriate, with representatives of other disciplines.

Drug preparation and dispensing shall be restricted to a licensed pharmacist, or to his designee under the direct supervision of the pharmacist. A pharmacist should review the prescriber's order, or a direct copy thereof, before the initial dose of medication is dispensed (with the exception of emergency orders when time does not permit). In cases when the medication order is written when the pharmacy is "closed" or the pharmacist is otherwise unavailable, the medication order should be reviewed by the pharmacist as soon thereafter as possible, preferably within 24 hours.

The use of floor stock medications should be minimized; the unit dose drug distribution system which permits identification of the drug up to the point of administration, is recommended for use throughout the hospital.

Written policies and procedures that are essential for patient safety and for the control, accountability, and intrahospital distribution of drugs be reviewed annually, revised as necessary, and enforced. Such policies and procedures shall include, but not be limited to, the following:

All drugs shall be labeled adequately, including the addition of appropriate accessory or cautionary statements, as well as the expiration date when applicable.

Discontinued and outdated drugs, and containers with worn, illegible, or missing labels, shall be returned to the pharmacy for proper disposition.

Only a pharmacist, or authorized pharmacy personnel under the direction and supervision of a pharmacist, shall dispense medications, make labeling changes, or transfer medications to different containers.

Only prepackaged drugs shall be removed from the pharmacy when a pharmacist is not available. These drugs shall be removed only by a designated registered nurse or a physician, and only in amounts sufficient for immediate therapeutic needs. Such drugs should be kept in a separate cabinet, closet, or other designated area and shall be properly labeled. A record of such withdrawals shall be made by the authorized individual removing such drugs and shall be verified by a pharmacist.

There shall be a written drug recall procedure that can be implemented readily and the results documented. This requirement shall apply to both inpatient and ambulatory care patient medications.

Drug product defects should be reported in accordance with the ASHP-USP-FDA Drug Product Problem Reporting Program.

Medications to be dispensed to inpatients at the time of discharge from the hospital shall be labeled as for ambulatory care patient prescriptions.

A system designed to assure accurate identification of ambulatory care patients at the time they receive prescribed medications should be established.

Unless otherwise provided by law, ambulatory care patient prescription labels should bear the following information:

Name, address, and telephone number of the hospital pharmacy;

Date and pharmacy's identifying serial number for the prescription;

Full name of the patient;

Name of the drug, strength, and amount dispensed;

Directions to the patient for use;

Name of the prescribing practitioner;

Name or initials of the dispensing individual; and

Any required Drug Enforcement Administration cautionary label on controlled substance drugs, and any other pertinent accessory cautionary labels.

In the interest of effective control, the distribution of drug samples within the hospital should be eliminated if possible. Sample drugs brought into the hospital shall be controlled through the pharmaceutical department/service.

Standard V

Written policies and procedures that govern the safe administration of drugs and biologicals shall be developed by the medical staff in cooperation with the pharmaceutical department/service, the nursing service, and, as necessary, representatives of other disciplines.

Written policies and procedures governing the safe administration of drugs shall be reviewed at least annually, revised as necessary, and enforced. Such policies and procedures shall include, but not necessarily be limited to, the following:

Drugs shall be administered only upon the order of a member of the medical staff, an authorized member of the house staff, or other individual who has been granted clinical privileges to write such orders. Verbal orders for drugs may be accepted only by personnel so designated in the medical staff rules and regulations and must be authenticated by the prescribing practitioner within the stated period of time.

All medications shall be administered by, or under the supervision of, appropriately licensed personnel in accordance with laws and governmental rules and regulations governing such acts and in accordance with the approved medical staff rules and regulations.

There shall be an automatic cancellation of standing drug orders when a patient undergoes surgery. Automatic drug stop orders shall otherwise be determined by the medical staff and stated in medical staff rules and regulations. There shall be a system to notify the responsible practitioner of the impending expiration of a drug order, so that the practitioner may determine whether the drug administration is to be continued or altered.

Cautionary measures for the safe admixture of parenteral products shall be developed. Whenever drugs are added to intravenous solutions, a distinctive supplementary label shall be affixed to the container. The label shall indicate the patient's name and location; the name and amount of the drug(s) added; the name of the basic parenteral solution; the date and time of the addition; the date, time, and rate of administration; the name or identifying code of the individual who prepared the admixture; supplemental instructions; and the expiration date of the compounded solution.

Drugs to be administered shall be verified with the prescribing practitioner's orders and properly prepared for administration. The patient shall be identified prior to drug administration, and each dose of medication administered shall be recorded properly in the patient's medical record.

Medication errors and adverse drug reactions shall be reported immediately in accordance with written procedures. This requirement shall include notification of the practitioner who ordered the drug. An entry of the medication administered and/or the drug reaction shall be properly recorded in the patient's medical record. Hospitals are encouraged to report any unexpected or significant adverse reactions promptly to the Food and Drug Administration and to the manufacturer.

Drugs brought into the hospital by patients shall not be administered unless the drugs have been identified and there is a written order from the responsible practitioner to administer the drugs. If the drugs are not to be used during the patient's hospitalization, they should be packaged and sealed, and either given to the patient's family or stored and returned to the patient at the time of discharge, provided such action is approved by the responsible practitioner.

Self-administration of medications by patients shall be permitted on a specific written order by the authorized prescribing practitioner and in accordance with established hospital policy.

Investigational drugs shall be properly labeled and stored, and shall be used only under the direct supervision of the authorized principal investigator. Such drugs should be approved by an appropriate medical staff committee. Investigational drugs should be administered in accordance with an approved protocol that includes any requirements for a patient's appropriate informed consent. On approval of the principal investigator, registered nurses may administer these drugs after they have been given, and have demonstrated an understanding of, basic pharmacologic information about the drugs. In the absence of an organized pharmaceutical department/service, a central unit should be established where essential information on such drugs is maintained.

Orders involving abbreviations and chemical symbols should be carried out only if the abbreviations/symbols appear on an explanatory legend approved by the medical staff. In the interest of minimizing errors, the use of abbreviations is discouraged, and the use of the leading decimal point should be avoided. Each practitioner who prescribes medication must clearly state the administration times or the time interval between doses. The use of "prn" and "on call" with medication orders should be qualified.

Drugs prescribed for ambulatory patient use in continuity with hospital care shall be released to patients upon discharge only after they are labeled for such use under the supervision of the pharmacist and only on written order of the authorized prescribing practitioner. Each drug released to a patient on discharge should be recorded in the medical record.

Individual drugs should be administered as soon as possible after the dose has been prepared, particularly medications prepared for parenteral administration, and, to the maximum extent possible, by the individual who prepared the dose, except where unit dose drug distribution systems are used.

Unless otherwise provided by the medical staff bylaws, rules and regulations or by legal requirements, prescribing practitioners may, within their discretion at the time of prescribing, approve or disapprove the dispensing of a nonproprietary drug or the dispensing of a different proprietary brand to their patients by the pharmacist.

Refer also to the Anesthesia Services, Emergency Services, Functional Safety and Sanitation, Home Care Services, Hospital-Sponsored Ambulatory Care Services, Infection Control, Medical Record Services, Medical Staff, Nuclear Medicine Services, Nursing Services, Respiratory Care Services, and Special Care Units sections of this *Manual*.[a]

Standard VI

As part of the hospital's quality assurance program, the quality and appropriateness of patient care services provided by the pharmaceutical depart-

---

[a]Accreditation Manual for Hospitals, AMH85, Joint Commission on Accreditation of Hospitals, Chicago, Ill. 60611.

ment/service are monitored and evaluated, and identified problems are resolved.

Required Characteristics

A. The pharmaceutical department/service has a planned and systematic process for the monitoring and evaluation of the quality and appropriateness of patient care services and for resolving identified problems.
1. The director of the pharmaceutical department/service is responsible for assuring that the process is implemented.
B. The quality and appropriateness of patient care services are monitored and evaluated in all major clinical functions of the pharmaceutical department/service. Such monitoring and evaluation are accomplished through the following means:
1. Routine collection in the pharmaceutical department/service, or through the hospital quality assurance program, of information about important aspects of pharmaceutical services; and.
2. Periodic assessment by the pharmaceutical department/service of the collected information in order to identify important problems in patient care services and opportunities to improve care.
   a) In B.1 and B.2, the pharmaceutical department/service agrees on objective criteria that reflect current knowledge and clinical experience.
      (1) These criteria are used by the pharmaceutical department/ service or by the hospital quality assurance program in the monitoring and evaluation of patient care services.
C. When important problems in patient care services or opportunities to improve care are identified,
1. actions are taken; and
2. the effectiveness of the actions is evaluated.
D. The findings from and conclusions of monitoring, evaluation, and problem-solving activities are documented and, as appropriate, are reported.
E. The actions taken to resolve problems and improve patient care services, and information about the impact of the actions taken, are documented and, as appropriate, are reported.
F. As part of the annual reappraisal of the hospital's quality assurance program the effectiveness of the monitoring, evaluation, and problem-solving activities in the pharmaceutical department/service is evaluated.
G. When and outside source(s) provides pharmaceutical services, or when there is no designated pharmaceutical department/service, the quality and appropriateness of patient care services provided are monitored and evaluated, and identified problems are resolved.
1. The chief executive officer is responsible for assuring that a planned and systemic process for such monitoring and problem-solving activities is implemented.

SELECTED READINGS

Black, B.L.: Competitive Alternatives to Hospital Inpatient Care. Am. J. Hosp. Pharm., *42*:3:545, Mar. 1985.
Brodie, D.C. and Smith, W.E.: Implications of New Technology for Pharmacy Education and Practice. Am. J. Hosp. Pharm., *42*:1:80, Jan. 1985.

REFERENCES

1. Cooke, E.F., and Martin, E.W.: *Remington's Practice of Pharmacy,* 10th Ed. Easton, The Mack Publishing Co., 1951.
2. Urdang, George: Foreword to Ten Years of the American Society of Hospital Pharmacists, The Bulletin, A.S.H.P., *9*:1:281, 1952.
3. A.H.A. Guide to the Health Care Field 1983 Ed. American Hospital Association, Chicago, Illinois.
4. Archambault, George F.: Needs for Hospital Pharmacists in the United States 1957–1970, Am. J. Hosp. Pharm., *15*:2:131, 1958.
5. Letourneau, Charles U.: The Hospital Pharmacist Needs Management Skills, Am. J. Hosp. Pharm., *16*:2:73, 1959.
6. Goals for Hospital Pharmacy, Am. J. Hosp. Pharm., *37*:1095 (Aug.) 1980.
7. ASHP Guidelines: Minimum Standards for Pharmacies in Institutions. Am. J. Hosp. Pharm., *42*:372, 1985.
8. ASHP Guidelines on the Competencies Required in Institutional Pharmacy Practice. Am. J. Hosp. Pharm., *32*:917, (Sept.) 1975.
9. A.S.H.P. Guidelines for Scientific Research in Institutional Pharmacy, Am. J. Hosp. Pharm., *35*:323–326, (Mar.) 1978.
10. Accreditation Manual for Hospitals 1985, Joint Commission on Accreditation of Hospitals, 875 No. Michigan Ave., Chicago, Ill. 60611.

2

The Hospital and Its Organization

"The hospital is a complex organization utilizing combinations of intricate, specialized scientific equipment, and functioning through a corps of trained people educated to the problems of modern medical science. These are all welded together in the common purpose of restoration and maintenance of good health.

The hospital, as an organization, provides special facilities and trained personnel to facilitate the work of the physician in his primary position involving care of the patient who is the focal point about which all activities of the hospital revolve. In the delivery of medical services to patients, therefore, the medical and associated technical staff of nurses, dietitians etc. become a most important factor. The character and extent of hospital services are adjusted continuously to keep abreast of changes and advances in medical science.

Although primary emphasis is placed on the care of bed patients, the frontier of the hospital in recent years has been extended from the sick person in the hospital bed, to the potentially sick person in his normal living situation. Hospitals have been assuming more and more responsibility for programs of preventive medicine. They serve as the medium in many communities through which the professional staffs and official health agencies pool their efforts for improvement of the public health."[1]

Because of the specific scope of this volume, only a general view of the complex organizational structure of a hospital will be presented.

CLASSIFICATION OF HOSPITALS

Hospitals may be classified in many different ways and any single institution may fall into more than one grouping. For example, the Peter Bent Brigham Hospital is a "private, non-profit, teaching hospital." The following is a brief general classification schedule which will serve to classify the great majority of hospitals.

HOSPITAL CLASSIFICATIONS

CLINICAL	OWNERSHIP & CONTROL
General Medical & Surgical	Governmental
Specialty	Army, Navy, Veterans
MEDICINE	Administration
Internal Medicine	Public Health Service
Psychiatric & Nervous Diseases	State
Tuberculosis	County
Communicable Diseases	City
Pediatrics	Non-Government
SURGERY	Private for profit
Orthopedic	Non-profit
Gynecologic	Church
Otolaryngologic	Fraternal order
MATERNITY	Community
Length of Stay	Non-profit private
Short term	BY ACCREDITATION*
Long term (Chronic)	Accredited
Custodial (Long term)	Non-accredited

*Joint Commission on Accreditation of Hospitals

What are teaching hospitals? A major teaching hospital is one which is used extensively for the clinical instruction of medical school students. A minor teaching hospital is used only for a limited amount of student instruction, such as occasional demonstrations or clinics.

Traditionally, teaching hospitals are places where the new medical graduate seeks postgraduate training. He almost always undergoes 1 year of hospital training as an intern. He may frequently spend 2 or more additional years in a hospital as a resident in some specialty, such as internal medicine, surgery, pediatrics or radiology. On the other hand, some community hospitals maintain intern and residency programs. When they exist, however, then tend to be far less complete than in the teaching institution.

Numerically, teaching hospitals represent approximately 400 of the nation's 6983 registered hospitals. However, they care for a little over one of every five hospitalized Americans.

Industry also recognizes the importance of the teaching hospital by virtue of the special coverage it receives from the company's medical service representatives as well as its desire to financially support both educational and research programs.

Because teaching hospitals act as referral centers for the more seriously ill patient, third party payors have been, in recent years, reimbursing these hospitals at a higher rate than small suburban institutions with no special programs for the care of these cases.

Most young physicians entering practice look for locations in a teaching hospital because such institutions assure them of the most contemporary educational opportunities coupled with broad experiences in the clinical care of patients, teaching and research.

ORGANIZATIONAL PATTERN

The organizational pattern of a hospital does not differ from that of any industrial plant. The apparent difference is superficial and deals only with the nomenclature of the positions. For example, the Director or Administrator of a hospital may be the Executive Vice-President or the General Manager of the commercial entity. Two organizational charts are presented in Figures 1 and 2. Obviously, the smaller the hospital the fewer the administrative positions of associate or assistant director and conversely, the large institutions may further sub-divide the general areas of clinical and administrative services into smaller units under the aegis of assistant directors. The corporation and the board of trustee segment of the organization is standard for all private hospitals. Governmental hospitals usually have a board of trustees but no corporate body.

GOVERNING BODY AND MANAGEMENT

Aside from licensure, most hospitals cherish recognition by the Joint Commission on Accreditation of Hospitals as "accredited" hospitals.

The Joint Commission on Accreditation of Hospitals (JCAH)[2] is an outgrowth of the *Hospital Standardization Program* established by the American College of Surgeons in 1918. Due to the fiscal drain which this program placed on the coffers of the College of Surgeons, participation by other national professional organizations was solicited in order to continue the program. In 1951, five major medical and hospital associations jointly created the JCAH. The founding members were the American College of Surgeons, the American College of Physicians, the American Hospital Association, the American Medical Association, and the Canadian Medical Association. The Canadian Medical Association continued its participation in the JCAH until 1959 when the Canadian Council on Hospital Accreditation activated its own program.

Recognizing that most of the nation's hospitals are eager to achieve a level higher than a required minimum, the Board of Commissioners, in 1966 voted "to review, re-evaluate, and re-write the hospitalization standards and their supplemented interpretations to attain the following two objectives":[3]

1. To raise and strengthen the standards from their present level of minimum essential to the level of optimal achievable and to assure their suitability to the state of the art.

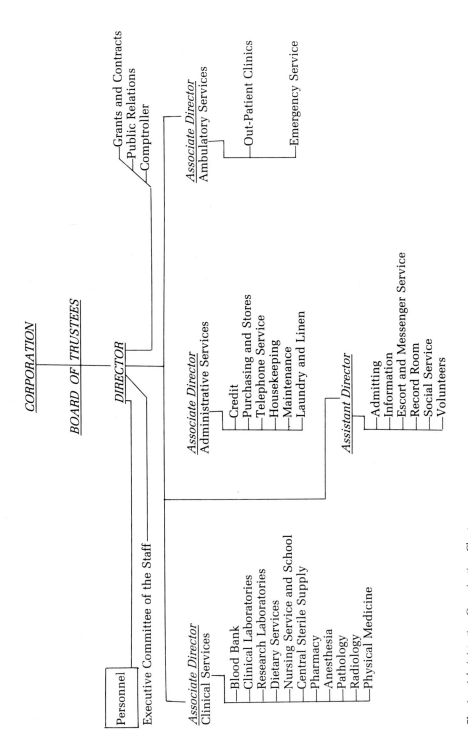

Fig. 1. Administrative Organization Chart.

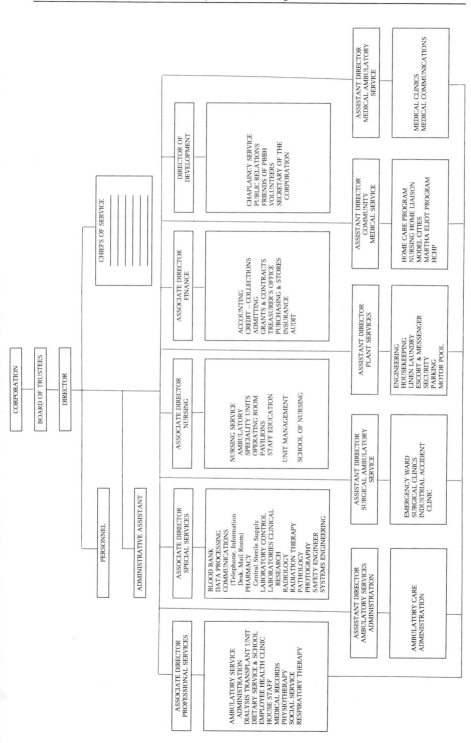

Fig. 2. Large Hospital Administrative Organization Chart.

2. To simplify and clarify the language of standards and interpretations to remove all possible ambiguities and misunderstandings.

With respect to the governing body, the JCAH adopted the following principle.[4]

There shall be an organized governing body, or designated person(s) so functioning, that has overall responsibility for the conduct of the hospital in a manner consonant with the hospital's objective of making available high quality patient care.

The resulting application of this principle is that hospitals, in general, are legally organized as CORPORATIONS according to the corporate laws of the State in which they operate, although a few of the privately owned and operated units still function under a partnership agreement. The total number of members in each corporation will vary from hospital to hospital.

Because the corporation may consist of a large number of people from widely scattered areas, a representative group, from within the corporation membership, is elected to a board of trustees. This group is also known as the governing board, board of governors, board of managers or board of directors.

Generally, the above board includes a broad representation of the community served by the hospital and its members are selected for their ability to contribute to its effective management.

It is required, both by State laws and the Joint Commission on the Accreditation of Hospitals, that the governing body adopt by-laws identifying the purposes of the hospital and the means of fulfilling them. Included in the by-laws are the following.[5]

(i)   definition of the powers and duties of the governing body officers, committees and chief executive officer.
(ii) qualifications for governing body membership.
(iii) method of selection of membership.
(iv) tenure.
(v)   committees—kinds, appointment and membership tenure.

The by-laws also describe the authority delegated to the chief executive officer (Director or Administrator) and to the medical staff. It should be clear to the student that such a delegation of authority does not preclude the governing body from exercising the control and authority required to meet its responsibility for the conduct of the hospital. The governing body always has the right to rescind any such delegation.

As part of the organizational process, the governing body elects its officers and causes to be appointed a wide variety of committees necessary for the discharge of its duties. These may include an Executive

Committee, Building Committee, Investment and Finance Committee and a Joint Conference Committee.

The governing body of the hospital has, through its chief executive officers, a number of obligations best exemplified by recording Standards I through X of the 1983 Accreditation Manual for Hospitals.[6]

Standard I

There shall be full disclosure of hospital ownership and control.

Standard II

The governing body shall adopt bylaws in accordance with legal requirements and its responsibility to the community.

Standard III

Governing body members shall be selected, unless otherwise provided by law, in accordance with the hospital's bylaws and, if applicable, articles of incorporation or charter.

Standard IV

The governing body shall provide for the selection of its officers, adopt a schedule of meetings, and define attendance requirements and the method of documenting governing body proceedings.

Standard V

The governing body shall provide mechanisms for fulfilling the functions necessary to the discharge of its responsibilities.

Standard VI

The governing body shall provide for institutional planning to meet the health needs of the community.

Standard VII

The governing body shall appoint a chief executive officer whose qualifications, responsibilities, authority, and accountability shall be defined in writing.

Standard VIII

The medical staff bylaws, rules and regulations shall be subject to governing body approval. This approval shall not be unreasonably withheld.

Standard IX

The governing body shall hold the medical staff responsible for making recommendations concerning initial medical staff appointments, reappointments, termination of appointments, the delineation of clinical privileges, and the curtailment of clinical privileges.

Standard X

The governing body shall require that the medical staff establish mechanisms designed to assure the achievement and maintenance of high standards of medical practice and patient care.

ADMINISTRATION

The active management of hospitals is delegated, by the board of trustees, to the administrator and his staff of associates, assistants, supervisors and department heads.

It should be noted that the Director of the Pharmacy Service (Pharmacist-in-Chief) reports to the assistant or associate director responsible for the clinical services of the hospital. Too often, the pharmacy is considered a business type of service and is assigned to the division of administrative services. Grouping the pharmacist with the housekeeper, laundry manager and maintenance group does irreparable harm to the professional stature of the pharmacist and damages his rapport with the other members of the clinical group.

The administrator of a hospital is especially trained for his position. Today, most of the new appointees to the top post in hospitals are graduates of special programs and hold the *Master of Hospital Administration* degree. The lack of such a degree does not preclude other qualified individuals from being appointed administrator. In addition, many boards of trustees require that the administrator be a *Fellow* of the American College of Hospital Administrators.

The main function of the administrator is to enforce trustee policy in the daily management routine. In addition, he is required to take all reasonable steps to assure that the hospital complies with applicable laws and regulations; establish an organizational structure to carry out the programs of the hospital and to meet the needs of the patients; to implement the governing body policy on the financial management of the hospital; and to develop and implement a comprehensive management reporting system throughout the hospital. The chief executive must also provide, maintain, and safeguard appropriate physical resources. In commenting upon the expanding role of the hospital administrator, Cordes[7] has stated . . .

". . . the hospital administrator of today must know and understand his community, its people, their historical traditions, the value structure that is at work, the resources available, and the weaknesses to be reckoned with in any course of action. Armed with this knowledge and understanding, he must educate the community to his enterprise, its goals, its problems, its needs, and its opportunities for contribution to the community. . ."

The modern hospital administrator can be described as a specialist in administration, as an educator, as a community adviser and as an organizer. Reporting to the governing body, he bears responsibility for the operation of the entire institution, assuring the medical and scientific staffs, the trustees and the patients of the highest possible standards of both service and economy. Within the hospital he plans, directs and coordinates activities which outside the institution would be complete entities in themselves: food service, laundry, pharmacy, out-patient clinic. The future of the institution depends, in significant measure, on the vision of the hospital administrator.[8]

MEDICAL STAFF

Because the medical staff is the backbone of any hospital, it is essential that it be well organized and controlled. Accordingly, the JCAH has set forth the following *Principle* and *Standard:*[9]

There is a single organized medical staff that has overall responsibility for the quality of the professional services provided by individuals with clinical privileges,[a] as well as the responsibility of accounting therefor to the governing body. There is a mechanism to assure that all individuals with clinical privileges provide services within the scope of individual clinical privileges granted.

Clearly, every hospital must have a medical staff that is responsible for the quality of all medical care provided to patients and for the ethical conduct and professional practices of its membership.

Generally, medical staff membership is limited to individuals who are fully licensed to practice medicine or dentistry. As a body, this group usually organizes itself to provide for the election or appointment of officers and committees whose function is to create and maintain an optimal level of professional performance of its membership.

The framework of the medical staff will vary from hospital to hospital due to the varying size and activities of the hospital and the staff. However, the staff may be divided into the following categories: active medical staff; associate medical staff; courtesy medical staff; consulting medical staff and honorary medical staff.

The active medical staff is responsible for the delivery of the preponderance of medical service within the hospital and is most involved in the organizational and administrative duties pertaining to the medical staff.

The associate medical staff consists of individuals who are being considered for advancement to the active medical staff. These practitioners are appointed and assigned to the various services in the same manner as are members of the active medical staff.

---

[a]**clinical privileges** Permission to provide medical or other patient care services in the granting institution, within well-defined limits, based on the individual's professional license and his experience, competence, ability, and judgement.

The courtesy medical staff consists of practitioners who are eligible for staff membership, who are given privileges to admit an occasional patient to the hospital. Courtesy staff members may neither vote nor hold office in the medical staff organizaiton.

The consulting medical staff consists of medical practitioners of recognized professional ability who are not members of the preceding categories of staff membership.

The honorary medical staff consists of former staff members, retired or emeritus, and of other practitioners whom the medical staff chooses to honor.

CLINICAL DEPARTMENTS

The degree of departmentalization of the clinical divisions of the hospital depends almost entirely upon the degree of specialization of the medical staff. In small communities, one would expect to find two major departments in a hospital—medicine and surgery. Supportive services such as radiology and pathology are also offered but are generally limited in their capability to provide service. In those areas where there are two or more small hospitals, it is common to have a single department of pathology or radiology servicing both institutions. However, in the large metropolitan areas the hospital staff is highly specialized and therefore greater subdivisions within a particular department.

Generally, the department of medicine includes the following subdivisions:

Internal Medicine	Pediatrics
Allergy	Gastroenterology
Cardiology	Nephrology
Infectious Diseases	Neurology
Dermatology	Psychiatry
Endocrinology	Pulmonary Diseases
Geriatrics	Rheumatology
Immunology	

The department of surgery is generally divided into the following:

General Surgery	Otolaryngology
Orthopedic Surgery	Plastic Surgery
Neurologic Surgery	Proctology
Obstetrics & Gynecology	Thoracic Surgery
Ophthalmology	Urology
Dental & Oral Surgery	

In addition there may be a division of general practice as well as a division of physical medicine and rehabilitation within the hospital.

Each of these sub-divisions usually has a chief-of-service who in turn is responsible to the department chief. In addition, the medical staff is organized in such a manner as to provide fair representation of each individual on the staff through to the administration and the governing body.

It should be clear to the student that the larger and more specialized medical staff is indicative of the fact that the institution is a teaching hospital. Because the description "teaching hospital" has been mis-used, the American Hospital Association describes such an institution in the following manner.[10,11]

A hospital that allocates a substantial part of its resources to conduct, in its own name or in formal association with a college or courses of instruction in the health disciplines that lead to the granting of recognized certificates, di-plomas, or degrees, or that are required for professional certification or licen-sure, is a teaching hospital.

The association also placed the following interpretation on the def-inition:

The allocation of resources and facilities, personnel, and funds must be ade-quate to demonstrate the discharge of teaching programs.

Educational programs or courses of instruction are "formal" when based upon published or recorded curricula covering specified periods of study and have faculty qualification and student admission require-ments established or agreed to by the hospital. They are not work and learn or on the job training assignments that primarily augment the hospital's capability to provide services. Further, the hospital controls, or agrees to, the appointment of faculty and selection of students except during the term of agreements that gives a college or medical school exclusive authority therefore.

Certificates, degrees or diplomas must be recognized and accepted by national educational agencies, professional qualifying bodies or state approving authorities. This implies that the courses of educational pro-grams meet standards generally recognized in the health field.

The teaching hospital affords the hospital pharmacists with innu-merable opportunities to participate in and to develop educational pro-grams. The literature is replete with articles describing endeavors by hospital pharmacists in the teaching of various subjects to student nurses, conducting inservice programs for graduate nurses and practical nurses, developing seminars on the pharmacology of drugs for interns, residents and senior staff physicians, training undergraduate and grad-uate students in hospital pharmacy and participating in the training of students in hospital administration.

Because of the unique training of the professional hospital pharmacist, he can make noteworthy contributions towards the fulfillment of the criteria required for an institution to qualify as a teaching hospital.

SUPPORT SERVICES

To those unfamiliar with the hospital environment, it would seem as though the hospital consisted of the clinical departments only. Actually, the clinical departments would not be able to function without the supporting services. Amongst the supporting services are the nursing department, the dietary service, laboratory services, the medical records department, the blood bank, the central sterile supply and the social service department.

There are other services clinically essential to the operation of the hospital such as the maintenance and engineering divisions. However, for the purpose of this text only the former will be discussed.

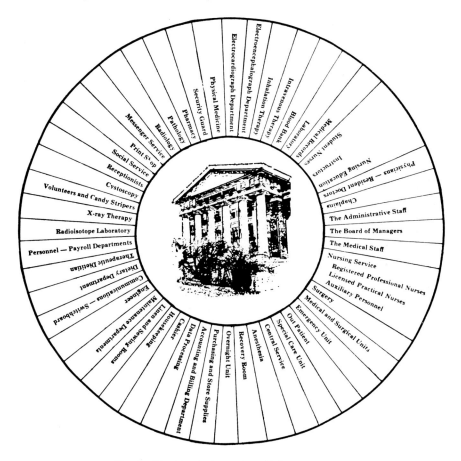

Fig. 3.   The Hospital . . . A Multiple Service Unit.

NURSING SERVICE

Much has been written relative to the progress that has been made in the field of medicine during the past decade. The revolution in medical care has had its effect on the other health professions. For nursing, keeping pace with medicine has meant many changes in practice. The nursing team, made up of workers with varying degrees of nursing skill and directed by a professional nurse, now replaces the single nurse who once did everything for the patient. Today's nursing practitioner recognizes social, psychological, or religious problems with the patient that might influence his physical well being and refer those that lie outside the province of nursing to the person most competent to deal with them. Helping the patients to help themselves is another new element of nursing practice, added because of increased emphasis on self care by the patient as an aid to early recovery. The new patterns of nursing service thus brought about are often misunderstood by the public when the changes and the reasons behind them are not explained. Thus in 1964, The National League for Nursing directed a statement concerning the basic assumptions which one could make about nursing care to those engaged in various aspects of nursing service as a means of improving service wherever it is given; to allied professions because nursing care is only a part of the total health provided by many groups, whose ability to work together improves the mutual understanding; and to consumers of nursing service who, as members of the community, share the responsibility for seeing that the care necessary for regaining and maintaining health is made available to themselves and to their families. The following are the basic assumptions.[12]

1. Nursing care encompasses health promotion, the care and prevention of disease or disability, rehabilitation, teaching, counseling, and emotional support as well as the care of illness.
2. Nursing care is an integral part of total health care and is planned and administered in combination with related medical, educational, and welfare services.
3. Nursing personnel respect individuality, dignity, and rights of every person; regardless of race, color, creed, national origin, social or economic status.

The nursing service is organized similarly to any other large service in the hospital. There is at its head a Director of Nursing who is generally an experienced nurse with administrative talent. The administrative nursing services carries ultimate administrative authority and responsibility in one or more health facilities for the nursing services provided individuals and families. As a member of the administrative staff, the administrative nursing service participates in formulating policy, and devising procedures essential to the achievement of objectives, and in developing and evaluating programs and services.

In some institutions, the Director of Nursing service is also responsible for the administration and operation of the School of Nursing. However, the modern trend is to separate the responsibility and assign it to an individual specifically trained in the educational aspect of nursing. In those institutions where the school of nursing has been separated from the nursing service, the individual heading the school assumes a position of responsibility similar to that of the Director of the Nursing Service and may be responsible directly to the Chief Executive Officer of the hospital.

DIETETIC SERVICES

An essential service of each institution is that of the dietary department. The JCAH requires that the dietetic service be organized in such a manner that it shall effectively apply the principles of the science of nutrition to the preparation of palatable and appropriate food. The services are generally directed by a qualified person and staffed by adequate numbers of dietitians and technical and clerical personnel. Qualified personnel in the dietary division are generally considered to be individuals who are registered by the American Dietetic Association or have met that Association's standards for qualification.

In addition to the purchasing, planning and preparation of menus, both for patients and employees, the dietitian is generally responsible for recording dietary histories of patients such as those with food allergies and those unable to accept a limited diet regimen; interviewing patients regarding their food habits; counseling patients and their families concerning normal or modified regimens, and encouraging patients to participate in planning their own normal or modified regimens; and participating in appropriate ward rounds and conferences.

MEDICAL RECORDS DEPARTMENT

Every hospital is required by law to maintain adequate medical records on their patients. These must be accurately documented, readily accessible and can be easily used for retrieving and compiling information.[13]

The purposes of the medical record are:

1. To serve as a basis for planning and for continuity of patient care;
2. To provide a means of communication among the physician and any professionals contributing to the patient's care;
3. To furnish documentary evidence for the course of the patient's illness and treatment during each hospital stay;

4. To serve as a basis for review, study and evaluation of the care rendered to the patient;
5. To assist in protecting the legal interest of the patient, hospital and responsible practitioner;
6. To provide data for use in research and education.

The medical record must contain all significant clinical information and should be sufficiently detailed to enable another practitioner to assume the care of the patient at any time, a consultant to give an opinion after his examination of the patient and the practitioner to give effective continuing care to the patient.

A complete medical record is one which includes identification and sociological data, personal family history, history of present illness, physical examination, special examination such as consultations, clinical laboratory data, x-ray and other examinations, provisional or working diagnosis, medical or surgical treatment, gross and microscopic pathologic findings, progress notes, final diagnosis, conditions on discharge, follow-up, and autopsy findings.

Identification data in the medical record are generally provided on what is known as the admission sheet. This sheet generally contains such perinent information as the unit record number, the patient's name, address, name of the patient's spouse, home telephone number, business telephone number, sex, date of birth, birth place, marital status, occupation, referring family physician's name and address, admission diagnosis, date and time of admission, and destination within the hospital. Attached to the admission sheet, one may generally find consent forms for the authorization for medical or surgical treatment, authorization for the release of information to insurance companies, and a general authorization for the release of information to other physicians or attorneys.

The admission history sheet usually provides space for recording the name of the informant as well as the name of the individual taking the history. The purpose of the admission history is to record the patient's chief complaint and a description of his present illness. In addition, it provides the opportunity of protecting the provisional or admitting diagnosis which is usually made on every patient at the time of admission.

The history and physical examination sheet provides the physician with such information as hospital admissions that have taken place in the past with their subsequent diagnosis, operations and major injuries that have been experienced by the patient, the history of childhood and adult infectious diseases, if applicable, pregnancies with dates, outcome and complications, immunization data, a history of transfusion with dates, reactions and complications, current medications, sociological data covering habits with alcohol or tobacco, diets, height, weight, date of birth, country of birth, education, military history, occupational history, marital status, health of spouse, family history.

The physical examination sheet consists of a routine systematic review of skin, head and neck, cardiorespiratory, breast, gastrointestinal, urinary, genitalia, endocrine-metabolic, lymph nodes and hematological, muscular skeletal and extremities, urologic, psychiatric, and allergy.

Once the physician has obtained all of this information, he then proceeds to record in the medical record a suggested program to be followed during the hospitalization of the patient.

Signed laboratory sheets are entered into the patient's medical record. The laboratory reports include those obtained from chemistry, hematology, microbiology, serology, pathology as well as radiology. For this purpose, hospitals have a preprinted form which permits for the recording of data under each of the specific sections. However, some hospitals find it practical to paste the original laboratory reports into the medical record.

All treatment procedures performed upon the patient are recorded in the medical record. Operative notes are also included in the record and contain both a description of the findings as well as a detailed account of the technique used and the tissue removed.

Progress notes are made in the medical record for the purpose of providing the physician with a chronologic picture and analysis of the clinical course of the patient.

Upon the completion of all of the diagnostic procedures to be performed, it is mandatory that the physician enter into the medical record a definitive final diagnosis which is based on the terms specified in the standard nomenclature of diseases and operations.

Upon discharge from the hospital, the patient's record will have entered into it a discharge summary. The purpose of this is to provide a recapitulation of the patient's hospitalization. In some hospitals, a copy of this discharge summary is forwarded with the patient whenever he is transferred either to another hospital or to an extended care facility or nursing home. Some of the items contained within the discharge summary include a brief history, results of the physical examination, laboratory data, a description of the patient's hospital course, the diagnosis, the present condition, medications that have been sent with the patient, a listing of the operations performed, complications, disposition, and an estimated length of diability.

If the patient has died while in the hospital, and an autopsy has been performed, the medical record will contain a complete protocol of the findings that have resulted from the autopsy.

PATHOLOGY SERVICES

The JCAH requires that the pathology services shall be directed by a physician who is qualified to assume professional, organizational and administrative responsibility for the facilities and for the services rendered and there shall be sufficient personnel who have had adequate training and experience to supervise and conduct the work of the laboratory. The Director of the Pathology Service is a member of the medical staff and has undertaken special training in pathology. Generally, he is certified by the American Board of Pathology or its equivalent. In addition to the cytologic and gross anatomic analysis performed within the department of pathology, most hospitals group clinical laboratories within this division. Laboratories such as clinical chemistry, microbiology, clinical microscopy, hematology, and serology are but a few examples.

BLOOD BANK

Because of the essential nature of blood as a therapeutic agent, most hospitals operate a blood bank. This service is generally under the supervision of a licensed physician who has a basic interest in hematology. However, some hospitals assign the blood bank to the department of pathology because of its laboratory-like operation. Most hospital's blood banks operate as an adjunct to the local Red Cross Blood Program.

RADIOLOGY

One of the most important of the scientific and therapeutic facilities of the hospital is the department of radiology. Radiology is that branch of medicine which deals with the diagnostic and therapeutic application of radiant energy, chiefly in the form of roentgen rays and radium. The department is under the supervision of a qualified physician who has also obtained adequate training and experience in general radiology.

Radiology services are performed only upon the written order of a member of the medical staff who has been granted clinical privileges in the hospital. The therapeutic use of radium or sealed radioactive sources in the hospital is limited to physicians, who have been granted this privilege, after consultation with, and consideration of, the recommendations of the radiologist and/or a radiation safety committee. Only persons who have suitable training and experience are permitted to handle radioactive materials.

The department of radiology generally consists of physicians who are trained as radiologists, physicists, technicians, radiotherapists, isotopepharmacists, nurses, orderlies, and secretarial personnel.

MEDICAL SOCIAL SERVICE DEPARTMENT

The Medical Social Service Department is an important liaison between the hospital and the patient and his community. The qualified social worker represents a discipline whose professional focus is on the social aspects of the patient and his family. Social service personnel generally provide information relating to medical social study of appropriate patients; social therapy and rehabilitation of patients; home environmental investigations for attending physician; cooperative activities with community agencies; social service summaries; and follow-up reports of discharged patients, confirming disposition, when obtained.

ANESTHESIA SERVICE

The Anesthesia Service of a hospital is generally directed by a physician member of the medical staff who has had special training and is responsible for the following: quality of anesthesia care rendered by anesthetist in the surgical and obstetrical areas; availability of equipment necessary for administering anesthesia and for related resuscitative effects; development of regulations concerning anesthetic safety; and retrospective evaluation of all anesthesia care.

Anesthesia care is usually provided by anesthesiologists, other qualified physician anesthetist, qualified nurse anesthetist, or appropriately supervised trainees in an approved educational program. Whenever nurse anesthetists are employed, they generally provide general anesthesia under the overall direction of the departmental director or his designee.

CENTRAL SERVICE DEPARTMENT

The Central Service Department furnishes all supplies required for the nursing units. These supplies include sterile linen, sterile kits, operating room packs, needles, syringes, and other medical surgical supplies. In addition the personnel in this department clean, inspect, repair, assemble, wrap, and sterilize special treatment trays for the various nursing units. Reference to Chapter 22 will provide the student with a greater insight as to the functions of this department.

PHARMACY'S ROLE IN THE HOSPITAL

Reference to the Administrative Organization Charts (Figs. 1 and 2) will quickly support the claim that a hospital is truly a "city within a city." Within its four walls there is in operation: a hotel which manifests itself by the patient's room accommodations; a dormitory for the student nurses, residents and interns; a school for the training of nurses, technicians, dietitians; laboratories; a pharmacy; food vending operations; a laundry and linen service; housekeeping services; engineering and power generating services; delivery services; a post office; a massive internal and external communications system; blood bank; accounting and credit services; a public relations department; a motor service and security patrols.

Although the pharmacy department is only one of the many divisions of a hospital, it exerts a great deal of influence on the professional stature of the hospital as well as upon the economics of the total operational costs of the institution because of its inter-relation with and the inter-dependency of these other services upon it.

In the community practice of pharmacy, the pharmacist is keenly aware of the doctor-patient-pharmacist triad. In this setting, the doctor diagnoses and prescribes, the pharmacist dispenses the medication and the patient administers the prescribed drug to himself or at most it is administered to him, under ordinary circumstances, by a member of his family.

This is not true in the hospital or in an extended care facility. In this setting we find interjected into the doctor-pharmacist-patient triad the professional nurse who assumes the major responsibility of administering all medications to the patient (unless the patient is on a self-medication regimen).

Clearly then, the pharmacist who practices his profession in an institutional environment must be aware of the forces operating around him, and he must learn not only to understand them, but to assist in marshalling them towards the ultimate goal of better patient care.

HOSPITAL CONTRACTUAL RELATIONS

Because of the high cost of delivering health care, governing boards of hospitals have resorted to various means of reducing operating costs. In some institutions this has been achieved via shared services agreement,[14] contract management,[15] and institutional management contracts.[16] Yet others have gone the corporate reorganization route.

SHARED SERVICES

Sharing of services offers a viable option to health care institutions in providing extensive and high-quality services in a cost-effective manner. Such services include both administrative and clinical activities. Shared services of an administrative nature can be defined as those support services that are not normally involved in the delivery of direct patient care and are not normally revenue producing. These services are easier to develop than clinical shared services programs because they do not directly involve the medical staff, have fewer external elements, and often can be implemented by the hospital's chief executive officer.[14]

Clinical shared services can be defined as those services that are normally involved with the delivery of direct patient care, are usually revenue producing, and may have a significant impact on the financial resources of the participating institutions.[14]

Hospitals may develop and participate in various types of arrangements to organize and operate shared services programs, including:

(a) Referral service—a service maintained by one member of a group of health care institutions.
(b) Purchased service—any service for which an institution pays directly.
(c) Multisponsored service—a service jointly controlled and operated by a group of institutions generally involving a legal agreement among the sponsoring hospitals.
(d) Regional service—a service sponsored by an association of institutions through a community hospital council, a state hospital association or a special association or organization formed for a specific purposes.[14]

CONTRACT MANAGEMENT

The past decade has seen the evolution of a new industry in the health care field—contract management of the hospital's pharmacy department. A departmental management contract (DMC) is a formal agreement between a health care institution and a contractor, under which the contractor provides to the institution various management functions and which may include other services, in return for a fee.

A DMC differs from consultative services in several respects. Consultative services are most frequently specific in nature, limited in scope, and used only periodically. On the other hand, DMCs are ongoing and comprehensive, relate to day-to-day operation of a department, and combine consultation with the authority and responsibility for action and implementation.[15]

Once a contract has been agreed upon, the hospital and contractor must develop plans to ensure a close day-to-day working relationship. The initiator's management should commit itself to regular monitoring of the contractor's performance under the contract, just as it would evaluate the performance of any of its internally provided services.

Most hospital trustees and administrators believe that, with proper organization and supervision, the well-qualified department head who is provided with adequate resources should be able to equal or exceed any advantages claimed by contractors for services provided by them and, or the same time, provide additional benefits to the hospital.

Advantages of maintaining in-hospital services include—greater employee loyalty; scheduling flexibility; better interdepartment cooperation and teamwork and lower overhead costs. Advantages of contracting for services include—reduced costs; provides skills not readily available to the hospital; improves efficiency of the department served and reduces the number on the payroll, thus lowering the cost of fringe benefits. Contractors claim that their services offer the following advantages: higher productivity, better supervision, custom designed services, familiarity with labor demands, research capability and provides equipment and supplies at a lower cost because he has the price advantage of a quantity discount.[15]

INSTITUTIONAL MANAGEMENT CONTRACTS

With tight fiscal constraints being placed on hospitals coupled with a shortage of highly trained business-type executives to management them, trustee have entered into institutional management contracts (IMCs).

The American Hospital Association defines an institutional management contract as one of many types of arrangements through which health care institutions can obtain the services of other organizations or provide services to other organizations. An IMC is a formal agreement in which a hospital or other organization contracts with the governing board of a hospital to assume the responsibility for general management of the hospital. This managing organization appoints the administrator and has overall day-to-day management authority and responsibility for the managed hospital, subject only to the direction of the governing body. Subject to the terms of the contract and local law, the managed hospital may retain total legal responsibility and ownership of the facility and its assets and liabilities.[16]

Potential contractors for this service include autonomous hospitals, tax-exempt multihospital systems, shared services organizations, investor-owned multihospital systems, hospital associations and firms specializing in management contracts.[16]

Among the reasons hospitals enter into management contracts are: economies of scale; access to specialized consultants in finance, reimbursement, and management systems; procurement of qualified management personnel; resolution of financial difficulties; and assistance in dealing with licensing, planning and related regulatory requirements.[16]

HOSPITAL REORGANIZATION

Regulatory and competitive pressures are requiring hospitals and other healthcare providers to examine their organizational structures, and to realign those structures to place themselves in a more flexible posture to compete on an as nearly equal basis as possible in a healthcare delivery system undergoing revolutionary changes.

Organizational and entity structure has come to be recognized as an important weapon in a healthcare facility's arsenal for confronting these regulatory and competitive pressures that will only intensify in the future.

As a result, institutions are now reassessing their modes of operations, and are restructuring or have restructured to protect present and future assets, develop and safeguard a wide variety of new sources of revenue, attract additional funds through philanthropy, and to raise venture and equity capital through cooperative ventures.

The pressures impelling reorganization are many but can be summarized as follows:

1. Regulatory pressures—best exemplified by the switch of Medicare/ Medicaid from "reasonable cost" to "prospective payment."
2. Pronouncements by the administration that more cuts in healthcare financing are to be expected.
3. The prospective/capital payment systems have forced greater cooperation between hospitals and physicians in an effort to control costs.
4. The oversupply of physicians and hospital beds have caused sharp competition among physicians, hospitals and often between hospitals and physicians.
5. Cost conscious party payors.

The response of the industry has been a realignment of corporate structure.

Essentially, this has involved (a) the transformation of the existing hospital corporation into a parent corporation, deprived of its authority to operate a hospital; (b) the creation of a new subsidiary corporation to operate the hospital; and (c) the creation of other subsidiary corporations to operate various business enterprises.

HOSPITAL FINANCES

All too often, the hospital pharmacist lacks a thorough knowledge of the ways and means by which the operation of a hospital is financed. This situation is brought about by the pharmacist's lack of interest or his belief that it is a subject which does not concern him or his department. In reality, the finances of the hospital affect every patient, employee, staff member, trustee and the community at large.

Accordingly, the following is a brief resumé of the sources from which income may be derived to meet operating expenses.

The primary source of revenue is derived from the billing of patients for services rendered. A patient receiving such a statement may either pay it in full himself or he may have *third party coverage* which may pay the bill in full or pay a specified portion with the patient serving as co-insurer. Since the phraseology "third party coverage" or "third party payor" is nonspecific in definition the student is reminded that it may mean that the bill, either in full or in part, will be paid by someone other than the patient. These "third party payors" may include agencies such as Welfare, Vocational Rehabilitation Services, Aid to Families of Dependent Children, Blue Cross, Medicare, Medicaid or private insurance carriers. Some of these payors pay charges as billed, while others reimburse the hospital on a fixed all-inclusive per diem rate.

HEALTH MAINTENANCE ORGANIZATIONS (HMO'S)

With the passage of the Health Maintenance Organization Act of 1973[17] Congress endorsed the Health Maintenance Organizations (HMO's) concept as a method of improving medical care efficiency. HMO's provide a uniquely competitive approach to health care delivery. The concept is based on the idea of providing comprehensive health services in exchange for prepaid annual fees. The management of HMO's and their affiliated medical staff strive to provide high quality care while eliminating wasteful and costly medical procedures. Because inpatient hospital charges constitute an HMO's largest expense, their greatest incentive is to reduce an enrollee's length of stay in a hospital.

HMO's differ from traditional fee for service insurance companies in two important respects. Insurance companies such as Blue Cross and Blue Shield reimburse hospitals and doctors for whatever medically reasonable hospital costs were incurred on behalf of the patients. HMO's on the other hand, are at risk for their enrollee's health costs; they receive a flat fee for all the medical treatments they provide. They achieve a competitive advantage by utilizing less expensive methods of treatment. The emergence of diagnostic related group (DRG) regu-latory systems threaten the viability of HMO's by eliminating their competitive advantage. State-adopted DRG systems require hospitals to charge a fixed rate to all patients with similar diagnoses thereby eliminating the HMO's advantage of reducing a length of stay.[17] (See also Chapter 31, p. 663.)

DIAGNOSIS RELATED GROUPINGS (DRG's)

One of the most significant changes in health care reimbursement legislation was the passage of Title VI of the Social Security Amend-ments of 1983 and the implementation of a prospective payment sys-tem. This drastic change was forced upon the health care industry by spiraling inpatient hospital expenses which, at times escalated to three times the inflation factor in the general economy. The cost to the federal government of the Medicare program alone increased by 17%.[18]

It is of prime importance for hospitals to give serious study to the programs established by the federal government for the payment of Medicare claims because these represent approximately 40 to 45% of the institution's income. Additionally, private insurers will follow with similar prospective pricing programs.

A patient's health problem is described by diagnosis using one of two coding schemes: the *International Classification of Diseases Adopted, 8th Revision,* (ICDA-8), and the *Hospital Adaptation of ICDA, 2nd Edition,* (HICDA-2). These schemes classify patients with similar ailments, and allow the development of data for medical and statistical reporting, medical research and utilization review. These schemes are used to identify the various diagnoses of the patient as determined by the patient's physician. Although these methods have proved satisfactory for medical reporting purposes, there are shortcomings. For examples, other factors which affect treatment modalities are secondary diagnosis, surgery, age, prognosis, other medical procedures, and socioeconomic factors.[19]

As a result thereof, the ICDA-8 and HICDA-2 schemes have been replaced by an updated version, *International Classification of Diseases, Clinical Modification*—9th Revision—Clinical Modification (ICD-9-CM). This scheme expands and, in some cases, changes the labeling definitions and the amount of data abstracted for each patient, and as of January 1, 1979, hospitals are required to use this system when preparing discharge abstracts for Medicare and Medicaid patients.[19]

DRG's have been used in several applications requiring a measure of hospital output by case type. Currently, DRG's are being used in utilization review programs, hospital reimbursement experiments, development of a case mix index and to ascertain cost per case limits.

TAX EQUITY AND FISCAL RESPONSIBILITY ACT (TEFRA)

Because of what health care economists perceive as continued escalation of medical care costs, the federal government undertook a regulatory approach to change the retrospective payment system. The established goals for such a changeover were: (1) to provide immediate restraints on the growth of federal payments for health care, (2) to correct the instability of the Medicare Hospital Trust Fund, (3) to provide reliable predictions of expenditures in order to stabilize budgetary predictions, (4) to encourage beneficiaries to be cost conscious and (5) to be easy to administer and understand.[20]

The result was the passage of the Tax Equity and Fiscal Responsibility Act (TEFRA) in August 1982. The new law restructured Medicare payment for hospital inpatient services to include not only routine operating costs, but also ancillary and special care unit services, establishing control over total inpatient costs, excluding capital and direct teaching costs. The method of calculating these costs was changed and is now based on a hospital's average total cost per case, rather than the average cost per diem. Thus, reimbursement is no longer dependent on the length of stay; instead, it has become a fixed payment per patient based on discharge diagnosis. Accordingly, hospital pharmacies will be affected and pharmacists will need to work closely with the administration and physicians to lower costs.

SELECTED READINGS

Naisbitt, John: Megatrends, New York, Warner Books Inc., 1982.
Starr, Paul: The Social Transformation of American Medicine, New York, Basic Books Inc./Harper Colophon Books, 1982.

REFERENCES

1. *Job Descriptions and Organizational Analysis for Hospitals and Related Health Services,* U.S. Government Printing Office, Washington, 1952.
2. *Accreditation Manual for Hospitals 1983.* Joint Commission on Accreditation of Hospitals, Chicago, Ill., 1983, page IX.
3. Ibid. page X.
4. Ibid. page 51.
5. Ibid. page 53.
6. Ibid. pages 51–56.
7. Cordes, D.W.: Radius of Administrative Responsibility, Hospitals, *38*:44, (June) 1964.
8. *The Hospital Administrator,* The Association of University Programs in Hospital Administration, Chicago, Ill.
9. Accreditation Manual for Hospitals 1985. Joint Commission on Accreditation of Hospitals, Chicago, 60611, p. 73.
10. Definition of a Teaching Hospital, American Hospital Association Memorandum, November 11–15, 1967.
11. Hassan, Wm. E.: The Teaching Hospital, Drug Topics, *112*:16:20, (Aug.) 5, 1968.
12. In Pursuit of Quality-Hospital Nursing Service, New York. National League for Nursing, 1964.
13. Hassan, Wm. E.: Clinical Pharmacy—The Medical Record, Drug Topics, *114*:16, (April), 1970.
14. American Hospital Association Guidelines for Shared Services for Hospitals Catalog No. G028, 1977. AHA. 840 N. Lake Shore Drive, Chicago, 60611.
15. American Hospital Association, Technical Adv. Bulletin, Department Management Contracts, Catalog No. 001703, 1979. AHA. 840 N. Lake Shore Dr., Chicago, 60611.
16. American Hospital Association, Technical Advisory Bulletin, Catalog No. T007, 1980. Institution Management Contracts, AHA. 840 N. Lake Shore Dr., Chicago, 60611.
17. Pub. L. No. 93-222,87 Stat. 931 (1973) Codified at 42 U.S.C. s.300e-10 (1973).
18. Diagnostic Related Groups, Their Evolution, Current Applications, and Future Implications. Ernst & Whinney Document No. J58341, 1980.
19. The Revised DRGs. Their Importance in Medicare Payments to Hospitals. Ernst & Whinney Document No. J58442, 1983.
20. Huffman, D.C., Jr. and Kilgore, Susan, M.: Changing Concepts in Hospitals Reimbursement. Curr. Concepts in Hosp. Pharm. Mgt.: *6*:3:13–18, 1984.

3

The Pharmacy—Its Organization and Personnel

A number of years ago, Francke et al.[1] stated:

"The dispensing function of the pharmacist, while important and even vital, is essentially a superficial practice of the profession which, by itself, does not require knowledge or skills basic to merit professional recognition to the depth that lies within the grasp of hospital pharmacists."

Clearly, the above observation was a forecast of pharmacy's future new role for, less than a decade later, pharmacists have assumed important new roles—those of clinical pharmacist and drug consultant. To be able to assume these positions, it has become necessary to alter the pharmacist's educational program and work habits.

The *Task Force on Prescription Drugs*[2] made the following comments on the new role of pharmacy:

"The pharmacy profession currently faces a dilemma which is partly though not entirely of its own making. Many other aspects of health care—the practice of medicine and surgery, hospital operations and particularly drug manufacture—have developed and adopted new devices and techniques which have remarkably improved the provision of health services. In contrast, the number of important new methods introduced to enhance the efficiency of retail pharmacy operations, at least during the past two or three decades, has not been noteworthy . . ."

The role of the community or retail pharmacist is viewed by many people as simply transferring pills from a large bottle to a small one—counting tablets, typing labels and calculating the price. Much of his time is seen as devoted to routine merchandising of cosmetics, shaving supplies, stationery and other commodities which have little or no relationship to health care.

This has raised doubts concerning the relevance of modern pharmacy education. As with other members of health professions, on the one hand, it would seem that much of the traditional education is not utilized, since a nonprofessional person—working under the supervision of a licensed pharmacist—can effectively perform many of the

60

routine tasks of counting, labeling and pricing. At the same time, many pharmacists are seeking a new role as drug information specialists, and thus their formal education has taken this into account.

SUPPORTIVE PERSONNEL

Experience in numerous pharmacies—military and hospitals—has demonstrated that individuals without formal pharmacy education can effectively undertake many of the routine activities of pharmacists, under the supervision of a licensed pharmacist. Such activities have stimulated many hospitals to develop training programs to meet this need. In recognition of this development, the ASHP distributed the following Statement on Supportive Personnel in Hospital Pharmacy.[3]

ASHP STATEMENT ON SUPPORTIVE PERSONNEL IN HOSPITAL PHARMACY[a]

The increasing complexity of health care in the modern hospital is creating ever greater demands for the hospital pharmacy to broaden its scope of services. New health care legislation and rapid changes in health care technology are imposing new demands on hospital pharmacy which result in a need for increased manpower. These demands dictate for the hospital pharmacist a multifarious role which he can assume only when there is an adequate number of personnel within the pharmacy.

There is a growing concern about the present shortage of hospital pharmacists and an even greater concern about future shortages. The scope of pharmaceutical services being provided in most hospitals is limited largely by personnel shortages. Studies have indicated that many of the tasks performed in today's modern hospital pharmacy could be delegated to supportive personnel under the supervision of a pharmacist and, in fact, such personnel have long been used in most hospitals.

If the hospital pharmacist could be freed to a greater extent from performing routine tasks which could be delegated with supervision to trained supportive personnel, he would be able to direct more of his attention to professional tasks only, thereby expanding professional pharmacy service in the interest of patient care. Other professions— notably medicine, nursing, and dentistry—are in the process of delegating more and more functions to technicians and to other supportive personnel. Hospital pharmacy must do likewise if it is to keep pace

[a]Approved by the ASHP Board of Directors October 26–27, 1970 and by the AACP Executive Committee December 1970.

with progress in the health field, meet the growing demand for hospital pharmacy manpower, make maximum use of the hospital pharmacists' unique body of knowledge, and provide an opportunity for developing a scope of pharmaceutical services yet undefined and unrealized in the institutional setting.

Observations

Careful consideration of this subject by representatives of the American Association of Colleges of Pharmacy and the AMERICAN SOCIETY OF HOSPITAL PHARMACISTS has led to the following observations:

1. Previous and current studies indicate a growing shortage of professional hospital pharmacy manpower now and in the future.
2. The performance by pharmacists of duties which might appropriately be assigned to supportive personnel results in a dilution of pharmaceutical talents and limits the scope of pharmaceutical services provided.
3. Supportive hospital pharmacy personnel are used in most hospitals today.
4. The accelerating development of expanded professional services by the hospital pharmacy emphasizes the need for supportive personnel to assume many of the routine, nonjudgmental duties traditionally associated with the delivery of pharmaceutical services.
5. There is a need to recognize and define several different levels, or categories, of supportive hospital pharmacy personnel.
6. There is a need to define those functions and responsibilities which can be assigned to each category of supportive hospital pharmacy personnel, as differentiated from those which can be carried out only by the pharmacist.
7. There is a need to define training requirements and to develop training programs for each category of supportive hospital pharmacy personnel.
8. There is a need to standardize nomenclature used in referring to supportive personnel in hospital pharmacy.

Recommendations

Based on these observations and consistent with the developments of pharmacy practice in hospitals, it is recommended that:

1. The term "supportive personnel" be adopted as standard nomenclature to be used in referring collectively to all nonprofessional personnel.
2. The American Association of Colleges of Pharmacy and the AMERICAN SOCIETY OF HOSPITAL PHARMACISTS give priority considerations to adopting standard nomenclature to be used in referring to the different levels, or categories, of supportive personnel.
3. The American Association of Colleges of Pharmacy cooperate with the AMERICAN SOCIETY OF HOSPITAL PHARMACISTS in developing hospital-based training programs for hospital pharmacy supportive personnel with consideration being given to the potential role of academic institutions and to the experiences of existing training programs.
4. The American Association of Colleges of Pharmacy continue to provide

consultation to the AMERICAN SOCIETY OF HOSPITAL PHARMACISTS to the development of training programs.
5. The American Association of Colleges of Pharmacy and the AMERICAN SOCIETY OF HOSPITAL PHARMACISTS support and participate in, where possible, projects defining the roles of, and the training requirements for, supportive personnel in hospital pharmacy.

Livengood and associates[4] conducted a regional survey to determine the utilization of hospital pharmacy supportive personnel. The survey showed that, within the region, a high percentage of the hospitals (92.4%) utilize pharmacy technicians and that, on the average, there is approximately one technician employed for each pharmacist.

PHARMACY SPECIALISTS

Major teaching hospitals require a diversified pharmacy staff. Professional personnel include clinical pharmacists (Chapter 11) and Drug Information Specialists (Chapter 25). The area of clinical pharmacy has undergone rapid change and its practitioners have undertaken to specialize in the sub-medical specialties of psychiatry, geriatrics, oncology, nuclear medicine and pediatrics. The ASHP has developed the appropriate supplemental standards and learning objectives for residency training in the sub-specialties of clinical pharmacy (Chapter 26).

Residencies in these specialties are defined as postgraduate programs of organized training that meet the requirements set forth and approved by the ASHP. The ASHP Accreditation Standard for Specialized Residency Training[6] together with special supplemental standards for each specialty are the basic criteria used in evaluating and accrediting these programs. For examples, see Chapter 26.

DRUG INFORMATION SPECIALISTS

At the other end of the spectrum, it is also becoming evident that appropriately trained pharmacists may become new and vital members of the total health team by serving as drug information specialists. Some hospitals—especially teaching institutions and those in major medical center complexes—are already using pharmacists as consultants on drug therapy. They serve not only as drug distributors, but also as sources of drug data for physicians, interns, residents and nurses. They may participate in ward rounds with the staff, providing valuable drug information on both old and new drug products. Although they do not prescribe for patients, they enable the physicians who do prescribe to keep up more effectively with drug information. While some pharmacists are already serving as drug information specialists, and others are probably competent to do so, not all pharmacists have adequate competency in this field. Some licensed pharmacists have received 5 or even 6 years of formal college training, but about 15% of those now in practice have received 2 years or less of formal pharmacy education, and nearly half of these have had courses lasting only about 5 months.

PHARMACY EDUCATION

The manner in which pharmacists, pharmacy associations, pharmacy schools and the pertinent state pharmacy agencies repond to increasing demands for pharmaceutical services will unquestionably determine in large measure how the pharmacy profession will evolve during the years to come. As a guide to the responses which should be made, there is a clear need for a broad study of pharmacy education similar to the famed Flexner study of medical education made half a century ago.

The Task Force therefore recommends that the Bureau of Health Manpower should support—

(a) The development of a pharmacist aid curriculum in junior colleges and other educational institutions.

(b) The development of appropriate curricula in medical and pharmacy schools for training pharmacists to serve as drug information specialists on the health team.

(c) A broad study of present and future requirements in pharmacy, adequacy of current pharmacy education, and the educational changes which must be made.

The department of pharmacy is typical of the majority of other departments in the hospital in that, depending upon its size and services rendered, it employs both professional and lay personnel. Therefore, it behooves the administrator or his pharmacist to ascertain the necessary number of employees in each category which will be required to render safe and prompt service. In addition, due to legal criteria the duties and responsibilities of each category of employee must be quite clearly defined.

JOB DESCRIPTIONS

The federal government, in a 1952 publication,[8] has clearly and adequately provided us with job descriptions for the positions of "Chief Pharmacist," "Pharmacist" and "Pharmacy Helper." Accordingly, the following is a direct excerpt of the job summary and performance requirements for the position of chief pharmacist.

"Compounds and dispenses medicines and preparations according to prescriptions written by physicians, dentists, and other practitioners authorized by law to prescribe. Prepares and sterilizes injectable medication manufactured in hospital, and manufactures pharmaceuticals. Furnishes information concerning medications to physicians, interns, and nurses. Plans, organizes, and directs pharmacy policies and procedures in accordance with established policies of hospital. Implements decisions of pharmacy and therapeutics committee of which he is a member. Performs related duties.

PERFORMANCE REQUIREMENTS

"RESPONSIBILITY FOR: Preparation and sterilization of injectable medication manufactured in hospital; manufacture of pharmaceuticals; dispensing of drugs, chemicals, and pharmaceutical preparations; filling and labeling of all drug containers issued to services; inspection of all pharmaceutical supplies on all services; maintenance of an approved stock of antidotes and other emergency drugs; dispensing of all narcotic drugs and alcohol and maintenance of a perpetual inventory of them; specifications for purchase of all drugs, chemicals, antibiotics, biologicals, and pharmaceutical preparations used in treatment of patients; furnishing information concerning medications to physicians, interns, and nurses; establishment and maintenance, in cooperation with accounting department, of a system of records and bookkeeping in accordance with policies of hospital for charges to patients, and control over requisitioning and dispensing of drugs and pharmaceutical supplies; planning, organizing, and directing pharmacy policies and procedures in accordance with established policies of hospital; cooperation in teaching courses to students in school of nursing and in medical intern training programs; implementing decisions of pharmacy and therapeutics committee; and preparation of periodic reports on progress of department.

"Accuracy in use of chemical and pharmaceutical equipment for compounding and dispensing drugs and medicines. Follows prescription in details, and is accurate in labeling of containers and indicating directions for use."

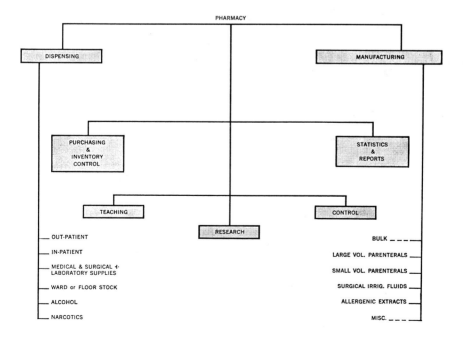

Fig. 4.   Departmental activity chart.

DETERMINING THE DEPARTMENTAL STAFF—PROFESSIONAL

The number of professional and lay employees necessary cannot be determined until some thought has been given to the scope of service to be rendered. Is the department to serve in-patients only? How many? Is there to be any out-patient service? If so, how many patients per day? Is there to be a manufacturing section of the pharmacy? Is the pharmacy going to stock and dispense surgical and laboratory supplies?

Once these questions are answered, the pharmacist must then determine which of the duties must, by law, be assigned to pharmacists and those which are within the scope of reasonably intelligent lay personnel who are herein referred to as pharmacy helpers.

In order to understand and to ascertain the personnel requirements, it is recommended that the department's major activities be dia-

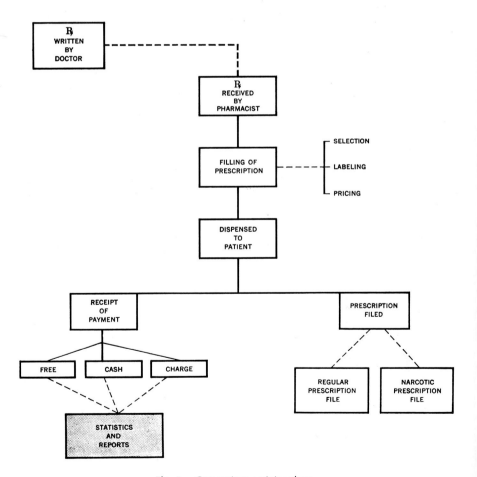

Fig. 5.   Out-patient activity chart.

grammed. Examples of such a process are provided in Figure 4 which represents the over-all functions of a department of pharmacy in a university teaching hospital, Figure 5 which briefly presents the activity involved in the dispensing of an out-patient's prescription and Figure 6 which provides a diagrammatic representation of the various processes involved in accommodating in-patient drug needs.

Once these charts are prepared, the hospital pharmacist is ready to evaluate the job, so diagrammed, through the preparation of a Flow Process Chart, Figure 7. By so doing, the pharmacist will be able to evaluate the time and motion involved in the performance of each job in the department. In addition, he will have a unique opportunity to utilize more efficiently the time of his personnel through simplification of the job by applying to it the various interrogatories of work simplification, namely:

What is its purpose?
Why is it necessary?

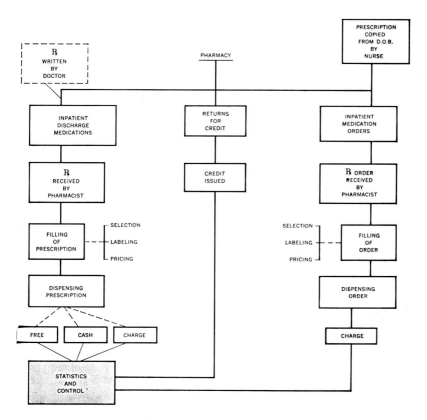

Fig. 6. In-patient activity chart.

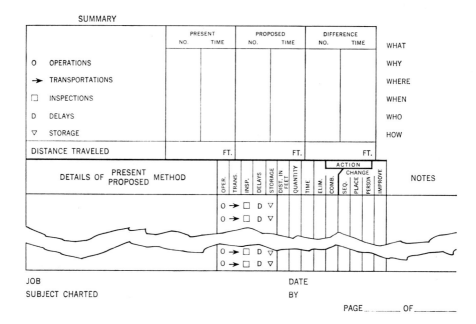

Fig. 7.   Flow process chart.

Where should it be done?
When should it be done?
Who should do it?
How should it be done?

Once each detail involved in the performance of a particular job has been challenged, each job will become sufficiently streamlined so as to require a minimal expenditure of the employee's time, motion, and energy thereby providing for maximal production without any increase in the labor force on hand.

As a result of the preparation of these flow charts, the pharmacist should be in a better position to visualize the volume of activity in each category as well as the number of assistants necessary to dispense the medications and supplies to the correct area in the hospital.

There are no standard rules for the staffing of a hospital pharmacy which can be quoted. However, in the publication *Mirror to Hospital Pharmacy* the following reference to staffing is made.[9]

"... in hospitals with from 100 to 500 beds and over, about 100 to 150 prescriptions or orders are processed daily for each full-time pharmacist employed. While it is difficult to make precise comparison of this workload with those reported by others, the number of prescriptions and requisitions filled falls within the range of those handled in pharmacies of the Public Health Services. For example, a report by Archambault (Division of Hospitals Bulletin No. 60–86 [1960]), states that the Pharmacy Branch considers a daily measurable workload of from 125 to 190 units plus a normal amount of non-measurable activities as reasonable for a pharmacist working with adequate non-professional assistance in hospitals utilizing 6 or less pharmacists. A daily range of 126 to 158 units per pharmacist is considered normal by Archambault for the one- or two-man pharmacies, while 168–181 units per man is considered normal in pharmacies employing 3 to 5 pharmacists."

Those individuals who are desirous of using the above quoted standards are reminded that the work units employed in the Public Health Service include a number of bulk compounded and pre-packaged items, as well as prescriptions and requisitions. In addition, the authors point out that the above standard omits consideration of a number of non-measurable workloads as well as the effect of non-professional assistance to the pharmacist.

Jeffries and Greenberg[10] in their study on prescription pricing, state that the average time required for the proper dispensing of a noncompounded prescription is 8 minutes and that 14 minutes is required for a compounded prescription.

Because the dispensing pattern within the hospital differs from that employed in the retail practice of pharmacy, a personally conducted survey of the dispensing time in the hospital pharmacy of a 300-bed teaching hospital was conducted. The results showed that a pre-packaged medication could be dispensed in an average time of 4 minutes (which coincides with the arbitrarily selected time of 4 minutes referred to in the *Mirror to Hospital Pharmacy*).[9] Accordingly, it should not be too difficult to ascertain the workload within the pharmacy and thereby arrive at the approximate number of pharmacists required. If this system is used, the reader is again cautioned to take into consideration the fact that not all of the services rendered by the pharmacist are reflected in the prescription or order workload. Time must be provided for administrative work, purchasing, teaching, sick time, and vacation time, to mention a few.

The following table, which may serve as a guide to those contemplating using this method of ascertaining staff needs, is reproduced from the *Mirror to Hospital Pharmacy*.[9]

Daily In-Patient Workload per Pharmacist

Bed Capacity Short-Term	Prescriptions	Other Orders	Combined Work Load
Under 50	10	10	20
50–99	45	17	62
100–199	96	44	140
200–299	101	50	151
300–399	100	52	152
400–499	89	38	127
500 and Over	61	35	96
Long-Term			
All sizes	39	38	77

Some investigators[11] have explored the applicability of the *queuing theory* as a mathematical tool in scheduling the pharmacist manpower needs of a hospital out-patient pharmacy. To apply this theory, it is necessary for the pharmacists to maintain time records to indicate "time in," "time start" and "time finish" or various types of prescriptions. The difference between "time in" and "time finish" is the waiting time (queue) of the patient.

Liebman *et al.*[12] suggest that the essential result of the use of the queuing theory is that the number of pharmacists on duty in the out-patient pharmacy should be synchronized to the fluctuations in the prescription order arrival rate.

With the introduction of clinical pharmacy activities into the institutional setting, the time spent on the product oriented services has decreased in favor of time devoted to clinical activities. This was borne out by a task analysis of a pharmacist's activities in a 45-bed rural hospital with comprehensive pharmaceutical services. The study[14] showed that almost one-third of the total work time was spent in clinical pharmacy activities. A major distinction between the activities of the pharmacist offering comprehensive services and those providing product-oriented services was the difference in the nonproductive amount of time. The latter group averaged 52.1% of its day in nonproductive time while the pharmacist in this study was nonproductive only 15% of the time.

DETERMINING THE DEPARTMENTAL STAFF—LAY PERSONNEL

Personnel falling into this category are secretarial or clerical workers, delivery men and hospital pharmacy technician-helpers.

The functions of secretarial or clerical workers would appear to be quite well defined and require no description here. Ascertaining the number of people required will depend on the amount of purchasing, inventory control and accounting procedures which are assigned to the pharmacy. Other factors which influence the need for secretrial assistance are the number of hospital committees upon which the pharmacist serves as secretary, the frequency of departmental publications such as pharmacy bulletins, frequency of updating the formulary, whether or not literature files are maintained and whether or not the pharmacist is active in teaching and research programs within the hospital.

Small hospital pharmacies usually have no need for delivery services or hospital pharmacy technician-helpers. The larger the unit, the more the need for this category of employee becomes. It can and has been argued that with modern means of communication, vertical conveyor systems and pneumatic tube devices, the pharmacy has little or no need for a delivery service. This is a sound argument and may be perfectly valid in departments which are located in new buildings with all of the above refinements. But even in those departments, certain types and sizes of products must be transported by human beings. If the volume is not great, the pharmacist may arrange to share the services of one messenger with other departments or may utilize the services of the *central transport* and *messenger service* of the hospital, if one exists. If, on the other hand none of the above mentioned modern conveyance devices are available, then the need for human transporters becomes obvious. Because of the shortage of nurses, pharmacists, technicians and other specially trained personnel, they should be spared the inconvenience and waste of time picking up and delivering supplies. Oftentimes hiring a delivery staff saves countless man-hours throughout the hospital.

Because of the acute shortage of pharmacists in many areas of the country, many hospitals have been forced to utilize hospital pharmacy technician-helpers.[13] As this trend developed, it became evident that some standards for such a category of personnel were needed. Thus, the Joint Committee on Hospital Pharmacy of the American Society of Hospital Pharmacists and the American Association of Colleges of Pharmacy met and agreed upon the following.[13a]

1. The worker classificaiton of hospital pharmacy technician-helper exists in most hospitals today;
2. There may be a need for more formal methods of training to improve the quality and quantity of technician-helpers;
3. Recent publications stress the dilution of pharmaceutical talents resulting from the performance of non-professional duties by pharmacists;
4. Previous and current studies indicate the possibility of a grave shortage of professional manpower in the near future;
5. Attempts to establish similar programs in the past resulted in emotional outbursts which damaged professional unity.

It was also the consensus that the details of such a training program should be developed by the American Society of Hospital Pharmacists because of the unique need of this type of employee within the hospital.

The use of hospital pharmacy technician-helpers is strongly advocated only if they are properly trained and supervised. It should be clear that these people may not perform a "dispensing act" for this would be in violation of a majority of the state pharmacy codes.

As has been previously stated, there is in existence a need for supportive personnel in hospital pharmacy to assist in the newer programs of strip packaging, unit of use distribution systems and intravenous additive programs. However, no definitive guidelines for this type of personnel were available until the American Society of Hospital Pharmacies released its original *Statement on Supportive Personnel in Hospital Pharmacy* and subsequently its Competency Standard for Pharmacy Supportive Personnel in Organized Health Care Settings which is reproduced[17] on page 61.

Beahm[15] in a study regarding the use of non-licensed personnel in pharmacy has reported that it is possible to ascertain which functions normally performed by a pharmacist may be done by a technician, those which may be done by a technician under supervision, and those which a technician is forbidden to do.

Among those which a non-licensed person is prohibited from doing are the following: take telephone orders for prescription refills from patients, weigh or measure ingredients to be used in compounding prescriptions, mix ingredients, already weighed or measured, to compound prescriptions, calculate percentages in prescription compounds, take telephone orders for new prescriptions, affix prescription labels to medication containers, provide information on use, precautions etc., to patients and professional personnel.

Those functions that may be done under supervision are as follows: type labels from prescription orders to be later attached to containers by pharmacist, assemble prescription ingredients immediately prior to pharmacist's filling of order, pre-package prescription drugs, print labels for pre-packaged drugs, affix pre-printed labels to containers of pre-packaged drugs, pre-package solid dosage forms in single unit packages, pre-package injectable dosage forms in single unit packages, pre-package all liquids in single unit packages, order and check in pharmaceuticals, calculate prices for prescriptions dispensed by pharmacists, maintain family prescription records, package finished dosage forms immediately prior to pharmacist's checking of prescription, weigh and measure ingredients in bulk compounding of pharmaceuticals, maintain narcotic drug inventory records, maintain drug inventory records.

Non-licensed personnel may perform the following duties independent of pharmacist's supervision: locate prescription order and file immediately prior to pharmacist's filling of prescription, routinely inventory supplies and re-stock prescription items, calculate the prices for prescriptions dispensed by pharmacists, clean bulk manufacturing and pre-packaging equipment, clean other prescription equipment, deliver prescription drugs to physicians and nurses in hospital or office for professional use, deliver prescriptions to patients but refer any quesitons to pharmacists, bill patients and/or third party and pay pharmacy accounts.

Although the foregoing classification is based upon responses from societies of hospital pharmacists, responses from colleges of pharmacy as well as boards of registration in pharmacy, it did not coincide with the entire breakdown. The variation in response relative to technician utilization in the various activities covered by the survey may have been due to the tradition of certain activities in hospital and/or community practice.

Unfortunately there are no reliable criteria whereby a formula may be arrived at which, when properly applied to a set of statistics, will reveal the magic number of pharmacy helpers required in any given situation. This, then, requires some serious planning and evaluation on the part of the pharmacist-in-chief.

PROFESSIONAL SERVICES RENDERED

The primary function of the hospital pharmacist is to dispense drugs to the in-patients and out-patients where hospital policy permits. However, there are a large number of important ancillary areas of pharmacy in which the pharmacist should exercise his skills. Again, depending upon the size of the hospital, the pharmacist may develop such areas as bulk compounding, sterile product manufacturing, control laboratory, distribution of laboratory and medical and surgical supplies, as well as expanding his role as a teacher, drug consultant and clinical pharmacist. Another service worthy of consideration is the after-hour pharmacy service which will be discussed later under methods of drug distribution.

The bulk compounding and sterile manufacturing program are two areas which offer the hospital great financial savings and the pharmacist pride and prestige. These two areas will be discussed in greater detail in a later chapter.

CHARTING OF PHARMACY ORGANIZATION

With the selection and categorizing of the employees, it now becomes essential to develop a chart showing the flow of administrative authority. Obviously, in the very small departments, this is usually generally understood and no problems arise. However, in the large units with assistant chief pharmacists, supervisors, and lay personnel, authority must be delegated by the chief pharmacist.

Sample distributions are depicted in Figures 8 and 9. Clearly this can and should be tailored to meet the specific requirements of the department and hospital. Once prepared and approved, it should be conspicuously posted for each of the departmental employees to read and adhere to.

In large hospitals, departments of pharmacy have a more complex organization. Note for example, the Ohio State University Hospital's Department of Pharmacy organizational chart. It should seem obvious to the student that each of the subdivisions of the department are assigned specific responsibilities. The following are some of the responsibilities of each division.

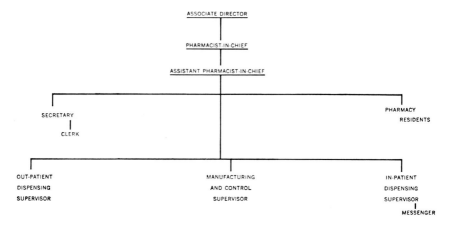

Fig. 8.   Departmental organization.

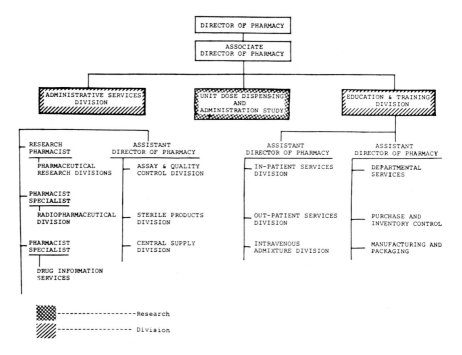

Fig. 9.   Departmental organization in a large university hospital pharmacy operation.

Administrative Services Division

1. Plan and coordinate departmental activities.
2. Develop policies.
3. Schedule personnel and provide supervision.

4. Coordinate administrative needs of the Pharmacy and Therapeutics Committee.
5. Supervise departmental office staff.

Education and Training Division

1. Coordinate programs of undergraduate and graduate pharmacy students.
2. Participate in hospital-wide educational programs involving nurses, doctors etc.
3. Train newly employed pharmacy department personnel.

Pharmaceutical Research Division

1. Develop new formulations of drugs, especially dosage forms not commercially available, and of research drugs.
2. Improve formulations of existing products.
3. Cooperate with the medical research staff of projects involving drugs.

In-Patient Services Division

1. Provide medications for all in-patients of the hospital on a 24-hour per day basis.
2. Inspection and control of drugs on all treatment areas.
3. Cooperate with medical drug research. See Chapter 7.

Out-Patient Services Division

1. Compound and dispense out-patient prescriptions.
2. Inspect and control all clinic and emergency service medication stations.
3. Maintain prescription records.
4. Provide drug consultation services to staff and medical students.

Drug Information Services Division

1. Provide drug information on drugs and drug therapy to doctors, nurses, medical and nursing students and the house staff.
2. Maintain the drug information center.
3. Prepare the hospital's pharmacy newsletter.
4. Maintain literature files.

Departmental Services Division

1. Control and dispense intravenous fluids.
2. Control and dispense controlled substances.
3. Coordinate and control all drug delivery and distribution systems.

Purchasing and Inventory Control Division

1. Maintain drug inventory control.
2. Purchase all drugs.

3. Receive, store and distribute drugs.
4. Interview medical service representatives. See Chapter 10.

Central Supply Services Division

1. Develop and coordinate distribution of medical supplies and irrigating fluids. See Chapter 15.

Assay and Quality Control Division

1. Perform analyses on products manufacturered and purchased.
2. Develop and revise assay procedures.
3. Assist research division in special formulations.

Manufacturing and Packaging Division

1. Manufacture wide variety of items in common use at the hospital.
2. Operate an overall drug packaging and prepackaging program.
3. Undertake program in product development.
4. Maintain a unit dose program.

Sterile Products Division

1. Produce small volume parenterals.
2. Manufacture sterile ophthalmologics, irrigating solutions etc.
3. Prepare aseptic dilution of lyophylizal and other "unstable" sterile injections for administration to patients.

Radiopharmaceutical Services Division

1. Centralize the procurement, storage and dispensing of radioisotopes used in clinical practice. See Chapter 23.

Intravenous Admixture Division

1. Centralize the preparation of intravenous solution admixture.
2. Review each I.V. admixture for physio-chemical incompatibilities.

ASHP COMPETENCY STANDARD FOR PHARMACY SUPPORTIVE PERSONNEL IN ORGANIZED HEALTH CARE SETTINGS[21]*

This Standard describes the *minimum* competencies which the technician category of pharmacy supportive personnel in organized health care settings should be expected to demonstrate. This is a companion document to the ASHP Training Guidelines for Hospital Pharmacy Supportive Personnel which outlines a suggested program for training technicians.

For purposes of this Standard, the definition of a pharmacy technician is the same as that given in the Training Guidelines, namely, someone who, under the supervision of a licensed pharmacist, assists in the nonprofessional (i.e., nonjudgmental) aspects of preparing and dispensing medications. Also, as in

---

*Approved by the ASHP Board of Directors, November 14–15, 1977. Originally drafted by the ASHP Council on Education and Manpower in response to a recommendation from the Council on Organizational Affairs.

the Training Guidelines, the duties of a "pharmacy technician" do not include those generally performed by secretaries, clerks, typists, delivery personnel or medication administration technicians. The Standard addresses itself to a "generalist" technician, one who can function appropriately in most hospitals, both small and large, in the kinds of activities for which there is generally the greatest need for supportive personnel manpower.

The competencies described in the Standard are representative ones and no attempt has been made to develop an exhaustive listing. It is believed that any technician who can demonstrate attainment of these competencies should be able to perform satisfactorily in any hospital or related health care facility after a reasonable period of orientation.

The competencies are described in behavioral terms; thus, it should be possible to evaluate the technician's attainment of each competency in the manner described in each statement. In some instances, this can be by paper and pencil tests, in other instances it can be by oral statement, and in yet other instances, by actually performing the activity or function under the observation of the evaluator. In the latter instances, it is extremely important that the evaluator judges the technician's performance strictly on the basis of the training objectives previously established for the respective training activity relating to the competency.

Omitted from most of the competency statements are references to time or error limits. Obviously, these must be taken into account in the evaluation process. It is suggested that reasonable time and error limits be imposed where indicated, based upon the evaluator's experience.

Standard 1

The technician shall demonstrate appropriate knowledge and understanding of the health care institution and its pharmacy department.

Competencies:
1. The technician will be able to interpret the institution's organizational chart in terms of the name and title of the administrative person to whom the director of pharmacy reports and the administrative and professional relationship of the pharmacy department to any other departments in the institution.
2. The technician will be able to describe the general responsibilities and job status of personnel in other institutional departments with whom he will have contact in carrying out his assigned duties and activities.
3. The technician will be able to interpret the organizational chart for the pharmacy department in terms of names and general responsibilities of all departmental supervisory and administrative personnel.
4. The technician will be able to describe the location of every department shown on the institutional organizational chart and will be able to escort another person to any department.
5. The technician will be able to state at least three valid reasons why information about patients must be kept confidential.
6. The technician will be able to state at lease five reasons for initiation of a disciplinary action in the institution (e.g., absenteeism, incompetency, dishonesty, etc.).

Standard 2

The technician shall demonstrate a thorough knowledge and understanding of the duties and responsibilities of his position.

Competencies:
1. The technician will be able to state all of his primary job responsibilities and the duties falling under each.
2. The technician will be able to state the institutional and departmental policies applicable to each of his primary job responsibilities and describe the procedures for each.
3. The technician will be able to define what is meant by "a decision requiring professional judgment" and will cite at least 10 examples.
4. The technician will be able to demonstrate the use of correct telephone communication technique and protocol both in receiving and in initiating calls.
5. The technician will be able to demonstrate the use of correct written communication by drafting a memorandum to his supervisor requesting a change in work assignment schedule to take care of personal business.
6. The technician will be able to state the general requirements of many local, state or federal laws which specifically affect any of his responsibilities.

Standard 3

The technician shall have a working knowledge of the pharmaceutical-medical terms, abbreviations and symbols commonly used in the prescribing, dispensing and charting of medications in the institution.

Competencies:
1. The technician will be able to interpret without error any 12 inpatient medication orders selected at random from at least four different patient units in the institution.
2. The technician will be able to define in lay terms the meaning of names of all the clinical, diagnostic and treatment units and services in the institution.

Standard 4

The technician shall have a working knowledge of the general chemical and physical properties of all drugs handled in manufacturing and packaging operations in the pharmacy department.

Competencies:
1. The technician will be able to designate from a list of 50 drug names those which are light-sensitive and those which must be refrigerated.
2. The technician will be able to list the titles of at least four reference books where he may find stability information on drug compounds.

Standard 5

The technician shall have a working knowledge of commonly used weight and volume equivalents and shall demonstrate an ability to carry out the arithmetic calculations required for the usual dosage determinations and solutions preparation.

Competencies:
1. The technician will be able to list without error the metric equivalents for the apothecaries doses and for household doses written in any 12 randomly selected medication orders.
2. The technician will be able to convert without error all metric or apothecary weights and volumes in at least four manufacturing formulas to the other system.
3. The technician will be able to perform the calculations necessary to prepare at least two different weight-in-volume and at least two different volume-in-volume solutions.

Standard 6

The technician shall demonstrate the ability to perform the essential functions relating to drug purchasing and inventory control.

Competencies:
1. The technician will be able to inventory a representative stock of pharmacy drugs and supplies using prepared forms and records.
2. The technician will be able to determine from existing reorder levels which inventoried items should be ordered and in what quantity.
3. The technician will be able to demonstrate an ability to check in a drug shipment using the packing list or invoice and purchase order, completing the receiving report, and adding the items to the inventory.
4. The technician will be able to demonstrate the ability to retrieve, without error, from the drug storeroom at least 10 randomly designated drug items.
5. The technician will be able to describe the procedure for returning outdated drugs to the manufacturer.

Standard 7

The technician shall demonstrate a working knowledge of drug dosages, routes of administration and dosage forms.

Competencies:
1. The technician will be able to list at least:
   a. Six routes of drug administration.
   b. Ten dosage forms and their respective routes of administration and
   c. Ten adverse effects encountered in drug therapy.
2. The technician will be able to state the lumen size, length and primary use for each of five different needles.
3. The technician will be able to identify, by name and use, each of five different syringes.

Standard 8

The technician shall have a working knowledge of the procedures and operation relating to the manufacturing, packaging and labeling of drug products.

Competencies:
1. The technician will be able to repackage and label 25 unit doses from a bulk supply of drugs and correctly complete all necessary control records.
2. The technician will be able to demonstrate for each of five randomly selected formulation and packaging requests:
   a. Correct selection of necessary equipment,

b. Proper assembly and use of the equipment,
c. Proper cleaning and storing of the equipment,
d. Proper selection of each ingredient,
e. Accurate calculation and measurement of each,
f. Proper completion of worksheet record of weights and volumes, manufacturers' lot numbers, and other required information,
g. Correct procedure for mixing and preparing product,
h. Proper selection and preparation of packages/containers and closures,
i. Proper packaging technique,
j. Correct selection and preparation of labels and
k. Proper quarantine procedure.
3. The technician will be able to identify from a list of 10 different steps in manufacturing and packaging operations, those functions which must be performed by a pharmacist only.

Standard 9

The technician shall have a working knowledge of the procedures and techniques relating to aseptic compounding and parenteral admixture operations.

Competencies:
1. The technician will be able to list five different possibilities for contamination of an injectable solution during its preparation and for each possibility a precaution which would prevent the contamination.
2. The technician will be able to demonstrate the proper technique for using a syringe and needle for aseptic withdrawal of the contents of:
   a. A rubber-capped vial, and
   b. A glass ampul.
3. The technician will be able to demonstrate the proper technique for aseptic reconstitution of an antibiotic injection.
4. The technician will be able to describe the occasions when hand washing is required and will demonstrate the proper technique.
5. The technician will be able to demonstrate the correct techniques and procedure for preparing at least three parenteral admixtures, including the proper preparation of the label and completion of the control records.
6. The technician will be able to identify the major components of a laminar air flow hood and state their functions.
7. The technician will be able to define and/or describe:
   a. Microbial growth and transmission,
   b. Origin, pharmacologic effect, and prevention of pyrogens,
   c. Sterility,
   d. Heat sterilization and
   e. "Cold" sterilization.
8. The technician will be able to designate from a list of 10 different sterile preparations those which may be safely heat-sterilized.
9. The technician will be able to demonstrate the proper technique for visual inpection of parenteral solutions.

Standard 10

The technician shall demonstrate the ability to perform the usual technician functions associated with a unit dose drug distribution system.

Competencies:
1. The technician will be able to prepare the drug profile for five newly admitted patients.
2. The technician will be able to pick all doses for one patient unit and complete the necessary dispensing records.
3. The technician will be able to describe the special dispensing and record-keeping procedures which apply to the dispensing of:
   a. Controlled drugs,
   b. Investigational drugs and
   c. Nonformulary drugs.
4. The technician will be able to list for each of 30 commonly prescribed drug trade names:
   a. The generic name,
   b. The common therapeutic use and
   c. The usual dose.

Standard 11

The technician shall demonstrate the ability to perform the manipulative and record-keeping functions associated with the dispensing of prescriptions for ambulatory patients.

Competencies:
1. The technician will be able to carry out the following functions for any 10 randomly selected ambulatory patient prescriptions:
   a. Correctly type the label,
   b. Select the proper drug from the dispensing rack,
   c. Accurately count or measure the product and place in the proper container,
   d. Complete the necessary records and documents and
   e. Calculate the charge for the prescription.
2. The technician will be able to describe the special procedures and documentation required in dispensing ambulatory patient prescriptions for:
   a. Controlled drugs,
   b. Investigational drugs and
   c. Alcohol.
3. The technician will be able to designate from a list of 10 steps involved in ambulatory patient prescription dispensing, those functions which only a pharmacist may carry out.

CONTROL OF PERSONNEL

This section is not intended as an invitation to the hospital pharmacist to subrogate the established personnel policies or procedures of the hospital. The purpose is to present a few relatively simple procedures whereby the pharmacist who is located in the smaller hospital and either functions alone or with lay help or who may be responsible for more than one department may maintain, in the absence of an active personnel director, reasonable employee records for accounting and administrative purposes.

The *Application for Employment* should elicit from the prospective employee vital information relative to his personal history, education, military service, office skills when applicable, previous employment record, interviewer's comments and the employment contract. It would seem necessary to obtain all of the above information in order to make an intelligent decision whether or not the applicant has the necessary qualifications for the position which he seeks or for which he is being interviewed. Certainly, if the question ever arose as to whether or not due care was used in the selection of the employee, a record, such as the one illustrated, properly completed, would serve as *prima facie* evidence.

It is essential that the director of pharmacy services evaluate the personnel in the department on a regular basis. In so doing, he must remain objective and impartial. To perform this important management responsibility the director should become familiar with such personnel appraisal systems as ranking, person-to-person comparison, grading, graphic scales, checklists, forced choice description, selection of critical incidents and management by objective.

Figure 10, the *Performance Rating Form,* can be used effectively in determining whether or not the employee is worthy of a pay increase. In addition, it can serve as a warning to the employee of his deficiency in certain areas. Many department heads in using this form assign a numerical value of 4 for each check mark under "excellent," 3 for "good," 2 for "fair" and 1 for "poor." A total is taken of the points and then divided by 10. The figure obtained determines where the category of "Overall Rating" is checked.

Figure 11, entitled *Paid Vacation,* is an example of a form which may be used within the department to keep an accurate record of those important fringe benefits due the employee, namely paid vacation or sick leave time. Improper records, particularly in the area of sick time, have been used to the detriment of the hospital in claims arising out of industrial accidents involving the employee or they may prove to be a great asset to him in his claim for insurance disability payments and income tax deductions.

HIRING OF PHARMACISTS

The hiring of pharmacy personnel is an extremely important function of the director of pharmacy service and requires special consideration.[16]

The State Board of Registration in Pharmacy is empowered to make rules and regulations for the enforcement of administration of the pharmacy law. Such regulatory and enforcement procedures must be in accord with the expressed or implied purposes of the enabling statutes. In view of the fact that the Board is an administrative, not legislative agency, it may not exercise any power of authority not delegated to it, or which, by reasonable implication is necessary to the proper functioning of the pharmacy law.

Brigham and Women's Hospital
EMPLOYEE PERFORMANCE REVIEW

Employee No. _____

Name _____ Department _____ Cost Center _____

Position _____ Review Date _____ Date Started in Present Position _____ ☐ Anniversary ☐ Transfer/Promotion

Please use Remarks Section for additional explanation of the areas evaluated below.

I. QUALITY OF WORK – Accuracy and neatness of work performed regardless of volume.

1. ___ Does very poor work.   2. ___ Work barely acceptable. Frequent errors.   3. ___ Usually does acceptable work.   4. ___ Better than average work. Very few errors.   5. ___ Outstanding work. Exceptionally accurate.

Remarks _____

II. QUANTITY OF WORK – Volume of work performed regardless of accuracy.

1. ___ Volume of work unsatisfactory. Seldom completes work on schedule.   2. ___ Barely passable volume of work.   3. ___ Usually accomplishes satisfactory volume of work. Average speed in producing results.   4. ___ Better than average volume of work.   5. ___ Outstanding volume of work. Completes jobs quickly.

Remarks _____

III. KNOWLEDGE OF JOB – Employee's knowledge in his particular field, his mastery of all phases of the job.

1. ___ Inadequate knowledge of job.   2. ___ Limited knowledge of job. Often needs explanation.   3. ___ Adequate knowledge of most phases of the job.   4. ___ Thorough knowledge of all phases of the job.   5. ___ Exceptional mastery of all phases of the job.

Remarks _____

VI. INTERPERSONAL RELATIONSHIPS – Ability to get along with fellow employees and his supervisor, i.e., disposition, tact, sincerity, thoughtfulness and courtesy.

1. ___ Frequently does not get along with others. Inclined to create friction. Cannot accept criticism.   2. ___ Indifferent to others. Cooperates occasionally. Fair teamworker.   3. ___ Accepts criticism with appropriate change in behavior. Gets along satisfactorily with others.   4. ___ Actively promotes harmony within a group. Flexible. Very good cooperation.   5. ___ Outstanding ability to create harmony in all situations. Goes out of way to cooperate.

Remarks _____

V. DEPENDABILITY – Reliability of employee and the extent to which employee can be counted on to carry out instructions.

1. ___ Completely unreliable. Has to be closely supervised.   2. ___ Not fully dependable. Needs more supervision than others.   3. ___ Dependable on routine work. Needs some supervision.   4. ___ Requires only occasional supervision.   5. ___ Needs no supervision.

Remarks _____

VI. ATTENDANCE – Attendance at work and work area. (Explain exact nature of any attendance problem.)

1. ___ Frequently absent.   2. ___ Some difficulty in attendance.   3. ___ Attendance is adequate.   4. ___ Consistently present.   5. ___ Attendance records are outstanding.

Remarks _____

VII. PUNCTUALITY – Arrival and departure for work and/or break periods.

1. ___ Frequently late.   2. ___ Sometimes late.   3. ___ Adequate punctuality.   4. ___ Consistently on time.   5. ___ Punctuality records are outstanding.

Remarks _____

VIII. GROWTH POTENTIAL – Ability to assume more responsibility and authority.

1. ___ Does not demonstrate ability to cope with present responsibilities.   2. ___ Does not demonstrate ability to grow and adapt.   3. ___ Demonstrates limited ability for growth and development in present job.   4. ___ Demonstrates considerable ability for growth and development in present job.   5. ___ Demonstrates ability to accept more responsibility and authority in other areas.

Remarks _____

(FOR SUPERVISORY EVALUATION OR PROMOTION TO SUPERVISORY POSITION ONLY)

JUDGMENT – Ability to make decisions by sound reasoning and the drawing of correct conclusions.

1. ___ Inclined to be illogical. Neglects and misinterprets facts.   2. ___ Makes frequent errors in judgment.   3. ___ Good common sense. Decisions seldom cause difficulty.   4. ___ Excellent judgment. Decisions are logical and sound.   5. ___ Outstanding ability to think quickly and logically and to use sound judgment.

Remarks _____

PLANNING AND ORGANIZING – Success in planning and organizing work to complete assignments on schedule.

1. ___ Inefficient. Work is poorly planned and organized.   2. ___ Planning ability is inadequate when under pressure.   3. ___ Effective under normal circumstances.   4. ___ Careful and effective planning.   5. ___ Exceptionally systematic. Inventive and creative.

Remarks _____

LEADERSHIP – Ability to train, supervise and get results through personnel.

1. ___ Antagonizes subordinates. Gets poor results.   2. ___ Fails to command respect and confidence.   3. ___ Meets minimum leadership requirements.   4. ___ Gets good results through motivation of subordinates.   5. ___ An extremely capable and forceful leader in directing and training subordinates.

Remarks _____

Additional Comments: _____

_____

_____

_____

Evaluator _____ Date _____ Department Head/Vice President/Assistant Vice President _____ Date _____

FOR EMPLOYEE ONLY

I understand that my signature neither confirms nor denies the validity of this performance rating but merely means that I have seen the report in its completed form. Upon inspection and discussion of this evaluation with my supervisor, my personal opinion:

_____ A Fair Evaluation _____ An Unfair Evaluation

Remarks: _____

Employee _____ Date _____ Reviewed by: _____ Personnel Representative _____ Date _____

Fig. 10.

PAID VACATION

Date of Employment _____

Name _____

Credit Balance 2/1/80
Starting 2/1/80
Period

Period	Dates	Added Credit	Paid Vac. Hours	Hours Balance
1	2/ 1/80– 3/ 7/80			
2	3/ 8/80– 4/11/80			
3	4/12/80– 5/16/80			
4	5/17/80– 6/20/80			
5	6/21/80– 7/25/80			
6	7/26/80– 8/30/80			
7	8/31/80–10/ 3/80			
8	10/ 4/80–11/ 7/80			
9	11/ 8/80–12/12/80			
10	12/13/80– 1/31/81			

VACATION DAYS

DATE TAKEN	HRS.	DATE TAKEN	HRS.	DATE TAKEN	HRS.

Fig. 11.

One of the clearly defined responsibilities of the State Board of Registration in Pharmacy is to establish the educational and experience qualifications which individuals must meet at the time of examination or registration.

Once an individual has successfully qualified for practice he is generally awarded a certificate of registration which enables him to practice pharmacy in the setting of his choice—community or institutional.

The American Society of Hospital Pharmacists through its Minimum Standard for Pharmacies in Hospitals prescribes that the department be under the direction of a "—professionally competent, legally qualified pharmacist—he shall be well trained in the specialized functions of hospital pharmacy and shall be a graduate of an accredited college of pharmacy or meet an equivalent standard of training or experience—."

Because of the fact that many of the approximately 7000 hospitals registered by the American Hospital Association are minus the services of a trained pharmacist, too many administrators are prone to overlook or ignore the mandates of good hiring procedure. The same applies to the overworked pharmacist in the larger hospital who is anxious to hire "another pair of hands" for peak periods in the operation of the department. Both of these "short-cuts" may prove to be disastrous from a legal point of view.

In practice, the hospital administrator, personnel director or director of pharmacy services, should insist that applications for pharmacist positions should show—

Proof of graduation from an accredited college/school of pharmacy.
Proof of licensure in the state in which the individual desired to practice.
Proof of professional competency.
Proof of good moral character.

In addition, a 6-month probationary period satisfactorily completed would be further evidence of the quality of the hiring procedures of the hospital in the selection of the pharmacist.

Should an unfortunate accident then occur, a charge of negligence might be defended successfully in some states.

State pharmacy laws, hospital licensing acts, Food and Drug laws, and state public health laws and agency regulations are clear on the issue that the use, as pharmacists, of those not skilled and experienced in the practice of pharmacy, as evidenced by state registration, is a criminal offense. In this connection, it should be borne in mind that neither the hospital administrator nor the director of pharmacy services are relieved by law of their responsibility where pharmacists are employed yet the work-load is so great that non-registered personnel must perform duties that the law limits to the registered practitioner of pharmacy.

DePiro et al.[15] studied the extension of unproductive and underproductive staff pharmacist activity to identify opportunities to improve use of pharmacists' time. The study noted the following percentages of time devoted to such areas as: (1) dispensing activities requiring professional judgment 19.5%; (2) dispensing activities not requiring professional judgment 37.8%; (3) therapy related activities 6.5%; (4) idle time 13.2%; (5) absent 8.9%; (6) communication and coordination 9.4% and (7) outpatient activities 0.5%.

As reasonable and prudent individuals, the hospital administrator and the director of pharmacy services know or should know the relationship between the work-load and the number of qualified staff necessary to handle it—expertly and on schedule.

Also of serious import is the civil liability that attaches to the institution in malpractice or negligence suits arising from injuries or deaths resulting from medication errors committed by a non-pharmacist acting in the capacity of a licensed pharmacist with the consent, implied or expressed, of the hospital management.

Accordingly, it behooves all pharmacists who are delegated the responsibility of managing the institution's pharmacy to exercise due care in the selection and hiring of personnel as well as the determination of acceptable work-loads and work assignments for the employees.

WOMEN IN PHARMACY

Although women are averaging 50% of pharmacy school enrollments, they represent only 15 to 20% of all practicing pharmacists. This segment of the work should not be ignored by hospital pharmacy directors when recruiting to fill vacant positions. Kirk[20] in a study of women in male dominated professions shows that even though women pharmacists are paid the same as men, have the same job responsibilities, and work the same hours, they are subconsciously stereotyped therefore precluding the occurrence of true equality for women pharmacists in many hospitals. Hospital pharmacy directors should make every effort to provide opportunities for female pharmacists to become actively involved in professional organizations to facilitate their gaining a professional identity. In addition, these women need to be encouraged to seek out managerial positions and to be given a clearer understanding that being a manager can be combined with family responsibilities.

SALARIES

At nearly every meeting of hospital pharmacists, the subject of salaries is discussed. Many of the state associations have conducted surveys amongst their membership in an attempt to determine the wage levels within the area and, when possible, to promote higher salaries.

The instigators of the salary survey movement are usually those individuals within the lower salary brackets. Some of these pharmacists may be doing an exceptionally fine job within their institutions but are harnessed by an unrealistic wage range within the hospital or even governmental salary structure.

On the other hand, there is a small segment of the profession which is continually advocating higher personal recompense even though they offer very little in return for the higher salary.

Because the hospital pharmacist is a highly trained professional member of the health team, his salary requirements should not be arrived at in the same manner as other members of the hospital staff. Neither should his salary be restricted by what other institutions in the area are paying.

It is generally agreed that no two hospitals are alike in their operation. By the same token, no two hospital pharmacists can be evaluated by what they do in neighboring institutions. They must be evaluated on their own performance standard within the particular institution they serve.

As a result of the economic pressures that are being exerted upon the hospital, many members of the professional staff are being subjected to unionization activities. Many pharmacists would prefer not to become involved with organizations whose sole goal is economic security but would demonstrate interest in a group combining both professional and economic goals.

Thus, the *Economic Status Program of the American Society of Hospital Pharmacists* came into being and is hereinafter reproduced.[18]

ECONOMIC STATUS PROGRAM OF THE AMERICAN SOCIETY OF HOSPITAL PHARMACISTS[a]

Policy on Economic Status

The professional and economic goals of the professional person are closely interrelated. Only in attainment of these goals can he assume the leadership role expected of him in the community by his colleagues, and by other health professions. When satisfactory economic status is achieved, the professional can realize his maximum potential and apply his full energies to the needs of the society.

The American Society of Hospital Pharmacists has, since its inception, concentrated on the professional responsibilities of hospital pharmacists through promotion of high standards of professional ethics, education and attainments. Nevertheless, the economic interests of members of the Society were acknowledged several years ago when the

[a]Approved by the Board of Directors on January 11, 1970.
Approved by the House of Delegates on March 29, 1971.

Mirror to Hospital Pharmacy and the Society's Commission on Goals counselled the ASHP to involve itself in activities dealing with the economic status of hospital pharmacists. Indeed one of the goals of the Society's statement, "Goals for Hospital Pharmacy" adopted in 1964, was to "Promote payment of realistic salaries to hospital pharmacists in both staff and managerial positions in order to attract and retain the services of career personnel." More recently, the Society conducted a salary survey to obtain factual data on the economic status of pharmacists in institutional practice.

The Society's concern for the economic welfare of its members complements the professional and scientific objectives presently set forth in the Constitution of the American Society of Hospital Pharmacists. Involvement by the Society in the economic well-being of its members is in the public interest since assurance of economic satisfaction tends to attract highly qualified pharmacists to institutional practice.

Salaries, working hours and fringe benefits of hospital pharmacists should be commensurate with professional education, responsibility and status and with the increased participation by hospital pharmacists in the actual planning and administration of pharmacy service and in the determination of policies which directly affect them. Both employers and employed pharmacists have an obligation to resolve employment issues fairly and in good faith.

The responsibility of the individual is primary. However, as institutions and the delivery of health care grow in size and complexity, collective effort may be necessary to solve group economic problems. With this view, the Society must meet the needs of its members by embarking on a broad program of economic status which may include such activities as the compilation of statistical data, the preparation of model contracts and, when necessary, mediation, conciliation and arbitration. When economic problems of employment cannot be resolved by the individual practitioner or the pharmacy staff of a hospital, the Society's Affiliated Chapters, with the legal and financial assistance of the ASHP, may find it necessary to engage in collective bargaining.

The Board of Directors of the American Society of Hospital Pharmacists, at its meeting of January 10–11, 1970 voted:

To engage in collective bargaining by assisting Affiliated Chapters, upon request, in accordance with policies and guidelines as established by the House of Delegates of the AMERICAN SOCIETY OF HOSPITAL PHARMACISTS; further,
To adopt the statement, "Economic Status Program of the American Society of Hospital Pharmacists."

In accordance with this action, the following are guidelines for individual members, Affiliated Chapters and the ASHP.

Guidelines for Collective Bargaining

Individual Members

1. Hospital pharmacists must recognize their obligation to the patient, the institution, the profession, the allied health professions and society.
2. Hospital pharmacists shall not deprive patients of pharmaceutical services by withholding their services in any form, including strikes, in support of economic demands.

Affiliated Chapters

1. Affiliated Chapters may engage in collective bargaining, preferably through the statewide Affiliated Chapter. Any such activity shall be conducted solely in the name of, and by, the Affiliated Chapter.
2. Affiliated Chapters may engage in collective bargaining when:
   a. professional prerogatives of the pharmacists are endangered by lack of effective representation; or
   b. wages or conditions of employment are below acceptable levels; or
   c. the environment in which the profession is practiced is not conducive to good patient care; and
   d. good faith attempts have failed to remedy the above situation(s).
3. Affiliated Chapters will make available the services of negotiating contracts to active ASHP members. All hospital pharmacists who practice at the contracting institution may be represented. Hospital pharmacists being represented who are not members of the Affiliated Chapter and the AMERICAN SOCIETY OF HOSPITAL PHARMACISTS must become members, if permitted by all applicable laws.
4. Affiliated Chapters will accept or reject contracts as determined by a majority of the members in the bargaining unit.
5. Affiliated Chapters will assess each hospital pharmacist a service fee for each contract negotiated, as determined by and paid to the ASHP, to the extent permitted by applicable laws.
6. Affiliated Chapters must follow procedures outlined by the ASHP.

American Society of Hospital Pharmacists

The SOCIETY will coordinate collective bargaining activities of Affiliated Chapters by providing:
   a. statistical information and research assistance;
   b. legal assistance; and
   c. financial assistance when necessary.

SELECTED READINGS

Stolar, M.: National Survey of Selected Hospital Pharmacy Practices, Am. J. Hosp. Pharm., *33*:225–230, (Mar.) 1976.

Dickson, W.M.: Measuring Pharmacist Time Use: A Note on the Use of Fixed-interval Work Sampling, Am. J. Hosp. Pharm., *35*:1241–1243, (Oct.) 1978.

Stolar, M.: National Survey of Hospital Pharmacy Technician Use, Am. J. Hosp. Pharm., *38*:1133–1137, 1981.

Mahoney, C.D., Gallina, J.N., Jeffrey, L.P.: A Comprehensive Program to Increase Job Satisfaction Among Pharmacy Technicians, Hosp. Pharm., *17*:547–550, 1982.

Shepherd, M.O. and Bouchard, J.M.: Pharmacist Financial Compensation 1979–82, Am. J. Hosp. Pharm., *41*:2390–2392, 1984.

REFERENCES

1. Francke, D.E., Latiolais, C.J., Francke, G.N., and Ho, N.F.H.: *Mirror to Hospital Pharmacy,* American Society of Hospital Pharmacists, Washington, D.C., 1964, p. 6.
2. Task Force of Prescription Drugs, U.S. Dept. of Health, Education and Welfare, Washington, D.C., 1968, pp. 54–58.
3. ASHP Statement on Supportive Personnel in Hospital Pharmacy, Am. J. Hosp. Pharm., *28*:516, (July) 1971.
4. Livengood, Bruce H., Kay, Douglas H., and Giannetti, Vincent, J.: Hospital Pharmacy Supportive Personnel Utilization: A Regional Survey, Hosp. Pharm., *19*:11:746–753, 1984.
5. ASHP Technical Assistance Bulletin on Outcome Competencies and Training Guidelines for Institutional Pharmacy Training Programs, Am. J. Hosp. Pharm., *39*:317–320, (Feb.) 1982.
6. ASHP Accreditation Standard for Specialized Pharmacy Residency Training, Am. J. Hosp. Pharm., *37*:1229–1232, (Sept.) 1980.
7. Accreditation Manual for Hospitals, 1985, p. 119–128. Joint Commission for the Accreditation of Hospitals, Chicago, Ill. 60611.
8. Descriptions and Organizational Analysis for Hospitals and Related Health Services, U.S. Government Printing Office, Washington, D.C., 1952.
9. Francke, D.E., Latiolais, C.J., Francke, G.N. and Ho, N.F.H.: *Mirror to Hospital Pharmacy,* American Society of Hospital Pharmacists, Washington, D.C., 1964, p. 103.
10. Jeffries, S.B. and Greenberg, J.: Prescription Pricing, J. Am. Pharm., Assoc. Pract. Pharm. Ed., *17*:383, (June) 1956.
11. Lamy, Peter P., Kitler, MaryEllen, Liebman, Judith S., LeSage, Paul J., Horn, Susan M. and Bolling, Thomas V.: Predicting Manpower Needs for Outpatient Pharmacy, Am. J. Hosp. Pharm., *27*:4:300, (Apr.) 1970.
12. Liebman, Judith S., Lamy, Peter P. and Kitler, MaryEllen: Further Investigation of the Use of Queuing Theory To Predict Manpower Requirements in an Outpatient Pharmacy, Am. J. Hosp. Pharm., *27*:6:480, (June) 1970.
13. Swartz, A.J.: Staff Evaluation, Am. J. Hosp. Pharm., *36*:187–193, (Feb.) 1979.
13a.Report of Joint Commission on Hospital Pharmacy: Hospital Pharmacy Technician-Helpers, Hospital Pharmacy, *1*:7:9, 1966.
14. Nelson, A.A., Gourley, D.R., Tindall, W.N., and Anderson, R.J.: Task Analysis of a Pharmacist's Activities in a 45-Bed Rural Hospital with Comprehensive Pharmaceutical Services, Am. J. Hosp. Pharm., *34*:1063–1068, (Oct.) 1977.
15. Beahm, Michael R.: A Survey of Opinion and Law Regarding the Use of Non-Licensed Personnel in Pharmacy, Am. J. Hosp. Pharm., *27*:9:713, (Sept.) 1970.
16. Hassan, Wm. E.: Hiring of Pharmacy Personnel, Drug Topics, *112*:24:11, (Nov.) 25, 1968.
17. Statement on Supportive Personnel in Hospital Pharmacy, Am. J. Hosp. Pharm., *28*:7:516, (July) 1971.
18. Economic Status Program of the American Society of Hospital Pharmacists, Am. J. Hosp. Pharm., *28*:7:517, (July) 1971.
19. DiPiro, J.T., Gousse, G.C. and Kubica, A.J.: Work Sampling To Evaluate Staff Pharmacist Productivity, Am. J. Hosp. Pharm., *36*:201–205, (Feb.) 1979.
20. Kirk, Kenneth W.: Women in Male Dominated Professions, Am. J. Hosp. Pharm., *39*:2089–2093, 1982.
21. ASHP Competency Standard for Pharmacy Supportive Personnel in Organized Health Care Settings, Am. J. Hosp. Pharm., *35*:449–451, (Apr.) 1978.

4

The Pharmacy and Therapeutics Committee

In these days of modern medicine when numerous agents are available for the treatment of disease, the judicious selection of drugs for use in the hospital has become an important administrative and therapeutic tool. During the last half century, there has been a dynamic change in the medical profession's attitude toward therapeutic agents. Fifty years ago there were few really worthwhile medicinal substances available; however, if one examines the formularies of that period, it is amazing to see the hundreds of preparations that were recommended. Perhaps one of the finest things that Sir William Osler did was to lead the endeavor to rid the profession of such valueless items.

Following Osler's period of clinical evaluation, there came a period of near therapeutic nihilism when most physicians were skeptical about nearly all therapeutic measures. As a consequence, it was difficult to get individuals deeply interested in the problems of reliable therapeutics. If an examination were made of the texts on therapy between 1920 and 1940, one notes that there was a definite lack of interest in therapeutics, and to a great extent, the use of various prescriptions and preparations was curtailed. Many of the medical graduates of this period had little idea about good therapy and received poor instruction in the subject during their clinical training in the hospital.

However, during this period, definite standards for improving drug therapy were established. Rules to guide manufacturers, as well as physicians, were established by the American Medical Association which did much to put drug therapy in a more desirable position. The Council on Pharmacy and Chemistry of the American Medical Association had been well established and was successfully operating when we were suddenly thrust into the modern era of therapeutics. This came about as a result of the discovery of the sulfa compounds and was quickly followed by the discovery of penicillin, streptomycin and the other antibiotics. In the 1950s, there was a flood of new substances of high potency and activity in many fields of pathologic physiology. This deluge of new therapeutic agents made it a nearly impossible task for the physician to become knowledgeable about more than a relatively few products.

Because of this profusion of agents, some excellent, some not so good, and some practically useless, it was necessary for the hospital to establish a system to bring the best medicinal agents to the attention of the staff, and thus assist them in the proper selection of therapeutic substances for the treatment of the hospitalized patient. This educational program was best brought about through the formation of a good Pharmacy and Therapeutics Committee whose responsibility was to include the preparations of a hospital formulary, the publishing of a pharmacy educational bulletin, the establishment of automatic stop orders for dangerous drugs, the supervision of investigational use drugs, the development of a program for reporting and investigating adverse drug reactions and assisting in the preparation of emergency kits or carts for medical emergencies.

Despite the creation of these hospital oriented committees, there appeared to be a need for a systematic evaluation of the entire drug system in the country. Thus, in May of 1967, acting upon a directive from the President, John W. Gardner—then Secretary of Health, Education, and Welfare—established the Task Force on Prescription Drugs. The charge to the Task Force was—

"Undertake a comprehensive study of the problems of including the cost of prescription drugs under medicare."

To achieve the goal set by the charge, the Task Force was obliged to seek objective data on the health needs of the elderly; the present patterns of drug use; the nature of drug research, production and distribution; current drug insurance programs in the United States and abroad; reimbursement methods and administrative approaches; legal and fiscal aspects; and the pharmacological and clinical aspects, including the intricate problem of chemical and clinical equivalency of generic products.[1]

In addition, a more drastic approach was taken. Under the authority granted to the Secretary of HEW by the Drug Amendments of 1962, the *National Academy of Sciences-National Research Council* (NAS-NRC) in 1966, at the request of the FDA, initiated a study to evaluate the effectiveness of new drugs marketed between 1938 and 1962. During that period of time, the law required only that a new drug be demonstrated to be safe. The requirement that a new drug be effective, as well as safe, was added by the Drug Amendments of 1962.

An advisory committee of the NAS-NRC created 27 panels of nongovernment experts to evaluate the efficacy of approximately 3000 drugs. On the basis of its findings, the *Drug Efficacy Study Group* classified the drugs as: *effective. probably effective, possibly effective, effective but,* or *ineffective.*

It has been stated[2] that the hospital Pharmacy and Therapeutics Committee is a tool for maintaining medical staff self-government. It is responsible to the medical staff as a whole and its recommendations are subject to medical staff approval. The Pharmacy and Therapeutics Committee is a mandatory committee under the **Conditions** of **Participation** of the Hospital Insurance Program—Medicare. Composed of physicians and the pharmacist, it serves as the organizational line of communication of liaison between the medical staff and the Pharmacy Department. This committee assists in the formulation of broad professional policies regarding the evaluation, selection, procurement, distribution, use, safety procedures and other matters relating to drugs in hospitals.

In 1959, the American Hospital Association and the American Society of Hospital Pharmacists approved a **Statement on the Pharmacy and Therapeutics Committee**[3] which has been superseded by the following ASHP Statement on the Pharmacy and Therapeutics Committee.

ASHP STATEMENT ON PHARMACY AND THERAPEUTICS COMMITTEE

The multiplicity of drugs available and the complexities surrounding their safe and effective use make it necessary for hospitals to have an organized, sound program for maximizing rational drug use. The pharmacy and therapeutics committee, or its equivalent, is the organizational keystone of the program.[a]

The pharmacy and therapeutics committee is an advisory group of the medical staff and serves as the organizational line of communication between the medical staff and pharmacy department. This committee is composed of physicians, pharmacists, and other health professionals selected with the guidance of the medical staff. It is a policy-recommending body to the medical staff and the administration of the hospital on matters related to the therapeutic use of drugs.

Purposes

The primary purposes of the pharmacy and therapeutics committee are as specified in the following.

---

[a]Approved by the ASHP House of Delegates, June 6, 1984. Approved by the ASHP Board of Directors, November 17–18, 1983. (The previous version was approved by the House of Delegates, May 15, 1978.) Revised by the ASHP Council on Clinical Affairs.

1. **Advisory.** The committee recommends the adoption of, or assists in the formulation of, policies regarding evaluation, selection, and therapeutic use of drugs in hospitals.
2. **Educational.** The committee recommends or assists in the formulation of programs designed to meet the needs of the professional staff (physicians, nurses, pharmacists, and other health-care practitioners) for complete current knowledge on matters related to drugs and drug use.

Organization and Operation

While the composition and operation of the pharmacy and therapeutics committee might vary from hospital to hospital, the following generally will apply:

1. The pharmacy and therapeutics committee should be composed of at least three physicians, a pharmacist, a nurse, and an administrator. Committee members are appointed by a governing unit or elected official of the organized medical staff.
2. A chairman from among the physician representatives should be appointed. A pharmacist usually is designated as secretary.
3. The committee should meet regularly, at least six times per year, and more often when necessary.
4. The committee should invite to its meetings persons within or outside the hospital who can contribute specialized or unique knowledge, skills, and judgments.
5. An agenda and supplementary materials (including minutes of the previous meeting) should be prepared by the secretary and submitted to the committee members in sufficient time before the meeting for them to properly review the material.
6. Minutes of the committee meetings should be prepared by the secretary and maintained in the permanent records of the hospital.
7. Recommendations of the committee shall be presented to the medical staff or its appropriate committee for adoption or recommendation.
8. Liaison with other hospital committees concerned with drug use (e.g., infection control, medical audit) shall be maintained.

Functions and Scope

The basic organization of the hospital and medical staffs will determine the functions and scope of the pharmacy and therapeutics committee. The following list of committee functions is offered as a guide:

1. To service in an advisory capacity to the medical staff and hospital administration in all matters pertaining to the use of drugs (including investigational drugs).
2. To develop a formulary of drugs accepted for use in the hospital and provide for its constant revision. The selection of items to be included in the formulary will be based on objective evaluation of their relative therapeutic merits, safety, and cost. The committee should minimize duplication of the same basic drug type, drug entity, or drug product.

3. To establish programs and procedures that help ensure cost-effective drug therapy.
4. To establish or plan suitable educational programs for the hospital's professional staff on matters related to drug use.
5. To participate in quality-assurance activities related to the distribution, administration, and use of medications.
6. To review adverse drug reactions occurring in the hospital.
7. To initiate or direct (or both) drug-use review programs and studies and review the results of such activities.
8. To advise the pharmacy in the implementation of effective drug distribution and control procedures.
9. To make recommendations concerning drugs to be stocked in hospital patient-care areas.

PURPOSE OF THE COMMITTEE

Pharmacy departments utilize the committee structure to coordinate and effectively integrate requisite aspects of planning, development, implementation, and control of designated activities. In both the interdepartmental and intradepartmental pathways, the resourceful hospital pharmacy manager will use the committee as an effective management tool.[4]

Longest[5] suggests the following as prerequisites for an effective committee:

1. The committee's tasks should be clearly defined.
2. Members should be selected from among those who have some definite relationship to the tasks to be accomplished.
3. For optimal effectiveness, superiors and subordinates should not serve on the same committee. Furthermore, the fact that a manager holds a position at a given level should not, in and of itself, be a basis for inclusion or exclusion.
4. Committees must have time to evolve interpersonal relationships before they can move on to effective problem-solving.
5. To function most effectively, committees require the support of the groups of individuals to whom the results of their deliberation are to be submitted.
6. Committees with a task to perform—for example, a pharmacy and therapeutics committee—should be clearly differentiated from staff groups whose major role is to communicate events and to develop the managerial competence of members.

The Pharmacy and Therapeutics Committee is a committee of the medical staff and serves as liaison between the medical staff and the pharmacy service on all matters pertaining to the use of drugs in the hospital. Its prime objective is to achieve optimal patient care and safety through rational drug therapy.

COMMITTEE NAME

The actual name given to this type of committee is irrelevant. For the sake of clarification, the following nomenclature has been applied to that committee acting in an advisory capacity to the hospital and its staff on all matters pertaining to drugs and pharmaceuticals: **Pharmacy Committee; Formulary Committee; Therapeutics Committee** and **Pharmacy and Therapeutics Committee.**

COMMITTEE MEMBERSHIP

Although the approved statement by the American Hospital Association and the American Society of Hospital Pharmacists provides for a membership of not less than three physicians and the pharmacist, the majority of the larger hospitals list committees which often include representatives of the following groups:

Surgery	*Medicine*
Anesthesiologist	Allergist
Urologist	Cardiologist
General Surgeon	Dermatologist
	Endocrinologist
	Gastroenterologist
Pharmacist	Pharmacologist
Administrator	Phychiatrist
Nurse	Internist

It is admitted that this constitutes a large committee; however, this is justifiable since no single individual is competent to rule on all categories of drugs which are being developed. A committee of these specialists can certainly provide a learned opinion as to the merit of any pharmaceutical agent.

Flack[6] has observed that too many hospitals had pharmacy and therapeutics committees with only two or three physician members and that such committees were not truly representative of all medical staff services. In describing the Pharmacy Committee of the attending medical staff at the Jefferson Medical College Hospital, it was shown to consist of three physicians, all of whom were department heads. However, there existed an Advisory Subcommittee to the Pharmacy Committee consisting of the head of each of the divisions of the department of medicine. Such an arrangement is beneficial in that it provides the parent committee with advisory input derived from a broad base of clinical expertise.

On occasion, the issue is raised as to whether or not the pharmacist should serve as a full voting member of the committee or serve in an *ex officio* capacity. The pharmacist should serve as a full voting member of the committee. Furthermore, he should serve as the secretary of the group and should, therefore, be fully responsible for developing the agenda and the preparation and distribution of the minutes of the meetings.

FREQUENCY OF MEETINGS

The number and frequency of meetings of this Committee depend upon the size of the hospital and the volume and variety of drugs used. Clearly, the Committee should meet at least once per quarter, and in the busier institutions at least monthly. Notices of the meeting date and accompanying agenda should be distributed by the secretary of the Committee in ample time to assure attendance and knowledgeable participation in the discussion of the agenda items.

THE COMMITTEE AGENDA

A successful meeting depends upon the preparation of an interesting agenda which is made available to the committee members reasonably far in advance of the scheduled meeting. Because of the broad scope enjoyed by this committee, many interesting subjects may, rightfully, be placed upon the agenda for discussion.

A typical agenda may consist of the following general categories:

1. Minutes of the previous meeting.
2. Review of a specified section of the Formulary for up-dating and deletion of products.
3. New drugs which have become commercially available.
4. Investigational use of drugs currently in use in the hospital.
5. Review of adverse drug reactions reported in the hospital since the last meeting.
6. Drug safety in the hospital.

FUNCTIONS OF THE COMMITTEE

Committees having as diversified a membership as the Pharmacy and Therapeutics Committee need to have a set of guidelines which delineate its activity. The following demonstrate this point:

A. To serve in an advisory capacity to the Medical Staff, to hospital administration, and to the Pharmacy Department on all matters pertaining to the use of drugs in the hospital. Actions taken by the Committee are subject to review and approval by the Executive Committee of the Medical Staff.
B. To assist the Pharmacy Department in the development and review of policies, rules, and regulations regarding the use of drugs in the hospital

in accordance with local, state, and federal regulatory and accreditation agencies.

C. To evaluate, approve, or reject drugs proposed for inclusion in or deletion from the Hospital Formulary.

D. To define categories of drugs used in the hospital and assign each drug to a specified category. (See section on "Policies" for a list of these categories.)

E. To review drug utilization in the hospital and promote optimum standards for rational drug therapy.

F. To collect and review adverse drug reaction reports.

G. To develop and disseminate pertinent educational materials and programs regarding drugs to members of the Medical and Nursing Staffs.

Policies of the Committee

In order that there be no misunderstanding amongst the membership and subsequently by the medical staff, it is essential that the Committee establish policies under which it proposes to control the use of drugs in the hospital. These policies should be comprehensive and should be reviewed periodically to ensure that they are current and are placed in the Pharmacy Procedural Manual.

The following are presented as an example of the thoroughness required:

A. Proposal of a new drug for the Hospital Formulary shall be submitted on a Formulary Request Form to the Pharmacy Department. These forms may be obtained from the Pharmacy. Such requests may be submitted by any member of the medical staff. The Committee will evaluate the request and notify the proposer as to acceptance or rejection. The proposer shall have the opportunity to appeal the decision of the Committee.

B. Drugs evaluated and approved by the Committee will be assigned to one of the following four categories:

1. *Formulary Drug*
    An FDA approved drug which is recommended as being essential for good patient care with a well established usage. Once accepted as a Formulary Drug, it may be prescribed by all members of the attending and house staffs.

2. *Drugs Approved on a Conditional Trial Period*
    A drug which has been approved by the FDA for general use but which the Committee will evaluate for a 6- or 12-month period before final consideration. During that period, the drug may be prescribed by all members of the attending and house staffs.

3. *Specialized Formulary Drug*
    An FDA approved drug which is recommended for use in specialized patient care. The drug may be placed in this category by the proposer or the Committee and either may designate those persons authorized to prescribe Specialized Formulary Drugs.

4. *Investigational Drugs*
    A drug which has been approved by the FDA for a specific use by its principal investigator and designated associates. Such drugs are not commercially available. They must be approved by the Human Sub-

jects Committee, the Pharmacy and Therapeutics Committe, and, if applicable, the Isotope Committee. A protocol of the study must be submitted to the Pharmacy if it is to be used in the hospital. The drug may be stored and dispensed by the Pharmacy if desired by the principal investigator.

C. Drugs which do not qualify for the four categories listed shall be considered as "Non-Formulary Drugs" and will not be stocked in the Pharmacy. A "Non-Formulary Drug" may be prescribed only by members of the attending staff and chief residents, or their designees in their absence. The Pharmacy will obtain and dispense a limited quantity of the drug.

D. The pre-signing of prescription blanks or drug orders for any purpose is prohibited.

E. The Pharmacy Department is authorized to dispense drugs according to policies and procedures of the Committee. According to the Formulary System, all drugs will be dispensed on the basis of generic names to avoid duplicate inventory and achieve a cost savings. Physicians may specify a specific brand name drug when deemed necessary. Authority for the routine selection of drug brands is delegated to the Pharmacy Department, utilizing a fair and equitable bid process when necessary.

F. The Committee is responsible for the rules and regulations which govern pharmaceutical company representative activities within the hospital. These rules and regulations are available from the Pharmacy.

G. *Drug Recall*

Drug recalls may emanate from manufacturers, regulatory agencies, or the Pharmacy Department, and may be of a general nature or a specific recall for one or more lot numbers. Once a recall notice is received, the drugs will be removed and replaced; and this information will be sent to staff and pertinent hospital departments. (See chart in Pharmacy and Policy Manual.) All recall drugs, if stocked, will be held in quarantine in the Pharmacy until directions for return or final resolution are received.

H. *Inpatient Prescribing*

1. *Routine Drug Orders*

A physician's medication order written on inpatient order form is deemed a legal prescription. A legible copy of the medication order must be forwarded to the Pharmacy and must include the following information:

a. The patient's addressograph information.
b. The name of the nursing unit.
c. The name and strength of each drug.
d. The directions for frequency of administration.
e. The route of administration.
f. The signature of the prescribing physician.
g. The date and time that the order was written.

Orders written by medical students must be countersigned by a member of the medical staff. Quantities of drugs to be dispensed need not be specified since the pharmacist will determine the optimum amounts in keeping with greatest economy to the patient and efficiency in handling and storage by the nursing and Pharmacy staffs.

2. *I.V. Orders*

Orders for intravenous medications must be written in the same manner as routine drug orders and must include the following additional information:

a. The exact quantity of the drug(s) which must be added.
b. The exact volume and name of the infusate solution.

    c. Specific directions for administration such as IV drip, IV bolus, IV push, etc.

    d. Specific times to hang infusate solution and drip rate.

    e. Specific directions for continuing or discontinuing any IV medications.

3. *Total Parenteral Nutrition (TPN)*

    a. TPN has been designed to serve as a nutritional infusion providing essential amino acids, carbohydrates, and electrolytes for patients incapable of ingesting, digesting, or absorbing food substances given by mouth. Since a standard hyperalimentation solution must always be prepared extemporaneously, the Pharmacy Department shall be responsible for the preparation of these solutions.

    b. *Ordering*

        (1) The TPN mixture may only be prescribed by an authorized House Staff physician in conjunction with a Dietician through consultation.

        (2) The written order must be sent to the Pharmacy for verification including the basic solution and all additives.

        (3) Following the original order, subsequent orders must be confirmed every morning and recorded on a card designated for that specific patient.

        (4) A 24-hour supply is to be ordered by the physician each morning.

        (5) Only electrolytes and vitamins may be added to hyperalimentation solutions.

4. *Self Medication*[8]

Only nitroglycerin and antacids may be left at the patient's bedside for self administration if so ordered by the physician. The quantity of nitroglycerin is limited to 10 tablets which must be counted by the nurse at the conclusion of each shift and charted in the patient's medical record. Antacids must be recorded and replenished in the same manner.

5. *Medication Brought to the Hospital by Patients*

Medications brought into the hospital by the patient may not be kept at the patient's bedside. Medications are shown to the physician, then sent home with a responsible family member or friend. If the latter is not possible, the medication container must be labeled with patient's name, locked in the medication cabinet and with physician's permission sent home with patient when discharged.

6. *Automatic Stop Orders*

Automatic stop-order requirements for medications are:

1. 24 hours for Schedule II Control drugs

2. 7 days for all other drugs

P.R.N. and standing orders for all medications except Schedule II Control drugs expire at 10:00 A.M. of the following Tuesday morning. All orders shall be renewed between the hours of 4:00 P.M. Monday and 10:00 A.M. Tuesday. Orders which are written on Monday become effective at 10:00 A.M. Tuesday.

7. A new medication order must be written by the physician if a change is wanted in route of administration or in dosage.

8. *Prescribing Schedule II Control Substances*

    a. Routine orders for Schedule II Control substances must be written on the inpatient's order form and signed by the physician. The physician's full name is required. The order must include the name of drug strength, route of administration, and frequency of administration.

    b. Pro Re Nata (prn) orders of Schedule II drugs are acceptable if a specific dose and a specific minimum interval is written.

    c. Telephone and verbal orders may be given by the physician in an emergency situation. The nurse will make the appropriate entry on the inpatient's order form, sign the physician's name, and initial the verbal or telephone order. It is the responsibility of the physician to sign the order prior to the next shift count.

    d. Discharge prescriptions for Schedule II drugs are restricted to a 30-day supply, no refills, patient's home address, and the physician's DEA number (See Discharge Prescriptions).

  9. *Prescribing Methadone*

    a. The FDA has issued new regulations governing the use of methadone for analgesia in severe pain and for detoxification and temporary maintenance treatment of heroin addicts.

    b. Methadone is permitted to be administered for analgesia in severe pain, detoxification, or temporary treatment of the acute withdrawal symnptoms for *hospitalized patients* for a period *not to exceed three weeks.* If the Hospital does not operate a maintenance program, an outside agency may be contracted. (See Outpatient Prescribing)

10. *Alcoholic Beverages*

Whiskey, wine, and other alcoholic beverages may be ordered from the Pharmacy. The order must specify the prescribed dose for the patient and bear the personal signature of the physician. The maximum quantity which may be dispensed on any one prescription is 240 ml. Alcoholic beverage prescriptions cannot be refilled. A new prescription must be written for each 240 ml quantity dispensed. Alcoholic beverages obtained from the Pharmacy may not be removed from the hospital. Unused quantities must be returned to the Pharmacy.

11. *Discharge Prescriptions*

A separate prescription is required for each medication which the patient is to take home. Each prescription must contain the following information:

    a. Patient addressograph information. (Home address for Schedule II drugs).

    b. Name of drug and strength.

    c. Quantity to be dispensed.

    d. Specific instructions for patient administration.

    e. Number of refills (none for Schedule II drugs).

    f. Signature and printed name of physician.

    g. For narcotic prescriptions, see Schedule II prescribing.

Discharge prescriptions must be received in the Pharmacy the day prior to discharge, so that they may be processed and returned to the nursing station. Delays may result in the patient having to wait which is not consistent with good patient care.

12. *Emergency (STAT) Orders*

Bona fide emergency (STAT) orders should be rare and in most cases obtained from the nursing station emergency drug supplies. When necessary, these orders should be transmitted in writing on the Pharmacy copy of the inpatient order form. This procedure prevents unnecessary delay and confusion which results from hurried verbal transmission orders. If it is necessary to phone the Pharmacy for emergency drugs, calls should be placed either by the physician or the nurse in order to avoid delay and error.

I. *Outpatient Prescribing*
1. The hospital requires that a prescription be written for any drug or medical supply which is to be dispensed for hospitalized patients at discharge, clinic patients, and employees. Such prescriptions may *only* be written on hospital prescription forms in compliance with all regulatory agencies.
2. Information required on prescriptions:
    a. Addressograph patient information
    b. Date
    c. Name and strength of medication
    d. Quantity to be dispensed
    e. Specific information for patient administration
    f. Specific number of refills
    g. Signature and printed name of the physician
3. Prescriptions for Control Drugs have special requirements, which are as follows:
    a. All Control Drug prescriptions require the physician's DEA number.
    b. Schedule II drugs (narcotics) are limited to a 30-day supply and *no* refills. These prescriptions are valid for 5 days and are not valid if there are crossouts, erasures, or any evidence of tampering.
    c. Schedule III drugs, such as paregoric and medium acting barbiturates, are limited to a 30-day supply and may be refilled up to 5 times within 6 months of issuance date.
    d. Schedule IV and V, such as benzodiazepines and cough preparations, may be refilled 5 times within 6 months of issuance date.

GENERIC VS. BRAND NAMED DRUGS[9]—A COMMITTEE DILEMMA

A quarter century ago, approximately 75% of all prescriptions were extemporaneously compounded by pharmacists. Today the reverse is true; nearly 90% are written for manufactured entities which usually bear a brand name. During this same 25-year period, material, labor and operational costs have steadily risen and industry has spent many millions of dollars in research for new drugs. Because of this increasing cost spiral, each newly released prefabricated brand name medication appeared to be closely associated with high prices. Thus the concept of brand name prescribing and dispensing has been erroneously linked with such descriptive adjectives as "expensive," "highly priced" and "exorbitantly priced" in comparison to generic prescribing and dispensing which is supposedly "inexpensive" and "money saving."

The advocates of generic prescribing and dispensing have been vociferous and have commanded much space in our drug journals. In addition, they have monopolized administrative and legislative sessions at both the federal and state levels. Their lobbyists have proposed that the government require generic prescribing and dispensing in all welfare programs. Others contend that the federal government offer the States a bonus payment with its Federal welfare payments whenever generic drugs are dispensed in state-operated programs. Still others suggest that the Federal government approach the issue by penalizing the State through lower welfare reimbursement rates if the State advocated the use of brand named drugs in its welfare programs. Some welfare departments have already succumbed to the pressure thus forcing pharmacists to become involved with the purchasing and dispensing of generic drugs.

Because hospitals with large active clinics usually carry a high welfare census in order to maintain an adequate resource of teaching cases, the hospital pharmacist will be faced with the problem of generic vs. brand named drug. Furthermore, the hospital administrator and many members of the medical staff will advocate generic prescribing and dispensing. They will do this in good faith and with good intentions. They want the clinic patients and the welfare agencies to pay as little as possible for medications.

At each meeting of the Pharmacy and Therapeutics Committee the hospital pharmacist will be, and in many institutions already has been, faced with the allegation that if several medications made by different companies conform to the standards of the U.S.P., then all of those medications will have identical effects on patients and the least expensive one will be just as good as the most expensive.

Hospital pharmacists know that this is not wholly true. Two preparations each labeled with the generic name and the symbol U.S.P. may be generic equivalents from a chemical point of view but the important question is whether the two products are *clinically effective equivalents.*

It should be noted at this point that clinicians advocate a comparison of the clinical effectiveness of a drug. Too often this is confused with a drug's pharmacologic activity which manifests itself by means of a specific physiologic response, whereas the clinical effectiveness of a drug includes not only its pharmacologic activity, but also such criteria as ease of application or removal, flavor and odor, allergic manifestations, tissue irritation, caloric values, disintegration and absorption rate to mention a few.

It should be common professional knowledge that the active ingredient alone does not make a medication. This chemical entity must be made into one of the accepted medicinal forms—tablet, capsule, injection, cream, ointment, elixir, syrup, a sustained release form or a suppository. This then means that other materials must be used to produce the pharmaceutical form desired. The choice of ingredients and method of combining is left to the judgment and experience of the manufacturer. The U.S.P. itself states that the actual formulating processes, by which the active ingredient becomes a medication, "are in general, beyond the scope of the Pharmacopeia."

Reference to any pharmacy textbook will show that the producer of a medication must concern himself with such things as potency, strength, purity, compatibility, solubility, particle size, choice of vehicle or base, pH, tonicity, melting point, surface tension, viscosity, storage factors, packaging and control. Deviation from accepted standard or omission of any of these may result in a product which because of its active chemical component is a generic equivalent but not a clinically effective equivalent.

By the same token, two products may both meet U.S.P. standards but, because of differences in composition or the way they are compounded, may not be clinically effective equivalents.

It should be emphasized at this point that all generic drugs are not being condemned. An observation is being made to the extent that if a manufacturer applies all of the standards of high quality ingredients, rigid manufacturing and control procedures, adequate packaging and supports medical research and development programs, the final product will be a generic equivalent with clinical effectiveness. However, its production cost will probably be the same as that of the brand name equivalent and therefore it will have the same retail price to the consumer.

Some hospital pharmacists operating in large metropolitan teaching and research hospitals may well be in a position to purchase generic products from manufacturers who are unfamiliar to them, because they have adequately staffed and equipped control laboratories and clinical testing programs in which they are able to make the assays necessary to ascertain the quality and effectiveness of the product purchased. It should be noted here that oftentimes when the cost of the hospital conducted analyses is added to the purchase price of the product, little financial advantages remains.

Pharmacists certainly realize that there are both high and poor quality pharmaceuticals available under both generic names and brand names.

The hospital pharmacist by virtue of this educational background and general familiarity with the reputation, integrity and facilities of pharmaceutical manufacturers is in an excellent position to evaluate the merits of brand named drugs vs. their generic equivalents. He should not relinquish this position of professional authority and competence to any administrator, physician, politician or welfare agency commissioner. He should, on the other hand, make himself available to all of these people to advise and teach them that the quality of a drug and its subsequent clinical effectiveness are quite independent of its name.

The hospital pharmacist can carry on his teaching program in a number of ways. As a member of the Pharmacy and Therapeutics Committee, he can make available to the Committee membership various articles dealing with the therapeutic implications of brand interchange, publications pertaining to clinical ineffectiveness of drugs due to faulty formulation and the various reports of the FDA in which they describe drug seizures due to faulty labeling or improper strengths.

As the editor of the hospital pharmacy newsletter, the hospital pharmacist should avail himself of the opportunity to editorialize his views on the subject.

As a lecturer in pharmacology in the school of nursing and as a lecturer in the in-service training programs for nurses and interns, the hospital pharmacist should deliver knowledgeable lectures on the subject in order that the doctors and nurses—particularly those in training—may keep in clear perspective the relationship between quality pharmaceuticals and therapeutic efficacy.

EVALUATION OF DRUGS

The evaluation, approval or rejection of drugs and biological agents from the hospital formulary is a time consuming task that dominates the committee agenda. Because no two institutional committees use the same drug evaluation criteria, it is suggested that the ASHP Technical Assistance Bulletin on the Scientific and Therapeutic Evaluation of Drugs for Hospital Formularies[7] be utilized.

ASHP TECHNICAL ASSISTANCE BULLETIN ON THE SCIENTIFIC AND THERAPEUTIC EVALUATION OF DRUGS FOR HOSPITAL FORMULARIES[a]

Preamble

One of the major roles of the Pharmacy and Therapeutics Committee is to develop and maintain a hospital drug formulary system. The hospital formulary can be used as the basis for promoting optimal pharmacotherapy because it contains only those drugs judged by the Pharmacy and Therapeutics Committee to be in the best interest of the patient's health needs in terms of efficacy and consideration of cost. The pharmacist is a key member of the drug evaluation team because of his knowledge of pharmacology, pharmacokinetics, toxicology, therapeutics, and drug purchasing.

The evaluation of comparative data associated with a drug's efficacy, adverse effects and cost, and the determination of its potential therapeutic advantages and deficiencies require specific attention by the

[a]Developed by the ASHP Council on Clinical Pharmacy and Therapeutics. Approved by the ASHP Board of Directors, April 30, 1981.

pharmacist. Products may be admitted to or rejected from entry into the hospital formulary based on the initial evaluation by the Pharmacy and Therapeutics Committee. Alternative recommendations might include either conditional approval for a specific time period, with subsequent re-evaluation, or temporary limitation of a drug's use to an individual medical service specialty with future reassessment.

Evaluation Process Considerations

Standardization forms should be developed for use in the evaluation process. It is recommended that each form should include the following information:

1. Generic Name
   - List the officially approved name of all chemical entities in the drug product.
2. Trade Name(s)
   - List the most common trade name(s) of the drug product, as used in the local area.
3. Sources(s) of Supply
   - Identify the pharmaceutical companies from which the drug product could be procured.
   - For a generic drug product, identify the actual manufacturer; if applicable, identify the pharmaceutical company marketing the product.
4. *American Hospital Formulary Service (AHFS)* Classification Number
   - List number for quick access and retrieval for information.
5. Pharmacologic Classification
   - State which pharmacologic class to which the drug belongs and any similar properties it possesses in comparison to existing drugs.
   - State the mechanism of action; if the mechanism of action is unknown, so state. If applicable, the mechanism of action may be compared with that of another drug or class of drugs.
   - List the potential nonapproved uses for the drug, based on an expanded description of its pharmacological activity (preferably in humans).
   - List bacterial spectrum and clinical effectiveness for an antimicrobial agent, comparing properties to existing formulary agents.
6. Therapeutic Indications
   - State the uses of the drug as approved by the Food and Drug Administration (FDA); indicate if use is prophylactic, therapeutic, palliative, curative, adjunctive or supportive.
   - Evaluate uses of the drug in comparison with other established forms of therapy using, if possible, human studies for comparison. Comparisons should emphasize therapeutics, i.e., efficacy, incidence of treatment success, remission, sansitivity, ease of monitoring and treatment periods required, and include critical analysis of clinical studies in such areas as patient population, methodology, statistics, and conclusion.
   - State potential drug-drug interactions.

- Identify non-FDA approved uses for the drug, and those uses that show promise in investigational studies.

7. Dosage Forms
   - List all dosage forms available as approved by the FDA; list unit costs.

8. Bioavailability and Pharmacokinetics
   - List bioavailability data for the most common route of administration and dosage of the drug. Other bioavailability data should be available upon request by the Pharmacy and Therapeutics Committee.
   - List pharmacokinetic data for absorption, distribution, metabolism, and excretion of drug.

   Absorption—Include information on the extent and rate of absorption of the drug by the usual routes of administration; the factors that might effect rate or extent of absorption; the therapeutic, toxic and lethal blood levels; the period of time required for onset, peak, and duration of therapeutic effect; the half-life and factors affecting it.

   Distribution—Include information on the usual distribution of the drug in body tissues and fluids; the drug's propensity to cross the blood-brain barrier, placenta, or appear in human milk; protein binding and volume of distribution.

   Metabolism—Include information on sites of metabolism and extent of biotransformation; metabolic products and their activity.

   Excretion—Include information on routes of elimination from the body; factors affecting elimination; form in which drug is eliminated.

9. Dosage Range
   - List dosage for different routes of administration of drug.
   - List initial, maintenance, maximum, and pediatric doses for the drug.

10. Known Side Effects and Toxicities
    - Discuss side effects of the drug and their frequency of occurrence from research data of human studies.
    - Discuss means or methods of prevention or treatment of side effects and toxicities. Benefits of disease treatment to risk of side effects should be emphasized.

11. Special Precautions
    - List precautions and contraindications for certain disease states or other conditions.
    - Compare all of the preceding with existing similar agents where applicable.
    - List potential drug-drug interactions if deemed clinically significant.

12. Advantages
    - Compare and list all advantages of the drug with existing products, using information from sections 5–10 as basis of comparison.

13. Disadvantages
    - Compare and list any disadvantages of the drug with existing products, using information from sections 5–10 as basis of comparison.

14. Comparisons
    - List therapeutic comparisons with other drugs or treatment regimens.
    - List cost comparison data of a standard treatment regimen with the new drug versus currently used drugs.

15. Recommendations
    - Formulate recommendations from analysis of all the preceding data, and consideration of other factors such as medical staff preference,

distribution problems, availability of drug, and manufacturer. Determine action to be taken in regard to hospital formulary status:

Uncontrolled—Available for use by all medical staff.

Monitored—Available for use by all medical staff, but use monitored by a department.

Restricted—Available for use by medical staff of a specific service or department.

Conditional—Available for use by all medical staff for a specific time period.

Deletion—Delete from current formulary.

RECOMMENDED REFERENCE MATERIALS

The development of a comprehensive data base is essential for evaluating drugs proposed for admission to a hospital formulary. A thorough review of the pharmaceutical and medical literature is necessary when accumulating these data. The list of recommended references include those sources that commonly provide useful information in drug evaluation; however, review of additional specialty journals may be required.

Texts:
1. *American Hospital Formulary Service*
2. *Drug Topics Redbook*
3. *Facts and Comparisons*
4. *Martindale—The Extra Pharmacopoeia*
5. *Physicians' Desk Reference*
6. *The Pharmacological Basis of Therapeutics*—Goodman and Gilman

Periodicals and Abstracting Systems:
1. *American Journal of Hospital Pharmacy*
2. *Annals of Internal Medicine*
3. *Archives of Internal Medicine*
4. *Antimicrobial Agents and Chemotherapy*
5. *Clinical Pharmacology and Therapeutics*
6. Drugdex
7. *Drugs*
8. Drug Intelligence and Clinical Pharmacy
9. *Hospital Formulary*
10. Iowa Drug Information Service
11. *International Pharmaceutical Abstracts*
12. *Journal of the American Medical Association*
13. *Lancet*
14. *Medical Letter on Drugs and Therapeutics*

15. *New England Journal of Medicine*
16. Paul de Haen Information Systems

RECOMMENDATIONS

"ASHP Guidelines for the Scientific and Therapeutic Evaluation of Drugs for Hospital Formularies" are supplementary to "ASHP Guidelines for Hospital Formularies"[1] and "ASHP Statement of Guiding Principles on the Operation of the Hospital Formulary System,"[2] which should be consulted for further information on the formulary system. These guidelines are recommended as an aid to the pharmacist responsible for the selection of drugs to be included in a hospital formulary.

REFERENCES

1. ASHP guidelines for hospital formularies. *Am. J. Hosp. Pharm.* 1978; *35*:326–8.
2. ASHP statement of guiding principles on the operation of the hospital formulary system. *Am. J. Hosp. Pharm.* 1964; *21*:40–1.

The Committee's Role in Drug Safety

With the advent of each new class of therapeutic agents, the scope, knowledge and responsibility of the hospital pharmacist increases conmensurately. Hand-in-hand with this increased responsibility goes the moral, legal, and professional obligation of insuring safety in the handling and administration of drugs.

Unfortunately, too many pharmacists and physicians take drug safety for granted. They are lulled into a false state of complacency by the fact that pharmacy "accidents" resulting in serious injury to or death of patients are relatively infrequent.

However, with the first press release describing a tragic drug "accident" in a neighboring hospital, every trustee, administrator, physician, and pharmacist suddenly awakens to the fact that their policies governing the pharmacy ought to be reviewed in the light of modern dispensing and prescribing trends.

This function could well be the responsibility of the Pharmacy and Therapeutics Committee and should be an on-going program. The following may serve as a guide to this Committee in ascertaining the safeness of the hospital pharmacy.[10]

1. Does the hospital employ a qualified registered pharmacist to supervise the pharmacy?
2. Does the hospital permit non-pharmacist personnel to dispense drugs and allied materials?
3. Does the hospital employ a sufficient number of qualified per-

sonnel to allow for adequate coverage of the pharmacy seven days per week?

4. Does the hospital employ personnel commensurate with the pharmacy work load?
5. Does the hospital provide adequate, safe work space, and safe storage facilities for the pharmacy?
6. Does the pharmacy have the equipment necessary to safely and adequately carry out the modern practice of pharmacy?
7. Does the hospital have an automatic stop order regulation for dangerous drugs such as narcotics, hypnotics and anticoagulants?
8. Does the hospital have a firm policy regarding the use of research drugs in the hospital and its clinics?
9. Does the hospital have a drug formulary? If so, is it periodically revised and kept up-to-date?
10. Does the hospital permit anybody other than a licensed pharmacist into the pharmacy "after hours"?
11. Are poisonous materials adequately segregated from non-poisonous materials in the pharmacy and on the nursing stations?
12. Are external use preparations separated from internal use medications in the pharmacy and on the nursing stations?
13. Does the pharmacy manufacture products for patient's use? If so, are these products checked for accuracy and asepsis by chemical and bacteriologic means?
14. Does the hospital allow the pharmacist sufficient help to permit him to engage in a teaching program to acquaint the nursing and resident staff with new drugs and to teach the student nurses the basic courses of pharmaceutical mathematics and pharmacology?
15. Are all nursing stations periodically inspected for the purpose of removing deteriorated and outdated drugs as well as to check all labels for legibility?
16. Does the pharmacy have an adequate reference library which contains texts on pharmacology, toxicology and posology?

COMMITTEE'S ROLE IN THE ADVERSE DRUG REACTION PROGRAM

A consequence of recent advances in drug therapy is the proportionate increase in drug reactions. In order to gain an understanding of these problems and to formulate competent opinions as to the best type of prevention and treatment, the Pharmacy and Therapeutics Committee must assume the responsibility for developing and instituting a procedure for the prompt reporting of an adverse drug reaction.

An adverse drug reaction has been defined by the Food and Drug Administration as follows:[11]

"An adverse drug reaction includes any pathological condition precipitated by a drug regardless of its nature or the circumstances of its occurrence, *i.e.,* toxicity caused by overdosage (therapeutic, accidental, homicidal); hypersensitivity; allergy; or injury from improper technique of administration, use of the wrong drug, error in compounding, labeling, or packaging, or from other error in the manufacture of the drug, or in its preparation for use in the hospital. Reactions caused by blood and plasma products need not be reported unless a chemical agent other than the basic substance is responsible."

An *Adverse Drug Reaction Report Form,* such as that shown in Figure 12, should be prepared by the Committee and made available on every nursing station.

A simple yet effective reporting program may be established by adopting the following criteria:

Every case of adverse drug reaction must be reported by the attending physician to the clinical pharmacologist, if one is available on the staff, otherwise to the Chairman of the Pharmacy and Therapeutics Committee. The attending physician should complete an *Adverse Drug Reaction Report Form* on any patient having an adverse reaction. The Medical Record Room will, upon the patient's discharge, remove the *Adverse Drug Reaction Form* from the medical record and forward it to the clinical pharmacologist or to the Chairman of the Pharmacy and Therapeutics Committee. Adverse drug reactions should be listed in the medical record as a diagnosis whenever such applies.

DRUG EXPERIENCE REPORTING

The FDA has in use a Drug Experience Report (Form FDA 1639 4/81) which seeks to gather information on drug defects and adverse drug reactions. The form states that the identity of the patient and the individual making the report will be held in confidence. The form is divided into three sections—Reaction Information, Suspect Drug(s) Information and Recent/Concomitant Drugs and Medical Problems. The forms are available from the FDA and it is recommended that Pharmacy and Therapeutics Committees make use of them in reporting drug incidents.

DRUG PRODUCT DEFECT REPORTING PROGRAM

In 1971, the ASHP, the USP and the FDA initiated a drug product defect reporting program. Since then, the program has been expanded to include, in addition to ASHP members who were in active practice,

Addressograph

ADVERSE DRUG
REACTION REPORT

Directions:

Every case of drug reaction (unusual or unexpected reactions), including acute poisonings by narcotics, barbiturates and amphetamines and industrial poisonings is to be reported by the attending physician to the Division of Pharmacology. The physician in charge of the patient is also responsible for notifying the allergist, dermatologist and others interested in the problem. Diagnostic procedures and therapy when such exist, will be instituted.

1. Drug or agent involved:_____

_____

_____

2. Type of reaction:_____

_____

_____

3. Therapy and Results:_____

_____

_____

4. Age	5. Sex:	6. Source of drug:
__Under 20	__M. __F.	__Prescription
__21–30		__Over the counter
__31–40	5A. Color:	__Other
__41–50	__Negro	
__51–60	__White	
__61 and Over	__Other	

Attending Physician

Fig. 12. Adverse Drug Reaction Report.

		Form Approved; OMB No. 57-R0059
		DO NOT USE THIS SPACE
HOSPITAL PHARMACIST'S DRUG DEFECT REPORT		DATE RECEIVED
		REFERENCE NO.

1. TRADE NAME, DOSAGE FORM, STRENGTH

2. LOT NUMBER(s)

3. DATE PURCHASED *(If known)*

4. SOURCE OF PRODUCT *(Where purchased, if known)*

5. NAME AND ADDRESS OF DRUG MANUFACTURER

6. REPORTING PHARMACIST'S NAME

7. NAME AND ADDRESS OF HOSPITAL *(Include ZIP Code)* 1/

8. PHONE NUMBER OF HOSPITAL *(Include Area Code)*

9. DEFECTS NOTED OR SUSPECTED

1/ *Additional forms and postage-paid envelopes will be mailed to you automatically at this address when this report is received.*

RETURN TO	United States Pharmacopeia 12601 Twinbrook Parkway Rockville, Maryland 20852 Attention: Dr. Joseph G. Valentino

FD FORM 2519 (2 '72)

Fig. 13.   Hospital Pharmacist's Drug Defect Report Form.

community pharmacists, the American Nurses' Association and hospital pharmacists who are not members of the ASHP.

Reporting forms (Fig. 13) are automatically sent to all those participating in the program. Reportable defects include inadequate packaging; confusing or inadequate labels or labeling; deteriorated, contaminated, or defective dosage forms; inaccurate fill or count of a drug product; faulty drug delivering apparatus etc. Obviously, the participants should report anything which, in their professional opinion, is considered to be defective or undesirably associated with the product.

The completed report forms are sent directly to the USP. The staff of the USP then forwards copies of the reports to the FDA and to the manufacturer or distributor involved for their information and use.

AUTOMATIC STOP ORDER FOR DANGEROUS DRUGS

The Pharmacy and Therapeutics Committee should develop a means whereby dangerous drugs may be properly administered under reasonable medical staff control.

The questionnaire for accreditation by the Joint Commission on Accreditation of Hospitals specifically determines whether or not the hospital has an automatic stop order in force.

The way two hospitals handle this matter is shown below. Either may be copied in principle by any hospital desiring to do so:

"All drug orders for narcotics, sedatives, hypnotics, anticoagulants, and antibiotics (administered orally or parenterally) shall be automatically discontinued after 48 hours, unless (1) the order indicates an exact number of doses to be administered, (2) an exact period of time for the medication is specified, or (3) the attending physician reorders the medication."

The second example of an automatic stop order is:

"All orders for narcotics, sedatives and hypnotics must be rewritten every 24 hours.

"All P.R.N. (pro re nata) and standing orders for all medications except narcotics, sedatives and hypnotics shall expire at 10:00 a.m. on the seventh day unless renewed."

COMMITTEE'S ROLE IN DEVELOPING EMERGENCY DRUG LISTS

Because in most true emergencies time is of the essence, it is imperative that emergency drug or "Stat" boxes containing drugs and supplies be readily available for use by the bedside. The Pharmacy and Therapeutics Committee should develop a list of supplies and drugs which ought to be in an emergency box and instruct the pharmacist and nursing service supervisors of their joint responsibility to have the box ready for use at all times.

Once the content of the box has been established and the responsibility for its stocking assigned, the units should be prepared and placed on each pavilion, in the clinic, in the emergency ward and in the special procedures room of the department of radiology.

After the emergency boxes have been placed on the wards, it is mandatory that a program be developed whereby they are checked daily either by the hospital pharmacist or by the nursing supervisor responsible for the ward.

The following list of contents is provided to serve as a guide.

Supplies to be Maintained in Emergency Box:

Syringes:
4– 2 ml
4– 5 ml
1–20 ml
1 insulin

Files, ampul.
Airway
Tourniquets

Needles:
2 #16
2 #18
2 #20
2 #23
2 cardiac, #20, 4"

Drugs for the Emergency Box:

Aminophylline 0.25 gm/10 ml
Amphetamine Sulfate 20 mg/ml
Amyl Nitrite Inhalation
Atropine Sulfate 0.4 mg/ml
Caffeine Sodium Benzoate 0.5 gm/2 ml
Calcium Gluconate 1 gm/10 ml
Chloroprophenpyrimadine Maleate
    50 mg/ml
Digoxin 0.25 mg/ml
Diphenylhydantoin Sodium 50 mg/ml
Epinephrine HCl 1:1000
Heparin 10,000 Units/ml
Hydrocortisone 100 mg
Isoproterenol 1:100
Magnesium Sulfate Injection 10% and
    50%

Metaraminol Bitartrate 10 mg/ml
Mannitol Injection 25%
Nalorphine HCl 10 mg/2 ml
Neostigmine Methylfulfate 0.25
    mg/ml
Nor-epinephrine Injection 0.2%
Pentobarbital 50 mg/ml
Pentylenetetrazol Injection 0.1 gm/ml
Phenobarbital 120 mg/ml
Phenylephrine HCl 10 mg/ml
Phytonadione Injection 50 mg/ml
Picrotoxin Injection 3 mg/ml
Procaine Amide 100 mg/ml
Protamine Sulfate 10 mg/ml
Saline for Injection 30 ml
Sodium Molar Lactate Solution
Water for Injection 50 ml

Supplies for Cabinet or Pavilion Utility Room:

1 Venous cannulization set
2 each—#14 and #17 venous
    catheters
2 6" shock blocks
2 Oxygen catheters

3 Sterile suction catheters
1 Sengstachen-Blakemore tube
1 Razor with blades
1 pkg. sterile gelatin sponge
1 Resuscitation tube

Other Emergency Supplies:

Resuscitation carts
Phlebotomy sets
Oxygen equipment

Tracheostomy sets
Dextran and tubing
Burn sheets

Drug Utilization Review

Drug utilization has been defined as the prescribing, dispensing, administering, and ingesting of prescription drugs.[12] Clearly, the magnitude of the problems associated with drug utilization is of great public concern and warrants the attention of health care practitioners. Yet, as a result of this study of the problem Brodie[12] concluded that "there is no organized mechanism for what can properly be called drug utilization review in the private sector of medical care."

Within the hospital, the Pharmacy and Therapeutics Committee provides the institutional authority for the formulary system of drug-use control as well as the mechanism for the continuing education of physicians, nurses and pharmacists. Thus, some institutions have initiated *patient drug utilization profiles* and medication history taking as part of their clinical pharmacy programs thereby enabling the pharmacists to monitor drug utilization within the hospital.

Medication histories are taken by pharmacists of every patient admitted to the hospital or seen in the ambulatory care section. These may be accomplished by personal interview or via a computerized questionnaire specifically designed for the purpose. In addition to personal identification and general diagnosis, the following information is elicited:

1. Medications being taken at time of admission.
2. Medications taken during the recent past. (Including antibiotics.)
3. Home remedies (OTC Drugs) used.
4. Drug allergies.
5. Laboratory tests performed out of the hospital during which diagnostic agents were ingested.
6. Idiosyncrasy towards food products.

The Patient Medication Profile (Fig. 14) is developed by the pharmacist for the following purposes.[13]

1. To help improve drug prescribing practices by promoting the safe and rational use of drugs.
2. To detect and help prevent potential drug interactions.
3. To help detect and prevent adverse drug reactions in sensitive patients.
4. To detect and prevent IV additive incompatibilities.
5. To detect drug-induced laboratory test abnormalities.
6. To detect possible drug-induced diseases.
7. To help detect and prevent potential drug toxicities.

When the Patient Medication Profile, Patient History and Laboratory Procedure Profile are compared, the pharmacist is in an excellent position to monitor proper drug utilization.

It should be obvious to the student that the compilation of drug utilization is a tedious responsibility that can be automated. A computer-based system provides for the entry of the information into the computer through the use of punch cards, magnetic tape, scanning device, or an electronic input terminal device. In the National Center for Health Services Research and Development Study[12] it was pointed

PATIENT MEDICATION PROFILE

Name_____Location_____Physician_____

Admitted_____Source of Admission_____Home_____Other hospital

_____Nursing   _____Emergency
Home   Service

Admission Diagnosis_____

Other Pathology_____

Operative Procedure Required_____

Pre-Op Medications Used_____

_____

_____

DRUG PROFILE
(includes I.V.'s)

DATE	MEDICATION	DOSE, ROUTE FREQUENCY	DISCONT. DATE	LAB. TESTS	PHARM. NOTE

DISCHARGED_____   PHARMACIST_____

Fig. 14. Patient Medication Profile for use by clinical pharmacists.

out that the ideal system should provide for both retrospective and prospective review.

Retrospective analysis is provided through the use of the punch cards and magnetic tapes whereas when electronic terminal devices are employed, both retrospective and prospective analyses are possible. Control of drug utilization by prospective review is possible when a computer read-out station is located on the patient pavilion. This device can display the profile of a patient's regimen (and others if desired) at the time a new drug is prescribed or when changes are made in therapy. In either case, the entry to the computer is made through an input station utilizing a typewriter keyboard, thereby making an instant entry into the on-line system.

Generally, the input information for an electronic data processing system is taken in a codified form from the source documents which, in this instance, are the prescription, medication order or doctor's order book. The following provides an idea of the type and scope of information utilized: patient's name, age, sex, ethnic background, diagnosis, drug product, manufacturer, therapeutic class, dosage form, strength, route of administration, directions for use, amount dispensed, days of therapy, drug effectiveness, toxicity, adverse reactions, reasons for termination of therapy, prescriber's name and specialty, etc.[12]

In those hospitals and nursing homes where it is not possible to develop patient drug profiles for the continuing surveillance of drug utilization, it may be advisable for the pharmacist to become a member of the Utilization Review Committee. Membership on this committee of a pharmacist is possible because it is required to be broadly representative of the entire scope of professional practice carried out in the institution. The pharmacist's training and experience in drug problems uniquely qualifies him to sit on such a committee and review patient drug utilization while physicians review clinical utilization of hospital services.

The ASHP has developed Guidelines on the Pharmacist's Role in Drug-Use Review and Patient-Care Audits[14] hereinafter reproduced.

ASHP GUIDELINES ON THE PHARMACIST'S ROLE IN DRUG-USE REVIEW AND PATIENT-CARE AUDITS[a]

Drug-use review (DUR) is "an authorized, structured, ongoing system for improving the quality of drug use within a health care organization."[1] This can be accomplished by the development of an evaluation process that uses predetermined criteria and leads to corrective measures that will improve use of drugs. DUR is a responsibility of the pharmacy and the medical staff; it is not unilaterally a pharmacy or medical staff function.[2]

DUR can either be a "freestanding activity"[3] or be incorporated in current patient-care audits performed by the medical staff. Patient-care audits use explicit and measurable process and outcome criteria applied to a sufficiently large number of patient records to evaluate the quality of care being provided for (most commonly) a certain disease state or

---

[a]Developed by the ASHP Council on Clinical Pharmacy and Therapeutics. Approved by the ASHP Board of Directors, April 30, 1981.

surgical procedure. Drug use is often an important component of the care provided and should be appropriately reviewed.

DUR may be performed retrospectively, concurrently, or prospectively, and can use patient outcomes or therapeutic processes or both as basis for judgments about the appropriateness of drug use. The basic requirements of a DUR program are as follows:

1. Authority for the program (This derives from the medical staff or hospital administration).
2. Adequate data bases for study.
3. Use of predetermined criteria.
4. Use of appropriate audit methodology in data retrieval.
5. Data analysis.
6. Education or corrective action or both (when appropriate).
7. Reaudit.
8. Documentation and report of all activities and results.

Responsibilities of the pharmacist in these activities include the following:

1. Preparing, in cooperation with the medical staff, drug use criteria and standards.
2. Obtaining quantitative data on drug use (e.g., information on the amounts and types of drugs used, prescribing patterns by medical services, and types of patients). These data will be useful in setting priorities for the review program.
3. Reviewing medication orders against the drug use criteria and standards.
4. Consulting with prescribers on the results from (3) above.
5. Participating in the follow-up activities of the review program (e.g., educational programs directed at prescribers, development of recommendations for the formulary, and changing drug control procedures in response to the results of the review process).

Quantitative data used to pick topics for qualitative studies can be found in such pharmacy records as: purchasing records, monthly usage data, drug profiles for inpatients and outpatient, patient charge, adverse drug reaction reports, and others. Review of these data bases usually leads to the study of drugs that are of substantial clinical or financial import.

The intent of these guidelines is to provide a framework for pharmacists to follow in developing individual DUR programs or participating in patient care audits at their own hospitals. Pharmacists should assume an active role in any quality assurance activities in their institution that deal with the use of drugs.

REFERENCES

1. The rationale for evaluating drug use through patient care audit. Interqual Manual. 1978; 1:3.

2. ASHP guidelines on hospital drug distribution and control (with references). *Am. J. Hosp. Pharm.* 1980; 37:1097–103.
3. Brodie, D.C., Hlynka, J.N., Smith, W.E.: Model for drug usage review in a hospital. *Am. J. Hosp. Pharm.* 1977; 34:251–4.

The following is offered as a starting point for the pharmacist to review the patient's drug therapy record in order to ascertain whether or not his stay was affected by drug therapy. Obviously, good therapy coupled with good clinical care can reduce the patient's length of stay whereas poor therapy, which leads to complications, may increase the patient's hospital stay.

I. Proper Choice of Therapeutic Agent
 1. Was the drug employed one with a special effect upon the diagnosed ailment? If not, why was it prescribed? If the medication prescribed was of multiple composition, was there contained therein a sufficient amount of the principal ingredient to produce a therapeutic effect?
 2. If the drug employed was a sulfonamide or antibiotic, were cultures of the infecting organism taken for the purpose of identification? Were sensitivities performed?
 3. Was any effort made to ascertain the patient's sensitivity to the drug?
 4. Did administration of the drug have any effect upon subsequent laboratory analyses essential to the diagnosis of the ailment?

II. Proper Choice of Dosage Form
 1. Did the patient receive his therapy via the parenteral route when the enteral should have been employed or vice versa?
 2. Were enteric coated tablets used when indicated?
 3. If time disintegrating dosage forms were employed, was there any evidence to indicate that the medication was being properly released?
 4. If intravenous fluids were employed, what drugs were administered simultaneously? Were they compatible with each other? With the intravenous vehicle?

III. Proper Route of Administration
 1. Was the route of administration preferable to another?
 2. If the oral route was selected, was the medication prescribed for administration at the recommended times, *i.e.* pre- or post-prandially?

IV. Drug Allergy
 1. Were there any manifestations of drug allergy?
 2. Were tests for predicting drug allergies done on patients with a suspicious history?
 3. Were the drug allergies subsequently managed adequately?

V. Drug Idiosyncrasy and Pharmacogenetics
1. If there was an abnormally prolonged drug effect, were steps taken to reduce dosage frequency?
2. If there was evidence of increased drug sensitivity, were steps taken to reduce dosage?
3. Were any novel or unusual drug effects noted?
4. If there was evidence of decreased responsiveness to the drugs employed, were counter measures taken?
5. Was there any evidence of the development of physical dependence upon the drug?

VI. Effect upon Utilization of Hospital Facilities
1. As a result of improper drug therapy, was the length of stay increased? How many days? At how much additional cost?
2. What additional laboratory tests were necessary? At how much additional cost?
3. What additional diagnostic and therapeutic measures were necessary due to the improper therapy? At what additional cost?
4. What additional medication was necessitated? At what additional cost?

VII. Follow-up and Discharge Medications
1. Were discharge medications prescribed?
2. Were they necessary? If yes, were the label instructions adequate to insure proper administration to the patient by law or semi-professional personnel?
3. If a follow-up visit is scheduled, were sufficient drug doses prescribed to carry the patient until the visit date? If not, does the prescription order indicate that a refill is permissible?

NURSING AND THE PHARMACY AND THERAPEUTICS COMMITTEE

In a large teaching hospital, it is not uncommon for members of the medical staff to request nurses to administer drugs with which they are not familiar.[15] More frequently than not the medication requires administration by the intravenous route. Because these requests invariably bring anxiety and frustration to the nurse, it is vital that the Pharmacy and Therapeutics Committee devise a system whereby these requests are reviewed and if appropriate the necessary educational and training programs be instituted.

It is suggested that any nurse or physician wishing to delegate to nurses the responsibility for the administering of an intravenous drug to a patient submit to the Pharmacy and Therapeutics Committee the following information on the drug or drug product.

Names
Method of Administration
  I.V. Push
  I.V. Bolus
  I.V. Drip
Dosage
Diluent
Administration Time
Necessary Blood Work and/or other laboratory data
Contraindications
Stability of the Drug
Incompatibilities
General Precautions
Special Indications Concerning Preparation
  a. By nursing
  b. By physician only
  c. By pharmacy only

If the Pharmacy and Therapeutics Committee approves, then the educational and training effort should include the above as part of the program.

DRG'S AND THE PHARMACY AND THERAPEUTICS COMMITTEE

The term, "DRG" refers to a methodology, developed at the Center for Health Studies, at Yale University, for compressing the entire range of inpatient diagnoses into a manageable and medically meaningful number of major categories according to certain patient attributes such as age, primary diagnosis, primary surgical procedure, secondary diagnosis (if present), and secondary surgical procedure (if present). DRG's are attracting intense interest from hospitals, regulators, PSROs, and planners because of their potential for describing hospitals' casemix on a common basis.

DRG's are used by hospitals for casemix accounting for budgeting and cost control, inhospital utilization review, reimbursement appeals and resource scheduling and control. Regulators use DRG for "per case" reimbursement determinations, interhospital groupings and cost comparisons and health planning. PSRO's use DRG's for concurrent review of utilization, length of stay profiles, focused review and national PSRO reporting.

With the acceptance of the DRG methodology, hospitals will be able to compare drug therapy for the major categories of diagnoses on an interhospital basis. Presumably, reinbursement by third party payors may be based upon a predetermined schedule of drugs for the respective diagnostic categories. Pharmacy and Therapeutics Committees should be aware of this development and should use it in performing drug utilization reviews as well as in the preparation of the hospital formulary.

SELECTED READINGS

Hellin, Dennis K., Norwood, G. Joseph, and Donner, John D.: An Assessment of Prescribing Using Drug Utilization Review Criteria. Drug Intel. and Clin. Pharm.,
   16:930–933, (Dec.) 1982.
Oakley, Robert S. and Bradham, Douglas, D.: Review of Quality Assurance in Hospital
   Pharmacy. Am. J. Hosp. Pharm., *40*:53–63, 1983.
Cohen, M.R., Klapp, D., Miller, K.B., Shaffer, V.L., and Miller, D.E.: Improving Pharmacy
   and Therapeutic Committee Operations. Am. J. Hosp. Pharm., *41*:1767–1777, (Sept.)
   1984.

REFERENCES

 1. ———: The Drug Prescribers, Task Force on Prescription Drugs, U.S. Department of
    Health, Education and Welfare, Washington, D.C. 20201, Dec. 1968.
 2. *Hospital Accreditation References,* Chicago, American Hospital Association, 1964,
    p. 120.
 3. ASHP Statement on the Pharmacy and Therapeutics Committee. Am. J. Hosp. Pharm.,
    41:1621, 1984.
 4. Peski, Lawrence J. and Pierpaoli, Paul G.: The Effective Committee. Cur. Concepts
    in Hosp. Pharm. Mgt., *4*:1:7, 1982.
 5. Longest, B.B. Jr.: *Management Practices for the Health Professional,* 2nd ed. Reston
    Va., Reston Publishing Co., Inc., 1980, pp. 170–180.
 6. Flack, Herbert L.: Goals for Hospital Pharmacists, Am. J. Hosp. Pharm., *18*:17:383,
    (July) 1961.
 7. ASHP Technical Assistance Bulletin on the Scientific and Therapeutic Evaluation
    of Drugs for Hospital Formularies. Am. J. Hosp. Pharm., *38*:1043–1044, (July) 1981.
 8. Madaio, A. and Clarke, T.R.: Benefits of a Self Medication Program in a Longterm
    Care Facility. Hosp. Pharm., *12*:72–75, (Feb.) 1977.
 9. Hassan, William E., Jr.: There is no General Equivalent for Quality, Drug Topics,
    110:30, (Oct.) 1966.
10. Hassan, William E. Jr.: Ensuring Safety in Drug Administration, Hospital Manage-
    ment, *84*:108, 1957.
11. Francke, Don E.: The Reporting of Adverse Drug Reactions as a Function of the
    Pharmacy and Therapeutics Committee, Am. J. Hosp. Pharm., *19*:10:533, (Oct.) 1962.
12. Brodie, Donald C.: Drug Utilization and Drug Utilization Review and Control,
    D.H.E.W. Publication No. (HSM) 72–3002, Dept. Health, Education, and Welfare,
    5600 Fishers Lane, Rockville, Maryland, 20852, May 1971.
13. Goldman, Laurence: The Pharmacist's Role in Monitoring Drug Therapy, Hospital
    Pharmacy, *6*:6:5, (June) 1971.
14. ASHP Guidelines on the Pharmacist's Role in Drug-Use Review and Patient-Care
    Audits. Am. J. Hosp. Pharm., *38*:1042–1043, (July) 1981.
15. Grotting, M.A., Latiolais, C.J. and Visconti, J.A.: Putting RN's in the IV Push Chem-
    otherapy Picture, Am. J. IV Ther., *3*:31–35, 38, 41, (Nov.) 1976.

5

The Hospital Formulary

American hospital and pharmaceutical literature is replete with both favorable and unfavorable comments and views on the use of the formulary system in hospitals. This chaotic state has been brought about because of the complete misunderstanding by certain minority groups of the purpose, scope and function of the hospital formulary system.

Those who denounce the system often cite the following reasons to make valid their claims:

(a) The hospital formulary system deprives the physician of his prerogative to prescribe and obtain the brand of his choice.

(b) The hospital formulary system, in many instances, permits the pharmacist to act as the sole judge of which brand of drug is to be purchased and dispensed.

(c) The hospital formulary system allows for the purchase of inferior quality drugs, particularly in institutions where there is no staff pharmacist.

(d) The hospital formulary system does not reduce the cost of drugs to the patient or to the third party payor because most institutions purchase large volumes of drugs at reduced rates but do not pass on to the patient any reductions in their cost.

The potential benefits of a formulary system are threefold: (1) therapeutic, (2) economic and (3) educational. The therapeutic aspect of a formulary system provides the greatest benefit to the patient and physician in that only the most efficient products are listed and available. The economic merit also has a double benefit in that the formulary eliminates duplication thus reducing inventory duplication and the opportunity for volume purchasing means lower charges to the patient. The passage of the Tax Equity and Fiscal Responsibility Act (TEFRA) and other cost containment laws and regulations will have major impact on the formulary system as hospitals seek an effective mechanism to reduce drug expenses. The educational benefit is also significant for the resident staff, nurses and medical students because many good formularies contain various prescribing tips and additional drug information of educational value.[1]

With the advent of Medicare, the hospital formulary system has taken on a new measure of importance in the hospital's economy. This is due to the fact that the Federal government will reimburse hospitals for the drugs administered or dispensed to a Medicare covered patient if the drugs were approved and listed in certain specified compendia or the hospital's formulary.

The concept of a hospital formulary system was endorsed by major health care associations in 1964 in the form of an ASHP Statement of Guiding Principles on the Operation of a Hospital Formulary System. This document has been retired in favor of the following ASHP Statement on the Formulary System.[2]

ASHP STATEMENT ON THE FORMULARY SYSTEM[a]

Preamble

The care of patients in hospitals and other health-care facilities is often dependent upon the effective use of drugs. The multiplicity of drugs available makes it mandatory that a sound program of drug usage be developed within the institution to ensure that patients receive the best possible care.

In the interest of better patient care, the institution should have a program of objective evaluation, selection, and use of medicinal agents in the facility. This program is the basis of appropriate, economical drug therapy. The formulary concept[b] is a method for providing such a program and has been utilized as such for many years.

To be effective, the formulary system must have the approval of the organized medical staff, the concurrence of individual staff members, and the functioning of a properly organized pharmacy and therapeutics committee[c] of the medical staff. The basic policies and procedures governing the formulary system should be incorporated in the medical staff bylaws or in the medical staff rules and regulations.

The pharmacy and therapeutics committee represents the official organizational line of communication and liaison between the medical and pharmacy staffs. The committee is responsible to the medical staff

---

[a]Approved by the ASHP House of Delegates, June 7, 1983. Approved by the ASHP Board of Directors, November 18, 1982. Developed by the ASHP Council on Clinical Affairs. Supersedes the "ASHP Statement of Guiding Principles on the Operation of the Hospital Formulary System" approved by the Board of Directors, January 10, 1964. This former ASHP statement had the endorsement of the American Hospital Association, the American Medical Association, and the American Pharmaceutical Association. At the appropriate time, ASHP will pursue approval of the new document by these organizations.

[b]The formulary system is adaptable for use in any type of health-care facility and is not limited to hospitals.

[c]For additional information, see the ASHP Statement on the Pharmacy and Therapeutics Committee, *Am J Hosp Pharm.* 1978; 35:813–4.

as a whole, and its recommendations are subject to approval by the organized medical staff, as well as to the normal administrative approval process.

This committee assists in the formulation of broad professional policies relating to drugs in institutions, including their evaluation of appraisal, selection, procurement, storage, distribution, and safe use.

Definition of Formulary and Formulary System

The *formulary* is a continually revised compilation of pharmaceuticals (plus important ancillary information) that reflects the current clinical judgment of the medical staff.[a]

The *formulary system* is a method whereby the medical staff of an institution, working through the pharmacy and therapeutics committee, evaluates, appraises, and selects from among the numerous available drug entities and drug products those that are considered most useful in patient care. Only those so selected are routinely available from the pharmacy. The formulary system is thus an important tool for assuring the quality of drug use and controlling its cost.

The formulary system provides for the procuring, prescribing, dispensing, and administering of drugs under either their nonproprietary or proprietary names in instances where drugs have both names.

Guiding Principles

The following principles will serve as a guide to physicians, pharmacists, nurses, and administrators in hospitals and other facilities utilizing the formulary system:

1. The medical staff shall appoint a multidisciplinary pharmacy and therapeutics committee and outline its purposes, organization, function, and scope.
2. The formulary system shall be sponsored by the medical staff based upon the recommendations of the pharmacy and therapeutics committee. The medical staff should adapt the principles of the system to the needs of the particular institution.
3. The medical staff shall adopt written policies and procedures governing the formulary system as developed by the pharmacy and therapeutics committee. Action of the medical staff is subject to the normal administrative approval process. These policies and procedures shall afford guidance in the evaluation or appraisal, selection, procurement, storage, distribution, safe use, and other matters relating to drugs, and shall be published in the institution's formulary or other media available to all members of the medical staff.
4. Drugs should be included in the formulary by their nonproprietary names, even though proprietary names may be in common use in the institution.

---

[a]For additional information, see the ASHP Guidelines for Hospital Formularies, *Am J Hosp Pharm.* 1978; 35:326–8.

Prescribers should be strongly encouraged to prescribe drugs by their nonproprietary names.

5. Limiting the number of drug entities and drug products routinely available from the pharmacy can produce substantial patient care and (particularly) financial benefits. These benefits are greatly increased through the use of *generic equivalents* (drug products considered to be identical with respect to their active components; e.g., two brands of tetracycline hydrochloride capsules) and *therapeutic equivalents* (drug products differing in composition or in their basic drug entity that are considered to have very similar pharmacologic and therapeutic activities; e.g., two different antacid products or two different alkylamine antihistamines.) The pharmacy and therapeutics committee must set forth policies and procedures governing the dispensing of generics and therapeutic equivalents. These policies and procedures should include the following points:

   • That the pharmacist is responsible for selecting, from available generic equivalents, those to be dispensed pursuant to a physician's order for a particular drug product.
   • That the prescriber has the option, at the time of prescribing, to specify the brand or supplier of drug to be disoensed for that particular medication order/prescription. The prescriber's decision should be based on pharmacologic or therapeutic considerations (or both) relative to that patient.
   • That the pharmacy and therapeutics committee is responsible for determining those drug products and entities (if any) that shall be considered therapeutic equivalents. The conditions and procedures for dispensing a therapeutic alternative in place of the prescribed drug shall be clearly delineated.

6. The institution shall make certain that its medical and nursing staffs are informed about the existence of the formulary system, the procedures governing its operation, and any changes in those procedures. Copies of the formulary must be readily available and accessible at all times.

7. Provision shall be made for the appraisal and use of drugs not included in the formulary, by the medical staff.

8. The pharmacist shall be responsible for specifications as to the quality, quantity, and source of supply of all drugs, chemicals, biologicals, and pharmaceutical preparations used in the diagnosis and treatment of patients. When applicable, such products should meet the standards of the *United States Pharmacopeia*.

Recommendation

A formulary system, based upon these guiding principles, is important in drug therapy in institutions, In the interest of better and more economical patient care, its adoption by medical staffs is strongly recommended.

ASHP TECHNICAL ASSISTANCE BULLETIN ON HOSPITAL FORMULARIES[4]*

The hospital formulary system is an ongoing process whereby a hospital's[a] medical staff, working through its pharmacy and therapeutics committee (or

---

*Approved by the ASHP Board of Directors, November 14–15, 1984. Revised by the ASHP Council on Clinical Affairs. Supersedes the previous version, which was approved on November 15, 1977.

[a]It should be noted that the formulary system is adaptable for use by any type of health care facility and is not limited to hospitals.

its equivalent), evaluates and selects from among the numerous drug products available in the market place, those it considers to be most useful in patient care. These products then are routinely available for use within the hospital. The formulary system is a powerful tool for improving the quality and controlling the cost of drug therapy, and its use is strongly encouraged. Central to the operation of the formulary system is the hospital formulary, a continually revised compilation of the drug products selected by the P & T committee, plus important ancillary information about the use of those drugs and relevant pharmacy policies and procedures.

Since the formulary is the vehicle by which the medical and nursing staffs make use of the system, it is important that it be complete, concise and easy to use. These guidelines are offered as an aid to pharmacists who will be preparing a formulary for their institution or who wish to improve an existing formulary. They do not deal with the specific drug products which might be included in a formulary or with the selection process, but, rather, with the formulary's format, organization and content.

"Guidelines for Hospital Formularies" is complementary to the "Statement of Guiding Principles on the Operation of the Hospital Formulary System"[a] which should be consulted for further information on the formulary system.

Formulary Content and Organization

The primary objectives of the formulary are to provide the hospital staff with: (1) information on what drug products[b] have ben approved for use by the pharmacy and therapeutics committee, (2) basic therapeutic information about each approved item, (3) information on hospital policies and procedures governing the use of drugs and (4) special information about drugs such as drug dosing rules and nomograms, hospital-approved abbreviations, sodium content of various formulary items, etc. In accordance with these objectives, the formulary should consist of three main parts:

Part One—Information on hospital policies and procedures concerning drugs,

Part Two—Drug products listing and

Part Three—Special information.

A more detailed look at each section follows.

Information on Hospital Policies and Procedures Concerning Drugs. The material to be included in this section will vary from hospital to hospital. Generally, the following items may be included:

1. Formulary policies and procedures, including such items as restrictions on drug use (if any) and procedures for requesting that a drug be added to the formulary.

2. *Brief description of the pharmacy and therapeutics committee,* including its membership, responsibilities and operation.

3. *Hospital regulations governing the prescribing, dispensing and administration of drugs,* including the writing of drug orders and prescriptions,

---

[a]Anon: Statement on the operation of the formulary system, *Am. J. Hosp. Pharm.,* *40*:1384–1385, 1983.

[b]"Drug product" refers to a specific drug entity/dosage form/strength/packaging/package size combination. Only certain dosage forms, for example, of a given drug entity might be included in a formulary.

controlled substances considerations, generic and therapeutic equivalency policies and procedures, automatic stop orders, verbal drug orders,
patients' use of their own medications, self-administration of drugs by
patients, use of drug samples, policies relative to "stat" and "emergency"
drug orders, use of emergency carts and kits, use of floor-stock items,
requests by staff for medications for their own use, rules to be followed
by medical service representatives, standard drug administration time
and the reporting of adverse drug reactions and medication errors. Other
topics should be included as deemed appropriate.

4. *Pharmacy operating procedures* such as hours of service, out-patient
prescription policies, pharmacy charging systems, prescription labeling
and packaging practices, inpatient drug distribution procedures, the handling of drug information requests, and specialized services of the pharmacy (e.g., patient education programs, pharmacy bulletins).

5. *Information on using the formulary,* including how the formulary entries
are arranged, the information contained in each entry and the procedure
for looking up a given drug product. Reference to sources of detailed
information on formulary drugs (e.g., *American Hospital Formulary Service,* pharmacy drug information service, etc.) should be included here.

Drug Products Listing. This section is the heart of the formulary and consists
of one or more descriptive entries for each formulary item plus one or more
indexes to facilitate use of the formulary.

Formulary Item Entries. The entries can be arranged in several ways: (1)
alphabetically by generic name, with entries for synonyms and brand names
containing only a "see (generic name)" notation; (2) alphabetically within therapeutic class, usually following the *American Hospital Formulary Service
(AHFS)* classification scheme; (3) a combination of the two systems whereby
the bulk of the drugs are contained (alphabetically) in a "general" section which
is supplemented by several "special" sections such as ophthalmic/otic drugs,
dermatologicals and diagnostic agents.

The type of information to be included in each entry will vary. At a minimum,
each entry must include:

1. Generic name of the basic drug entity or product; combination products
may be listed by generic, common or trade name;

2. Common synonym(s) and trade name(s); there should be a note in the
"directions for use" section of the formulary explaining that inclusion
or omission of a given brand does not imply that it is or is not stocked
by the pharmacy;

3. Dosage form(s), strength(s), packaging(s) and size(s) stocked by the pharmacy;

4. Formulation (active ingredients) of a combination product; and

5. *AHFS* category number.

Additional information which may be part of the drug entries includes:
1. Usual adult or pediatric dosage ranges, or both;
2. Special cautions and notes such as: "do not administer i.v." or "refrigerate";
3. Controlled substances symbol; and
4. Cost information; this generally will be most useful where the therapeutic
classification system is used or, alternatively, lists of similar drugs (e.g.,
oral steroids) may be presented showing relative cost data.

Indexes to the Drug Products Listing. There are two indexes which can be included at the beginning or end of this section which will facilitate the use of the formulary. They are:

1. *Generic Name-Brand/Synonym Cross Index.* The proper page number reference should be included in each entry. An example of this type of index is:

   Ophthaine: brand of proparacaine, p 114
   Ophthetic: brand of proparacaine, p 114
   Opium tincture, camphorated: synonym for paregoric, p 103
   Paragoric: p 103
   Proparacaine: p 114

   This index also could be integrated into the drug products listing rather than being a separate entity. The listing, in this event, must be arranged alphabetically.

2. *Therapeutic/Pharmacologic Index.* This index is a listing of all formulary items within each therapeutic category. It is useful in ascertaining what therapeutic alternatives exist for a given situation such as patient allergy to a particular drug. An example of this type of index is:

   4:00 Antihistamine drugs
         Brompheniramine maleate, p 14
         Chlorpheniramine maleate, p 14
         Diphenhydramine HCl, p 14
         Promethazine HCl, p 20
   8:00 Anti-infective agents
   8:04 Ambecides
         Chloroquine, p 43
         Diiodohydroxyquin, p 22

The entries should include the *AHFS* code number.

Special Information. The material to be included in this section will vary from hospital to hospital. However, what is included should be of general interest to the hospital staff and not readily available from other sources. Examples of the type of items often found in the special information section of hospital formularies are:

1. Nutritional products list.
2. Tables of equivalent dosages of similar drugs (e.g., corticosteroids),
3. List of hospital-approved abbreviations,
4. Rules for calculating pediatric dosages,
5. Table of the sodium content of antacids,
6. List of sugar-free drug products,
7. List of items available from central supply,
8. List of the contents of emergency carts,
9. Lists of dialyzable poisons,
10. Pharmacokinetic dosing and monitoring information,
11. Metric conversion scales and tables,
12. Examples of blank or completed hospital forms such as prescription blanks, request for nonformulary drug forms and adverse drug reaction report forms.

13. Tables of drug interactions, drug interferences with diagnostic tests and parenteral drug incompatibilities, and
14. Poison control information.

FORMAT AND APPEARANCE OF THE FORMULARY

The physical appearance and structure of the formulary is an important influence on its use. Although elaborate and expensive artwork and materials are unnecessary, the formulary should be visually pleasing, easily readable, and professional in appearance. The need for proper grammar, punctuation, correct spelling, and neatness is obvious.

There is no one single format or arrangement which all formularies must follow. A typical formulary must have the following composition:

1. Title page
2. Names and titles of the members of the pharmacy and therapeutics committee
3. Table of contents
4. Information on hospital policies and procedures concerning drugs
    4.1 The pharmacy and therapeutics committee of XYZ hospital
    4.2 Objectives and operation of the formulary system
    4.3 Hospital regulations and procedures for prescribing and dispensing drugs
    4.4 Hospital pharmacy services and procedures
    4.5 How to use the formulary
5. Products accepted for use at XYZ hospital
    5.1 Items added and deleted since the previous edition
    5.2 Generic-brand name cross reference list
    5.3 Pharmacologic/therapeutic index with relative cost codes
    5.4 Descriptions of formulary drug products by pharmacologic therapeutic class
6. Appendix
    6.1 Central service equipment and supply list
    6.2 Rules for calculating pediatric doses
    6.3 Nomogram for estimating body surface area
    6.4 Schedule of standard drug administration times

Several techniques can be used to improve the appearance and ease of use of the formulary. Among these are:

1. Using a different color paper for each section of the formulary,
2. Using an edge index,
3. Making the formulary pocket size (approximately 4" × 7") and
4. Printing the generic name heading of each drug entry in boldface type or using some other method for making it stand out from the rest of the entry.

DISTRIBUTION OF THE FORMULARY

Copies of the formulary should be placed at each patient care unit, including clinics and other outpatient care areas such as the emergency room. Each division of the pharmacy (inpatient dispensing, outpatient dispensing, drug information service, etc.) should receive a copy. Heads of departments providing direct patient care should receive a copy as should hospital administration. Each member of the medical staff should receive a copy.

The necessary steps should be taken to insure that the nursing and medical staffs are familiar with the formulary and know how to use it.

Enough formularies should be printed to allow for replacement of copies which become lost or worn.

KEEPING THE FORMULARY CURRENT

Generally, the formulary will need to be revised annually. Additions and deletions to the formulary, changes in drug products, removal of drugs from the marketplace and changes in hospital policies and procedures all will necessitate periodic revision of the formulary. There should be a system for including "between revision" changes in the current edition of the formulary. One method is to attach formulary supplement sheets to the inside back covers of the formulary books.

Another means of keeping a formulary current is through an organized system of soliciting changes in the formulary from the medical staff. One institution[3] utilizes a form as exhibited in Chart A.

USE OF NON-FORMULARY DRUGS

In many institutions, a non-formulary drug will not be dispensed from the out-patient pharmacy. The patients are instructed to obtain the medication from their local pharmacy.

With respect to in-patients, a physician is allowed to order a non-formulary drug for a specific patient by the use of a special non-formulary drug request form Chart B.

PATIENT PACKAGE INSERTS (PPI)

The Food and Drug Administration has proposed regulations requiring that prescription drugs be accompanied by a non-technical explanation informing patients about the drug. The purpose of this is to promote the safe and effective use of prescription drugs by patients. In addition, this proposal would ensure that patients have the opportunity to be informed of the risks/benefits involved in the use of the prescription drug. It has been estimated that the cost of the system will be $90 million.[5] Industry and pharmacy costs will be 97% of that total or 6.3¢ per prescription.[2] Pharmacy costs will be $20 million initially and within 5 years rise to $75 million.[5]

Because PPI's distributed to hospitalized patients would create many logistical and practical problems, the hospital association and the professional pharmaceutical society have compaigned to exempt hospitals from compliance. The FDA took into consideration the facts that hospitalized patients may be too ill to read the labeling; that many institutions already have programs providing drug information; that patients have hospital staff readily available to them to answer questions about drugs; and that patients often take several drugs at once. Because of these problems, the FDA exempted hospitals from the labeling distribution requirement if the patient (or patient's agent) is

DEPARTMENT OF PHARMACY SERVICES
REQUEST FOR FORMULARY CHANGE

Request for: . . . .   Admission . . . . Deletion

Generic Name: Trade Name(s):

Manufacturer:

Pharmacologic Class:

Dosage Form(s):

Oral: . . . . Parenteral: . . . . Topical: . . . . Other: . . . .

                                                                 (Specify)

Strength:

List vehicles, preservatives, and solubilizers where applicable.

Similar products currently stocked:

Similar products by other manufacturers:

Justification with references:

Will new drug be used:
   A.   Widely for inpatients?
   B.   Widely for outpatients?
   C.   On a limited basis?

Requestor's Name Printed: . . . .   Signature . . . .

Department: . . . .   Telephone: . . . .

                                              Date: . . . .

Cost of drug (to be completed by Pharmacy Services):

Completed forms should he directed to the Department of Pharmacy Services

   1. Accepted   a) For general formulary
                    b) For conditional formulary
                    c) For restricted use
   2. Restricted: Reason
   3. Deferred: Reason
   4. Date action taken: . . . .

. . . .
Secretary, Pharmacy & Therapeutics Committee

Chart. A.   Request for formulary change initiated by members of the medical staff.

informed at the time of admission—or as soon thereafter as possible—
that drug descriptions are available on request. Further, institutions are
not required to provide patients with personal copies of any specific
information. However, the information ought to be available to the
patient. Some suggested ways are to maintain the information in a
compendium, a file or via the use of audio or audio-visual tape
recordings.

Other exemptions include instances of: legally incompetent patients;

BRIGHAM & WOMEN'S HOSPITAL
NON-FORMULARY MEDICATION REQUEST

This form must accompany a copy of physician's order sheet for each non-formulary drug ordered.

This form is to be used by house officers only when attending physicians or chief resident countersigns.

THIS FORM IS FOR INPATIENT DRUG ORDERS ONLY.

Patient Name:

Floor and Room: Use addressograph or print.

Drug Name:

Manufacturer:

Dosage Schedule and Route:

Number Doses Required (Approximate):

.... M.D.   Date: ....
Signature of House Officer

.... M.D.   Date: ....
Signature of Attending Staff or Chief Resident

NOTE: By ordering a non-formulary drug, you are obliging your patient to pay for the entire package of medication. *Twenty-four hours* may be required to obtain a non-formulary drug.

Completed forms should be directed to Pharmacy Administrative Office.

....
Pharmacist Sending Form   Date & Time Form Sent

....
Pharmacist Receiving Completed Form   Date & Time Completed Form Received

Chart. B.   Form used by members of the medical staff to obtain a non-formulary drug for use by their patient.

a specific request by the doctor that the information be withheld; emergency treatment; blind patients and those whose primary language is not English.

In the preparation of the hospital formulary, the Pharmacy and Therapeutics Committee should give serious consideration to limiting the number of drugs admitted to the formulary in the light of the PPI regulations. Further, it is incumbent upon the committee members to give consideration to the content and preparation of the non-technical brochure which would be given to the patient should it be requested.

THE LEGAL BASIS OF THE FORMULARY SYSTEM

A written and signed prescription or a written and signed medication order in the Doctor's Order Book constitutes the only legal permit to dispense or administer a prescription legend drug. If the physician in writing the prescription or medication order uses a generic or chemical name for the desired preparation, the pharmacist may then dispense the brand which, in his professional judgment, meets the therapeutic need, and there will arise no legal problems irrespective of whether or not the hospital has adopted a formulary system.

The problem usually arises when the hospital has in effect a formulary system yet the prescriber continues to use a proprietary name for the drug desired. In many instances, the prescriber is aware of the fact that the hospital is operating under the formulary system but, through habit, writes for brand-named drugs. Under these circumstances, if the prescriber had previously agreed to the policy that all prescriptions and medication orders will be dispensed without reference to brand identity, then the pharmacist may so dispense. On the other hand, if there had been no previous consent to the policy by the physician, the pharmacist is professionally and morally duty bound to honor the prescriber's wishes as to brand.

In general, this system of prior **blanket consent** is no longer recommended because it is established upon unsound legal principles.

In order to avoid such situations, hospitals have devised many ways of obtaining the prescriber's consent to the hospital formulary system of dispensing.

One common method is the use of a suitably worded imprint on the prescription form. Examples of such wording are: *"Generic Equivalent Permitted"* or *"Dispensed in accord with the hospital formulary system."* Any physician not desirous of the generic equivalent may obtain the selected brand merely by drawing a line through the permissive statement. In some hospitals, the consent statement is often followed by a check box with a "Yes" or "No," thereby giving the physician an option each time he prescribes. Although both methods are acceptable, I prefer the former since it takes the positive permissive approach and places the responsibility upon the physician of giving notice to the pharmacist of the deviation from accepted policy.

The second method of obtaining prior medical consent to the operation of a hospital formulary system is to incorporate the basic policy and procedures governing its use in the medical staff by-laws or in the rules and regulations. Therefore, as each physician accepts appointment or reappointment, he accepts the formulary system. It is strongly recommended that the acceptance of the appointment and the willingness to abide by the by-laws or the rules and regulations be executed in writing. Members of the intern and resident staffs who normally do not sign documents to abide by the by-laws or rules and regulations of the medical staff should be requested to execute separate consent agreements. Since this method is a modification of the blanket prior consent policy, it should be used with caution.

The third method of obtaining prior medical consent to the operation of a hospital formulary system is to express the policy and procedures governing the formulary system in a separate document and request that all physicians sign it.

The second and third methods have long been criticized on the basis that they abrogate the professional prerogatives of the clinician. This is no longer a valid argument since the adoption of the Statement of Guiding Principles on the Operation of the Hospital Formulary System which provides a means whereby a physician who, for clinical reasons, desires the brand-named product may still obtain it for his patient.

It is the opinion of some attorney[6] that whenever a physician accepts an appointment to a hospital staff, he "commonly yields to the medical staff as a whole, so far as his practice in that hospital is concerned, certain professional decisions which he is otherwise free to make for himself." It should be quite clear that if the physician does not wish to conform to all of the rules of the particular hospital, he is free to take his patients elsewhere and practice as he chooses. However, so long as he admits to and treats patients in the hospital, he may not disregard or willfully circumvent the accepted by-laws of the staff or the institution.

ANTISUBSTITUTION LAWS AND THE FORMULARY

The movement to modify state antisubstitution laws which interfere with the pharmacist's ability to exercise his professional judgment has gained momentum. As each state legislature has formulated its own approach to the problem, a wide variety of solutions have evolved. Hospital pharmacists should certainly be knowledgeable about the legislation affecting pharmacy practice in their state, and they may even wish to consider modifying the language in their hospital formulary systems to comply with that of the state legislation regarding physician specification of a certain brand; however, this would not appear to be an absolute necessity. The legal basis of the hospital formulary system remains intact regardless of the changes in state antisubstitution laws.[12]

PREPARATION OF THE FORMULARY

The preparation of the hospital formulary, although the prime responsibility of the Pharmacy and Therapeutics Committee, rests upon the Pharmacist-in-Chief. This is desirable for the sake of expediency. The Committee is here free to make the necessary decisions relative to the materials to be included in the formulary and the pharmacist undertakes the production aspects of preparation.

The initial step in the development of a formulary for any hospital, irrespective of size, specialty, or control, is the selection of a competent

Pharmacy and Therapeutics Committee. Because of the importance of this Committee, a separate chapter has been devoted to its organization, membership and functions. Suffice it to say here that, once established, this Committee must take the initial step in the preparation of the formulary.

Some of the decisions which must be reached by this Committee concern themselves with the following:

a. What type of publication will best suit the needs of the hospital?
  1. A hospital owned formulary?
  2. A simple drug list or catalogue?
  3. A purchased formulary service?
b. Irrespective of what decision is reached in the above, it will be necessary to promulgate a series of rules or guides which the Committee may use to evaluate drugs for admission to the formulary or drug list.
c. If the desirable end product is to be a formulary, a decision must be reached as to possible contents other than the sections on various therapeutic agents.
  1. Section on prescription writing?
  2. Section governing the use of drugs?
  3. Tables of metric weights and apothecary and household equivalents?
  4. Table of common laboratory values?
  5. Section on the calculation of dosages for children based on established rules and by use of the body surface method?
  6. Pharmacological index?
  7. Section on reagents?
d. What type of format should the formulary take?
  1. Size?
  2. Loose leaf or bound?
  3. Printed or mimeographed?
  4. Categorizing and indexing—to what extent?

Once answers to the above have been provided for the Pharmacist-in-Chief, the preparation of the formulary becomes a routine matter requiring diligence to detail, accuracy and perseverance.

FORMULARY VS. DRUG CATALOGUE OR LIST

Unfortunately, too many people use the terms *formulary* and *drug list* interchangeably. This is erroneous in view of the fact that there exists a vast difference in the scope and preparation of a formulary over a drug list.

A formulary usually consists of a listing of therapeutic agents by their generic names followed by informaiton on strength, form, posology, toxicology, use, and recommended quantity to be dispensed, whereas a drug list usually consists of a listing of therapeutic agents by their generic names followed by data on strength and form. There may or may not be any additional information although some drug lists may provide the prescriber with recommended quantities to be dispensed.

Clearly then, the formulary is the more information type of publication and may exert an influential role in the educational aspects of drug therapy particularly in hospitals with an active intern and residency training program and a school of nursing.

If a formulary type of publication is desirable, then the Committee ha the option of either preparing a private formulary for the hospital or to subscribe to a perpetual drug monograph service such as the *American Hospital Formulary Service,* a publication of the American Society of Hospital Pharmacists.

Either a well-prepared private formulary or the *American Hospital Formulary Service* will provide the hospital with adequate information concerning drugs. Each has its own merits.

Some of the advantages of the private formulary are that it is prepared locally by the hospital's own clinical staff and thereby engenders in them a sense of pride and loyalty as well as a determination to make the system succeed; its contents with respect to the amount of information provided under each monograph is subject to local needs and desires; it may include sections on related clinical matters which are characteristic to the local hospital; it may be published in a more convenient size and format; drugs may be added or deleted with greater frequency; and finally certain drugs may be added to the formulary before they have attained sufficient stature to be considered on a national level.

Some of the advantages of the *American Hospital Formulary Service* are that it is a continuing drug monograph subscription service published by a national professional society of means; it has the official approval of the American Pharmaceutical Association, the Catholic Hospital Association, and the American Hospital Association; it is prepared by a reference panel of the nation's outstanding clinicians, pharmacologists and pharmacists; each monograph contains a complete rundown on drugs including physical and chemical properties, pharmacologic responses, uses, toxicology, contraindications, posology and preparations; and the drugs are classified and coded according to pharmacologic action and therapeutic indications by a system of numbers which can be adapted to the filing of all informative drug literature in the pharmacy library.

SELECTION OF GUIDING PRINCIPLES FOR ADMISSION OR DELETION OF DRUGS

Of all the tasks which face the Pharmacy and Therapeutics Committee, the selection of criteria by which to gauge the worthiness of a drug for admission to the formulary is the most difficult and troublesome. This is due to the fact that no single member of the Committee is qualified to evaluate the therapeutic efficacy of every drug in every area of clinical specialization. Accordingly, from the outset, the Committee should feel free to invite staff specialists to attend specific committee meetings for the purpose of evaluating preparations commonly used in his specialized practice for inclusion into the formulary.

Thus one of the first criteria to be established is whether or not the local general and specialty staff consider the drug to be of proven clinical value based upon their experience with it.

A second may be that the drug must be recognized by the *United States Pharmacopeia,* the *National Formulary,* or their supplements.

A third may be that the manufacturer of the drug must be one of proven integrity and dependability as well as having the reputation of initiating and supporting research activities of merit.

A fourth criterion may be that no preparation of secret composition will be considered or admitted to the formulary.

A fifth criterion may deal with products of multiple composition. Some hospitals have adopted the policy that no preparation of multiple composition may be admitted if the same therapeutic effect can be achieved through the use of a single drug entity.

On the same subject, the **Drug Efficacy Study** considered questions of efficacy peculiar to combination drug products and in its 1969 Final Report to the FDA, the National Academy of Sciences stated:[7]

It is a basic principle of medical practice that more than one drug should be administered for the treatment of a given condition only if the physician is persuaded that there is substantial reason to believe that each drug will make a positive contribution to the effect he seeks. Risks of adverse drug reactions should not be multiplied unless there be overriding benefit. Moreover, each drug should be given at the dose level that may be expected to make its optimal contribution to the total effect, taking into account the status of the individual patient and any synergistic or antagonistic effects that one drug may be known to have on the safety or efficacy of the other.

One these grounds, multiple therapy using fixed dose ratios determined by the manufacturer and not by the physician is, in general, poor practice."

This general opinion of combination drugs is shared by other expert bodies. The Council on Drugs of the American Medical Association in a letter accompanying the first edition of AMA Drug Evaluation says:[7]

"The effects of drugs are intrinsically so complex that it is generally advisable to administer multiple agents separately in order that the dosage and frequency of administration of the individual drugs may be varied in accordance with a patient's requirements. Therefore, most fixed-ratio combinations listed are not recommended. This reflects a long-standing policy of the Council."

The FDA is not opposed to combination drug products; it recognizes that many are safe and effective and provide important advantages to patient and physician.

For a combination to be approved under the law there must be substantial evidence that each active component contributes to the claimed effect of the product, a requirement since 1962. If this requirement is satisfied, two or more drugs may be combined in a single dosage form when, in good medical practice, they would be given concurrently and when putting them together in the same product in no way detracts from their safety and efficacy. Such a combination product should provide appropriate dosage for a significant patient population that can be defined in the labeling. A special case of this general rule is the addition of an ingredient that enhances the safety or effectiveness of the principal active component or minimizes its abuse potential.[7]

Obviously, the above criteria are merely presented as sample guides and should be either elaborated upon or restricted in their scope depending upon the requirements of the local committee and hospital.

Once the Pharmacy and Therapeutics Committee agrees upon a set of principles to guide them in their decisions relative to admissions or deletions from the hospital formulary, it is recommended that these principles be published and included in the finished formulary. In addition, it may be desirable to circulate these amongst the medical staff in order that they may have prior knowledge of them and therefore acquire an understanding of why a particular preparation may not have been included in the final publication.

CONTENTS

The decision as to the contents of the private formulary rests with those responsible for its publication. There are no published requirements for such which are established by an accrediting agency or professional association.

It would, therefore, appear that the Pharmacy and Therapeutics Committee should be guided and influenced by the role which they foresee or expect the formulary to take. If the formulary is to function merely as a control of what drugs may be used in the hospital by the staff, then all that is required is a listing of the drugs with whatever ancillary informaiton the Pharmacy and Therapeutics Committee deems desirable.

On the other hand, if it is the intent that the formulary in addition to its control value is to function as a useful helpful informative tool in the clinician's daily practice, then its contents should be expanded to meet this goal.[8]

Experience has demonstrated the fact that a section on prescription writing is a valuable asset to the young physician joining the intern staff, for throughout his medical school education this facet of his training is relatively skimpy. The section should be brief yet should cover the important parts of the prescription, the use of the metric system, a list of acceptable abbreviations, and the essentials of a narcotic prescription. The following is a briefly written section on prescription writing which may serve as a guide to those contemplating such a chapter in a hospital formulary.

PRESCRIPTION WRITING

All prescriptions must be written clearly and correctly. Every prescription must bear the following information:
Name and address of the patient.
The date.
The medication prescribed.
(This should be written for in the terminology listed in the formulary.)
The strength of the medication prescribed.
(This must be given in the metric system, *e.g.* milligrams [mg.], grams [gm.], milliliters [ml.] or micrograms [μg. or mcg.].)
The total amount to be dispensed should be clearly indicated.
The signa, containing the instructions to the patient, should be in clear, concise and simple terminology. The physician hould avoid mixing Latin and English abbreviations. The term, "As directed," should seldom, if ever, be used.
When refills are desired, the number wanted should be indicated. If this is not done, the prescription will not be refilled.
Prescriptions calling for a controlled substance must have, in addition to all of the above information, the DEA number of the prescribing physician.
It is essential that all prescriptions be signed by the physician issuing them.
Schedule II drugs are limited to a 30-day supply and no refill. These prescriptions are valid for 5 days and are not valid if there are crossouts, erasures, or any evidence of tampering.
Schedule III, IV, and V drugs are limited to a 30-day supply and may be refilled up to 5 times within 6 months of issuance date.

Other important data such as normal laboratory values; tables of heights and weights; tables for the calculation of percentages, milliequivalents and dosages; formulas of the various diagnostic stains and reagents in common use in the hospital as well as a myriad of other factual informaiton may be considered for inclusion. Obviously, all of this material cannot be included without making the publication unwieldy and expensive. Therefore the judicious evaluation of each entry by the Pharmacy and Therapeutics Committee is vital.

FORMAT

The format is extremely important since it will determine the practicality of daily use of the formulary as well as the publishing costs.
Prior to commencing work on the development of the hospital formulary format, it is suggested that the hospital pharmacist gather for-

mularies from various hospitals. The hospital pharmacist may also obtain a representative sample of formularies from many different types of hospitals merely by requesting same from the American Society of Hospital Pharmacists. Needless to say, once the local hospital formulary is published, two copies should be forwarded to the Society in order that their collection continue to expand and therefore be of assistance to other pharmacists seeking ideas.

SIZE

Experience has shown that a formulary which is sufficiently small in size to permit its being carried in a uniform or laboratory coat pocket will, in all probability, enjoy widespread use in the hospital. A small-sized book also can be carried in the doctor's bag along with his prescription blanks. Many physicians who have become accustomed to using the formulary in their hospital practice often use the hospital formulary in their private office practice.

No specific size can be recommended at the present time, and therefore this determination must be arrived at after careful study of the local need as well as the formularies gathered from the Society and local hospitals.

LOOSE-LEAF VS. BOUND

Whether or not the hospital formulary should be loose-leaf or bound will depend upon a number of factors. The most important of these is the ease by which a loose-leaf formulary can be kept current. A bound volume is difficult to keep up-to-date and therefore requires more frequent revision. In comparison, a loose-leaf formulary can be revised at will simply by printing, distributing and inserting the necessary page or pages.

The type of loose-leaf binder is immaterial and is left to the decision of the Pharmacy and Therapeutics Committee. The local stationer, if consulted, will be able to provide sample binders in all price ranges.

Those desiring a permanently bound volume also have many selections to choose from ranging from paper to cardboard to plastic to leather or its substitutes. The controlling factor here will, in all probability, be the cost involved.

PUBLICATION

A printed hospital formulary is obviously more esthetic in appearance, easier to read, and imparts to the user the impression that the hospital considers the formulary as an extremely important document and therefore worthy of the cost of printing. This does not mean that a mimeographed formulary will not be used or is not good. A study of a number of formularies will show that some of the better units are mimeographed. However, where it is possible, it is recommended that printing be the selection of choice.

Some formularies appear to have been developed by individuals with a flair for public relations or advertising. Drawings, colored ink, and colored paper should be avoided. The formulary is a professional publication and should reflect the high ethical standards of the hospital and its staff. Therefore, a white or slightly off-white paper should be used. Black ink is always in good taste.

Many authors have been concerned about the use of electronic data processing equipment in preparing and publishing the hospital formulary.[9-11] Reasons generally given for the utilization of the computer for this task are *(a)* to take advantage of the computer process to lower the cost of producing the formulary and *(b)* to adopt the formulary information for future applications resulting from computerized hospital information systems.[8]

Generally, the program has two phases. Phase-I produces the drug information file which is maintained on magnetic tape. Punched cards prepared from the source documents are used as the input to the drug information file. Phase-II produces the printed formulary using the magnetic tape drug information file.

A coding technique must be either developed or adopted for the purpose, as well as data concerning choice of paper, printing technique and photoreduction if necessary.

The American Society of Hospital Pharmacists has developed a computer-processable *Drug Products Information File* which is available to hospitals and nursing homes and from which a hospital formulary can be prepared. Because of the comprehensive nature of the Drug Products Information File (DPIF) it also may be used in drug-drug interaction and drug-laboratory interaction programs.

FORMULARY DRUG LISTING SERVICE

"FDLS" refers to the Formulary Drug Listing Service of the American Society of Hospital Pharmacists (ASHP). The service provides reproducible copy of a hospital's drugs in two parts: A Drug Listing Section and a Pharmacologic-Therapeutic Index. The hospital uses the printout to reproduce as many copies of its formulary drug list as are required for distribution to the hospital's professional staff, nursing units, outpatient clinics and libraries.

The Drug Listing Section contains each of the drug products selected by the subscriber, including the nonproprietary name of the drug; selected trade names, synonyms and/or abbreviations; the therapeutic category of the drug; and the specific dosage forms and strengths of the drug selected by the hospital. Package sizes are included for injectable preparations. The ingredients of combination products are listed in tabular form. The section is alphabetically arranged by non-proprietary drug names. Trade names and synonyms are cross-referenced in alphabetical sequence. The Pharmacologic-Therapeutic Index consists of the non-proprietary drug names categorized according to the classification system of the American Hospital Formulary Service (AHFS). Only those drugs and categories included in the Drug Listing Section are included in the index.

All hospitals should have a list of drugs which the medical staff considers acceptable for use in the hospital (i.e., a formulary). Both the Conditions of Participation for "Medicare," and the Standards for Pharmaceutical Services of the Joint Commission on Accreditation of Hospitals (JCAH) stipulate the existence or development of a formulary or drug list.

Since the development of a formulary drug list requires a substantial investment in professional personnel time and because of limited budgets or staff shortages, many hospitals have not prepared a formulary drug list or have not revised an out-of-date edition. The amount of professional personnel time required, annually, to revise a formulary drug list can easily exceed 300 hours!

Under these circumstance, it behooves the hospital administration to approve a subscription to the ASHP's Formulary Drug Listing Service. By so doing, a substantial reduction in cost of personnel time can be realized by the hospital thereby permitting this valuable professional time to be allocated to other hospital programs.

FORMULARY DRUG LISTING SERVICE PREPARATIONS

The ASHP sends to the hospital a checklist containing about 3,000 "core" drugs—those found to be the most frequently approved by Pharmacy and Therapeutics Committees for use within the nation's hospitals. The description of these core drugs on the checklist includes nonproprietary name, trade name, route of administration, dosage form and strength. The format of the checklist includes an access number for ASHP use and a "check" column for use by the subscribing hospital. The checklist is arranged alphabetically by nonproprietary name.

The hospital pharmacist reviews and marks the checklist. Checks on the appropriate lines assure that the products so identified will be included in the drug list for that individual hospital.

The subscribing hospital writes in those additional drug products to be listed in its formulary drug list which do not appear on the checklist.

The checklist, with individual additions, is returned to the ASHP where the input codes for the products designated by the hospital are punched into machine readable form. The input data for a number of uniquely identified hospitals are run against the ASHP's computerized Drug Products Information File and individualized formulary drug lists are output.

Each subscribing hospital receives a listing of only those drugs it has selected. The hospital receives a single computer printout of its formulary drug list.

The hospital then reproduces the desired number of copies required for distribution within the institution.

The reproduction masters (printout) provided by FDLS can be reproduced in any desirable page size. The masters can be reproduced at exact size (*e.g.,* xerography) on standard 8½" × 11" pages. If necessary the masters can be photo-reduced for the printing of pocket-sized lists.

CATEGORIZING AND INDEXING

The ease by which a physician may locate an item in the formulary will have an impact upon its usability. Too often, the formulary contains all of the desired information, but due to poor indexing data are not readily found. Therefore, since the index is the key to a good formulary, it behooves the pharmacist to expend effort on it.

Most formularies have a general index located at the end of the text. This index is usually alphabetical by generic name and is cross-indexed with brand names of drugs used in the text portion of the formulary. Although the general index is an essential and integral part of any text and cannot be eliminated, it presumes that the user knows what he is looking for. In a formulary, this presumption is not always valid. Here the physician knows that he has need for an anticholinergic drug and he obviously has knowledge of the generic or brand names of a number of drugs which bear this pharmacologic classification. This now means that he must search the index to find a familiar anticholinergic drug. Because this is a burdensome and time-consuming procedure, it is strongly suggested that the general index be implemented with a pharmacologic index which will alleviate similar occurrences.

SAMPLE PHARMACOLOGIC INDEX

The following pharmacologic classification represents main headings only and the pharmacist in conjunction with the Pharmacy and Therapeutics Committee should classify the drugs which are to be listed in the hospital formulary under each heading. This complete index should then be placed in the front or rear of the formulary.

Amebicides
Analgesics
  1. Narcotic
  2. Non-narcotic
Anesthetics
  1. General
  2. Local
Anthelmintics
Antiallergenics
Antibacterials
  1. Antibiotic
  2. Chemotherapeutic
Antiepileptics
Antihistaminics
Antihypertensives
Antimalarials
Antiparkinsonism Agents
Antisyphilitics
Antituberculous Agents
Cardiovascular Agents
  1. Cardiac Drugs
    a. Accelerators
    b. Depressants
    c. Glycosides
  2. Vascular Drugs
    a. Constrictors
    b. Dilators
    c. Sclerosing Agents
Central Nervous System Drugs
  1. Depressants
    a. Analgesics
    b. Anesthetics
    c. Antispasmodics
    d. Hypnotics
    e. Sedatives
  2. Stimulants
  3. Tranquilizers
Dermatological Agents
  1. Anhydrotics
  2. Antipruritics
  3. Antiseborrheics
  4. Antiseptics
  5. Astringents
  6. Bactericides
  7. Caustics
  8. Cleansers
  9. Emollients
  10. Fungicides
  11. Keratolytics
  12. Parasiticides
    a. Lice
    b. Scabies
  13. Protectives
Deterrent Therapy
Diuretics
  1. Mercurial

  2. Thiazide Derivatives
  3. Other
Gastrointestinal Agents
  1. Anorexogenics
  2. Antacids
  3. Antidiarrheals
  4. Antinauseants
  5. Antispasmodics
  6. Cathartics
  7. Choleretics
  8. Digestives
  9. Emetics
  10. Emulsifiers
  11. Spasmogenics
Genitourinary Agents
  1. Antibacterials
    a. Antibiotic
    b. Chemotherapeutic
  2. Antiseptics
  3. Antispasmodics
  4. Diuretics
  5. Oxytocics
  6. Spasmogenics
Hematics
  1. Antianemics
  2. Anticoagulants
  3. Coagulants
  4. Expanders
  5. Hemostatics
  6. Neoplastics
Hormones and Synthetic Substitutes
  1. Adrenal hormones
  2. Ovarian hormones
  3. Pancreas hormones
  4. Parathyroid hormones
  5. Pituitary hormones
  6. Placental hormones
  7. Testicular hormones
  8. Thyroid hormones
    a. Depressants
    b. Stimulants
Muscular Relaxants
Nutritional Aids
  1. Albumin preparations
  2. Amino acid preparations
  3. Carbohydrate preparations
  4. Choline preparations
  5. Fat preparations
  6. Gustatory aids
  7. Mineral preparations
  8. Nutritives
  9. Protein hydrolysates
Parasiticides—Internal
  1. Amebicides
  2. Malaria Therapy
  3. Spirochete

4. Trichomoniasis
5. Worms
Respiratory Agents
  1. Antihistaminics
  2. Bronchial dilators
  3. Cough preparations
    a. Depressants
    b. Expectorants
  4. Respiratory stimulants

Sedatives and Hypnotics
  1. Barbiturates
    a. Short duration
    b. Moderate duration
    c. Long duration
  2. Non-barbiturates
Serums and Vaccines
Vitamin and Vitamin Mixtures

In addition to the general and pharmacologic index, the formulary may be divided into specific sections with each section segregated by a divider. A suggested subdivision of the formulary is as follows:

Ear

Eye

Nose

Rectal

Throat

Vaginal

Skin

Nutritional Aids

Oral and Injectable

By such a subdivision, the clinician can easily refer to the agents specifically used for either the anatomic entity or to the broad category of drugs used orally or by injection.

TEXT

Finally, the selection of the scope of the text material under each generic named drug should be given serious consideration. The amount of material published will depend upon the goals established by the Pharmacy and Therapeutics Committee. The membership of the committee is hereby cautioned that insufficient information does not enhance the use and acceptance of the formulary by the staff. On the other hand, the busy practitioner will also shy away from the formulary if it develops into a miniature text on pharmacology. The ideal situation obviously lies somewhere in between these extremes. As an aid to the hospital pharmacist, three examples are presented.

Figure 15 represents a sample page from the American Hospital Formulary Service. The important point to notice here is the detailed nature of the text material.

Figure 16 represents a sample page from the Formulary of the Peter

SEDATIVES AND HYPNOTICS *28:24*

Aprobarbital **Alurate®**

Aprobarbital, 5-allyl-5-isopropylbarbituric acid, is classified as a short-acting barbiturate. It occurs as a bitter, white, crystalline powder and is very slightly soluble in water and soluble in alcohol.

Aprobarbital is useful as a hypnotic and for the treatment of conditions in which mild sedation is desirable, as in hypertension, preoperative apprehension, functional gastrointestinal disorders, anxiety neuroses, and coronary artery disease.

For the mode of action, cautions, and contraindications in therapy with aprobarbital, and for the treatment of acute or chronic toxic reactions, see the general statement on The Barbiturates 28:24.

Dosage

Aprobarbital is administered orally. The recommended sedative dosage for adults is 20 to 40 mg three times daily. The adult hypnotic dose is usually 80 to 160 mg. Dosage for children has not been established but, as for adults, the smallest effective dose should be used.

Preparations

APROBARBITAL
  Elixir, 40 mg per 5 ml
  Tablets, 20 mg and 40 mg

Only those Preparations underlined or checked above are included in the Formulary of this hospital
© Copyright, December 1963, American Society of Hospital Pharmacists

Fig. 15. Sample page from the American Hospital Formulary Service.

NICOTINIC ACID
(Niacin)

FORMS AVAILABLE:
Tablet: 50 mg
                      100 mg
Injection: 100 mg/10 ml
USUAL DOSE: 25 to 50 mg
DAILY DOSE: 50 to 100 mg
ROUTE: Orally.
                      Intravenously.
                      Intramuscularly.
CAUTION: High doses produce a flushing of the skin.
PRESCRIBE: 25 Tablets (1) either strength.
                      1 Ampul (1).
USE: Vasodilator, correct nicotinic acid deficiency.

NITROFURANTOIN
(Furadantin)

FORM AVAILABLE:
Tablet: 100 mg
USUAL DOSE: 5 to 10 mg per kg of body weight per 24 hours;
                      given in 4 doses with meals and at bedtime.
PRESCRIBE: 25 Tablets (6).
USE: Urinary antibacterial.

Fig. 16.   Sample page from the Formulary of the Peter Bent Brigham Hospital,
Boston, Massachusetts.

Bent Brigham Hospital. Note here the fact that although brief in nature, the practitioner is provided with all of the necessary information.

Figure 17 represents a sample page from the Formulary of the Massachusetts General Hospital. Note here the interesting presentation of each drug in the form of an individual prescription.

Figure 18 represents a sample page from the Formulary of the Newton-Wellesley Hospital. This presentation is of interest due to the fact

AUTONOMIC DRUGS

SYMPATHOMIMETIC DRUGS

(Adrenergic)

Ephedrine Sulfate Injection
  1 ml. contains 50 mg
Disp.:   1 ml
Route: Subcutaneous, intramuscular
Dose: 25 to 50 mg every 4 hours

Epinephrine Injection
  1 ml contains 1 mg
Disp.:   1 ml
Route: Subcutaneous
Dose: 0.2 to 1 mg every 4 hours

Epinephrine in Oil Injection, Suspension
  1 ml contains 2 mg
Disp: 1 ml
Route: Intramuscular, only
Dose: 2 mg every 8 or 12 hours

Levarterenol Bitrate Injection
  4 ml contains 4 mg Levarterenol
Disp: 4 ml
Route: Intravenous only, by infusion
Dose: 4 mg is added to 1000 ml 5% Dextrose solution. Each 1 ml of this dilution contains 4 mcg Levarterenol.

Metaraminol Bitartrate Injection
  1 ml contains 10 mg
Disp: 10 ml
Route: Intramuscular, intravenous, not subcutaneous
Dose: Intramuscular 2 to 10 mg. Intravenous 15 to 100 mg added to 200 ml isotonic sodium chloride solution or 5% dextrose in water. Administered by drip.

Phenylephrine Hydrochloride Injection
  1 ml contains 10 mg
Disp.:   1 ml
Route: Subcutaneous
Dose: 1 to 10 mg every 8 hours.

Fig. 17. Sample page from the Formulary of the Massachusetts General Hospital, Boston, Massachusetts.

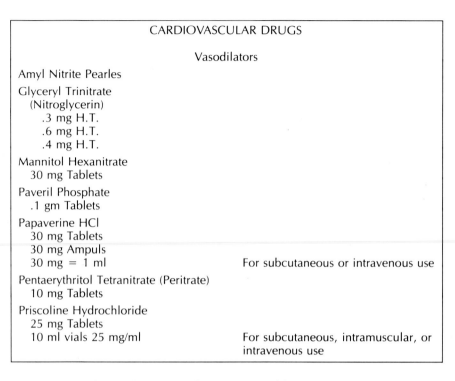

Fig. 18.   Sample page from a Formulary (Drug List) of the Newton-Wellesley Hospital, Newton, Massachusetts.

that it combines the brevity of a drug list with a pharmacological classification and the routes of administration for injectable preparations.

Figure 19 represents a sample page from the Commonwealth of Massachusetts formulary entitled *The Massachusetts Drug Formulary.* This formulary was prepared by a state drug formulary commission consisting of physicians, nurses and pharmacists and must be used for the prescribing of medications for patients on state welfare plans.

SPECIALTY FORMULARIES

With the increasing use of enteral nutrition products in hospitals and hospital-based home care programs, one university hospital has developed a formulary for use of the medical and dietetic staffs.[13]

The formulary reports product variables such as osmolality, caloric density, protein content and source, fat content and source, freedom

---

THE MASSACHUSETTS DRUG FORMULARY

Brand Name
Generic Name

Acidulin OTC	Glutamic Acid Hydrochloride
Acon OTC	Vitamin A Water Soluble USP
Acthar	
Acthar Gel	Corticotropin Gel USP
Adrenalin OTC	Epinephrine Hydrochloride USP
Adrenalin Injection	Epinephrine Hydrochloride USP
Adrenotrate	Epinephrine Bitartrate USP
Albolene OTC	Mineral Oil, Light NF
Alcon-Efrin OTC	Phenylephrine Hydrochloride USP
Almocarpine	Pilocarpine Hydrochloride USP
Alphalin OTC	Vitamin A USP
Alurate	Aprobarbital NF
Ambodryl	Bromodiphenhydramine Hydrochloride NF
Amnestrogen	Esterified Estrogens USP
Amphicol	Chloramphenicol USP

Fig. 19. Sample page from the Massachsetts Drug Formulary of 1972.

from lactose, and, for oral supplements, flavors. The products are categorized as follows: liquid supplemental feedings, isotonic supplemental feedings, isotonic tube feedings, high caloric/high nitrogen tube feedings, high nitrogen tube feedings and blenderized tube feedings.

SELECTED READINGS

Rucker, T.D. and Visconti, J.A.: How Effective Are Drug Formularies? A Descriptive and Normative Study, ASHP Research and Education Foundation, Inc., Washington, D.C. 20014, 1978.
Chase, Kathy, Meyer, John D., and Kelly, William N.: Total Formulary Review-the Easy Way. Hosp. Pharm., *19*:159–162, 1984.
Rucker, T.D.: Superior Formularies: A Critical Analysis. Hosp. Pharm., *17*:465, 1982.

REFERENCES

1. Hoffman, Richard P.: Perspectives on the Hospital Formulary. Hosp. Pharm., *19*:5:359–364, 1984.
2. ASHP Statement on the Formulary System. Am. J. Hosp. Pharm., *40*:1384–1385 (Aug.) 1983.
3. Formulary of the Brigham & Women's Hospital. Boston, Mass. 02115.
4. ASHP Technical Assistance Bulletin on Hospital Formularies. Am. J. Hosp. Pharm., *42*:375–377, 1985.
5. The Voice of the Pharmacist, *21*:10:3, (Oct.) 1979.
6. Willcox, Alanson W.: The Legal Basis of the Hospital Formulary System. Hospitals, J.A.H.A., *34*:55, (Oct.) 16, 1960.
7. Fixed Combination Prescription Drugs, FDA Bulletin, June 1971, U.S. Dept. HEW, Food and Drug Administration, 5600 Fishers Lane, Rockville, Md. 20852.
8. Pellegrino, E.D.: A Physician Appraises the Formulary System. Hospital, J.A.H.A., *39*:1:77, 1965.
9. Lamy, P.P., Bourn, I.F., and Flack, H.L.: Applications of Data Processing Equipment to the Hospital Formulary. Am. J. Hosp. Pharm., *18*:11:642, (Nov.) 1961.
10. Flack, H.L., Downs, G.E., and Lanning, L.E.: Electronic Data Processing and the Hospital Formulary. Am. J. Hosp. Pharm., *24*:1:15, (Jan.) 1967.
11. Frankenfeld, F.M., Black, H.J., and Dick, R.W.: Automated Formulary Printing from a Computerized Drug Information File. Am. J. Hosp. Pharm., *28*:3:154, (Mar.) 1971.
12. Fink, Joseph L. III: Antisubstitution Law Changes and the Hospital Formulary System. Am. J. Hosp. Pharm., *34*:1:90, (Jan.) 1977.
13. Hopefl, A.W. and Herman, V.M: Developing a Formulary for Enteral Nutrition Products, Am. J. Hosp. Pharm., *39*:1514–1517, (Sept.) 1982.

6

Pharmacy Communications

It is a well-documented fact that the majority of the hospitals in this country lack a good method of communicating with the staff and patients. The methods employed to disseminate interdepartment information are usually well prototyped, namely, bulletins, memoranda, bulletin board notices and committee meetings. In most instances, this form of communication is adequate even though it is limited in its scope.

The department of pharmacy, because its method of operation brings it into close contact with the major hospital services, departments and the entire medical staff, is in a position to alleviate that portion of the problem that relates to the dissemination of data concerning drugs and related supplies.

As has been stated earlier, one of the duties of the Pharmacy and Therapeutics Committee is to assist the pharmacist in conducting a teaching program within the hospital via a pharmacy publication. The membership of this committee can be extremely helpful by preparing brief lead articles concerning the latest therapeutic advances in their specialty and by reviewing the materials by the pharmacist for publication.

With today's emphasis on clinical pharmacy, the publication may be edited by the clinical pharmacist members of the department and therefore the direction of the effort will be in the area of therapeutics, pharmacokinetics, toxicology and drug interactions. Also of importance is the fact that the nursing service constitutes a large segment of the readership and therefore the editor should invite contributions from the nursing group as well as to include articles of interest to them.

The individual assigned the reponsibility for pharmacy communications must be alert to the fact that other groups in the hospital have an interest in drugs and drug therapy. A good example would be the interest of the therapeutic dietician in food-drug interactions.

Another interested party with whom the clinical pharmacist comes into daily contact is the patient. Since no two patients are alike, it is the pharmacist's duty to devise different methodologies for disseminating drug information.[1] After developing these, it is of great importance to ascertain the patient's evaluation of the method and its content.[2]

The preparation of a worthwhile pharmacy publication requires a great deal of time and forethought. The purpose of this chapter is to provide some ideas relative to possible contents, format, duplication, and distribution of such an educational and informative medium.

SELECTION OF A TITLE

The title selected for the publication should be specific, short and of such a nature that it identifies the publication as well as its contents.

Too often, a title is selected which imparts the impression that the publication is a collegiate gossip paper rather than a professional journal.

Examples of good titles are: Pharmacy Bulletin, Pharmacy News, Therapeutic Notes, Pharmacy Review, and Pharmacy Newsletter.

Examples of titles which are not acceptable are: The Mortar and Pestle, The Pill Roller News, Drug Store News, News Capsules, etc.

CONTENTS

Since the purpose of this publication is to educate as well as to inform, it is imperative that its contents be of such a nature.

In general, the publication should be divided into five categories. They are as follows:
A. Editorial.
B. New Drug Section.
C. Abstract of the Pharmacy and Therapeutics Committee Meeting.
D. Lead articles by prominent members of the medical staff.
E. General.

The *editorial,* prepared by the Pharmacist-in-Chief or other interested member of the Pharmacy and Therapeutics Committee, should be a means whereby new procedures relative to ordering, prescribing, storage or administration of drugs within the hospital are introduced and publicized. It may also be used to focus attention on infractions of established procedures and to editorialize therapeutic trends and opinions.

The *new drug section* should contain the major data on each drug accepted for use within the hospital by the Pharmacy Committee. Major information in this instance includes a brief description of the drug, its range of usefulness indications, side effects, administration and dosage and how supplied by the pharmacy. The format employed in the presentation of this information may be in a number of forms.

The *abstract of the minutes* of the Pharmacy and Therapeutics Committee meeting is a worthy inclusion in the publication in that it keeps the entire staff aware of the constantly changing trend of therapeutics within the institution. In addition, it allows those members of the staff who have had reason to communicate with the Pharmacy and Therapeutics Committee to note that their recommendations have received attention.

Each issue should have a *lead article* by a prominent member of the staff. The article should not be lengthy and should be restricted to an evaluation of current pharmaceuticals or trends of therapy within the author's field of specialization or to topics of current interest to the staff.

The section categorized as "General" may include anything the editor feels is of interest to the medical staff, nursing service or laboratory staff. Samples of the type of information that might well be placed in this category are abstracts of releases from the state department of public health, abstracts of articles of interest on current situations such as the recurrence of an outbreak of Asian influenza and abstracts from the various journals relative to unusual sources of poisoning in humans, drug research news or drug warnings.

This section can be particularly helpful to the medical and nursing staffs, when, due to a change of suppliers, medications arrive on the floor in new colors, shapes, sizes and packages. By planning ahead, nurses can be alerted to the proposed changes and can be assured that although medication appearances and brands may change as new suppliers are integrated into the system, drug content and quality remain constant.

FORMAT AND DUPLICATION

The format of the publication will vary with the originality of the pharmacist; therefore, the following description is provided as a basis for further development by the individual concerned.

The paper should be a good quality paper measuring 8½″ × 11″. In view of the fact that the first page should be inviting to the potential reader, it is recommended that the heading be preprinted. By so doing, you will have the advantage of being able to use stock cuts of pharmaceutical symbols which the printer can obtain for you in order to decorate the publication. In addition, you will be able to have the heading of each issue printed in a different colored ink on the white or colored paper stock. Neither of the above suggestions would cost much, but would serve to draw the attention to the potential reader (Fig. 20).

Some authors have suggested that the page be longitudinally split in half and the data typed in columns. The advantage of this being that many of the readers like to clip out the data on a new drug and affix

PHARMACY

R̠   # BULLETIN   R̠

PETER BENT BRIGHAM HOSPITAL   BOSTON, MASS.

Fig. 20

it to a page in their Formulary or, in the case of the nursing service, 3″ × 5″ cards in their new drug file.

DISTRIBUTION

The completed issue should be distributed to the following areas and individuals, provided they exist in the particular hospital:

A. Every member of the medical staff and to the staff library.
B. Administration.
C. Nursing Service.
    1. A copy to each station
    2. Several copies to Nursing School Office
    3. Nursing School Faculty
    4. Nurses' Library
D. Laboratories.

ADVANTAGES

The preparation of a pharmacy publication requires the time, effort and imagination of the pharmacist who undertakes such a project. On the other hand, a well-prepared issue can save the pharmacy a great deal of time by reducing the number of telephone calls concerning new drugs or newly instituted procedures.

In addition, it will add to the professional stature of the pharmacist within the institution and give him the satisfaction of having made a contribution towards better self communication between his department and the professional staff.

The ASHP, in recognition of the pharmacist's role in teaching patients about their drug therapy, has caused to be prepared and distributed a series of guidelines[3] to assist hospital pharmacists in this endeavor.

ASHP GUIDELINES ON PHARMACIST-CONDUCTED PATIENT COUNSELING[a]

It is well-documented that safe and effective drug therapy most frequently occurs when patients are well-informed about medications and their use. Knowledgeable patients exhibit increased compliance with drug regimens, resulting in improved therapeutic outcomes. Therefore pharmacists, as well as other health professionals, have a responsibility to properly inform patients about their drug therapy.

Pharmacists' drug consultations with patients should be aimed at improving therapeutic outcomes by maximizing proper use of medications. Pharmacists, in conjunction with other health team members whenever possible, must make appropriate value judgments to determine the specific information and counseling required in each patient care situation.

Using suitable verbal, written or audio-visual communication techniques and methods, the pharmacist should inform, educate and counsel patients (or their representative or guardian) about the following items for each medication in the patient's drug regimen:

1. Name [trademark, generic, common synonym or other descriptive name(s)];
2. Intended use and expected action;
3. Route, dosage form, dosage and administration schedule;
4. Special directions for preparation;
5. Special directions for administration;
6. Precautions to be observed during administration;
7. Common side effects that may be encountered, including their avoidance and action required if they occur;
8. Techniques for self-monitoring of drug therapy;
9. Proper storage;
10. Potential drug-drug or drug-food interactions or other therapeutic contraindications;
11. Prescription refill information;
12. Action to be taken in the event of a missed dose; and
13. Any other information peculiar to the specific patient or drug.

These thirteen points are applicable to nonprescription drugs as well as those ordered by a physician or other prescriber. In addition, pharmacists must counsel patients in the proper selection of nonprescription drugs as well as when and if they should be used.

---

[a]Approved by the ASHP Board of Directors at its meeting of November 17–18, 1975, and by the ASHP House of Delegates on April 7, 1976.

AUDIOVISUAL COMMUNICATIONS

Pharmacy communications should not be limited to printed materials. Today, most major teachng hospitals have on their staff individuals who are well versed in the science and art of audio and audiovisual educational materials. Slides, film strips and sound movies are an excellent means to communicate new techniques in drug administration, treatments and to highlight special reactions attributable to drug therapy. These educational materials can then be distributed by the pharmacy to the house staff, school of nursing, college of pharmacy and to small pharmacies in neighboring hospitals. These hospitals that do not have this in-house capability might give consideration to contracting for such service with an outside firm specializing in this type of work.

With the advent of the concept of the prescription package insert (PPI) hospitals might very well consider the preparation of a set of audio-visual materials on these drugs. By so doing patients will be able to study the material on the scene and thereby ask any questions that they may have prior to leaving.

SELECTED READING

Baker, David: A Study Contrasting Different Modalities of Medication Discharge Counseling. Hosp. Pharm., *19*:8:545, (Aug.) 1984.

REFERENCES

1. deHaen, P.: Drug Information for the Patient—Different Approach. Drug Inf. J., *11*:141–145, (July–Sept.) 1977.
2. Stefani, E.: Consumer's Evaluation of Available Drug Information. Drug Inf. J., *11*:158–163, (July–Sept.) 1977.
3. ASHP Guidelines on Pharmacist-Conducted Patient Counseling. Am. J. Hosp. Pharm., *33*:644–645, (July) 1976.

7

Investigational Use Drugs

By definition, research or investigational use drugs are those compounds or mixtures which have not been released by the Federal Food and Drug Administration for general distribution and use. These drugs usually bear the following statement on their labels:

Caution: New Drug—Limited by Federal Law to Investigational Use

They are released only to physicians who sign the proper Federal Food and Drug Release form for the manufacturer.

With the increased use of the clinical facilities of teaching hospitals for the therapeutic evaluation of investigational use drugs, it has become necessary to define the responsibility for the use of these products and to centralize pertinent information concerning them.

A lack of control and information relative to investigational use drugs in a hospital obviously can lead to chaos. This can induce drug administration "accidents" as well as deter suit-conscious, yet competent, clinical investigators from carrying out this important phase of medicine within the hospital.

Prior to 1950, the literature describing methods of controlling this class of preparations was sparse. As the tempo for the clinical evaluation of new drugs increased, so too did the literature describing methods employed by various hospitals to control the drugs and disseminate information concerning them to the proper personnel.

THE U.S. PUBLIC HEALTH SERVICE POLICY

The U.S. Public Health Service now requires assurance that the rights, privacy and welfare of human beings involved as subjects in research or training activities are protected, and that their informed consent has been obtained before subjecting them to any research procedure, and that any protocol involving human subjects has received *a priori* review and approval by a committee of the staff of the hospital.[1]

Thus each hospital has found it necessary to establish a Committee on Human Use in Research.

The Committee on Human Use in Research, a standing committee of the hospital, is charged with the responsibility of considering the problems associated with the use of human subjects for clinical research and other biomedical (including psychological) investigations, to establish guiding principles with respect to these matters, and to advise the Administrative officers with respect to policy issues that may arise. In accordance with the recommendations of this Committee, mechanisms are established to assure that every proposal for clinical research or investigation involving human subjects will receive the best possible review and guidance.

Any investigation that proposes to apply to human subjects a procedure of protocol potentially hazardous or uncomfortable (or which may invade his rights of privacy) and is not clearly for the individual's benefit, is to be reviewed prior to its initiation by the Committee on Human Use in Research at the hospital with reference to (1) the risks and potential medical benefits of the investigation, (2) the rights and welfare of the individuals involved, and (3) the appropriateness of the methods used to obtain informed consent. The committee's comments and any recommended changes in protocol or procedure should be reported to or discussed with the principal investigator and his chief of service. Appropriate written records should be maintained. A signed and dated report of the committee's recommendation on each application submitted by the hospital to outside sources of support for research or training should be forwarded to the proper administrative office and kept on file.

All research involving the use of human subjects must be approved by the appropriate chief of service, who is responsible for maintaining over-sight as the investigation proceeds. Any significant changes in protocol or emergent problems which would alter the experimental situation or adversely affect the rights or welfare of the subjects should be promptly referred to the Committee on Human Use in Research for Review and advice.

In order to ensure continuing surveillance of the research project by the Committee of Human Use in Research, each principal investigator should prepare a Continuing Surveillance Report, on a quarterly basis, and forward it to the Secretary of the Committee on Use of Humans in Research.

FDA Amendments of 1966

The Federal Food, Drug and Cosmetic Act was amended in 1966 by the addition of a new statement of policy as follows.

Consent for use of investigational new drugs on humans; statement of policy.[2]

(a) Section 505(i) of the act provides that regulations on use of investigational new drugs on human beings shall impose the condition that investigators "obtain the consent of such human beings or their representatives, except where they deem it not feasible or, in their professional judgment, contrary to the best interest of such human beings."

(b) This means that the consent of such human beings (or the consent of their representatives) to whom investigational drugs are administered primarily for the accumulation of scientific knowledge, for such purposes as studying drug behavior, body processes, or the course of a disease, must be obtained in all cases and, in all but exceptional cases, the consent of patients under treatment with investigational drugs must be obtained.

(c) "Under treatment" applies when the administration of the investigational drug for either diagnostic or therapeutic purposes constitutes responsible medical judgment, taking into account the availability of other remedies or drugs and the individual circumstances pertaining to the person to whom the investigational drug is to be administered.

(d) *"Exceptional cases,"* as used in paragraph *(b)* of this section, which exceptions are to be strictly applied, are cases where it is not feasible to obtain the patient's consent or the consent of his representative, or where, as a matter of professional judgment exercised in the best interest of a particular patient under the investigator's care, it would be contrary to that patient's welfare to obtain his consent.

(e) "Patient" means a person under treatment.

(f) *"Not feasible"* is limited to cases where the investigator is not capable of obtaining consent because of inability to communicate with the patient or his representative; for example, where the patient is in a coma or is otherwise incapable of giving informed consent, his representative cannot be reached, and it is imperative to administer the drug without delay.

(g) *"Contrary to the best interest of such human beings"* applies when the communication of information to obtain consent would seriously affect the patient's disease status and the physician has exercised a professional judgment that under the particular circumstances of this patient's case, the patient's best interest would suffer if consent were sought.

(h) *"Consent"* or *"informed consent"* means that the person involved has legal capacity to give consent, is so situated as to be able to exercise free power of choice, and is provided with a fair explanation of all material information concerning the administration of the investigational drug, or his possible use as a control, as to enable him to make an understanding decision as to his willingness to receive said investigational drug. This latter element requires that before the acceptance of an affirmative decision by such person the investigator should make known to him the nature, duration, and purpose of the administration of said investigational drug; the method and means by which it is to be administered; all inconveniences and hazards reasonably to be expected, including the fact, where applicable, that the person may be used as a control; the existence of alternative forms of therapy, if any; and the effects upon his health or person that may possibly come from the administration of the investigational drug. Said patient's consent shall be obtained in writing by the investigator. (See Figures 25 and 26, pp. 175 and 176, for sample Consent Forms.)

The Office of Grant Administration Policy

The Office of Grant Administration Policy, Department of Health and Human Services has issued its Manual, Chapter 1–40, entitled "Protection of Human Subjects." The stated purpose of the new manual is to establish uniform policies for the protection of human subjects involved in research, demonstration and other activities supported by the Department's grants and contracts.

Chapter 1–40 attributes broad definitions to the terms "subject" and "at risk" to include anyone exposed to the possibility of physical, psychologic, sociologic, or other adverse effect as a consequence of any activity which goes beyond the application of standard and accepted methods to meet individual needs. The determination of when an individual is at risk is a matter of the application of common sense and sound professional judgment to the circumstances of the activity in question.[3]

Emphasized in the policy is the responsibility of the grantee or contractor to safeguard the rights and welfare of human subjects. To provide for the proper discharge of this responsibility, the Department of Health and Human Services will not require the grantee or contractor to carry out initial and continuing committee review of all activities involving human subjects. The review must establish that the rights and welfare of the subject are adequately protected, that the risks to him are outweighed by the activity's potential benefit, and that informed consent is to be obtained by methods that are adequate and appropriate.[4]

This review is expected to take into consideration such matters as local standard of professional practice, applicable laws, practical aspects of community acceptability, and to benefit from the committee's knowledge of the personnel involved and of the conditions under which the study is to be carried out. The policy also requires a review of the grant application by a committee of the Department of Health and Human Services.[4]

The manual chapter further spells out procedures for certifying institutional review of applications, for institutional review of cooperative activities, for documentation of institutional committee actions, and for Department of Health and Human Services administration of policy. Responsibility for administration of the policy has been delegated to the Division of Research Grants, National Institute for Health because of its experience in the administration of a similar Public Health Service Policy.

Principles Involved in the Use of Investigational Drugs in Hospitals

The following *"Guidelines for the Use of Investigational Drugs in Hospitals"* was approved by the Board of Directors of the American

Hospital Association and has been published in the February 1979 issue of the *Journal of the American Society of Hospital Pharmacists* and is reprinted here for convenient reference.[5]

ASHP GUIDELINES FOR THE USE OF INVESTIGATIONAL DRUGS IN INSTITUTIONS[a]

Hospitals and related health care facilities, the primary centers for clinical studies on investigational drugs,[b] must ensure that policies and procedures for the safe use of these drugs are established and followed. This document is designed to help institutions to develop these policies and procedures and evaluate those presently in use.

Basic Principles

Procedures in the use of investigational drugs should be built around these basic principles:[c]

1. An institution that is the setting for investigational drug studies must assure that such studies contain adequate safeguards for itself, its staff, the scientific integrity of the study and, especially, the patient. In doing so, the institution must have written policies and procedures for the approval, management and control of investigational drug studies. Equally important, all involved staff must be fully informed about, and comply with, these policies and procedures.
2. All investigational drug studies must meet accepted ethical, legal and scientific standards and be conducted by appropriately qualified investigators.
3. All patients who participate in investigational drug studies must freely consent[d], in writing, to treatment with the drugs. This consent must be obtained from the patient or his legally authorized representative before treatment is begun, and only after the patient has been fully informed about the study objectives and the risks and benefits associated with the study drugs. No exhorbitant inducements should be offered to patients to encourage their participation in the study.

Guidelines for Institutions

The following recommendations will serve as a guide to develop investigational drug procedures in keeping with the aforementioned basic principles.
1. As required by federal regulation, institutions in which clinical research is conducted must have an Institutional Review Committee (IRC), often titled a "Committee on Human Investigations" or "Clinical Research

---

[a]Approved by the ASHP Board of Directors, December 12, 1978; revised November 18, 1982, based on the recommendation of the ASHP Council on Clinical Affairs. Originally developed by the ASHP Council on Professional Affairs.

[b]In this document, investigational drugs are defined as those which are being considered for, but have not as yet received, approval by the federal Food and Drug Administration for human use.
[c]It should be noted that the principles and procedures described here are applicable to *all* clinical drug studies, not just those involving investigational drugs.
[d]There are certain emergency situations in which a priori consent may be waived.

Committee." This committee must evaluate each proposed clinical research study in terms of its compliance with recognized ethical, legal and scientific standards. No clinical study may be initiated unless approved, in writing, by the committee. The committee must also monitor approved studies to ensure they are carried out appropriately. The Director of Pharmacy or the director's designee should be a member of the IRB or be consulted by the committee whenever drug studies are involved.

2. Investigational drugs must be used only under the supervision of the principal investigator or authorized co-investigators, all of whom must be members of the institution's professional staff.

3. The principal investigator is responsible for obtaining the written, informed consent of the patient to participate in the study. The informed consent process must conform to current federal and state regulations. Approval of the consent document by the IRB is required; review by the institution's legal counsel may be desirable also. The following items must be addressed, either in the document or its accompanying oral explanation by the investigator:

   a. A fair representation of the nature and purpose of the study, the expected benefits, and the risks or discomfort (or both) involved. The name of the person(s) to contact for answers to questions about the study or drug should be provided. Any compensation or treatment that will be furnished in the event of injury should be described.

   b. A balanced description of the alternative treatments available (including their respective risks and benefits).

   c. A general description of the study procedures and the expected length of therapy with the drug.

   d. A statement to the effect that: (1) the patient may withdraw from the study at any time without penalty; and (2) the principal investigator may remove the patient from the study if circumstances warrant.

   e. The name of the drug(s), name and signature of the patient and name and signature of the principal or co-investigator.

   f. A statement of who will have access to any study records that contain the patient's name.

   The consent form should be as detailed as is practical, minimizing the amount of information that must be presented orally. For non-English speaking patients, the consent form should be in the patient's own language when feasible or adequate interpretation provided. The patient (or his representative) must have adequate time to read the consent form before signing it and should receive a copy of the signed form.

4. The principal investigator is responsible for the proper maintenance of the case report forms and all other records required in the study by the drug sponsor, institution or Food and Drug Administration.

5. The institution's drug control system must contain the following elements regarding investigational drugs:

   a. Drugs must be properly packaged in accordance with all applicable standards and regulations (e.g., FDA, USP, Poison Prevention Packaging Act).

   b. Drugs must be labeled properly so as to ensure their safe use by the nursing staff and patient (see item 4 under "Guidelines for Pharmacists").

   c. There must be a mechanism to assure that sufficient supplies of the drugs are always available in the institution for the duration of the studies.

    d. Nurses called upon to administer investigational drugs must have adequate written information about their pharmacology (particularly adverse effects), storage requirements, method of dose preparation and administration, precautions to be taken, authorized prescribers, patient monitoring guidelines and any other material pertinent to the safe and proper use of the drugs. They also should be informed about the overall study objectives and procedures.

    e. Bulk supplies of the drug must be properly stored.

    f. There must be a method to assure that only authorized practitioners prescribe the drug and that all patients who receive it have provided the necessary consent.

    g. Records of the amounts of drug received from the sponsor and of its disposition (amounts dispensed to patients, returned to sponsor, etc.) must be maintained. These records should be retained for two years or as required by regulation.

    h. If the patient is to receive the drug at another facility, suitable arrangements for its transfer must be made. Sufficient information for safe use of the drug (see item d above), including a copy of the patient's signed consent form and the study protocol, must accompany the drug. The facility to which the drug is transferred should have written procedures governing the proper handling of investigational drugs.

    i. The institution's records on investigational drug studies should be designed so that various statistical reports (e.g., the names of all drugs under study, the names of those patients who have received a drug, etc.) may be generated conveniently and expeditiously.

The pharmaceutical services standards of the Joint Commission on Accreditation of Hospitals[a] and the ASHP Minimum Standard For Pharmacies in Institutions[b] note that the pharmacy is the area to which the drug control responsibilities described above should be assigned. This is to the advantage of the principal investigator, who will be relieved of many of the technical aspects of drug control, and therefore will have more time for the clinical concerns of the study. In addition, the pharmacy may be able to assist in protocol development, drug procurement, preparation of codes for blinded studies, patient monitoring, education of nursing and personnel, data collection and analysis, and special dosage form and packaging development.

GUIDELINES FOR PHARMACISTS

The pharmacist is reponsible to the institution and the principal investigator for seeing that procedures for the control of investigational drug use as described above are developed and implemented. Suggestions to accomplish this are as follows; however, each facility must develop procedures specific to its own needs and organization.

---

[a]Joint Commission on Accreditation of Hospitals. Accreditation manual for hospitals. Chicago, IL: Joint Commission on Accreditation of Hospitals; 1982.

[b]American Society of Hospital Pharmacists. ASHP minimum standard for pharmacies in institutions. *Am. J. Hosp. Pharm.* 1977; *34*:1356–8.

1. A copy of the IRB-approved research protocol should be kept in the pharmacy.

2. Using the protocol and additional information (if needed) supplied by the principal investigator, the pharmacy should prepare an Investigational Drug Data Sheet which concisely summarizes for the medical, nursing and pharmacy staffs information pertinent to use of the drug. This form should contain, at the minimum: (a) drug designation and common synonym(s); (b) dosage form(s) and strength(s) available; (c) usual dosage range, including dosage schedule and route of administration; (d) indications; (e) expected therapeutic effect; (f) expected and potential untoward effects (including symptoms of toxicity and their treatment); (g) contraindications; (h) storage requirements; (i) instructions for dosage preparation and administration; (j) instructions for disposition of unused doses; (k) names and telephone numbers of principal and authorized co-investigators. The drug data sheet should be reviewed by the principal investigator and included with the study protocol submitted to the IRC. Copies should be distributed to the appropriate pharmacy staff and all patient care units where the drug will be used. It is the responsibility of the involved staff to become familiar with the information on these data sheets.

3. Investigational drug supplies must be kept only in the pharmacy. The pharmacy should maintain an Investigational Drug Inventory Record where a perpetual inventory of the drug is kept. This form[a] should contain the drug's name, dosage form and strength, lot number and the name, address and telephone number of the sponsor and any other information needed for ordering the drug. It should provide for recording data on the disposition of the drug (amounts dispensed, data, names of patients and prescribers) and the amount currently on hand.

4. The dispensing of investigational drugs should be integrated with the rest of the drug distribution system with respect to packaging, labeling, order review, profile maintenance, delivery and so forth. However, prescription labels for investigational drugs should be distinguishable from other labels by an appropriate legend (e.g., "investigational drug"). There must be a method to verify that a valid, signed consent form has been received from the patient prior to dispensing the initial supply of drug. The drug must be dispensed only upon the order of an authorized investigator.

5. Patient education and monitoring of therapy are two clinical functions which are particularly important and applicable to investigational drugs. These functions should be provided in a coordinated fashion by the pharmacy and nursing staffs and the authorized investigator(s).

6. At the conclusion of the study, the pharmacy should return all unused drugs to the principal investigator or sponsor.

7. The pharmacy should prepare for the institution's administrator an annual or semiannual statistical summary of investigational drug use, including such information as the number of drug studies in progress and a listing of all drugs studied during the previous year.

8. Drug costs and other expenses associated with investigational drug studies (e.g., costs of record-keeping, drug administration) should be properly allocated and reimbursed.

---

[a]Stolar, M.H., ed.: Pharmacy-coordinated investigational drug services. Bethesda, MD: American Society of Hospital Pharmacists; 1982.

Elaboration on these guidelines and further information on investigational drug studies is in the book *Pharmacy-Coordinated Investigational Drug Services.*

Classification of Drugs

Summarized, the *Statement of Principles Involved in the Use of Investigational Use Drugs in Hospitals* espouses four distinct purposes:

1. To establish a drug classification.
2. To centralize pertinent information concerning drugs available for research use.
3. To define the availability of such drugs to staff members.
4. To establish a single stocking and dispensing unit within the hospital.

In order to attain the above goals, it is necessary for the Pharmacy and Therapeutics Committee to establish a drug classification system within the hospital. By establishing drug categories, a more definitive approach to the control, distribution and utilization of drugs, within each category, may be realized.

One simple classification which can be adapted to any hospital research program is to categorize all drugs in the institution into four classes: Classes A, B, C, and D.

Class A should contain all investigational use drugs that are in a preliminary experimental stage. The use of drugs in this category is usually restricted to the principal investigator. With regard to the storage and dispensing of drugs in Class A, there are two schools of thought. One group believes that products in this category should be stocked and dispensed by the principal investigator; the other group firmly holds that all drugs should be stored and dispensed through the pharmacy by pharmacists. The advantages of the latter are obvious; however, both systems will work if the interested parties, the clinical investigator and the pharmacist, will cooperate in a united endeavor.

Class B should consist of investigational use drugs which have passed through the preliminary research stage. Usually, drugs in this category are supplied to the department of pharmacy by the principal investigator and are dispensed only upon his written prescription or those of his duly designated co-investigators.

Class C is limited to drugs approved by the United States Pharmacopeia, National Formulary, or passed by the Federal Food and Drug Administration for commercial distribution.

Drugs in this category may be used within the hospital or its clinics if the physician complies with the following procedure:

If the product is to be used by a single patient, the prescriber must obtain the consent of the Chief-of-Service or his duly designated alternate (usually the Chairman of the Pharmacy and Therapeutics Committee) before the product may be obtained by the pharmacist.

A Class C preparation, which various members of the Staff feel has therapeutic promise, may be introduced into the hospital on a six-month trial. A request for such drug must be made to the Pharmacy and Therapeutics Committee which may then authorize the pharmacist to purchase, stock, and dispense the product. Pertinent data, concerning this special drug, are to be gathered and filed in the pharmacy office. At the completion of the trial period, the clinical experience is reviewed by the Pharmacy and Therapeutics Committee along with the clinician. If the results are favorable, the product is accepted into the hospital formulary; if the evidence is not favorable, the product is barred from further use within the hospital.

Class D drugs are preparations which have been accepted for use in the hospital and are listed in the hospital formulary.

Information concerning these products is to be kept in the general literature file in the pharmacy library.

Preparations in this class may be precribed routinely by any licensed physician on the hospital staff.

Another simple classification which can be adapted to any hospital pharmacy operation again classifies each drug into three categories: General, Conditional and Investigational.

1. **General**—An FDA-approved drug which as recommended as essential for good patient care with a well established usage, once accepted, may be prescribed by all members of the attending and house staff.
2. **Conditional**—Certain drugs may be approved for a conditional period of trial. A drug approved by the FDA for general use, but which the Committee wishes to evaluate for a given period before final consideration, may be prescribed by all members of the attending and house staff.
3. **Investigational**—Drugs which are not approved by the FDA for use other than under controlled clinical settings must be approved by the Research Advisory/Human Subjects Committees. Radioisotopes must also be approved by the Radiation Safety Committee. A protocol of any study involving drugs must be submitted to the Pharmacy.

CONTROL OF INVESTIGATIONAL USE DRUGS

All investigational use drugs should be registered with the Pharmacy and Therapeutics Committee. This may be accomplished by a letter from the principal investigator which provides the following information on each drug.

1. New Drug Number	7. Pharmacology
2. Generic Name	8. Toxicology
3. Manufacturer	9. Dose Range
4. Proprietary Name (if any)	10. Method of Administration
5. Chemical Name	11. Antidote (if known)
6. General Chemistry	12. Therapeutic Uses

The above data are usually found in the brochure prepared by the manufacturer and supplied to each investigator. Therefore, the brochure may be sent to the Pharmacy and Therapeutics Committee with a letter indicating the investigator's intent to use such a product.

Many pharmacists have developed various forms which may be used to disseminate the above information on an investigational use drug to the various staff doctors and nurses. These forms are usually titled *"Physician's Data Sheet on Investigational Drugs," "Nurse's Data Sheet on Investigational Drugs"* and *"Pharmacist's Data Sheet on Investigational Drugs."* Figures 21, 22 and 23 illustrate these various data sheets which have been used by the Pharmacy Service of the Veterans Administration Hospital in Albany, New York.[6] Under this system, the pharmacist completes the necessary form or portion of a form and sends it to the appropriate physician or pavilion each time a new investigational drug is prescribed. Although this method does offer control and proper dissemination of information, it is burdensome upon the phar-

PHYSICIAN'S DATA SHEET ON INVESTIGATIONAL DRUGS

1. Name of Investigational Drug _____

2. Manufacturer or Other Source _____

3. Strength and Form of Investigational Drug _____

4. Amount Received _____

        Date Received _____

        Control or Batch No. _____

5. *Pharmacologic and Therapeutic Properties, Dosage, Precautions:*
6. *Arrangements Which Have been Made for its Administration:*

                                                _____
                                                  Investigator

Registered:

_____
        Date

Fig. 21

NURSE'S DATA SHEET ON INVESTIGATIONAL DRUGS

1. Name of Investigational Drug: _____

2. Manufacturer or Other Source: _____

3. Strength and Form of Investigational Drug: _____

4. Pharmacologic, Therapeutic Properties and Precautions to be Observed:

5. *Arrangements Which Have Been Made for its Administration:*

_____

Chief Pharmacist

Fig. 22

macist since three different forms bearing similar information must be prepared.

Figure 24 illustrates a *New Drug Report Form.* This form, as designed, provides all of the data required for the proper handling of the investigational use drug by physician, pharmacist and nurse.

The *New Drug Report Form* may be placed on each pavilion, where it is readily available to any investigator. Each time a clinician desires to prescribe an investigational use drug, he must complete the *New Drug Report Form* in duplicate, place the original in the patient's medical record folder, and have the carbon copy sent to the pharmacy with the drug order slip appended. By so doing, the pharmacist is aware that the new drug is being used on a particular patient in a specific area, the nurses have the necessary information, and physicians on the pavilion also have all the necessary data. This same procedure should be followed irrespective of the number of patients using the drug on

PHARMACIST'S DATA SHEET ON INVESTIGATIONAL DRUGS

Investigational Drug: _____Manufacturer: _____

Chief Investigator: _____

DATE	PHYSICIAN	PATIENT	℞ No.	AMOUNT	WARD
———	—————	—————	———	—————	———
———	—————	—————	———	—————	———
———	—————	—————	———	—————	———
———	—————	—————	———	—————	———
———	—————	—————	———	—————	———

Fig. 23

PETER BENT BRIGHAM HOSPITAL

NEW DRUG FORM

Addressograph Use Only

New Drug No.: _____

Generic Name: _____   Date & Time of 1st Dose: _____

Trade Name (If Any): _____

Chemical Name: _____

Chemistry:

Pharmacologic Action:

Dose: _____   Method of Administration: _____

_____   _____

_____   _____

Toxicity: Antidote(s):

Therapeutic Uses: Names of physicians from whom drug
_____   is available:

_____   _____

_____   _____

Fig. 24

the same pavilion. In order to save the clinician's time in such a situation, he may complete one form in detail and permit either the medication nurse or resident to complete similar forms for each of the other patients on the same pavilion.

In hospitals where the research load may not be quite so heavy, the pharmacist may undertake to complete each set of *New Drug Report Forms* each time he receives an order for an investigational use drug.

The fact that carbon copies are used saves time and provides the identical information to both clinician and nurse. A separate file for prescriptions for each investigational use drug readily serves the purpose of tracing the drug and accounting for each dose consumed.

Identification of Investigational Use Drugs

Whenever Class A or Class B drugs are dispensed from the pharmacy, they should be labeled in such a manner as to differentiate them from routine prescription drugs. In some hospitals, investigational use drug labels are printed in red ink on white paper stock. In addition to the commonly required label information of patient's name, data, prescription number, doctor's name and directions for use a space for the research drug number is provided. This double set of numbers, the prescription number and the manufacturer's research drug number, provides a two-day control relative to the identity of the product dispensed.

Charge Policy for Handling and Dispensing

Because it is usually difficult to convince drug investigators that investigational use drugs should be stored and dispensed from the pharmacy, many hospital pharmacists waive a charge for this service, the consensus being that it serves as an inducement to the investigator to avail himself of the pharmacist's service. In these institutions a charge is made when a special dosage form is prepared in the pharmacy. The basis of the charge is arrived at by determining the cost of materials and labor involved.

In hospitals where there is a potent Pharmacy and Therapeutics Committee, a routine nominal charge is made for handling and dispensing research drugs. This charge is usually passed on to the patient but, where sufficient funds are available to the investigator, he may wish to assume the total cost of the project and accordingly requests the pharmacy not to charge the patient but to bill his research grant or fund on a monthly basis.

Personnel in the department of pharmacy at Ohio State University Hospital have studied the administrative aspects of a pharmacy coordinated investigational drug service and its related cost.[7] It was demonstrated that an average of 5 hours is required to coordinate pharmacy participation in a drug study. A drug information specialist spends about 1.5 hours developing a data sheet on the investigational drug and recordkeeping consumes 11 hours per study. After ascertaining personnel and space charges, the director of pharmacy services should institute a departmental fee for the pharmacy's involvement in investigational drug studies.

Authorization for Treatment with Drug Under Clinical Investigation

The Law Department of the American Medical Association[8] states that drugs under clinical investigation should be administered only where:

1. the informed consent of the patient or his authorized representative has been obtained;
2. the physician is convinced of the reasonable accuracy of his di-

agnosis and, if necessary, has confirmed it by adequate consultation; and

3. existing methods of treatment have proven unsatisfactory.

The voluntary participation of the patient will not excuse a deviation from the physician's obligation to exercise his best skill in rendering the care required of a reasonable practitioner. Furthermore, the physician is advised to confine his clinical investigations of new drugs to those furnished by reputable sources who have supplied him with comprehensive written information concerning:

1. animal experimentation;
2. previous clinical investigations, if any;
3. recommended dosages;
4. contraindications;
5. possible side effects to be watched for, and
6. the safety and possible usefulness of the drug from existing data.

Since oral consent is not sufficient, the American Medical Association has developed medicolegal form number 29 (Fig. 25).

Another example of a consent form which does not limit itself to the use of investigational use drugs is that used on the Clinical Center of the Harvard Medical School at the Peter Bent Brigham Hospital (Fig. 26).

Since this text material is not intended to offer legal advice due to the fact that state laws vary from state to state, the hospital pharmacist is urged to consult the hospital's legal counsel for the law applicable to the area in which the hospital is located.

Role of the Pharmacist in the Clinical Evaluation of a Drug

Once the pharmacologist has demonstrated a new compound to be effective and safe in animal tests, clinical trials are invariably commenced. These trials usually proceed in two steps—preliminary and extended.

During the preliminary stage, the principal investigator cautiously administers the drug to a limited number of selected patients and closely follows the results. After having gained experience and confidence in its use, the investigator is generally ready to conduct an extended comprehensive evaluation of its efficacy.

It is during this stage that the pharmacist can play an important role by assisting in the development of the protocol and the control of a double blind study. Such tests are devised by having the experimental drug and the placebo prepared in exactly the same dose form. The

AUTHORIZATION FOR TREATMENT WITH DRUG
UNDER CLINICAL INVESTIGATION

A.M.

Date _____ Time _____P.M.

I authorize Dr. _____, the attending physician, to

treat _____with the drug presently
(Name of Patient)

identified as _____for the following condition:

_____

_____

_____

(Describe symptoms of disease to be treated)

It has been explained to me that the safety and usefulness of the drug in the
treatment of patients for the above condition are now being investigated and
that the manufacturer or distributor has supplied the drug for the purpose of
providing further evidence of its safety and usefulness.

I voluntarily consent to treatment with the drug and release the attending
physician from liability from any results that may occur.

Signed _____
(Patient or person authorized
to consent for patient)

Witness _____

Fig. 25

identified products are then entrusted to the pharmacist to dispense
according to a predetermined pattern and to maintain an exact record
of which patient received the true drug and which received the placebo.
Neither the patient nor the physician is informed as to whether the
placebo or potent article is being tried in any individual patient. All
information for breaking double blind codes must be kept in the pharmacy. Should an emergency arise requiring the breaking of the code,
the pharmacist on duty or on call is authorized to provide the necessary
information.

In addition to the above role, the hospital pharmacist can render a
valuable service to the new drug researcher by formulating new dosage
forms from the pure chemical. A word of caution should be interjected
at this point—since time is of the essence in a research project, many
investigators will attempt to speed up the pharmacist by waiving certain
control tests. The pharmacist should insist upon the time necessary to

CONSENT FORM

Patient's Name: _____Date: _____

Project Title:

Description of procedure to be undertaken:

I have fully explained to the patient _____
the nature and purpose of the procedure described above and such risks as are
involved in its performance.

_____

Physician's signature

I have been fully informed of the risks and possible consequences involved in the
peformance of the procedure described above, have been advised that unforeseen
results may occur and, nevertheless, hereby authorize Dr. _____
and such assistants as he may designate to perform the procedure upon me and
hereby release and forever discharge him, such assistants, the Peter Bent Brigham
Hospital, its officers, agents and employees, and all persons on its medical and
surgical staff who are in any way connected with the procedure from liability from
injury which may result directly or indirectly from the performance of the procedure.

_____

Patient's signature

_____

Witness

Fig. 26

develop a scientifically sound formulation as well as for the performance of chemical and bacteriological tests for potency and sterility.

As the Colleges of Pharmacy train more and more clinical pharmacists, these individuals become available to participate in the clinical
evaluation of new drug products. Because of their training in biopharmaceutics, pharmacokinetics and in the use of modern instrumentation
techniques of analysis, clinical pharmacists can monitor the blood and
tissue levels of the new drugs as well as their excretion rates and thereby
advise the clinical pharmacologist relative to the need for dosage adjustment, mode of administration or product formulation.

CLINICAL TESTING FOR SALE AND EFFECTIVE DRUGS

Investigational Drug Procedures[9]

Before 1962, there was no requirement that the Food and Drug Administration by notified that drugs were being tested on humans.

The 1962 Kefauver-Harris Amendments to the Federal Food, Drug, and Cosmetic Act greatly strengthened the Government's authority over clinical (human) testing of new drugs.

With this new regulatory authority, the Food and Drug Administration has taken steps to:
1. Provide added safeguards for those on whom drugs are tested.
2. Improve reports by drug investigators.
3. Establish investigative procedures to supply substantial scientific evidence that a drug is safe and effective.

First Steps

Before a new drug may be tested on humans, the sponsor (usually a pharmaceutical firm, sometimes a physician) must give the FDA the information specified as a "Notice of Claimed Investigational Exemption for a New Drug" (Forms FD 1571, 1572, and 1573), known as an "IND." Copies of these IND forms may be obtained from:

> Document and Records Service Section
> (HFD-106)
> Bureau of Drugs
> Food and Drug Administration
> 5600 Fishers Lane
> Rockville, Maryland 20852

The IND should include the following information:
a. Complete composition of the drug, its source, and manufacturing data, to show that appropriate standards exist to insure safety.
b. Results of all preclinical investigations, including animal studies. Initially, these should be directed toward defining the drug's safety, rather than its efficacy. The data must demonstrate that there will not be unreasonable hazard in initiating studies in humans. Further animal studies may be conducted concurrently with clinical studies. The Bureau of Drugs will, on request, comment on the adequacy of the proposed animal studies. The FDA generally requires as a minimum: (i) pharmacological profile, (ii) acute toxicity be determined in several species of animals and that the route of administration be that which will be used in the animal trials, (iii) short term studies ranging from two weeks to three months depending upon the proposed use to evaluate toxicity. Additional animal studies are frequently necessary.

c. A detailed outline (protocol) of the planned investigation.
d. Information regarding training and experience of the investigators. (See "Qualifications of Investigators.") Investigators are responsible to the sponsor and are required to submit, to the sponsor (not the FDA), either Form FD 1572 for clinical pharmacology or Form FD 1573 for clinical trials.
e. Copies of all informational material supplied to each investigator. (The type of information is listed in Form 1571.)
f. An agreement from the sponsor to notify the FDA and all investigators if any adverse effects arise during either the animal or human tests.
g. The investigator's agreement to obtain the consent of the person on whom the drug is to be tested before the test is made.
h. Agreement to submit annual progress reports and commitments regarding disposal of the drug when studies are discontinued.

Physician-Sponsored IND

When an investigator wishes to act as sponsor for the use of a drug solely as a research tool or for early clinical investigation of a drug of therapeutic or diagnostic potential (clinical pharmacology—phases 1 and 2) a simpler abbreviated form of submission is acceptable. An example would be the study of a drug that no manufacturer is interested in sponsoring. An outline of such a study should provide the following information:
1. The identity of the compound or compounds, together with the facts that satisfy the investigator that the agent may be justifiably administered to man as intended.
2. The purpose of the use and the general protocol.
3. Appropriate background information, including a brief statement of the investigator's scientific training and experience and the nature of the facilities available to him.

The physician sponsoring this form of IND deals directly with the FDA. The FDA has no authority over the practice of medicine and cannot require a physician to prescribe or not to prescribe for a drug for a particular illness. But physicians are encouraged to submit an IND when they use a drug for purposes other than those approved by the FDA, when the drug was marketed. This enables the FDA to accumulate data on the safety and efficacy of the drug for that kind of treatment and to share the information with other physicians.

The Clinical Investigation

The kind and extent of the investigational drug tests are crucial to producing the substantial scientific evidence of safety and effectiveness needed to approve the drug for marketing. This evidence is obtained in three phases:

Phase I

Pharmacology studies are used to determine toxicity, metabolism absorption and elimination, and other pharmacological actions; preferred route of administration, and safe dosage range. These studies involve a small number of persons and are conducted under carefully controlled circumstances by persons trained in clinical pharmacology.

Phase II

Initial trials are conducted on a limited number of patients for a specific disease treatment or prevention. Additional pharmacological studies performed concurrently on animals may be necessary to indicate safety.

Phase III

Proposals for this phase, involving extensive clinical trials, are in order if the information obtained in the first two phases demonstrates reasonable assurance of safety and effectiveness, or suggests that the drug may have a potential value outweighing possible hazards. The phase III studies are intended to assess the drug's safety, effectiveness and most desirable dosage in treating a specific disease in a large group of subjects. The studies should be carefully monitored, no matter how extensive.

The FDA receives constant reports on the progress of each phase. If the continuation of the studies appears to present an unwarranted hazard to the patients, the sponsor may be requested to modify or discontinue clinical testing until further preclinical work has been done.

30-Day Delay

After the sponsor submits his IND, he must wait 30 days before beginning clinical tests. This delay enables the FDA to review the protocol to make certains it contain all of the necessary information and to assure that patients are not exposed to unwarranted risks. The 30-day period may be extended if the FDA feels additional time is needed for the sponsor to correct deficiencies in the protocol. The FDA also may waive the delay requirement if it feels such action is justified.

Sponsors may discuss their protocols at any time either before or during the tests with the Office of Scientific Evaluation, Bureau of Drugs.

Test in Institutions

Drug tests on persons in hospitals, prisons, research facilities, and other institutions must be carefully supervised by institutional review committees.

The committees must be composed of persons with varying backgrounds, such as lawyers, clergymen or laymen, as well as scientists. They are appointed by the institution involved in the study. The FDA inspects the institutions periodically to determine if the committees are operating properly.

Qualifications of Investigators

The sponsor of an investigational new drug (usually the manufacturer) will ask the clinical investigator to supply the following information on Form FD 1572 (for the clinical pharmacologist engaged in phase 1 or 2 trials) or Form FD 1573 (for the physician engaged in phase 3 clinical trials):

1. A statement of his education, training and experience.
2. Information regarding the hospital or other medical institution where the investigations will be conducted; special equipment and other facilities.

The training and experience needed will vary, depending upon the kind of drug and the nature of the investigation. In phase 1, the investigator must be able to evaluate human toxicology and pharmacology. In phase 2, the clinicians should be familiar with the conditions to be treated, the drugs used in these conditions and the methods of their evaluation. In phase 3, in addition to experienced clinical investigators, physicians not regarded as specialists in any particular field of medicine may serve as investigators. At this stage, a large number of patients may be treated by different physicians to get a broad background of experience.

Obligations of Investigators

The investigator must keep careful records of his study and retain them for at least two years after the NDA is approved. The records must be made available promptly to the drug sponsor and to the FDA when required. Regular progress reports must be sent to the sponsor.

Reports must be sent to the sponsor immediately when dangerous adverse effects are observed, so the FDA and the other investigators can be notified, and the study stopped if the hazard warrants.

The regulations regarding consent of human beings given investigational drugs must be observed.

Patient Consent

The law requires that before using investigational drugs on human beings, the physician must "obtain the consent of such human beings or their representatives except when it is not feasible or when in his professional judgment it is contrary to the best interest of such human beings."

The consent for use of an investigational new drug in phase 1 and phase 2 must be in writing. In phase 3, it is the responsibility of the investigator, taking into consideration the physical and mental state of the patient, to decide when it is necessary or preferable to obtain consent in other than written form.

If written consent is not obtained, the investigator must obtain oral consent except as provided above, and record that fact in the medical record of the person receiving the drug.

Causes for Termination of Investigation

The FDA may direct the sponsor to terminate an investigation at any stage under certain conditions. These include:

Evidence of significant hazard.

Convincing evidence that the drug is ineffective.

Submission of false data.

Omission of material information.

Unsatisfactory manufacturing practices.

Failure to conduct the investigation in accordance with the plan submitted by the sponsor and approved by the FDA.

Commercialization of the drug. The IND regulations are not intended to provide a way of marketing a drug for profit without an approved NDA.

Failure to submit progress reports at intervals not exceeding one year.

Failure to report serious or potentially serious adverse reactions.

Failure to meet requirements for patient consent.

The Commissioner may notify the sponsor of any of the above conditions and invite immediate correction. A conference may be arranged. If the corrections are not effected immediately the Commissioner may require the sponsor to terminate the investigation and recall unused supplies of the drug. The drug in question may not be reintroduced into clinical testing in man until additional data have been submitted to the FDA and the Commissioner has approved the proposed resumption of the study.

The Investigator and "Promotion"

The regulations forbid manufacturers or any persons acting for or on their behalf to disseminate any promotional material concerning a new drug prior to completion of the investigation.

This is not intended to restrict the full exchange of scientific findings in scientific or other communications media. Its purpose is to restrict promotional claims by the sponsor until the safety and effectiveness of the investigational drug have been established. Violation of the regulations by an investigator may result in FDA action to deny him further supplies of the drug. The manufacturer may also jeopardize his right to sponsor the investigation.

Special Preclearance before Human Trials

Before starting an investigation in any of the following categories, FDA approval is required for:

a. Substances controlled under Schedule I of the Controlled Substances Act (PL 91–513).
b. Investigations of drugs so toxic that their use may be justified only under special conditions.
c. Substances proposed for treatment of drug dependence.
d. Reinstitution of drug investigations which have been terminated by the Commissioner.

Use of Drugs for Laboratory Procedures

New drugs used only for studies in vitro (test tubes) or in laboratory animals are being exempted from the new-drug provisions of the Act provided they are labeled "Caution—Contains a new drug for investigational use only in laboratory research animals, or for tests in vitro. Not for use in humans."

The exemption does not apply, however, for a new drug used in vitro when this use will influence the diagnosis or treatment of disease in a human patient—for example, discs to determine the sensitivity to antibiotics of bacteria in culture, or a stick or strip of paper incorporating a reagent to test for sugar in the urine. Apparent ineffectiveness of an antibiotic sensitivity disc or a false negative test for glycosuria might well lead to an incorrect diagnosis and deprive the patient of appropriate treatment.

Before such a preparation can be marketed there must be certification (in the case of antibiotics) or approval of a New Drug Application (in the case of other drugs). For that reason, it is necessary to submit adequate proof of the effectiveness of these preparations before they can be marketed.

INVESTIGATIONAL USE DRUGS AND THE PHARMACY AND THERAPEUTICS COMMITTEE

In view of the fact that all drugs used in the hospital are subject to review by the Pharmacy and Therapeutics Committee, it is this group's responsibility to develop procedures for the introduction of investigational drugs into the institution. The following policies are in force in one major teaching hospital.[10]

Investigational drugs are defined as those which have been filed with the Food and Drug Administration (FDA) in the form of a Notice of Claimed Investigational Exemption for a New Drug (IND) under the provisions of Section 505 of the Federal Food, Drug and Cosmetics Act and paragraphs 312.1 of Title 21 of the Code of Federal Regulations. Such drugs must be approved by the FDA and assigned an IND number. An investigaitonal drug must be approved by the Human Subjects Committee, the Pharmacy and Therapeutics Committee, and, if applicable, the Isotope Committee before it can be administered to Peter Bent Brigham Hospital patients.

In emergency situations, for the use of investigational drugs or an approved drug for a non-approved indication which has not been assigned an IND number by the FDA, the policy is as follows:

a. The physician must notify the Chairpersons of the Human Subjects and Pharmacy & Therapeutics Committees for their approval. When the Chairpersons cannot be reached, (holidays, nights or weekends) the physician may contact the Hospital administrator on call.

b. The physician shall be informed that neither the hospital nor other hospital personnel will be reponsible for any legal liabilities which may result from the use of the drug(s). Further, the physician shall hold these persons harmless and indemnify them against any legal action or payments made in connection therewith.

c. Patient, or legally responsible person, must sign a hospital approved consent form.

d. The physician is responsible to register the drug(s) in the Pharmacy and provide all pertinent drug information such as pharmacological action, contraindications, adverse reactions, dosage range and route of administration, who may administer the drug, where the drug will be stored and the name of the principal investigator.

Hospital pharmacists should know that there are a number of ways in which a physician may introduce an investigational drug into the institution. They are:

a. Obtain an IND individually

b. Become a co-investigator under another physician's IND and

c. Become an investigator for a pharmaceutical or chemical company under that firm's IND.

In those situations where a physician wishes to prescribe an investigational drug in one hospital but the drug is under a IND in another, the physician may be granted an emergency IND after telephoning the FDA and presenting the case for such special consideration.

INVESTIGATIONAL DRUG CIRCULAR

Because hospital pharmacists have great interest in investigational use drugs, it is suggested that they subscribe to the *Investigational Drug Circular.* This publication is issued by the Bureau of Medicine of the Food and Drug Administration. It is stated that the purpose of this *Circular* ". . . is to answer questions asked by drug sponsors and clinicians regarding requirements of the Food, Drug and Cosmetic Act. . . ."

SELECTED READINGS

Benfell, Kathleen, Powell, Stephen H., and Kaul, Alan F.: Comprehensive Pharmacy-Based Investigational Drug Service. Am. J. Hosp. Pharm., *40*:64–67, (Jan.) 1983.

Anon, The Maintenance of High Ethical Standards in the Conduct of Research (1982). Association of American Medical Colleges, One Dupont Circle, Washington, D.C. 20036.

Young, L.M., Haakenson, C.M., Weber, J.H., and Tosch, T.J.: National Survey of Pharmacy Coordinated Investigational Drug Services. Am. J. Hosp. Pharm., *41*:1792–1796, (Sept.) 1984.

REFERENCES

1. Surgeon General's Memorandum of July 1, 1966, Policy and Procedure Order No. 129, Revised.
2. Title 21, Subchapter C, Part 130 Section 130–57 Federal Register, *31,* No. 168, August 30, 1966.
3. Manual Grants Administration 1–40-10B, Chapter 1–40, Protection of Human Subjects, Dept. Health, Education and Welfare, Washington, D.C.
4. DHEW Policy on Protection of Human Subjects, DRG Newsletter, p. 3, May 1971.
5. ASHP Guidelines for the Use of Investigational Drugs in Institutions. Am. J. Hosp. Pharm., *40*:449–451, (Mar.) 1983.
6. Teplitsky, B.: American Professional Pharmacist, *22*:11:1018, 1956.
7. Ngu, B., Schneider, P.J., and Kilarski, D.: Establishing a Fee for Handling Investigational Drug Studies. Am. J. Hosp. Pharm., *39*:1308–1310, (Aug.) 1982.
8. *Medicolegal Forms with Legal Analysis,* Chicago, American Medical Association, 1961.
9. DHEW Publication No. (FDA) 74–3015, U.S. Dept. Health, Education, and Welfare, Food and Brug Admin., Rockville, Md., 20852.
10. Formulary of the Peter Bent Brigham Hospital, 1978–79 Edition, Boston, Mass. 02115.

8

Developing the Budget

One of the most important tasks in the fiscal operation of the department is the preparation of the annual budget. Too often, many administrators and chief pharmacists take the development of the budget too lightly and thereby arrive at a document which does not serve its true purpose.

Hahn[1] describes the budget as an instrument

". . . through which hospital administration, management at departmental levels, and the governing board can review the hospital's services in relationship to a prepared plan in a comprehensive and integrated form expressed in financial terms."

In order that the over-all hospital budget complies with the above definition, each and every departmental budget must be accurately prepared and submitted.

Hahn[1] further states that—

"A properly developed and used budget should have as its goals (1) development of standards of performance, (2) comparison of actual results with these standards thus identifying deviations, and (3) subsequent analysis of deviations to determine whether they are controllable or uncontrollable."

Larson[2] in writing on the political aspects of budgeting in hospitals believes that, the pharmacist, in order to participate more effectively in the budgetary process, must be cognizant of the political aspects of the process. Among these political considerations are
1. Personal considerations,
2. Development of confidence among other officials,
3. Institutional-philosophical pressures, and
4. Demographic pressures.

Each of these factors affects the power base of a department and, consequently, the strength of its bargaining position in the budgetary process.

Personal considerations, in the form of individual reputations, are important in any political process. An individual who has acquired a reputation for having submitted previous budgets that have been thoroughly researched and supported by substantial justification stands a better chance of having his budget submittal approved.

Since most pharmacy programs affect other hospital departments, it is important for the Director of Pharmacy Services to obtain their collaboration and support. This support from the other departments provides the clout necessary to win administrative approval of the proposed program.

The institutional-philosophical considerations in the budgetary process consist of the goals and objectives of the hospital and its divisions. Since many state planning agencies require hospitals to submit 1- and 5-year plans outlining the institution's short- and long-range programs, it is of vital importance that the programs of the pharmacy service coincide with the overall plan of the institution.

In view of the fact that most hospitals are community based, the consumer public has made inroads into the decision making process of the institution. Today, many boards of trustees have consumer representatives from the local community serving on them. With a knowledge of the demographic, epidemiologic and attitudinal characteristics of the communities they serve, pharmacists are able to delineate the services desired and needed by the people.[2]

A budget is a short-range plan for future operations. The meaning and appropriate use of a budget must be clearly understood by those in managerial positions since their participation is required in its preparation and their cooperation is essential if it is to serve the function of a control device over operations. Prior to embarking upon a plan, management must first define the purpose of the unit, establish policies for its operation, and project the hospital's growth.

The plan should be reasonable and, through the concientious efforts of all personnel, attainable. It should not forecast results that are not possible under current and anticipated conditions. Students must not be misled when first exposed to the jargon "estimated results" during a discussion of a budget. This does not mean guesswork but rather carefully determined values based upon a knowledge of current financial and operating conditions and their relationship to future periods. The budget must not be construed as a tool to restrict initiative or to be impervious to the effects of changing conditions.

Between 1976 and 1979, hospital costs rose at an average annual rate of 14.1%, which turned out to be higher than the total inflation rate of all cost indicators.[3] Health-related expenditures in 1980 accounted for approximately 10% of the gross national product, compared with 8.5% in 1975.[4]

Supplies and other expenses usually comprise 60 to 70% of a pharmacy department's operating budget; drugs and intravenous solutions account for more than 95% of the category. The remainder of the operating budget is assigned to salaries (approximately 27%) and capital equipment.[5]

In 1978, the federal government began giving serious consideration towards price control and cost containment legislation in an effort to control spiraling health care costs. Not desirous of further governmental intrusions into an already over-regulated industry, a coalition of business, industry, labor, insurance and health care associations was formed and identified as "The Voluntary Effort to Contain Health Care Costs" commonly referred to as the "VE" program. Among the organizations joining to form the coalition were the American Hospital Association, American Medical Association, Federation of American Hospitals, Health Industry Manufacturers Association, Health Insurance Association of America and the Blue Cross and Blue Shield Associations.

The purpose of the "VE" program was to decelerate the rapidly rising cost of health care by instructing all providers to redouble their commitment to cost containment and to specifically request institutions to keep their operating and capital budgets at the lowest possible level.

The type of reimbursement that a hospital operates under is of great importance. Knowing the potential for increasing revenue over costs will affect the type of budget developed. For example, if the hospital is basically cost-reimbursed with little charge reimbursement, budgeting increased revenue is meaningless. On the other hand, projections showing expenditures that are within the cost restraints of the institution, or which actually decrease costs are desirable.[6]

In the preparation of the budget, it is important to consider the impact of reimbursement under the Tax Equity and Fiscal Responsibility Act (TEFRA), Diagnostic Related Groupings (DRGs) and Health Maintenance Organizations (HMOs) amongst others. For example, with the implementation of Social Security's Prospective Payments for Medicare Inpatient Hospital Services, hospitals must conform to a prospective payment system to replace the former cost-based reimbursement system for short-term acute care hospitals. The prospective payment system provides for a fixed price for DRG's that will be paid to hospitals.[6]

SECTIONS OF THE BUDGET

Every budget consists of three separate parts, *(a)* Revenue Accounts, *(b)* Expense Accounts and *(c)* Capital Equipment Requests.

The Revenue Account

The *Chart of Accounts and Definitions for Hospitals*[7] provides as follows.

PHARMACY

Account Number

Revenue	Expense
4070	7070

"This department produces, preserves, stores, compounds, manufactures, packages, controls, assays, dispenses, and distributes medications (including intravenous solutions) for inpatients and out-patients under the direction of a licensed pharmacist. Pharmacy services include the maintenance in designated areas of separate stocks of commonly used items. Additional activities can include, but are not limited to: development and maintenance of formularies established by the medical staff, consultation with and advice to medical and nursing staff on drug therapy, adding drugs to intravenous solutions, determining incompatibility in drug combinations, and stocking floor drugs and dispensing machines.

This responsibility center should be credited or charged with all the direct revenues and expenses incurred in maintaining a pharmacy under the direction of a licensed pharmacist. Appropriate subaccounts should be established to accumulate the expenses of this center under the natural classification—salaries and wages, supplies, and so forth. The cost of supplies and equipment that are not billed to patients and are issued at invoice cost to other areas represented by responsibility centers should be transferred to the accounts of the consuming responsibility centers on a monthly basis."

A commonly used method is whereby either the department of pharmacy or the accounting department maintains a daily, weekly, monthly or annual total of the cost of the pharmaceuticals issued to the various patient services as well as to the special service departments. This total, when added to that obtained from the processing of patient prescriptions and requisitions, represents the true income of the department.

In addition, there are other statistics that are of value in assisting management to accurately predict the volume of activity of the department of pharmacy. They are:

a. Number of prescriptions according to subcategories.
b. Number of prescriptions dispensed per pharmacist.
c. Hours of service.
d. Prescription volume per hour of service.
e. Medication cost per patient day.
f. Medication cost per clinic visit.
g. Average drug cost per prescription.
h. Average salary cost per prescription.
i. Average supply cost per requisition.

Although, "income" is considered as a single figure by the beginner, it is important to understand the derivation of the figure. Generally, income in the hospital pharmacy is limited to the sale of drugs to inpatients, ambulatory patients and departments of the hospital. However, the sale of drugs to patients may be sub-divided further based upon the patients' ability to pay or to their employment status if they are employed by the hospital. The following sub-division is but one example:

a.	Full pay.	*d.*	Physicians
b.	Part pay.	*e.*	General employee.
c.	Non-pay		

If income is generated from a combination of the above, it is desirable to separate the data so as to lead to more accurate appraisal and evaluation.

In some hospitals, the Controller may choose to treat income from the sale of drugs to other hospital departments as a "deduction" from the Purchase Account rather than added to the Income Account on the premise that such a maneuver enables a better evaluation of drug purchase costs for patient use.

THE EXPENSE ACCOUNTS—GENERAL INFORMATION

Expense accounts may be divided into four general categories— *Administration and General; Professional Care of Patients' Out-Patient and Emergency* and *Other Expenses.*

The department of pharmacy is listed under the category of Professional Care of Patients and is assigned code number 4070 for revenue and 7070 for expenses. (This code need not be used by all hospitals.) Each subdivision under this expense code number is coded by the addition of a dot and another digit, *e.g.,* 7070.1 is the code for Salaries and Wages; 7070.2 for Supplies and Expenses.

Although the hospital pharmacist will not be involved with the establishing of expense codes for his department (this being the prerogative of the comptroller), he should have a general understanding of what expenses belong under each section expense code.

Accordingly, the following is a sample categorization and contents.[8]

Salaries and Wages
Salaries and wages of pharmacists, assistants, clerks and other employed in the hospital pharmacy department.

Supplies and Expense

Drugs and Pharmaceuticals
Drugs and pharmaceuticals dispensed by prescription or otherwise from the hospital pharmacy department. Drugs and pharmaceuticals used in the out-patient and emergency departments should be charged there and not to this account.

Purchaed Services
This account should include the cost of prescriptions (excluding those in-

tended for out-patients) purchased from an outside pharmacy in the event the hospital does not have its own pharmacy.

Miscellaneous Supplies and Expense

Bottles, labels, glassware, narcotic and alcoholic permit fees, printed forms and stationery, pharmacists' uniforms, reference books, etc. Parts required to repair and maintain equipment used by this department and repairs made by outside concerns to such equipment also should be charged to this account, to separate sub-accounts if significant in amount.

It should be clearly understood that the above codes and designations are not intended to provide the ideal system of segregating costs. At most, it is a guide and should be modified by the individual hospital to meet its particular need.

EXPENSE ACCOUNT—SALARIES AND WAGES

In order to arrive at an accurate determination of the salaries and wages, it is recommended that the Pharmacist-in-Chief prepare a break-down of the personnel in the department of pharmacy into the following categories:

    a. Authorized permanent full-time positions—filled.
    b. Authorized permanent full-time positions—vacant.
    c. Authorized permanent part-time positions—filled.
    d. Authorized permanent part-time positions—vacant.
    e. Authorized temporary positions.
    f. Proposed new positions.
    g. Overtime requested.

It may also be of value to the Pharmacist-in-Chief if he further subdivided the above positions into three sub-categories, *i.e.,* administrative, professional and non-professional staff. It may be useful to prepare a table of all full-time administrative, professional and non-professional pharmacy staff and a similar table for the part-time employees in each category. Once the proposed annual salary for each employee is determined, the cost of new positions is added and finally any overtime which, according to past experience may be necessary, is also added. This, then, represents the total anticipated salary and wage expenditure for the next fiscal year.

EXPENSE ACCOUNT—SUPPLIES AND MATERIAL

In developing the supplies and expense portion of the budget, it is important for the department head to have available the dollar amount budgeted for each expense code for the fiscal year. It is also necessary to have available the latest financial statement showing the present actual cost of materials and supplies. From this, it is a relatively simple mathematical process to estimate what the actual expense will be for the present fiscal year. If the budgeted figure and the estimated actual figure agree, then the previously prepared budget was well done. On the other hand, if these two figures are too far apart, it indicates that either there was an error in the calculation of the previous year's expense budget or something has occurred or is occurring in the present fiscal year which was not anticipated and, therefore, needs investigation and evaluation.

If the department is to be involved in an expansion program of service, *i.e.,* dispensing to new clinics, opening of a new wing, etc., then the Pharmacist-in-Chief should ascertain the cost of the materials and supplies to be consumed by the new program and so provide for it in the new budget.

From the above discussion, it would appear that the department of pharmacy is required to keep rather detailed records in order to arrive at the figures requested by the budget. Although it is highly desirable to accumulate one's own statistical data, it is common practice for the pharmacist to rely upon the accounting department for many of his base figures. Therefore, there should be developed a close rapport between the Pharmacist-in-Chief and the Comptroller.

EQUIPMENT AND CONSTRUCTION BUDGET

In hospitals where funding of the depreciation of physical plant and equipment is practiced, the actual cash for replacement or remodeling is usually readily available. In those hospitals where funding is not a policy, then construction and purchase of equipment creates a major financial burden requiring the development of a comprehensive and detailed budget.

However, irrespective of the policy with regard to funding, an equipment and construction budget must be prepared. Many hospitals require that any price of equipment with a unit cost of $500 or more is considered to be "capital equipment" and must be included in this portion of the budget. By the same reasoning, any construction with a total cost which exceeds $500 is considered "major" and must also be included in this section of the budget. Although the figure of $500 appears to be quite low, it is usually intentionally set at this level in order to exert greater control.

For the convenience of the reader, the following is a check list of depreciable equipment commonly found in the department of pharmacy[8] and which provides an indication of the "life" of the item.

DEPRECIABLE EQUIPMENT CHECK LIST

Professional Equipment	Life in Years	Professional Equipment	Life in Years
Balances	10	Meters, conductivity	25
Cabinets		Mixers, electric	10
Metal	20	Prescription cases, cabinets	15
Wood	15	Pumps, vacuum and pressure	10
Capsule machines	15	Refrigerators	10
Chemical hoods	10	Rinsers	10
Cleaners, pressure	15	Safe, Narcotic	25
Distilling apparatus	15	Scales	15
Drum hoists	15	Sterilizers	20
Filters (except glass)	10	Tanks	15
Homogenizers	15	Typewriters	5
Hot plates	10	Worktables	10
Labels, cabinet	15		

Administrative Equipment	Life in Years		
Adding machines	10	Clocks	15
Bookcases, metal	20	Desks, wood	15
Bulletin Boards	10	Filing Cabinets, metal	20
Calculators	10	Lockers, metal	20
Cash Registers	10	Worktables	10

During the budget preparation process, it is essential to prepare work papers that can be used to eliminate confusion and provide a good set of reference documents for later use. One way is to produce simple work sheets, for example, the supplies and expenses detail sheet (below). While there are far too many items to be listed individually, the central storeroom listing of inventory items will provide useful groupings, i.e., instruments, office supplies etc. for which an average cost and approximate usage can be determined.

SUPPLIES & EXPENSE DETAIL

Department _____ Account Code _____ Date _____

Item	Unit Cost ×	Inflation = Index	Projected × Unit Cost	Projected = Ann. Usage	Projected Ann. Cost

Another example is the travel budget request form which provides an accurate record of this type of activity for use by the department after it has ceased to be useful in the budget preparation.

TRAVEL BUDGET REQUEST

Department ————————— Account No.   ————————— Date ———————

Prepared By: ——————————————————

Name and Position of Traveler	Destination	Purpose of Trip	Days Away	Budget Request

SELECTED READINGS

Silverman, H.M.: Financial Fundamentals for the Hospital Pharmacist. Current Concepts in Hospital Pharmacy Management, 4:2:9, (Summer) 1982.

Poniatowski, J.J., Hanan, Z.I., and Mason, R.H.: A Method of Substantiating the Projections for a Drug Budget. Current Concepts in Hospital Pharmacy Management, 4:1:15, (Spring) 1982.

REFERENCES

1. Hahn, Jack, A.L.: Budgetary Reporting and Management Action, Hospitals. J.A.H.A., 37:46, (Mar.) 1963.
2. Larson, L.N.: Political Aspects for Budgeting in Hospitals. Am. J. Hosp. Pharm., 34:4:387, (Apr.) 1977.
3. Bicket, W.J. and Gagnon, J.P.: Purchase and Inventory Control for Hospital Pharmacies. Topics in Hospital Pharmacy Management, 111–15, 1981.
4. Hawkins, B.: Nature Of and Reasons for Cost Increases Under Scrutiny. Hospitals, 51:113–116, 1977.
5. Lilly Hospital Pharmacy Survey '81. Indianapolis, Eli Lilly Company, 1981.
6. Sok, J.E.: DRGs: Whats In For Pharmacy. Current Concepts in Hospital Pharmacy, 6:3:9, (Fall) 1984.
7. Chart of Accounts for Hospitals, 1976, Chicago, American Hospital Association.
8. Uniform Chart of Accounts and Definition for Hospitals, Chicago, American Hosp. Association, pp. 117, 163 and 168.

9

Purchasing and Inventory Control

The purchase and inventory control of pharmaceuticals is a special and important phase of the operation of a successful hospital pharmacy.

A portion of the purchases, controlled drugs and alcohol, is rigidly controlled by Federal regulations which in reality provide the means for accurate purchase and inventory control. These two classes of products, however, constitute a relatively small portion of the over-all purchases of an institutional pharmacy. Therefore, the purchase and control of the largest segment of the inventory is left to the administrative staff of the hospital or its duly authorized delegates.

In most general hospitals with an out-patient clinic operation, a pharmacy inventory of $100. to $200. per bed may be considered reasonable. However, many pharmacies, particularly those associated with the large teaching hospitals, include in their inventory parenteral and irrigating fluids, surgical dressings, rubber goods, sutures, surgical instruments, syringes and laboratory supplies. Clearly then, the dollar value of the inventory when expressed in dollars per bed may vary depending upon the variety of the inventory as well as the activity of the institution. In general, the pharmacy inventory should be adapted to the individual hospital's needs taking into consideration its distance from a source of supply, storage facilities, and rapidity of inventory turn-over.[1]

In view of the fact that, throughout this discussion, three words "purchase," "inventory" and "control" will be in constant use, it is felt that these terms should be defined.

The word *purchase*, as defined in the dictionary, has numerous meanings, the most appropriate being—"to obtain by paying money or its equivalent; to buy for a price."

The word *inventory* is defined as—"an itemized list of goods with their estimated worth; specifically an annual account of stock taken in any business."

The word *control* is defined as follows—"to exercise, directing, guiding, or retraining of power over."

193

Purchasing Agent vs. Pharmacist

The hospital literature is replete with articles dealing with the question, "Should pharmaceutical and related products be purchased by the purchasing agent or the pharmacist?"

One school believes that all institutional purchasing should be centralized under the aegis of the purchasing agent. According to this system the pharmacist, like all other department heads, requests, on a special form, the item to be purchased. The selection of the brand and vendor is thereby left to the discretion of the purchasing agent, unless the pharmacist has prepared a list of specifications which may or may not restrict the selection to the product of a particular manufacturer. This system has certain control and economic merits and can function within the hospital. It must, however, depend upon the close cooperation between the pharmacist and purchasing agent. Each must be aware of the definite contribution which he can make to such a specialized purchase.

The other school believes that pharmaceuticals and related items constitute specialties which require the technical skills of a formally trained individual for their proper selection and purchase.[2]

A leading advocate of this school was Dr. Malcolm T. MacEachern who in his text[3] stated:

". . . the purchase of drugs and pharmaceuticals is a specialty which can be carried out to the best advantage by a pharmacist trained in managing a hospital pharmacy. . . . This is the only department in the hospital in which it is usually *not* advisable to have purchasing done by a general purchasing agent."

One of the principles enunciated in the American Society of Hospital Pharmacist' *Minimum Standard for Pharmacies in Hospitals*[4] is that ". . . the pharmacist in charge shall be responsible for specifications both as to quality and source for purchase of all drugs, chemicals, antibiotics, biologicals and pharmaceutical preparations used in the treatment of patients. . . "

This same document under the section on *Elaboration of Responsibilities* goes on to state that

. . . . "The pharmacist should furnish specifications for the purchase of all drugs, chemicals and pharmaceutical preparations even though a purchasing agent may do the actual procurement through a centralized department.

Since the pharmacist has the responsibility for the compounding, dispensing and manufacture of the drugs used in the hospital he should also have the authority to specify the drugs to be purchased. In large institutions with centralized purchasing, the pharmacist and the purchasing agent should work hand-in-hand, each recognizing the importance of the function of the other. In such a system it is essential that the pharmacist state the specifications for drugs to be purchased and to have authority to reject any article below standard or not complying with specifications so that the purchasing agent may be guided and assisted in his function. The pharmacist will also, in certain instances, wish to consult with the Pharmacy and Therapeutics Committee concerning specifications for drugs."

Franck[5] writing editorially states that "in the application of this principle, the pharmacist is made, in effect, the agent of the medical staff and of the hospital for the specification of medicinal agents. Justification for this lies in the fact that since the pharmacist has the responsibility for the compounding, dispensing and manufacturing of drugs in the hospital, he should also have the authority for the specifications of drugs to be purchased."

The hospital may follow the intermediate plan whereby the actual function of purchasing is retained by the purchasing department, and yet utilize the benefits of the technical knowledge of the pharmacist by permitting him to develop the necessary specifications for the purchase of the drugs and allied products.

The importance of a policy governing the procurement, drug selection and purchasing authority are clearly stated in the following excerpt from the ASHP Technical Assistance Bulletin on Hospital Drug Distribution and Control.[6]

PROCUREMENT: DRUG SELECTION, PURCHASING AUTHORITY, RESPONSIBILITY AND CONTROL

The selection of pharmaceuticals is a basic and extremely important function of the hospital pharmacist, who is charged with making decisions regarding products, quantities, product specifications and sources of supply. It is the pharmacist's obligation to establish and maintain standards assuring the quality, proper storage, control, and safe use of all pharmaceuticals and related supplies (e.g., fluid administration sets); this responsibility must not be delegated to another individual. Although the actual purchasing of drugs and supplies may be performed by a nonpharmacist, the setting of quality standards and specifications requires professional knowledge and judgment and must be performed by the pharmacist.

Economic and therapeutic considerations make it necessary for hospitals to have a well-controlled, continuously updated formulary. It is the pharmacist's responsibility to develop and maintain adequate product specifications to aid in the purchase of drugs and related supplies under the formulary system. The *USP-NF* is a good base for drug product specifications; there also should be criteria to evaluate the acceptability of manufacturers and distributors. In establishing the formulary, the pharmacy and therapeutics committee recommends guidelines for drug selection. However, when his knowledge indicates, the pharmacist must have the authority to reject a particular drug product or supplier.

Though the pharmacist has the authority to select a brand or source of supply, he must make economic considerations subordinate to those of quality. Competitive-bid purchasing is an important method for achieving a proper balance between quality and cost when two or more acceptable suppliers market a particular product meeting the pharmacist's specifications. In selecting a vendor, the pharmacist must consider price, terms, shipping times, dependability, quality of service, returned goods policy, and packaging; however, prime importance always must be placed on drug quality and the manufacturer's reputation. It should be noted that the pharmacist is responsible for the quality of all drugs dispensed by the pharmacy.

Records. The pharmacist must establish and maintain adequate record-keeping systems. Various records must be retained (and be retrievable) by the pharmacy because of governmental regulations; some are advisable for legal protection; others are needed for JCAH accreditation, and still others are necessary for sound management (evaluation of productivity, workloads and expenses, and assessment of departmental growth and progress) of the pharmacy department. Records must be retained for at least the length of time prescribed by law (where such requirements apply).

It is important the pharmacist study federal, state, and local laws to become familiar with their requirements for permits, tax stamps, storage of alcohol and controlled substances, records, and reports.

Among the records needed in the drug distribution and control system are:

- Controlled substances inventory and dispensing records.
- Records of medication orders and their processing.
- Manufacturing and packaging production records.
- Pharmacy workload records.
- Purchase and inventory records.
- Records of equipment maintenance.
- Records of results and actions taken in quality assurance and drug audit programs.

Receiving Drugs. Receiving control should be under the auspices of a responsible individual, and the pharmacist must ensure that records and forms provide proper control upon receipt of drugs. Complete accountability from purchase order initiation to drug administration must be provided.

Personnel involved in the purchase, receipt, and control of drugs should be well-trained in their responsibilities and duties and must understand the serious nature of drugs. All nonprofessional personnel employed by the pharmacy should be selected and supervised by the pharmacist.

Delivery of drugs directly to the pharmacy or other pharmacy receiving area is highly desirable; it should be considered mandatory for controlled drugs. Orders for controlled substances must be checked against the official order blank (when applicable) and against hospital purchase order forms. All drugs should be placed into stock promptly upon receipt, and controlled substances must be directly transferred to safes or other secure areas.

Drug Storage and Inventory Control. Storage is an important aspect of the total drug control system. Proper environmental control (i.e., proper temperature, light, humidity, conditions of sanitation, ventilation, and segregation) must be maintained wherever drugs and supplies are stored in the institution. Storage areas must be secure; fixtures and equipment used to store drugs should be constructed so that drugs are accessible only to designated and authorized personnel, such personnel must be carefully selected and supervised. Safety also is an important factor, and proper consideration should be given to the safe storage of poisons and flammable compounds. Externals should be stored separately from internal medications. Medications stored in a refrigerator containing items other than drugs should be kept in a secured, separate compartment.

Proper control is important wherever medications are kept, whether in general storage in the institution or the pharmacy or patient care areas (including satellite pharmacies, nursing units, clinics, emergency rooms, operating rooms, recovery rooms, and treatment rooms). Expiration dates of perishable drugs must be considered in all of these locations and stock rotated as required. A method to detect and properly dispose of outdated, deteriorated, recalled, or obsolete drugs and supplies should be established. This should include monthly audits of all medication storage areas in the institution. (The results of these audits should be documented in writing.)

Since the pharmacist must justify and account for the expenditure of pharmacy funds, he must maintain an adequate inventory management system. Such a system should enable the pharmacist to analyze and interpret prescribing trends and their economic impacts, and appropriately minimize inventory levels. It is essential that a system to indicate subminimum inventory levels be developed to avoid "outages," along with procedures to procure emergency supplies of drugs when necessary.

ROLE OF PURCHASING AGENT IN DRUG PROCUREMENT

The role of the purchasing agent in drug procurement may vary markedly from small to large hospitals. In the small hospital, the purchasing function may be a part-time one and may be handled by the administrator, an administrative assistant or the storekeeper. This, therefore, means that lack of time or pressure from other duties will cause the individual to restrict his activities in this function to a minimum.

In a large hospital, where the purchasing function is of such magnitude that it is a full-time position for one or more individuals, the purchasing agent may assume the following duties in relation to drug purchases:

1. issues purchase orders
2. maintains purchase records
3. follows-up on delayed orders
4. initiates competitive bidding procedures
5. obtains quotations from specified sources

ROLE OF PHARMACIST IN DRUG PROCUREMENT

The National Survey of Hospital Pharmacy Services[7] shows that in 87% of the hospitals surveyed pharmacists had the authority to select the brand supplier of the drugs dispensed; this is about 20% higher than in the 1975 survey. In addition, 72% of the hospitals were involved in group purchasing. This is nearly double the percentage in 1975.

Pharmaceuticals for hospital use may be purchased in one of the following ways:

1. by direct purchase from the manufacturer
2. by direct purchase from a wholesaler
3. by bid from either manufacturer or wholesaler[8]

4. by purchase from a local retail pharmacy (emergency purchases only)
5. by a contract purchase arrangement with the manufacturer (*e.g.* ampul contract or solutions contract)
6. by a contract purchase through a hospital purchase bureau or corporation.

The hospital pharmacist should acquaint the purchasing agent with the above avenues of drug purchasing. The choice of one over the other may be made by the pharmacist or left to the discretion of the purchasing agent.

With regard to bid purchasing, a word of caution needs to be interjected. If the bids for drugs are released to a select group of reputable manufacturers, then the lowest bidder should receive the purchase order and the hospital may be assured of receiving first-quality merchandise. If, on the other hand, the bids are released to all vendors requesting them, the lowest price does not always mean quality merchandise. Therefore, if this type of bid release program is to be employed, it is strongly recommended that some arrangement be made for the analytical and clinical testing of samples of the product. This testing program may be carried out by a local laboratory or by the hospital.

In addition to the above, the hospital pharmacist should, in collaboration with the purchasing agent, assume the following duties:

1. maintain a list of the names, addresses and telephone numbers of drug manufacturers, wholesalers, and their local representatives
2. prepare detailed specifications for drugs, chemicals and biologicals
3. prepare Request for Purchase Forms
4. prepare Receiving Memo if drugs are received directly by the pharmacy
5. prepare Return Goods Memo, whenever applicable.

With regard to the development of drug specifications, the hospital pharmacist should make liberal use of the latest editions of the *United States Pharmacopeia,* the *National Formulary* and their supplements. These compendia are officially referred to as the "U.S.P." and the "N.F."

PURCHASING PROCEDURE

The plan of purchasing procedures herein described assumes that there exist in the hospital a qualified pharmacist and a hospital purchasing agent who have been instructed to cooperate in the purchasing of pharmaceuticals and allied products. The plan further assumes that specifications have been drawn and that all supplies ordered will be received and stored either in the pharmacy or in the storeroom exclusively controlled by the pharmacist.

The pharmacist, or a person authorized by him, should complete a **Purchase Request Form** (Fig. 27) for the product desired. Drugs coming from the same vendor may be grouped upon a single form. This form provides the purchasing department with the data concerning the description, specification, packaging, price, quantity needed as well as information concerning the inventory balance and anticipated monthly use. In addition, this form also is the source document for information which is of importance to the accounting office, namely the cost center to be charged and the discount which may or may not be earned upon payment for the merchandise. The original of this form should be forwarded to the administrative officer responsible for the department. Upon his approval, the form is then forwarded to the purchasing agent. The copy is retained by the pharmacist as a record of the fact that the merchandise is in the process of being procured.

Upon the receipt of the approved Purchase Request, the purchasing agent should then prepare the official **Purchase Order** (Fig. 28). This form utilizes the data from the source document, the Purchase Request. The purchase order may take the form of any number of different types—it may consist of a two-page or a many page snap-out form. The majority of institutions prefer the multi copy snap-out form since it provides a copy for the vendor, accounts payable department of the

DATE TODAY

PURCHASE OR REPAIR REQUEST

PETER BENT BRIGHAM HOSPITAL   № 6605

☐ REPAIR OF EQUIPMENT
☐ PURCHASE

DEPARTMENT NAME | Account NAME - Charge to:

CHARGE CODE | SUGGESTED VENDOR

DATE NEEDED

PURCHASE DEPARTMENT USE ONLY
TERMS | PURCHASE ORDER NO. NO.

COMMODITY NO.	DESCRIPTION — SPECIFICATIONS — PACKAGING	PRICE PER UNIT	UNITS NEEDED	TOTAL PRICE	QUANTITY ON HAND DATE	QUANTITY USED PER MONTH

REQUESTED BY ______________ APPROVED BY ______________

Form 90

FORWARD WHITE COPY TO PURCHASING/MAINTENANCE. RETAIN PINK COPY.

Fig. 27. Purchase Request Form.

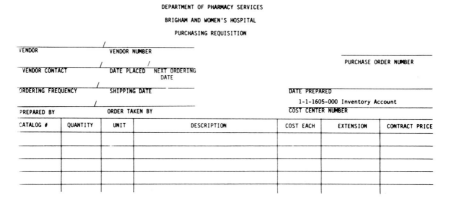

Fig. 28. Purchase Order Form.

hospital, purchasing number file, initiating department, two receiving reports and a history copy.

The vendor's copy is either mailed or given to the vendor's representative.

The accounts payable copy is forwarded to the accounting office where it is held until the invoice is received from the vendor and the completed receiving reports from the initiating department. Then and only then may the invoice be processed for payment.

Copy 3 is retained by the purchasing agent for his "number file." This will serve as a source of information to him whenever a question is raised relative to the issuance of the order.

Copy 4 is returned to the initiating department, in this case, the pharmacy. This copy should be matched with the Request for Purchase to check for accuracy.

Copies 5 and 6 serve as receiving reports and are sent to the receiving department. If the order is received in full, only copy 5 is required to be completed and forwarded to the accounting office. Should merchandise be back ordered, the second receiving report (copy 6) is utilized.

Copy 7 is known as the history copy and is retained by the purchasing agent for use in ascertaining rates of use, etc.

Some hospitals prefer to use a separate purchase order form and a separate Receiving Notice. The disadvantage in the use of this system is that the individual receiving the merchandise must record by hand the name of each item. This may cause error and, if rushed by the load of work, a delay in receiving the completed memo in the accounting office, thereby causing a loss of the discount for prompt payment.

This form also provides for copies for the accounting department, purchasing agent, initiating department, and storeroom files.

Whenever merchandise that has been received by the hospital is to be returned to the vendor for any cause, a Returned Goods Memorandum must be prepared, for it is by this means that the hospital can be assured of receiving credit for the merchandise. This form is of the snap-out type and provides for copies for the accounting department, purchasing agent, storeroom, initiating department and the vendor.

Once the merchandise is received, it is the duty of the pharmacist to record upon a **Purchase Record** (Fig. 29) the transaction for each item purchased. By so doing, he will have available a source of reference for determining rate of use, cost of drug, source, etc. Some pharmacists feel that this card should be maintained by the purchasing agent and made available to them whenever necessary. Whichever way the situation is to be handled is irrelevant so long as the card is prepared and kept up to date. The final decision as to whose responsibility it is rests with the desires of the administrator.

On occasion, merchandise may be ordered from the pharmacy at a time when it is out of stock. This may happen quite frequently in pharmacy departments handling surgical and laboratory supplies as well as drugs. When this happens, an **Out-of-Stock Form** (see Chapter 15, Fig. 62) should be prepared in duplicate and one copy sent to the initiating pavilion or laboratory. The other copy is retained in the pharmacy. This form serves a dual purpose in that it speeds the delivery of merchandise to the floor upon its arrival and it prevents the pavilion or laboratory from reordering and creating a false sense of heavy demand which could result in over ordering by the pharmacy.

CONTROLS ON PURCHASES

Many administrators attempt to exercise a power of control over the volume of purchases by the pharmacist by placing a dollar limitation on the purchase order. This method is archaic and is easily circumvented by the issuance of multiple small orders which in the long run is more costly for the hospital.

A more modern and reliable means is the *computation* of *inventory turnover.* Inventory turnover is computed by dividing the cost of goods

No.	VENDOR	No.	VENDOR	No.	VENDOR	No.	VENDOR
1		4		7		10	
2		5		8		11	
3		6		9		12	

Mo.	Yr.	Ven.	Ordered Quantity	Dept.	Price Per	Total Cost	RATE OF USE		
							From	To	Months

Fig. 29. A sample of a Purchase Record Form.

sold during the fiscal period by the average of opening and closing inventories. This gives the number of times the inventory has been "turned" during the fiscal period.[9]

A low turnover indicates:

1. duplication of stock
2. large purchases of slow-moving items
3. dead inventory

A high turnover of inventory may be due to small volume purchasing which is indicative of a failure to take advantage of the maximum quantity discounts.

A turnover of six to eight times a year is considered satisfactory for most institutions. However, those in short supply of cash reserves may wish to increase their turnover rate. This is a policy decision and should be arrived at by discussion with the administrator.

The Lilly Hospital Pharmacy Survey for 1984 revealed the following:[10]

a. the estimated turnover rate increased from 6.6 to 7.2 times.
b. hospital pharmacy managers have improved their turnover rate more than two full turns since 1977 (from 5.1 to 7.2 in 1983) suggesting that managers are continuing to exercise more control over inventory.
c. inventory investment rose 47.4% for an annual growth rate of about 6% for the recent 8-year period.
d. purchases grew at an annual rate of 15%.

Hospital pharmacists might well try to control purchase volume and inventory by the time of the EOQ (Economic Order Quantity) and RQL (Reorder Quantity Level).

The RQL is stated to be the inventory level that must be reached before additional stock can be ordered. Ideally, the remaining inventory should be almost depleted before the arrival of the new shipment. Obviously, zero stock level must be avoided because it can cause serious problems. This can usually be avoided by building into the system safety factors for various vendor lead times. Sapp[11] makes utilization of the following table:

SAFETY FACTORS FOR VARIOUS VENDOR LEAD TIMES

Vendor Lead Time (VLT)	Safety Factor
0 to 2 weeks	1.0
2 to 5 weeks	1.5
5 to 8 weeks	2.0
8 to 11 weeks	2.5
11 to 15 weeks	3.0

To determine the RQ, divide the **average usage** rate per month in units of issue (AU) by thirteen weeks; then multiply this figure by the average **vendor lead time** (VLT) plus the safety factor.

In the application of the above formula, Sapp[11] stressed the following points:

(1) Unanticipated large increases in usage.
(2) Shelf life of the items involved.
(3) Unusual delays in delivery caused by strikes or storms.
(4) Necessity for rechecking the RQL periodically to allow for a change in usage rate.

The determination of how much to order is the EOQ factor. In determining the EOQ factor it is important to ascertain the *cost of ordering* and the *cost* of *carrying inventory.*

The following must be considered in arriving at the *cost* of *ordering.*[11]

(1) All labor in purchasing except the purchasing manager.
(2) The labor cost in supporting areas such as the stockroom, receiving and material control.
(3) The cost applicable to payment of invoices generated by the purchasing section should apply to ordering cost.
(4) Cost of general operating supplies such as pencils, paper, forms etc.
(5) Freight and telephone costs.

After all of the above are applied to total cost, divide the resulting figure by the total number of purchase orders to obtain the *ordering cost* in *dollars per order.* Ordering cost per order can vary from $5.00 to $8.00.

To obtain item cost, divide average number of line items on purchase order into total ordering cost.

To determine carrying charges consideration must be given to the following.[11]

(1) Interest on the dollar value of the inventory.
(2) Space charge (rent) for the storage area.
(3) Labor costs for storage operations.
(4) Cost of supplies for storage operations.
(5) Insurance.
(6) Taxes (if applicable).
(7) Obsolescence.
(8) Deterioration.
(9) Pilferage.

Dividing the value of the average inventory by the total of the above costs results in the *inventory holding* or *carrying cost* for the particular inventory item. Thus, it may be advantageous to order expensive items on a monthly basis and inexpensive items annually. In general, carrying charges may range from 18 to 30%.

Thus the formula for determining Economic Order Quantity is the following:

$$EOQ = \sqrt{\frac{2 \times 12 \times \text{monthly usage} \times \text{cost of ordering}}{\text{Unit cost} \times \text{Holding Cost}}}$$

On the basis of the above equation, purchasing agents have developed nomographs to simplify figuring the EOQ.

QUALITY OF DRUGS

As has been stated above, the pharmacist should draw freely upon the specifications detailed in the *United States Pharmacopeia*, the *National Formulary* and their supplements.

Both the U.S.P. and the N.F. are designated as official compendia by the terms of the Federal Food and Drug Law and the Federal Food, Drug, and Cosmetic Act.

The *Pharmacopeia* and the *National Formulary* render "a distinct service to pharmacists and pharmaceutical manufacturers by providing specifications for the procurement of drugs used in dispensing, prescription compounding, and manufacturing, and supplying formulas and working directions for the preparation of dosage forms."[12]

During recent years, there has been a move towards the acceptance and use of the initials A.R.B. (Any Reliable Brand). Certainly, if there exists a situation where the prescriber believes in the use of these initials, well and good; however, these symbols should never be used by a hospital pharmacist or a hospital purchasing agent as a specification for quality merchandise. What one individual considers to be "reliable" may oftentimes be far from the truth. If any symbols are to be used as a means of specification then those of U.S.P. and N.F. are the safest and most reliable.

Oftentimes a hospital pharmacist may desire assistance in the selection of a product for use by the hospital. If the hospital has an active Pharmacy and Therapeutics Committee, this committee may serve as an advisor to the pharmacist. Because of the background and experience of the membership, it behooves the hospital pharmacist to give a great deal of weight to their suggestions.

Certain large hospitals in this country feel that it is more economical to purchase drugs from manufacturers who might not be listed in the "Class A group." The consensus being that these small firms do not have to support expensive research and large sales staffs, the savings can be passed along to the purchaser. This premise can be dangerous and should not be followed unless the hospital is in a position to establish a small control laboratory for the purpose of analyzing products purchased from these firms. Oftentimes the cost of operating such a laboratory will far exceed the cost of purchasing under tight specifications from a reliable manufacturer.

Some pharmacists utilize a *Qualified Suppliers List* which is based upon their personal knowledge and experience with the manufacturer and his products.[9]

Other pharmacists make use of a *Suppliers Application Form* to obtain information about prospective suppliers. The information requested includes the company's annual sales, a list of other accounts, the number of employees, type of operation, description of quality control procedures and the company's location and facilities. The use of this form is stated to discourage marginal suppliers and serves as a screening technique for the hospital pharmacist.[13]

DISCOUNTS

There are three ways in which merchandise may be purchased at a discount or savings: (1) volume contract, (2) "deals," and (3) discounts.

Volume contracts are usually offered by a majority of the manufacturers and include contracts to cover total purchases of parenteral solutions, ampoules, tablets or even gallon goods. Under this system, the institution approximates its annual consumption of the particular class of product and signs an agreement with the company to purchase this amount. At the end of the contract period, usually a year, if the goal has been reached, the manufacturer will issue a rebate check based on a percentage of the value of the total purchase. A hidden benefit of this type of purchase is the fact that the contract price is usually protected from an increase yet any reduction in price is passed on to the hospital.

"Deals" represent that type of transaction that involves the purchase of a specified volume and receiving certain merchandise at no additional cost (*e.g.* "Three free with the purchase of a dozen"). There is nothing wrong with this type of purchase if the "free goods" remain in the pharmacy inventory. In order that the inventory not be understated, the entry into the hospital inventory records should indicate that fifteen units were received for the price paid.

"Deals" which are created by the representative and the pharmacist without the full sanction of the manufacturer should be either avoided or carefully scrutinized by the Administrator or Comptroller since these offer a great temptation for dishonesty.

Discounts may accrue to the institution for the prompt payment of its drug bills. Because of the large volume of drug consumption, these discounts amount to a sizeable sum of money at the end of a year.

Other types of discounts are also available from the manufacturers, *e.g.,* discounts to government institutions or to educational institutions. Obviously, the hospital pharmacist should immediately investigate the discount policy of every new firm with which he deals.

CENTRAL STORAGE VS. PHARMACY STORAGE

The dichotomous storage arrangements of supplies is prevalent in many hospitals, although it is common knowledge that central storage is ideal.

The proponents of centralized storage facilities are quick to demonstrate the reduction in labor and record keeping, as well as the tight control afforded by centralization.

In contrast, it should be pointed out that the responsibility for the storage of drugs should be placed with competent individuals who have been educated, trained and licensed to handle pharmaceuticals. These individuals are the pharmacists.

In order that the pharmacist may properly supervise the storage of drugs, they should be stored in an area directly under his control. This allows him the freedom of stock arrangement, instituting of inventory controls, the adjustment of inventory based upon his knowledge of the prescribing trends of the staff and the preparation of inventory cost reports to management.

Therefore, all merchandise ordered by or for the pharmacy should be shipped directly to the pharmacy receiving area. Should the merchandise be received by the hospital post office or central storeroom, it should immediately be forwarded to the pharmacy in the unopened state.

Upon the receipt of the merchandise in the pharmacy receiving area, the department personnel then process it in the routine manner, namely, checking the receiving slip with the copy of the purchase order and preparing a receiving memorandum.

STOREROOM ARRANGEMENT

There is no definite rule specifying how a pharmacy storeroom should be arranged. Each individual may so arrange the area to meet both his and the institution's needs.

In general hospitals handling a variety of supplies, the storeroom is divided into the following areas.

1. Alcohol and Liquors
2. Capsules and Tablets
3. Chemicals
4. Gallon Goods
5. Narcotic Vault
6. Ointments
7. Biologicals and other cold room inventory
8. Laboratory Instruments
9. Surgical Instruments
10. Rubber Goods
11. Sutures
12. Medical and Surgical Supplies

Alphabetical arrangement is followed, where possible, within the section. Each shalf, drawer, or bin within the section is numbered to facilitate location of the item during the taking of a physical inventory as well as to locate the item for new personnel.

"SHELF-STRIPPING" AND "FLOOR-MARKING"

"Shelf-stripping" consists of applying a strip of tape to the front run of the shelf and marking upon it pertinent information relative to the product being stored. The usual information placed on the tape consists of the name and strength of the product, unit size, maximum level and minimal level, the re-order point being the minimal level.

Where adequate funds are available plastic or metallic strips may be applied to the shelving which will permit the insertion of a card bearing the essential data.

Another means of accomplishing the same goal is to attach the data card to the wooden shelf by means of a thumbtack or stapler.

"Floor-marking" consists of preparing a stencil with the necessary information and painting it on the storeroom floor. This is best done on concrete or wooden floors. In areas where the floor is tiled or marking the floor is not desirable, a good quality tape with adherability may be employed.

By so marking and identifying the storage areas, one provides a definite space for the storage of a particular product, induces orderliness and provides another means of checking inventory to prevent shortages.

MARKING OF MERCHANDISE

Management consultants all agree that money invested in drug inventories should have a turnover of four to five times a year. A turnover of less than four indicates overstocking and a turnover of more than five may indicate understocking.

One means of sound inventory control is to date and price each item when it is received into inventory. This may be accomplished by the utilization of a marking machine to print small adhesive-backed tags that contain the following information: date received, cost price, and the selling price.

The date is placed on the first line and consists of the month and year. This is usually numerically indicated as "6/80."

The second line represents the cost price of the particular unit. This figure is usually coded in order to preserve confidential price quotations. This figure is of great value in institutions where supplies are sent to areas at cost for it enables the dispensing pharmacist to immediately price the charge slips. In addition, the availability of this figure is of great value in taking and pricing a physical inventory.

The third line represents the retail price to the patient. By placing this figure on the tag, it is possible to save a great deal of time by having the dispensing pharmacist price the charge ticket without having to refer to a charge or rate book.

CONTROL OF DATED OR PERISHABLE INVENTORY

Dated inventory such as biologicals or antibiotics requires special control in order to insure potency at the time of dispensing and to be sure that the pharmacy is not carrying in inventory worthless stock.

This can be accomplished by the use of a form such as the **Record of Dated Pharmaceuticals** (Fig. 30).

Each dated product is entered on this sheet which provides the name of the product, the date of purchase, the manufacturer, the control number and the expiration date. By placing a check mark in the box of the appropriate month, the pharmacist can tell at a glance which product is expiring and should be replaced or returned for credit.

Some pharmacists prepare a separate sheet for each dated product. This modified sheet eliminates the need for re-writing the name of the product each time it is purchased. The remaining information and format remains the same.

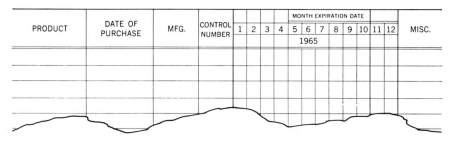

Fig. 30.

TAKING OF A PHYSICAL INVENTORY

The taking of a total physical inventory in the pharmacy is usually required by the auditing firm employed to audit the hospital's fiscal operation. Since the pharmacy inventory usually is the largest in dollar value, it receives a great deal of attention.

On the other hand, some auditing firms will require only a spot check type of inventory on 10 or 20% of the high-cost, fast-moving items.

The actual taking of a physical inventory cannot be undertaken without a great deal of planning and attention to detail. Anything less than one's maximum effort will lead to a faulty inventory and thus to a repeat performance.

Approximately 2 months before the taking of an inventory, the pharmacist should review his stock and remove from it all merchandise which has not moved since the last inventory. In addition, any merchandise should be removed which has been purchased during the year but has not moved appreciably during the preceding three months. These items should be returned for credit whenever possible; if such a move is not feasible, they should be written off the inventory via an adjustment in the books of account in the business office.

Once this has been accomplished, the inventory should be recorded on the inventory sheets. This recording should consist of only the name of the item, or other identification. The sheets upon which the recording is to take place should be in duplicate, and should have proper spaces to show the date, location, recorder and caller (Fig. 31).

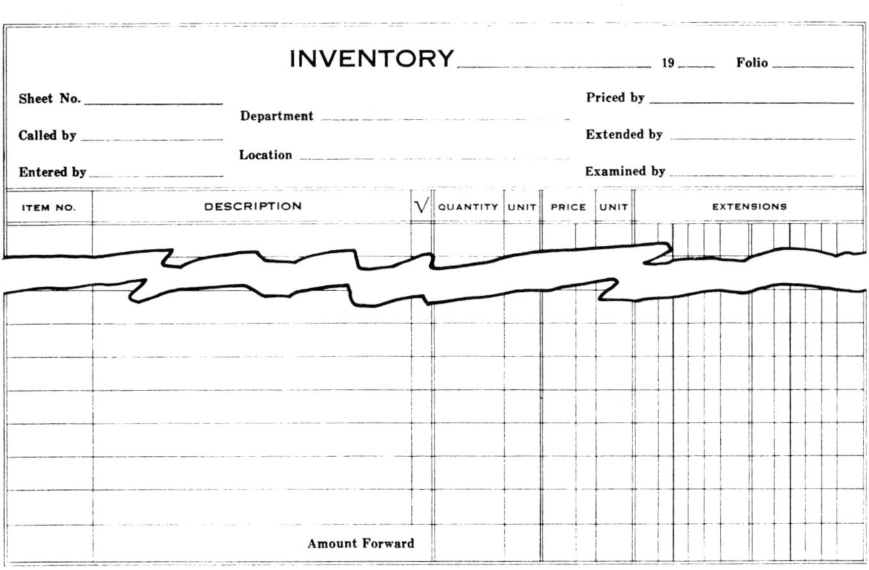
INVENTORY ______ 19___ Folio ______

Sheet No. ______
Department ______
Called by ______
Location ______
Entered by ______
Priced by ______
Extended by ______
Examined by ______

ITEM NO.	DESCRIPTION	√	QUANTITY	UNIT	PRICE	UNIT	EXTENSIONS
	Amount Forward						

Fig. 31. Sample form for the recording of the inventory.

The actual taking of the inventory may start at the close of a business day or at a time when there is no movement of merchandise. At this time the pharmacy staff and its helpers may arrange themselves into teams of two—one to record and the other to call out the name of the item, price, and count. As each sheet is completed, it is handed to the auditor supervising the inventory. It is the prerogative of the supervising auditor as to how many entries he wishes to check out. The usual procedure is to check all large dollar volume items and to random check the less valuable entries.

At the close of the inventory, the sheets may be turned over to the comptroller for extension, or this operation may be delegated to the pharmacist.

Any merchandise ordered prior to the date of inventory and received on the day of inventory or shortly thereafter need not be counted. The invoices pertaining to these purchases should be clearly marked with the fact that they were received "post inventory." The accounting office will make the appropriate adjustment in the final inventory figure to account for this merchandise.

THE PERPETUAL INVENTORY

The maintaining of a perpetual inventory is, of course, an ideal situation if the record-keeping can be kept up to date. In many small hospital pharmacies, the pharmacist, at the end of each day, summarizes all drug charge slips and makes the proper posting in the perpetual inventory file. The process of tabulation may be accomplished by either the pegboard method or the use of punched cards.

The pegboard method merely requires a pegboard and requisition forms with holes evenly spaced and punched along the top. The forms are then aligned on the board so that the first sheet is entirely visible and subsequent sheets covering all but the section showing the quantities ordered. The forms are then summarized across into one master requisition form which is used for posting the inventory records.

The larger and more complex operations require mechanized equipment such as that provided by the International Business Machine Corporation or the Remington Rand Corporation. The basic operations performed on this specialized equipment are key punching, verifying, sorting, collating, interpreting, calculating, tabulating and reproducing. These systems may utilize a punched card whereby the data are punched in the various fields in the body of the card.

By using this type of system it is possible to have purchase orders, receiving reports and disbursement requisitions forwarded to the tabulating department daily, where transaction cards are punched. These cards are then fed into calculators and tabulators which issue a comprehensive stock status report. This report may be produced on a daily, weekly or monthly basis.

The latest and most sophisticated system for electronic data processing is the computer.

With one of these systems, a hospital can readily obtain a record of all inventory items, and their balances in quantity and dollar value is maintained. Using item numbers already in use, the inventory record can show the following:

1. item number	6. disbursements
2. description	7. vendor number
3. unit size	8. price
4. quantity on hand	9. general ledger number
5. receipts	

The installation of either of these mechanized systems is highly technical as well as costly and therefore the institutional officers, comptroller and pharmacist should avail themselves of the counsel and advice of the various reputable manufacturers or consulting services before embarking upon such a program.

MATERIALS MANAGEMENT

To this point, purchasing and inventory control have been discussed from the viewpoint of the department of pharmacy—that is, complete control over the drugs by the pharmacist from purchase to disposition. In the operation of a modern hospital, it is still possible to provide the control feature even though part of the responsibility may rest in another person—the Director of Materials Management. In some hospitals, the Department of Materials Management has operational responsibility over purchasing, receiving, inventories, print shop, central sterile supply, laundry, distribution, messenger service, traffic and disposal activities.

Simply defined, materials management encompasses all materials and their movement from point of origin to point of use, and then to their final breakdown back into the environment.[14]

In those hospitals utilizing the materials management concept, it is not uncommon to find that the hospital pharmacist plays an important role in developing the program associated with the acquisition, storage, distribution and disposition of biologicals, radioisotopes, drugs and chemicals.

SELECTED READINGS

Anonymous: GAO Report on Hospital Purchasing and Inventory Management, Am. J. Hosp. Pharm., *36*:1169–1179, (Sept.) 1979.

Johnson, L.H. and Herrick, J.D.: Evaluating Group Purchasing Through a Prime Vendor. Am. J. Hosp. Pharm., *41*:1783–1788, (Sept.) 1984.

Rubin, H. and Keller, D.D.: Improving a Pharmaceutical Purchasing and Inventory Control System Am. J. Hosp. Pharm., *40*:67–70, (Jan.) 1983.

Daniels, C.E.: Managing the Inventory Control System. Am. J. Hosp. Pharm., *42*:346–551, 1985.

Lindley, C. and Mackowiak, J.: Methods of Inventory Control. Am. J. Hosp. Pharm., *42*:122–128, 1985.

Basic Techniques For Inventory Management, Technical Advisory Bulletin—1980, American Hospital Association, Chicago, Ill. 60611.

REFERENCES

1. Ambrose, J.M.: Organizing Pharmacy Purchases in a Small Hospital. Hosp. Pharm., *15*:1:17, (Jan.) 1980.
2. Hassan, William E. Jr.: Purchase and Inventory Control of Pharmaceuticals. Hospital Progress, October, 1958.
3. MacEachern, Malcolm T.: *Hospital Organization and Management,* 3rd Ed. Chicago, Physicians' Record Co., 1957.
4. Minimum Standard for Pharmacies in Hospitals. Am. J. Hosp. Pharm., *15*:11:992, 1958.
5. Francke, D.E.: Editorial, Am. J. Hosp. Pharm., *13*:2:107, 1956.
6. ASHP Technical Assistance Bulletin on Hospital Drug Distribution and Control. Am. J. Hosp. Pharm., *37*:1097–1103, (Aug.) 1980.
7. Stolar, M.H.: National Survey of Hospital Pharmacy Services—1978. Am. J. Hosp. Pharm., *36*:316–325, (Mar.) 1979.
8. Swift, R.G.: Bid Purchasing of Pharmaceuticals. Am. J. Hosp. Pharm., *35*:1390–1392, (Nov.) 1978.
9. Bowles, G.C. Jr.: Consulting with Bowles. Am. J. Hosp. Pharm., *15*:9:818, 1958.
10. *Lilly Hospital Pharmacy Survey 1984,* Indianapolis, Eli Lilly & Co.
11. Sapp, Donald E.: How We Use EOQ and RLQ for Better Inventory Control. Health Institution Purchasing, *2*:3:24, (Oct.) 1971.
12. *The National Formulary,* 12th Ed., Easton, Mack Printing Co., 1965.
13. Drake, Charles E. and Kabat, Hugh F.: A Quality Assurance Program for Pharmaceutical Purchases. J.A.Ph. A., NS*11*:11:612, (Nov.) 1971.
14. Miller, James G.: Materials Management: Some Guidelines. Hospital Care, *3*:3:17, (Nov.) 1972.

10

Medical Service Representative-Pharmacist Relationship

Each year the pharmaceutical industry budgets millions of dollars for the purpose of promoting their products. A sizeable portion of this allocation is devoted to providing the profession with well-trained detailmen or medical service representatives. One of the duties of these people is to carry on a large-scale educational program relative to the use of the latest therapeutic agents. This is usually achieved in hospitals through the media of drug exhibits and "detailing" of the chief of the pharmacy service and physicians.[1]

In a recent survey, it was shown that 92% of the physicians interviewed stated that they saw "some" or "all" detailmen.[2] Of interest to the hospital pharmacist is the further statistic that in answer to the question—Has the Detailman's Contribution Increased or Lessened in the Past Five Years?—30 physicians answered "increased," 29 answered "lessened" and 28 answered "same."[2]

By the same token, there must be rapport between the pharmacist and the detailman. That this does not always exist is supported by such derogatory opinions as—"nothing but order takers"; "detailmen have generally poor attitude"; and "not told what is being detailed."[3]

Although it behooves the manufacturer to exercise extreme care in the selection of his field representative, it is imperative that the hospital pharmacist develop appropriate rapport with the detailman in order that the hospital and medical staff might benefit from his specialized knowledge.

Hospital displays are desirable since they offer a convenient means of contacting a large number of staff physicians in a minimal amount of time. Furthermore, there is, by this approach, a saving of the physician's valuable time when compared to an office visit by the same medical representative.

Many hospital administrators frown upon drug exhibits on the grounds that they promote an aura of commercialism in an otherwise highly professional atmosphere. To avoid the "taunt of commercialism," it behooves the hospital pharmacist to develop basic policies for the conduct of detailmen within the hospital and guiding principles for scheduling drug exhibits.

The relationship between the hospital and the manufacturer can be enhanced if the pharmacist responsible for the purchasing function will take the time to review with the marketing representative the following ASHP Guidelines for Selecting Pharmaceutical Manufacturers and Distributors.[4]

ASHP GUIDELINES FOR SELECTING PHARMACEUTICAL MANUFACTURERS AND DISTRIBUTORS[a]

Preamble

Pharmacists are responsible for selecting, from the hundreds of manufacturers and suppliers of drugs, those that will enable them to fulfill an important obligation: assuring that their patients receive pharmaceuticals and related supplies at the lowest cost consistent with high quality. These guidelines are offered as an aid to the pharmacist in achieving this goal.

Obligations of the Supplier

Pharmacists may purchase with confidence the products of those companies meeting the critera presented below. It should be noted that other factors such as credit policies, delivery times, and the breadth of a company's product line must also be considered in selecting a supplier.

Technical Considerations

1. Upon request of the pharmacist (via the ASHP Drug Product Information Request Form[b]), the supplier should furnish analytical control, sterility testing and bioavailability data, descriptions of testing, procedures for raw materials and finished products, or any other information which may be indicative of the quality of a given finished drug product. This information should be supplied at no charge.
2. There should be no history of recurring product recalls indicative of deficient quality control procedures.
3. The company should permit visits (during normal business hours) by the pharmacist to inspect its manufacturing and control procedures.

---

[a]Approved by the ASHP Board of Directors at its meeting of November 17–18, 1983. Supersedes an earlier version approved by the Board of Directors in 1975. Developed initially and revised by the ASHP Council on Clinical Affairs.

[b]Available from the American Hospital Formulary Service, 4630 Montgomery Avenue, Bethesda, MD 20814.

4. All drug products shipped to the hospital should conform to the requirements of the most recent USP-NF unless otherwise specified by the pharmacist. Items not recognized by the USP-NF should meet the specifications set forth by the pharmacist.
5. All single unit packages of drugs should conform to the ASHP Technical Assistance Bulletin on Single Unit Packages of Drugs.
6. The name and address of the fabricator of the final dosage form should be present on the product labeling.
7. Expiration dates shall be clearly indicated on the package label and, unless stability properties warrant otherwise, should be dated January or July.
8. Therapeutic, biopharmaceutic, and toxicologic information should be available to the pharmacist upon request. Toxicity information should be available around the clock.
9. Patient and staff educational materials that are important for proper use of the product should be routinely available.

Distribution Policies

1. Whenever possible, delivery of a drug product should be confined to a single lot number.
2. Unless otherwise specified or required by stability considerations, not less than a 12-month interval between a product's time of delivery and its expiration date shall be present.
3. The supplier should accept for full credit (based on purchase price), without prior authorization, any unopened packages of goods returned within 12 months of the expiration date. Credits should be in cash or applied to the institution's account.
4. The supplier should ship all goods in a timely manner, freight prepaid, and enclose a packing slip with each shipment. All items "out of stock" should be noted and the anticipated availability of the item should be clearly indicated. There should be no extensive recurrence of back orders.
5. The supplier should warrant title to commodities supplied by him, warrant them free from defects and imperfections, and fit for any rational use of the product, and indemnify and hold the purchaser harmless against any and all suits, claims and expenses, including attorneys' fees, damages and injuries or any claims by third parties relating to his product.

Marketing and Sales Policies

1. The supplier should furnish, upon written request of the pharmacist, proof of any claims made regarding the efficacy, safety, and superiority of its products.
2. The supplier shall not, without the written consent of the pharmacist and administrator, use the pharmacist's or institution's name in any advertising or other promotional materials or activities.
3. A reasonable quantity of the supplier's products should be available, for evaluative purposes, upon request of the pharmacist, at no cost to the institution.
4. The supplier's sales representatives shall comply with the institution's regulations governing their activities if such regulations are in force at the institution.
5. The supplier shall not offer cash, equipment, or merchandise to the institution or its staff as an inducement to purchase its products.

6. Discounts should be in cash, not merchandise, and should be clearly indicated on invoices and bills, rather than consisting of end-of-year rebates or similar discount practices.
7. In entering into a contract to supply goods to the institution, the supplier should guarantee to furnish, at the price specified, any minimum amount of products so stated. If the supplier is unable to meet the supply commitment, he should reimburse the institution for any excess costs incurred in obtaining the product from other sources. If, during the life of the contract, a price reduction is announced, the lower price shall prevail.
8. All parties to the bidding process should respect the integrity of the process and the contracts awarded thereby.

Responsibilities of the Purchaser

It may be desirable to purchase drugs or other commodities on a competitive bid basis. The pharmacist should insure that competitive bidding procedures conform to the guidelines below:

1. Invitations to bid should be mailed to the companies' home offices with copies to their local representatives (if any), unless the company specifies otherwise.
2. Potential bidders should be given no less than three weeks to submit a bid.
3. The opening date for the bids shall be specified and adhered to by the institution.
4. The language of the invitation to bid form should be clear and concise, and the form should include the specific name and phone number of the person the bidder should contact in the event of questions or problems. Specifications should be complete with respect to products, packagings, and quantities desired.
5. If the bidder is to return the form to the institution, it should contain adequate space for the bidder to enter the information requested.
6. The winning bidder should be notified in writing and the unsuccessful bidders may be informed of who won the award and at what price, if they so request.
7. The quantities specified in the invitation to bid should be a reasonable estimate of the institution's requirements.
8. If the invitation to bid is offered on behalf of a group of institutions, the individual members should not engage in bidding procedures of their own and should purchase the goods in question from the winning bidder.

APPOINTMENTS

In order to carry on a successful professional relations program and to service hospital inventory requirements, it is necessary for the manufacturer's representative to make periodic visits to the pharmacy. Faced with a heavy work-load, a shortage of staff, or an unforeseen event, the pharmacist is prone to dismiss him with an "I'll see you the next time around." In other instances, the visit of the detailman is taken too lightly and the time devoted to the interview is rapidly utilized with needless "chit-chat."

After consideration of the above, it should be clear that the direct loser is the hospital pharmacist and the indirect loss is shared by the entire hospital staff. The hospital pharmacist must avail himself of the opportunity to draw upon the specialized knowledge of the detailman.

There are many ways in which this can be accomplished. Those most commonly employed are to arrange the detailman's visit on an "appointment only" basis, the use of a product information sheet, and the development of a controlled method of allowing demonstration and sales promotional displays within the hospital.

While it is relatively easy for the pharmacist to schedule appointments, it may place an undue hardship upon the detailman unless the scheduling is given some forethought.

One method of scheduling appointments is to divide the list of detailmen into three categories: (1) Those on a monthly basis, (2) Those on a bi-weekly basis, and (3) Those to be interviewed whenever they are in the territory.

For each representative in categories 1 and 2, a definite time should be assigned which coincides with the hours he expects to be in the particular section of the community in which the hospital is located. Once the schedule is established, it behooves each party to be prompt, and when necessary to cancel the appointment in advance.

Representatives in the third category must realize that they are being accorded a special privilege. They, therefore, have special obligations which are relatively simple. These entail the courtesy of notifying the pharmacist in advance of the approximate date and hour of the intended visit, and, conversely, the pharmacist should inform the representative of his ability to keep the appointment. Either of the above can be easily accomplished by postcard or telephone.

PROPER UTILIZATION OF APPOINTMENT TIME

Having established the routine for visitation, the pharmacist should use the time to best advantage. The nature of the division of time and the topics to be discussed rests with the pharmacist. As a guide, the allocated time may be divided into two units: (1) to discuss inventory needs, and (2) new products. It is in connection with the latter that the greatest amount of time can be saved. This can be accomplished through the use of a *Product Information Sheet* (Fig. 32). The required information can be recorded by the pharmacist while he is being "detailed" by the representative. Since the data on the sheet are concise, it serves as a valuable quick reference for pharmacists and medical staff. It may also serve the worthy purpose of providing the members of the Pharmacy and Therapeutics Committee with an "abstract" of a new product.

PRODUCT INFORMATION SHEET

Name _____   Mfg. _____

Generic Name _____

Chemical Name _____

Synonyms _____   _____   _____

Composition (if a combination)   Therapeutic Uses

_____ _____   _____

_____ _____   _____

_____ _____   _____

_____ _____   _____

_____ _____   _____

Contraindications and Cautions   Toxicology and Antidote

_____   _____

_____   _____

_____   _____

Dosage and Administration   Forms Available   Similar Products

_____   _____   _____

_____   _____   _____

_____   _____   _____

Package Sizes and Prices   Literature   ____Yes   ____No

_____   _____   Samples   ____Yes   ____No

_____   _____   Date:_____

This Space Reserved for Pharmacy and Therapeutics Committee.

Fig. 32

PROMOTIONAL DISPLAYS

The sponsoring of sales promotional displays within the hospital by pharmaceutical and medical supply representatives can be an interesting and worthwhile venture if properly controlled and supervised. One way to regulate these exhibits is to prepare a set of guiding principles governing displays; develop an application form which requests permission to conduct an exhibit; and finally place the total responsibility for the notification of the clinical and nursing staff of the exhibit as well as the supervision of the display upon the hospital pharmacist.

The rules for conducting the exhibit may vary with each institution, therefore, the following guiding principles are suggested as a model:

1. Demonstration and sales promotional displays by pharmaceutical and hospital supply representatives may be arranged by completing and having approved the "Request for Display Form" available from the pharmacy.
2. Displays or exhibits, for which application is made in the pharmacy, must be of a professional and ethical nature and must be related to hospital function.
3. All displays, not to exceed one per week, are presented in the staff room. Special group meetings, including film presentations, require arrangement through the executive offices.
4. Sales representatives and exhibitors are not permitted entrance to the various hospital departments without administrative approval: this includes the clinics, nursing stations, pavilions and operating suite.
5. Exhibitors must remain by their displays, and shall not solicit orders or approach persons who do not wish to view the displays.
6. Distribution of advertising in the form of samples and brochures must be confined to the display area, and only during the time reserved for the display or exhibit. Distribution of prescription legend items is allowed to physicians only.
7. Notices of any kind are not to be posted throughout the hospital by an exhibitor.
8. Displays and exhibits of each supplier are limited to two annually, and each to one-half day from 9:00 a.m. to 1:00 p.m.
9. Pharmaceutical products to be displayed are limited to those officially included in the latest revisions and supplements of the hospital formulary or those products accepted by the therapeutics committee for clinical trial in the hospital.
10. Representatives should have available a supply of reprints of clinical studies by qualified investigators of each product displayed.

The Request for Display forms (Fig. 33) should always be used because they serve a number of valuable control purposes. From the completed form, the pharmacist may determine exactly what is to be displayed and who is going to conduct the exhibit. In addition, reference to the copy of the Request for Display form will enable the pharmacist to determine whether or not the display of any particular product coincided with its increased use; the frequency of displays by any particular firm; and the frequency which an individual therapeutic category was featured.

Once the display is scheduled, the pharmacist should notify all clin-

REQUEST FOR DISPLAY

I, (We) do hereby agree to abide by the rules and regulations covering displays in the hospital, and request the following date to feature the items listed below in a display.

Date of Application:_____

Company:_____

Representative(s) Covering Display: _____

_____

_____

Display Date Requested:

    1st Choice_____   2nd Choice_____

Do You Need Display Equipment?   _____Yes   _____No

Products to be Displayed:

_____   _____   _____

_____   _____   _____

Display Approved By_____ Date:_____
Please prepare in duplicate. Return *both* copies to the Pharmacy. The approved copy will be returned to you and is your authorization to conduct the display.

Fig. 33

ical and nursing personnel of the date, hour and products to be exhibited. This notification can be accomplished in any number of ways.

1. General memo to clinical and nursing staffs.
2. Posting of a list of displays for the month or season in the Nursing Office and Staff Room.
3. Publication of the display dates in the Pharmacy Bulletin.
4. Specific letter to the Chief-of-Staff and to the Director of Nursing.

On occasion, the question arises as to whether or not the hospital should charge the manufacturer for the right to conduct displays on the hospital premises. The argument advanced is that a certain amount of administrative time is utilized in the scheduling and announcing of displays; guard services are utilized to deter unauthorized personnel or visitors from entering the display area; parking facilities are utilized; and hospital equipment such as tables or small trucks are used by the representative.

There is no single answer to the question. Certainly the above reasons are valid and if it is the policy of the hospital to rent space for various functions, then a rental for a pharmaceutical display is warranted. On the other hand, the donation of the above services and the space for a display provides a return to the hospital in the form of a well-informed staff on the latest developments in pharmacology and therapeutics.[1]

DEFINITION OF DRUG SAMPLES

The words "drug sample" would appear to be clearly self-explanatory, however, in order that there be no misunderstanding, the following definition is presented.

A drug sample may be considered as a quantity of any form of a chemical, drug or drug product which is made available by the manufacturer to an individual legally qualified to receive it. It makes no difference whether the drug is made available in an original trade package, or in a clearly identifiable sample package.

USE OF SAMPLES IN THE HOSPITAL

Any discussion governing the use of drug samples must, of necessity, be divided into two parts—for their use by the hospital and secondly, the use of samples by the manufacturer or his representative.

The use of drug samples in the hospital may be as varied as the imagination of the pharmacist in charge. One type of program that falls into this category and is worthy of mention is the pharmacist and the student nurse association "adopt" a hospital located in some remote part of the world and undertake to accumulate and ship the samples of its medical staff for distribution to their indigent patients.

In some hospitals, sample drugs are used in the care of the intern and resident staff as well as the students enrolled in the various nursing, dietary or technician training programs.

One pharmacist has gone on record[5] as recommending the availability of drug samples as a means of inducing widespread clinical use. Another[6] has described a method whereby drug samples are utilized in the care of the indigent ill irrespective of whether they were ambulatory clinic patients or admitted to the hospital.

Insofar as the manufacturer is concerned, drug samples are used as a means of introducing the physician to a new product and to induce him to try it clinically.

USE OF SAMPLES IN COMPETITIVE BUYING

Some manufacturer's representatives have used drug samples as a means of offsetting the company's higher price for a particular product, especially when competitive prices are lower. Whether or not this is ethical conduct on the part of the medical service representative and the hospital pharmacist is a difficult point to debate. Certainly those pharmacists who do not permit such transactions are to be commended and those who are prone to permit this practice under the guise that they are doing their job—namely, obtaining the best drugs available for the lowest net cost—should be cautioned to make every aspect of the negotiation open to the scrutiny of those in authority lest their individual integrity became the object of question.

CONTROL OF DRUG SAMPLES

Hospital mail rooms are deluged with drug samples. Often these samples are addressed to doctors no longer on the staff, and unfortunately the samples are often carelessly handled by the mail room personnel or the physician himself. It should be clear that any unsolicited drug sample entrusted to the general mail has a good chance of being discarded by the physician in such a manner that it unintentionally creates a hazard.

The hazard can be of many different types. (1) By disposing of the drug material into a wastebasket, it becomes readily available to cleaning personnel who may salvage it for the purpose of self-medication or for the illegitimate drug traffic. (2) Improper disposition of the baskets may mean that they could fall into the hands of children with disastrous results and (3) if incinerated by housekeeping personnel an explosion hazard is incurred, particularly if many vials or sealed containers of various drugs have been discarded.

The best place to control sample distribution in the hospital is at the source of the sample's entry into the institution—the detailman, drug displays and in the mail receiving room.

All detailmen or medical service representatives whether on private calls to physicians in the hospital or conducting displays should be fully informed of the hospital's policy governing the distribution of drug samples. Although a conscientious medical service representative will acquaint himself with the rules, it behooves the hospital pharmacist to call them to the attention of the representatives prior to each display request.

In brief, a good drug sample control policy would dictate that no samples may be left in the clinics, on the pavilions or nursing stations, nor may large quantities be left with physicians for the purpose of being dispensed by him for clinical trial.

Any physician desirous of using sample drugs for clinical trial should arrange to have the material deposited in the pharmacy from whence his prescriptions for the material will be honored. In this case the hospital may or may not collect a small handling fee from the patient.

Furthermore, the policy should also prohibit the distribution of drug products to hospital personnel even though the particular product to be distributed may have an over-the-counter status.

Some manufactureres have adopted an excellent policy in requiring the physician to write a prescription for the material requested, whereas others do not distribute samples during a display but will mail samples of the requested products directly to the physician.

Mass mailings to physicians in hospitals create problems in drug control, as these samples are or may be carelessly discarded and thereby fall into the wrong hands, or they are easily pilfered which awaiting distribution.

One way of mastering this problem is to have all mass handlings of drugs delivered directly to the pharmacy. Here, under the control of pharmacists,[7] the samples may be sorted and properly stored or, if necessary, adequately destroyed or discarded. Any physician desiring the sample material may obtain a reasonable supply from the pharmacy.

CATALOGUING OF DRUG SAMPLES

Once the packages of drug samples are delivered to the pharmacy, they should be sorted, exterior mailing cartons removed, catalogued and properly stored in a sample section. The pharmacist is reminded that sample drugs, like their purchased counterpart, should not have their control number identification removed as it may be the only means of identifying a particular batch of drug being recalled due to untoward side effects or reactions or possible error in preparation.

The cataloguing procedure should be reasonably detailed and accurate if it is to serve its purpose. The recording may be done on cards for storage in a card file or punched paper suitable for storage in a binder. Irrespective of the choice, the following data should be recorded for each drug sample received:

(a)	Trade Name	*(f)*	Control Number
(b)	Generic Name	*(g)*	Expiration Date (if any)
(c)	Manufacturer	*(h)*	Date Received
(d)	Strength	*(i)*	Quantity Received
(e)	Pharmaceutical Form	*(j)*	Location: Shelf #_: Drawer #_

Once catalogued and stored, any pharmacist removing a portion or the entire supply of sample must then record on the back of the page or card the following information concerning its disposition:

(a)	Date	*(c)*	To Whom
(b)	Amount Dispensed	*(d)*	Signature of dispensing pharmacist.

If the sample material is given to a physician his name is placed in the space after "*(c)* To Whom;" if a patient on a physician's prescription, then the prescription serial number is entered; if to a house patient, his name and hospital number should be entered.

EFFECT OF SAMPLES ON FISCAL OPERATIONS

Drug samples that are not obtained in the process of competitive buying are not usually considered a part of the pharmacy inventory.

However, if a relatively large volume of sample material is solicited and dispensed from the pharmacy, two obvious results may be immediately noted: (a) there will usually be a reduction in pharmacy income and (b) the volume of purchases will decline. The long range effect will invariably manifest itself by a reduction in the "turn-over rate" of the inventory.

On the other hand, if the drug samples are being dispensed to indigent patients, there should be a corresponding decrease in the allowances associated with the patient's inability to pay the hospital's bills for drugs.

Both aspects of the effect of the use of large amounts of drug samples on income, inventory and allowances have been briefly presented in order that the pharmacist may be forewarned of these possible repercussions.

CONTROLLED SUBSTANCES ACT OF 1970 ON SAMPLES

The Controlled Substances Act of 1970 amends the Federal Food, Drug and Cosmetic Act by placing additional controls over *stimulant and depressant drugs* through increased record keeping and inspection requirements providing control over intrastate traffic in these drugs, and making possession of them illegal except under certain specified conditions. (See Chapter 16.)

SELECTED READINGS

Burkholder, D.: The Role of the Pharmaceutical Detailman in a Large Teaching Hospital. Am. J. Hosp. Pharm., *20*:6:274, 1963.

Eno, D.M. and Sperandio, G.J.: Drug Samples in Hospital Pharmacy: A Study of Distribution and Control. Am. J. Hosp. Pharm., *17*:11:679, 1960.

Grimm, John E.: Practical Aspects of Selecting a Pharmaceutical Purchasing Group. Topics in Hosp. Pharm. Mgt., *1*:2:49, (Aug.) 1981.

Yost, R. David and Flowers, David, M.: New Roles for Wholesalers in Hospital Drug Distribution. Topics in Hosp. Pharm. Mgt., *1*:2:61, (Aug.) 1981.

Gouveia, W.A.: Hospital Pharmacy and Industry—Conflict and Collaboration. Am. J. Hosp. Pharm., *41*:1391–1394, 1984.

REFERENCES

1. Hassan, William E., Jr.: Pharmaceutical Detailman—Liability or Asset? Hospital Management, *88*:1:40, 1959.

2. Anonymous: The Physician and the Detailman. Medical Marketing & Media, *4*:4:8, (April) 1969.
3. Lecca, Pedro J., Gold, Stuart, and Smith, Mickey C.: Pharmacists' Response to a Program to Improve Pharmacist-Manufacturer Relations. J.A.Ph.A., NS*11*:11:592, (Nov.) 1971.
4. ASHP Guidelines for Selecting Pharmaceutical Manufacturers and Distributors. Am. J. Hosp. Pharm., *41*:331–332, 1984.
5. Moravec, D.F.: Drug Samples. Hosp. Management, *86*:102, (Nov.) 1958.
6. Jeffrey, L.P.: A Method for the Control of Drug Samples. Bull. Am. Soc. Hosp. Pharm., *14*:415, (July–Aug.) 1957.
7. Accreditation Manual For Hospitals—AMH 85, p. 119, Joint Commission on Accreditation of Hospitals, Chicago, Ill. 60611.

11|

The Pharmacy Procedural Manual

Journals and texts concerned with the broad subject of management are replete with articles and chapters on the importance of written policies as a managerial control tool. The hospital, in general, and the pharmacy, in particular, should have written policies for a number of reasons:

(a)   They serve as a guide for the training of new employees.
(b)   They prevent error resulting from the verbal transmission of the policy from one employee to another.
(c)   They insure the fact that the same policy will apply in all like situations.
(d)   They serve as a control tool in ensuring a defined procedure for performing a task, thereby eliminating waste of materials through error or carelessness.
(e)   In the hands of the supervisor, they serve as a means of evaluating job performance.
(f)   In a legal suit, they may serve as an important element in the hospital's defense of an action in tort arising out of a pharmacy error.

The management of the department of pharmacy in the hospital utilizes the same concepts which are commonly utilized in industry; namely, the pharmacist-in-chief as the manager or supervisor must coordinate people, supplies and equipment in such a manner as to produce efficiently an end-product which in the case of a hospital pharmacy is efficient and economical drug service.

Because of the number of people who may become involved, as well as the myriad of processes which must be utilized and controlled, the manager should, for the sake of uniformity and control, record the policy and technics in a manual.

Unfortunately, too many hospital pharmacists do not develop a policy manual for a number of reasons, the most common of which may be simple procrastination or lack of appreciation of its value. In other instances, it may be due to a false sense of security resulting from the belief that if no one else knows how to do a particular job, the individual who does know how is an indispensable being. And finally, the plain truth in many instances is the fact that many pharmacists do not even know what a procedural manual is nor how to commence work for its development.

The importance of a policy and procedural manual is stressed by the following excerpt from the ASHP Technical Assistance Bulletin on Hospital Drug Distribution and Control.[1]

POLICY AND PROCEDURES MANUALS' STATEMENT FROM ASHP TECHNICAL ASSISTANCE BULLETIN ON HOSPITAL DRUG DISTRIBUTION AND CONTROL

Policy and Procedure Manuals. The effectiveness of the drug control system depends upon adherence to policies (broad, general statements of philosophy) and procedures (detailed guidelines for implementing policy). The importance of an up-to-date policy and procedure manual for drug control cannot be overestimated. All pharmacy staff must be familiar with the manual; it is an important part of orientation for new staff and crucial to the pharmacy's internal communication mechanism. In addition, preparing written policies and procedures requires a thorough analysis of control operations; this review might go undone otherwise.

Drug control begins with the setting of policy. The authority to enforce drug control policy and procedures must come from the administration of the institution, with the endorsement of the medical staff, via the pharmacy and therapeutics (P&T) committee and/or other appropriate committee(s). Because the drug control system interfaces with numerous departments and professions, the P&T committee should be the focal point for communications relating to drug control in the institution. The pharmacist, with the cooperation of the P&T committee, should develop media such as newsletters, bulletins, and seminars to communicate with persons functioning within the framework of the control system.

In-service Training and Education. Intra- and inter-departmental education and training programs are important to the effective implementation of policies and procedures and the institution's drug control system in general. They are part of effective communication and help establish and maintain professional relationships among the pharmacy staff and between it and other hospital departments. Drug control policies and procedures should be included in the pharmacy's educational programs.

Standards, Laws, and Regulations

The pharmacist must be aware of and comply with the laws, regulations, and standards governing the profession. Many of these standards and regulations deal with aspects of drug control. Among the agencies and organizations affecting institutional pharmacy practice are those described below.

Regulatory Agencies and Organizations. The U.S. government, through its Food and Drug Administration (FDA), is responsible for implementing and enforcing the federal Food, Drug and Cosmetic Act. The FDA is responsible for the control and prevention of misbranding and of adulteration of food, drugs, and cosmetics moving in interstate commerce. The FDA also sets label requirements for food, drugs, and cosmetics; sets standards for investigational drug studies and for marketing of new drug products, and compiles data on adverse drug reactions.

The U.S. Department of the Treasury influences pharmacy operation by regulating the use of tax-free alcohol through the Bureau of Alcohol, Tobacco and Firearms. The U.S. Department of Justice affects pharmacy practice through its Drug Enforcement Agency (DEA) by enforcing the Controlled Substances Act of 1970 and other federal laws and regulations for controlled drugs.

Another federal agency, the Health Care Financing Administration, has established Conditions of Participation for hospitals and skilled nursing facilities to assist these institutions to qualify for reimbursement under the health insurance program for the aged (Medicare) and for Medicaid.

The state board of pharmacy is the agency of state government responsible for regulating pharmacy practice within the state. Practitioners, institutions, and community pharmacies must obtain licenses from the board to practice pharmacy or provide pharmacy services in the state. State boards of pharmacy promulgate numerous regulations pertaining to drug dispensing and control. (In some states, the state board of health licenses the hospital pharmacy separately or through a license that includes all departments of the hospital.)

Standards and guidelines for pharmaceutical services have been established by the Joint Commission on Accreditation of Hospitals (JCAH)[2] and the American Society of Hospital Pharmacists (ASHP).[3] The United States Pharmacopeial Convention also promulgates certain pharmacy practice procedures as well as official standards for drugs and drug testing. Professional practice guidelines and standards generally do not have the force of law, but rather, are intended to assist pharmacists in achieving the highest level of practice. They may, however, be employed in legal proceedings as evidence of what constitutes acceptable practice as determined by the profession itself.

In some instances, both federal and state laws may deal with a specific activity; in such cases, the more stringent law will apply.

The Joint Commission on Accreditation of Hospitals has created a standard for pharmaceutical services which mandates the preparation of written policies and procedures that pertain to the intrahospital drug distribution system.[2] The interpretation of this standard provides the hospital pharmacist with an appropriate guideline as to what must be included in the procedural manual in order for the hospital to be accredited. These are hereinafter reproduced but the student is referred to other sections of this chapter for concepts in format and sample policies.

Drug preparation and dispensing shall be restricted to a licensed pharmacist, or to his designee under the direct supervision of the pharmacist. A pharmacist should review the prescriber's order, or a direct copy thereof, before the initial dose of medication is dispensed (with the exception of emergency orders when time does not permit). In cases when the medication order is written when the pharmacy is "closed" or the pharmacist is otherwise unavailable, the medication order should be reviewed by the pharmacist as soon thereafter as possible, preferably within 24 hours.

The use of floor stock medications should be minimized; the unit dose drug distribution system, which permits identification of the drug up to the point of administration, is recommended for use throughout the hospital.

Written policies and procedures that are essential for patient safety and for the control, accountability, and intrahospital distribution of drugs shall be reviewed annually, revised as necessary, and enforced. Such policies and procedures shall include, but not be limited to, the following:

- All drugs shall be labeled adequately, including the addition of appropriate accessory or cautionary statements, as well as the expiration date when applicable.
- Discontinued and outdated drugs, and containers with worn, illegible, or missing labels, shall be returned to the pharmacy for proper disposition.
- Only a pharmacist, or authorized pharmacy personnel under the direction and supervision of a pharmacist, shall dispense medications, make labeling changes, or transfer medications to different containers.
- Only prepackaged drugs shall be removed from the pharmacy when a pharmacist is not available. These drugs shall be removed only by a designated registered nurse or a physician, and only in amounts sufficient for immediate therapeutic needs. Such drugs should be kept in a separate cabinet, closet, or other designated area and shall be properly labeled. A record of such withdrawals shall be made by the authorized individual removing such drugs and shall be verified by a pharmacist.
- There shall be a written drug recall procedure that can be implemented readily and the results documented. This requirement shall apply to both inpatient and ambulatory care patient medications.
- Drug product defects should be reported in accordance with the ASHP-USP-FDA Drug Product Problem Reporting Program.
- Medications to be dispensed to inpatients at the time of discharge from the hospital shall be labeled as for ambulatory care patient prescriptions.
- A system designed to assure accurate identification of ambulatory care

patients at the time they receive prescribed medications should be established.

- Unless otherwise provided by law, ambulatory care patient prescription labels should bear the following information:

  · Name, address, and telephone number of the hospital pharmacy;
  · Date and pharmacy's identifying serial number for the prescription;
  · Full name of the patient;
  · Name of the drug, strength, and amount dispensed;
  · Directions to the patient for use;
  · Name of the prescribing practitioner;
  · Name or initials of the dispensing individual; and
  · Any required Drug Enforcement Administration cautionary label on controlled substance drugs, and any other pertinent accessory cautionary labels.

- In the interest of effective control, the distribution of drug samples within the hospital should be eliminated if possible. Sample drugs brought into the hospital shall be controlled through the pharmaceutical department/service.

Written policies and procedures governing the safe administration of drugs shall be reviewed at least annually, revised as necessary, and enforced. Such policies and procedures shall include, but not necessarily be limited to, the following:

- Drugs shall be administered only upon the order of a member of the medical staff, an authorized member of the house staff, or other individual who has been granted clinical privileges to write such orders. Verbal orders for drugs may be accepted only by personnel so designated in the medical staff rules and regulations and must be authenticated by the prescribing practitioner within the stated period of time.
- All medications shall be administered by, or under the supervision of, appropriately licensed personnel in accordance with laws and governmental rules and regulations governing such acts and in accordance with the approved medical staff rules and regulations.
- There shall be an automatic cancellation of standing drug orders when a patient undergoes surgery. Automatic drug stop orders shall otherwise be determined by the medical staff and stated in medical staff rules and regulations. There shall be a system to notify the responsible practitioner of the impending expiration of a drug order, so that the practitioner may determine whether the drug administration is to be continued or altered.
- Cautionary measures for the safe admixture of parenteral products shall be developed. Whenever drugs are added to intravenous solutions, a distinctive supplementary label shall be affixed to the container. The label shall indicate the patient's name and location; the name and amount of the drug(s) added; the name of the basic parenteral solution; the date and time of the addition; the date, time, and rate of administration; the name or identifying code of the individual who prepared the admixture; supplemental instructions; and the expiration date of the compounded solution.
- Drugs to be administered shall be verified with the prescribing practitioner's orders and properly prepared for administration. The patient shall

be identified prior to drug administration, and each dose of medication administered shall be recorded properly in the patient's medical record.

- Medication errors and adverse drug reactions shall be reported immediately in accordance with written procedures. This requirement shall include notification of the practitioner who ordered the drug. An entry of the medication administered and/or the drug reaction shall be properly recorded in the patient's medical record. Hospitals are encouraged to report any unexpected or significant adverse reactions promptly to the Food and Drug Administration and to the manufacturer.
- Drugs brought into the hospital by patients shall not be administered unless the drugs have been identified and there is a written order from the responsible practitioner to administer the drugs. If the drugs are not to be used during the patient's hospitalization, they should be packaged and sealed, and either given to the patient's family or stored and returned to the patient at the time of discharge, provided such action is approved by the responsible practitioner.
- Self-administration of medications by patients shall be permitted on a specific written order by the authorized prescribing practitioner and in accordance with established hospital policy.
- Investigational drugs shall be properly labeled and stored, and shall be used only under the direct supervision of the authorized principal investigator. Such drugs should be approved by an appropriate medical staff committee. Investigational drugs should be administered in accordance with an approved protocol that includes any requirements for a patient's appropriate informed consent. On approval of the principal investigator, registered nurses may administer these drugs after they have been given, and have demonstrated an understanding of, basic pharmacologic information about the drugs. In the absence of an organized pharmaceutical department/service, a central unit should be established where essential information on such drugs is maintained.
- Orders involving abbreviations and chemical symbols should be carried out only if the abbreviation/symbols appear on an esplanatory legend approved by the medical staff. In the interest of minimizing errors, the use of abbreviations is discouraged, and the use of the leading decimal point should be avoided. Each practitioner who prescribed medication must clearly state the administration times or the time interval between doses. The use of "prn" and "on call" with medication orders should be qualified.
- Drugs prescribed for ambulatory care patient use in continuity with hospital care shall be released to patients upon discharge only after they are labeled for such use under the supervision of the pharmacist and only on written order of the authorized prescribing practitioner. Each drug released to a patient on discharge should be recorded in the medical record.
- Individual drugs should be administered as soon as possible after the dose has been prepared, particularly medications prepared for parenteral administration, and, to the maximum extent possible, by the individual who prepared the dose, except where unit dose drug distribution systems are used.

Unless otherwise provided by the medical staff bylaws, rules and regulations or by legal requirements, prescribing practitioners may, within their discretion at the time of prescribing, approve or disapprove the dispensing of a nonproprietary drug or the dispensing of a different proprietary brand to their patients by the pharmacist.

DEFINITION

A procedural manual may be defined as a series of administrative and professional policies which may serve as guide to the hospital pharmacist in the development and execution of effective and proficient pharmaceutical services in the hospital.

SCOPE

Of necessity, the scope of the pharmacy procedural manual must be as broad as that of the department which it is to serve.

Berenice[3] in describing operational manuals in hospital pharmacy provides an example of the comprehensiveness of a good manual:

"The first operational manual of any pharmacy department must contain the recorded development of the operation of the department from its very beginning, its objectives, philosophy, motivation, policies, regulations, departmental procedures, staffing pattern, job specifications, organizational plan and chart, floor plans, plot plans, description of the department, listing of physical facilities and library holdings, its intradepartmental, and interdepartmental relationships, description of its Formulary System, its Pharmacy and Therapeutics Committee and its activities, guidance manual for Internship and/or Residency Program in Hospital Pharmacy when such a program is offered. At the outset, one should give a short history of the institution and also state the purpose of the manual itself."

CONTENTS AND FORMAT

The organization of the wealth of administrative and professional policy material requires a great deal of thought and planning, for to do otherwise will result in a chaotic presentation which may complicate rather than elucidate matters.

Latiolais[4] has suggested that the procedural manual be divided into four general sections: Organization; Facilities; Personnel; Services and Activities, with this section being subdivided into an Administrative and a Professional division.

This concept is adequate and is recommended to those who may wish to organize and develop a procedural manual for their hospital pharmacy. One must, however, bear in mind that no two manuals or hospitals will have the exact same policy and, therefore, in some instances even this general classification will not suffice. For the purpose of this chapter, the four sections suggested above will be developed in order that the student may have some insight into the subject.

The following is a presentation of a format which may be readily adapted to a specific operation by any pharmacist.

The main sections are identified by a numeral from 1 to 4. Therefore, each subject under each main section is identified by the section number plus a second number to identify the subject. For example, the first topic under Organization would be identified by the numerals 1-1; the second by 1-2, etc.

In addition, the student is provided with a reasonably comprehensive check list under each main heading which will serve as a guide, as well as a reminder as to the type of subject material which might well fall within the scope of a particular section.

1. *ORGANIZATION*
    1-1. Organization of the hospital
    1-2. Organization of the pharmacy
    1-3. Services offered by the department
    1-4. Intra and Interdepartmental Relationships
    1-5. The Pharmacy and Therapeutics Committee
    1-6. The Antibiotics Committee

2. *EQUIPMENT and PHYSICAL PLANT*
    2-1. General policies relating to the use, maintenance and repair of equipment
        2-1-1. The distilled water still
        2-1-2. Ointment mill
        2-1-3. High speed mixer
        2-1-4. Variable speed mixer
        2-1-5. Homogenizer
            etc.
    2-2. Policy and procedure governing the loan of pharmacy equipment.
    2-3. Obtaining maintenance department services for the pharmacy.
    2-4. Obtaining engineering department services for the pharmacy.
    2-5. Policy governing the use of Central Sterile Supply Department autoclaves and sterilizers.
    2-6. Policy governing the use of laboratory equipment in control procedures.

3. *PERSONNEL POLICIES*
    3-1. Job descriptions
    3-2. Fringe benefits—General Policy
        3-2-1. Sick leave
        3-2-2. Vacation
        3-2-3. Holidays
        3-2-4. Jury duty
        3-2-5. Attending institutes, seminars or conventions
            etc.
        3-3-1. Hospital Employee Relations
        3-3-2. Discipline—Criteria for Warning, Probation and Dismissal

4. *SERVICES and ACTIVITIES*

  4-1. *ADMINISTRATIVE*
- 4-1- 1. Hours of operation
- 4-1- 2. Purchasing procedure
- 4-1- 3. Pricing policy
- 4-1- 4. Refund policy
- 4-1- 5. Handling of cash receipts
- 4-1- 6. Requisitioning of charge floor stock
- 4-1- 7. Requisitioning of non-charge floor stock
- 4-1- 8. Requisitioning of special patient charge drugs
- 4-1- 9. Requisitioning of ancillary surgical and medical supplies
- 4-1-10. Alcohol records and controls
- 4-1-11. Controlled substances records and controls
- 4-1-12. Inventory taking and its records
- 4-1-13. Compounding records
- 4-1-14. The monthly and annual report.
- 4-1-15. Drug Recall Program
- 4-1-16. Capital Expenditure Budget
- 4-1-17. Competitive Bid Policy
- 4-1-18. Policy re: Pharmaceutical Company Representatives
- 4-1-19. Policy re: After Hours Procurement of Drugs
- 4-1-20. Policy re: Drug Defects
- 4-1-21. Use of Approved Abbreviations in the Hospital
- 4-1-22. Policy re: Prescriptions—New and Discharge
- 4-1-23. Policy re: Prescription Refills
- 4-1-24. Policy re: Forged or Altered Prescriptions
- 4-1-25. Policy re: Nursing Responsibilities for the Management of Narcotics and Other Controlled Substances

  4-2. *PROFESSIONAL*
- 4-2- 1. Narcotic regulations
- 4-2- 2. Use of research drugs
- 4-2- 3. Automatic stop orders
- 4-2- 4. The Formulary System
- 4-2- 5. Policy governing drugs brought to the hospital by patients
- 4-2- 6. Labels and labelling
- 4-2- 7. Use of the metric system
- 4-2- 8. Prepackaging of bulk drugs
- 4-2- 9. Dispensing policies
- 4-2-10. On-call service
- 4-2-11. Bulk compounding (Formula, procedure, etc. for each product.)
- 4-2-12. Sterile compounding (Formula, procedure, etc. for each product.)
- 4-2-13. The residency training program in the hospital pharmacy
- 4-2-14. Poison Control Center
- 4-2-15. Information Services
    - 4-2-15-1. Pharmacy Library
    - 4-2-15-2. Pharmacy Bulletin
    - 4-2-15-3. Lecture Service
    - 4-2-15-4. Drug Displays
- 4-2-16. The addition of drugs to intravenous solutions by nurses.

SAMPLE BULLETINS FOR A MANUAL

The style of writing the procedural manual need not be restricted; it may be in outline form or in text style. The language used should be simple and direct. Verbosity should be avoided for the sake of clarity, brevity and safety.

Division 1–16
Bulletin -5-

Requisitions for Pharmacy Supplies

In order to account accurately for the distribution of Pharmacy supplies issued to the various hospital departments the proper requisition must be completed.

Ward Stock Medications must be requisitioned on Form No. 16.

Laboratory and Medical and Surgical Supplies must be requisitioned on Form No. 16a.

Prescription drugs for personal use must be requisitioned on Form 29-12-59.

All of the above requisition forms must be legibly and completely filled out including the proper code number to which the charge is to be made.

Division 1–16
Bulletin -6-

Hospital Prescriptions

Hospital policy requires that a prescription be written for any drug, prescribed for clinic patients, discharge patients, or employees regardless of its nature, which is to be issued from the Hospital Pharmacy.

As the Hospital Pharmacy is not a licensed retail drug outlet, and in order that the hospital may meet fully the requirements of the State Board of Registration in Pharmacy, all such prescriptions must be written on Hospital prescription blanks (white for discharge patients, yellow for clinic patients and employees).

Division 1–16
Bulletin -7-

Automatic Stop Order for Dangerous Drugs

1. *Controlled Substances:* Orders are automatically discontinued after 72 hours.
2. *Anticoagulants:* Low dose subcutaneous heparin (defined as less than 5000 units of heparin administered 2 hours before surgery and repeated every 8 to 12 hours thereafter) for primary prophylaxis of deep vein thrombosis is automatically discontinued after 7 days. Orders for all other anticoagulants are discontinued after 24 hours unless the physician indicates otherwise.
3. *Oxytocics:* Parenteral drugs are automatically discontinued after 24 hours unless physician indicates otherwise. Oral drugs are automatically discontinued after 72 hours.
4. *Post-operative medications:* All standing orders are cancelled when a patient undergoes surgery and must be reordered post-operatively.
5. *Other drugs:* All other drugs are automatically discontinued after seven days unless the physician indicates otherwise.

Your compliance with this policy will insure that your patient's drug therapy will continue uninterrupted and will obviate the need for a pharmacist to inform you that a medication is about to expire.

Division 1–16
Bulletin -8-

Separation of Internal Use Preparations from Those for External Use

The licensure rules and regulations for hospitals in Massachusetts specifically state that "poisons and medications for external use shall be kept in a separate compartment."

Accordingly, all drug supplies shall be arranged in such manner as to comply with the above regulation.

If you have any question as to what products should be classed in the category "poisons and medications for external use," please call the Pharmacist-in-Chief, Ext. xxx or the Associate Director, Ext. xxx.

Division 1–16
Bulletin   -10-

Pharmacy Hours

The Pharmacy is open during the following hours for use by both clinic and house patients.

Monday–Saturday . . . . 8:00 A.M.–9:00 P.M.
Sunday and Holidays . . . . 9:00 A.M.–9:00 P.M.

House patients requiring special medications after these hours may have them dispensed by the Nursing Supervisor from the Emergency Drug Cabinet.

The Nursing Supervisor may not mix or compound medications. Should this be necessary, the Nursing Supervisor shall call in the "on call" pharmacist.

A list of the "on call" pharmacists is maintained by the switchboard operator.

Division 1–16
Bulletin -11-

Intravenous Solutions, the Addition of Drugs by Nurses

1. The addition of drugs for intravenous administration to intravenous solutions is often most conveniently and expeditiously performed by the Nursing Service and may thereby facilitate patient care.
2. In all circumstances this may be performed only under specific written order in the appropriate order book by the doctor responsible for the patient's care.
3. This addition may be performed only by graduate nurses and senior class nursing students under supervision of a graduate nurse.
4. No medication may be given by the Nursing Service directly intravenously, *i.e.,* without further dilution by an appropriate and specified volume of intravenous fluid.
5. Also excluded specifically are phenolsulfonphthalein (PSP), sulfobromophthalein sodium (Bromsulphalein, BSP), similar testing drugs and solutions commonly used without dilution, and experimental drugs and solutions not yet accepted for routine use by the Pharmacy and Therapeutics Committee.
6. The following medications and solutions in preparations specifically for intravenous use may be added under the rules of this bulletin.

    a. Antibiotics

    b. Electrolyte solutions, *e.g.,* sodium bicarbonate, potassium chloride, sodium lactate, sodium iodide, sodium chloride and all other intravenous electrolyte solutions

    c. Vasopressors, *e.g.,* Phenylephrine (Neo-Synephrine), 1-arterenol (Levophed) and other such agents

    d. Vitamins

    e. Aminophylline

    f. Barbiturates

    g. Diphenylhydantoin (Dilantin)

    h. Hormonal preparations for intravenous use, *e.g.,* hydrocortisone

7. The following drugs may be administered by a graduate nurse provided that the initial dose has been administered by a physician, the dosage and its dilution are specifically written in the Doctor's Order Book and the medication order is re-written on a *daily basis.*

    a. 5-fluouracil

    b. Heparin

Division 1–16
Bulletin -12-

Medications, Preparation and Administration by Nurses

Purpose: To prepare and administer medications as ordered by the physician safely, accurately and efficiently.

Responsibilities of the Nurse

1. The nurse must know the nature of the drug, the desired effect, the average dose, the mathematical preparation of the dose, the toxic symptoms, the method of preparation and administration and the antidote before administering any medication.

2. The nurse must clearly understand all medication orders before carrying them out.

3. The nurse must administer and chart only those medications which she herself has prepared.

4. Medications poured but not administered must be discarded and may not be returned to the drug bottle.

5. See Bulletin 1–16–2 for reporting adverse drug reactions

    1–16–3 for reporting drug intoxication

    1–16–4 for emergency drugs

    1–16–5 and 1–16–6 for ordering from Pharmacy

    1–16–7 for automatic stop orders

    1–16–8 for the storage of internal and external preparations

Regulations Concerning Narcotics

1. See Bulletin 1–16–1 for federal and hospital regulations.
2. All narcotics must be counted at each change of shift by two nurses, one from each tour of duty. Both nurses must sign that the count was made and was correct. Errors in the count must be reported to the supervisor.
3. All narcotics obtained from the Pharmacy are to be counted and signed for by a professional nurse. Any discrepancy is to be reported to the pharmacist at once.

Medications at Bedside

1. Nitroglycerin tablets may be left at the bedside if so ordered by the doctor. No more than ten tablets should be left with the patient. At 7 A.M. and 7 P.M., the tablets are to be counted, the number used by the patient recorded and additional tablets added to the bedside supply to maintain the supply of ten.
2. Medication brought to the hospital with the patient is not kept at the bedside. It is shown to the physician, then sent home with a responsible family member or friend. If this is not possible, the medication is labeled with the patient's name, locked in the medication cabinet and, with the permission of the physician, sent home with the patient at the time of his discharge.
3. No medication other than nitroglycerin is maintained or left at the bedside of any patient.

Administration of Medications

1. *Policies*
   a) Medication cards are made out by the nurse in charge, noting the patient's name, full name of the drug, dose, route of administration, times ordered or frequency of administration. Each card is initialled by the nurse who makes it out. All 'stat' and single dose orders are written on red cards; all other medications on white cards.
   b) The medicine card is checked against the Kardex and/or Doctor's Order Book for drug, route, patient's name, date and time.
   c) The drug label is checked with the medication card at least three times: before removing the bottle from the shelf, before pouring, when returning to the shelf.
   d) At the bedside, before the medication is administered, the patient is identified by checking the medication card against the name on the wrist band, with the name on the bed card and by asking the patient to state his name if he is able to do so.
   e) The nurse remains at the bedside until the patient has taken the medication; medication is never left at the bedside.

f) The medication is charted immediately after administration.

g) Any untoward situation (patient refuses medication, is absent from the pavilion etc.) is reported to the Head Nurse and noted on the Kardex.

2. *Intravenous Medication*

No medication may be given intravenously by nurses at this hospital.

3. *Liqid Medications*

a) Spirits and tinctures must be kept tightly capped since the strength of the drug increases as the solvent evaporates.

b) Acids are to be given through a straw to avoid discoloration of the teeth.

c) Iodine preparations are to be given in milk or well diluted with fruit juice or water.

4. *Rectal Medications*

a) Rectal medications may be administered by retention enema or by suppository.

b) It is explained to the patient that the medication is to be given rectally and to be retained. The patient is assisted to turn on his left side.

c) If medication is given by suppository, the nurse puts on a glove or finger cot, lubricates the tapered end of the suppository and inserts it well beyond the sphincter.

d) If medication is given by retention enema, the least amount of solution which will dissolve the drug and provide safe dilution is used and the solution is allowed to run in slowly.

e) The patient remains quietly on the left side for a few minutes to aid in retention.

5. *Parenteral Medications*

a) Policies—Graduate Nurses

Nurses may give parenteral medications (subcutaneous, intramuscular, intradermal) if they have had adequate instruction and supervision in the method used and have adequate knowledge of the drug.

Nurses may not administer tetanus anti-toxin.

Special restrictions may be imposed on non-formulary drugs. The nurse must check with her immediate superior (head nurse or supervisor) before administering these drugs.

No more than 5 ml of medication may be injected intramuscularly into one site at any one time.

b) Policies—Student Nurses

Student nurses may not administer narcotics without first obtaining the permission of the head nurse. The student must be prepared to give the following information: patient's full name, medication and dose ordered, frequency with which medica-

tion may be given, time medication was last given, pulse and respiration of the patient.

Student nurses may never administer medication intravenously or into the I.V. tubing.

Student nurses may add medication to intravenous solutions only under the direct supervision of an instructor.

c) Administration of Parenteral Medications

Medication is prepared in the syringe. With a transfer forceps, a sponge moistened with benzalkonium chloride (Zephiran) 1:750 is removed from the container and placed in a medicine cup. The cup and syringe with needle protected by a needle guard are carried to the bedside.

Disposable needles are bent after use to prevent re-use and discarded *only* in the container provided for needles.

Injection sites and methods:

Subcutaneous—injected at a 45° angle into the lateral aspect of the upper arm.

Intramuscular—injected at a 90° angle. The injection is given in the upper portion of the upper outer quadrant of the buttocks, two inches below the crest of the ileum. The deltoid or the lateral aspect of the thigh may also be used. Sites of injection should be rotated.

Intradermal—injected as nearly parallel as possible in the skin of the anterior forearm. Only the tip of the needle should be inserted in the skin and a wheal should appear as soon as the medication is injected.

SPECIAL MANUALS

Hospital pharmacies within large teaching hospitals generally require, in addition to the standard procedural manual, a special manual to cover specific aspects of the operation. These may be for use in such areas as the control laboratory, sterile technics laboratory, manufacturing laboratory, hyperalimentation unit and unit dose section.

In preparing the sections of the special manuals, it is essential that specific detail be provided in order that the special manual be useful.[6]

After all is said and done with regard to this topic of procedural manuals, the student as well as the seasoned hospital pharmacist will benefit greatly from the wisdom afforded by the following excerpt from an editorial.[4]

"Procedural manuals can be a great asset in the proper management of the Pharmacy Department and the coordination of its activities with other departments and the professional and administrative staffs. Hospital pharmacists will

find them valuable tools, tools however, which can never replace the professional judgment of the pharmacist."

SPECIAL SECTION ON CLINICAL PHARMACY

All institutional practitioners recognize the need and value of a procedural manual, yet they do not always recognize the needs of clinical pharmacists operating within that hospital unit recognized in the organizational chart as the Pharmacy Department or Pharmaceutical Service. Too often the procedural manual deals with the departmental operations and excludes the functions of the clinical pharmacist which are predominantly external to the central pharmacy. These services are patient-oriented and as such will require acceptance by the medical and nursing staffs. As a start in this direction, it is suggested that the procedural manual give consideration to the scope and degree of clinical pharmacist functions in the hospital.

Accordingly consideration should be given to including in the departmental manual the responsibilities of the clinical pharmacist via a review of two very important ASHP Guidelines which are hereinafter reprinted.[7]

ASHP STATEMENT ON CLINICAL FUNCTIONS IN INSTITUTIONAL PHARMACY PRACTICE[a]

Contemporary pharmaceutical services include clinical functions such as drug-related decision making and patient-care activities as well as drug preparation, distribution, and control. These clinical functions often are performed in patient-care areas in association with or in support of physicians and other health-care practitioners. They are an integral component of a pharmaceutical service program and consist primarily of drug-therapy monitoring, consultation, and patient education.

The scope and degree of clinical pharmacy services should be commensurate with the goals of the institution. Each director of pharmaceutical services is responsible for establishing and maintaining an appropriate clinical services program.

The American Society of Hospital Pharmacists believes that pharmacists must be able to develop and provide clinical pharmacy services, and it supports and endorses the following clinical functions:

1. Preparation of medication histories for the patient's permanent medical record or other database or both.

---

[a]Approved by the ASHP House of Delegates, June 7, 1983. Approved by the ASHP Board of Directors, November 19, 1982. Developed by the ASHP Council on Clinical Affairs. Supersedes an earlier version approved by the House of Delegates on May 15, 1978.

2. Monitoring of drug therapy by direct involvement with the patient and routine evaluation of the patient's drug regimen, medical problems, laboratory data, and special procedures, and communicating relevant findings and recommendations to other clinicians who are also responsible for the patient's care.
3. Patient education and counseling.
4. Participation in management of medical emergencies, adverse drug reactions, and acute and chronic disease states.
5. Provision of written consultations in such areas as drug therapy selection, pharmacokinetics, nutritional support, and determination of therapeutic endpoints.
6. Initiation and participation in research, including clinical drug investigations.
7. Control of medication administration and drug distribution in the patient-care area.
8. Detection and reporting of adverse drug reactions.
9. Participation in the education of health-care practitioners.
10. Participation in drug-use review and other quality-assurance programs.

In addition to providing the aforementioned services, pharmacists have a responsibility to communicate advances in development and delivery of clinical pharmacy services to the health-care community through appropriate publications, presentations, and programs.

ASHP STATEMENT ON THE ROLE OF THE PHARMACIST IN CLINICAL PHARMACOKINETIC SERVICES[8]*

Clinical pharmacokinetics is a health science discipline that applies the principles of pharmacokinetics to the development of safe and effective drug therapy. Pharmacists involved in this discipline must understand and apply those pharmacokinetic principles of drug absorption, distribution, metabolism, and excretion, as well as the physicochemical properties of drugs, in the selection of appropriate doses and dosage intervals of medications for individual patients. Since drugs must be looked at in terms of their pharmacokinetic behavior, pharmacists must understand how the pharmacokinetic characteristics can be profoundly changed by disease or altered pathophysiological states.

As previously defined in the ASHP Statement on Clinical Functions in Institutional Pharmacy Practice,[1] pharmacists' clinical functions include monitoring of drug therapy and the provision of clinical pharmacokinetic consultations. Specific training or experience is required to fulfill pharmacokinetic functions. Pharmacists involved in the application of clinical pharmacokinetics to drug therapy management should strive to participate in the following.

*Developed by the ASHP Council on Clinical Affairs. Approved by the ASHP Board of Directors, November 19–20, 1981, and by the ASHP House of Delegates, June 7, 1982.

1. Design of individualized drug dosage regimens based on the pharmacokinetic principles of the drug, the purpose of the medication, concurrent diseases and drug therapy, and the patient's clinical data base.
2. Adjustment of dosage regimens in response to drug concentrations of other biochemical or clinical markers.
3. Evaluation of unusual patient responses to drug therapy for possible pharmacacokinetic explanations.
4. Recommendation of procedures and assays for the analysis of drug concentrations in order to facilitate the evaluation of dosage regimens.
5. Formation of collaborative relationships with individuals and departments involved in drug therapeutic monitoring services to encourage the development and appropriate use of these services. When such collaboration is not feasible, pharmacists should participate in the administrative, technical, and quality control activities involved in providing analytical services.
6. Development of effective written and oral communication skills to relate to physicians, nurses, and other health-care practitioners, information on the individualized drug therapy of patients they serve.
7. Education of pharmacists, physicians, nurses, and other clinical practitioners on pharmacokinetic principles to improve drug safety and efficacy and to encourage the development and application of those principles in therapeutic drug monitoring programs provided by pharmacists and other clinical practitioners.
8. Design and conduct of research that will expand the clinical pharmacokinetic data base and contribute to the documentation, assessment, and expansion of clinical pharmacokinetic services.

The responsibility of the pharmacist to contribute to drug therapy knowledge in the management of the patient increases as the pharmacokinetic characteristics of drugs become clearly defined and therapeutic concentrations are established. Education, training, and experience should prepare the pharmacist to accept the challenges and opportunities of providing clinical pharmacokinetic services.

REFERENCE

1. American Society of Hospital Pharmacists. ASHP statement on clinical functions in institutional pharmacy practice. *Am. J. Hosp. Pharm.* 1978; *35*:813.

ASHP GUIDELINES FOR OBTAINING AUTHORIZATION FOR PHARMACISTS' NOTATIONS IN THE PATIENT MEDICAL RECORD[9a]

Introduction

The clinical influences and functions of pharmacists are well established and accepted in many health care settings. To develop and provide patient-oriented services, pharmacists must communicate with physicians, nurses and other health care practitioners about the patients they serve. One important

---

[a]Approved by the ASHP Board of Directors, November 16–17, 1978. Originally developed by the ASHP Council on Clinical Pharmacy and Therapeutics.

means of communication is the written notation in the patient medical record. While it is understood that information placed in the patient medical record should be selective, specific drug information influencing patient care should become a permanent part of the patient record. It is also understood that some information may be better provided orally or in such a manner which does not become a permanent part of the patient record. Written communication should complement, not replace, oral communication.

Authority

The Joint Commission on Accreditation of Hospitals (JCAH) regulations specify that "entries in medical records may be made only by individuals given this right as specified in hospital and medical staff policies." Pharmacists, as responsible health care providers involved in patient care, should communicate in writing with other members of the health care team, when appropriate, by notations in patient medical records.

In settings where no such authority exists, the following steps are recommended:

1. Development of a statement by the department of pharmacy services which defines the types of solicited entries or unsolicited entries or both, the pharmacist should make in the patient medical record; identifies the location of such entries; describes the format in which the entries will be made; defines the types of entries that should not be included in the patient medical record; and outlines a procedure for periodic review of entries made by the pharmacist in the medical record.
2. Submission of the statement to the pharmacy and therapeutics committee for review and approval. The statement also should be submitted to other committees of the medical staff responsible for granting the right of staff members to make written notations in patient medical records.
3. Attainment of authorization of the pharmacist's written notations in the patient medical record. A recommendation from the appropriate committee of the medical staff should be submitted to the medical staff executive body for authorization of the pharmacist's written notations in the patient medical record according to the guidelines contained in the statement of the department of pharmacy service.
4. Submission of the statement to hospital administration.

Types of Entries

Examples of information a pharmacist may wish to document in the patient medical record include, but are not limited to:

1. Admission medication history summary.
2. Drug therapy consultations, including pharmacokinetic monitoring data.
3. Documentation of clinical pharmacy services (e.g., drug-related patient education and discharge counseling).
4. Recording physicians' drug orders—reducing physicians' oral drug orders to written form.
5. Potential drug-related problems which should be called to the attention of medical care providers.
6. Patient progress notes—documentation of patient assessments (e.g., blood pressure measurements, urine sugars) which are performed by the pharmacist in the determination of therapeutic outcomes.

SELECTED READINGS

Anon. Policy and Procedural Manual: Discipline. Current Concepts in Hosp. Pharm. Mgt., *5*:4:20, (Winter) 1983.

Anon. Policy and Procedural Manual: Medication Quality Assurance Rounds. Current Concepts in Hosp. Pharm. Mgt., *5*:3:20, (Fall) 1983.

Anon. Policy and Procedural Manual: Competitive Bid Policy. Current Concepts in Hosp. Pharm. Mgt., *6*:1:15, (Spring) 1984.

Anon. Policy and Procedural Manual: Drug Recall Program. Current Concepts in Hosp. Pharm. Mgt., *6*:3:19, (Fall) 1984.

REFERENCES

1. ASHP Technical Assistance Bulletin on Hospital Drug Distribution and Control. Am. J. Hosp. Pharm., *37*:1097–1103, (Aug.) 1980.
2. Accreditation Manual for Hospitals—AMH-85, Joint Commission on Accreditation of Hospitals, 875 No. Michigan Ave., Chicago, Ill. 60611.
3. Berenice, Sr. Mary: Operational Manuals in Hospital Pharmacy. Am. J. Hosp. Pharm., *16*:6:269, 1959.
4. Latiolais, Clifton J.: Pharmacy Procedure Manual, Hospitals. J.A.H.A., *33*:13:77, 1959.
5. Francke, Don E.: An Editorial Procedural Manuals as Administrative Tools. Am. J. Hosp. Pharm., *16*:6:267, 1959.
6. Avis, Kenneth E., Carlin, Herbert S., Flack, Herbert L.: Procedure Manual for Parenteral and Other Sterile Preparations (1960), Sterile Technics Laboratory, Jefferson Medical College, Philadelphia, Pa.
7. ASHP Statement on Clinical Functions in Institutional Pharmacy Practice. Am. J. Hosp. Pharm., *40*:1385–1386, (Aug.) 1983.
8. ASHP Statement on the Role of the Pharmacist in Clinical Pharmacokinetic Services. Am. J. Hosp. Pharm., *39*:1369, (Aug.) 1982.
9. ASHP Guidelines For Obtaining Authorization for Pharmacists Notations in the Patient Medical Record. Am. J. Hosp. Pharm., *36*:222–223, (Feb.) 1979.

12|

Policy and Procedure for Drug Distribution and Administration

The pharmacist's responsibility for drugs in the institutional setting does not end with the dispensing or distribution of the medication. Practitioners must provide for special labeling and packaging to meet the needs of the physicians and nurses in the areas where the drugs are to be administered. In addition, pharmacists should work closely with the Nursing Service to develop policy and procedure for drug distribution and administration.

PRESCRIBING OF FLOOR STOCK DRUGS

There are three techniques employed in transmitting drug order information from the nursing stations to the pharmacist. They are:

(i)   Prescription order is written on a separate blank by the physician (Fig. 34).
(ii) A copy of the chart order (Physician's Order Sheet) is sent to the pharmacist.
(iii) Chart order is transcribed by hospital personnel assigned to the nursing station.

In hospitals where the pharmacy operation is a decentralized one, pharmacy personnel pick-up physicians' orders at the nursing stations at predetermined intervals and deliver the medication to the floor. This provides the patient with therapy until the next unit dose cart exchange. Some hospitals use their on-line computer to transmit the drug order to the pharmacy and also create a hardcopy for subsequent use. See Chapter 13 for details concerning entering the patient into the system. When a physician's order is received in the pharmacy and the order appears to be incorrect, for whatever reason, it is the responsibility of the dispensing pharmacist to clarify the problem with the physician and so notify the nursing station of the correction. It is also good policy

247

	PHYSICIAN'S ORDERS	John Doe Hosp. #12-34-56 Location B25 Dr. Smith

Date Ordered	Date Discontinued	ORDERS
1/1/80		Digitoxin 0.1 mg one at 7:00 a.m.
		Hexavitamin Capsule one daily
1/2/80		Secobarbital 100 mg one h.s. prn
1/3/80	1/5/80	Potassium Chloride 1 gm one daily in a.m.

Fig. 34. An example of a Physician's Order Sheet found in the patient's medical record. The orders shown here are typed. Under normal circumstances, these are written by the physician in ink.

to have the prescribing physicians telephone the nursing unit with the corrected order and follow-up with a written order for confirmation.

Some of the smaller hospitals continue to require separate prescriptions for all medications. The student must bear in mind that there is nothing wrong with this in that it establishes the same professional relationship and fosters the same practice existing in the community practice of pharmacy. In the larger hospitals, this system is not favored by the physicians.

A second method consists of using a copy of the doctor's written order as a prescription order. In this system the pharmacist receives a copy of the original medication order. No transcribing or copying is required of hospital personnel assigned to the nursing station in order to obtain prescribed medication as initially ordered. It has been demonstrated that this system reduces medication errors because of the review by pharmacists of all drug orders for each patient in the original handwriting of the physician ordering the medication.

In one version of this system, physicians are allowed to mix all types of orders for the patient on one sheet. Although this has the advantage of providing the pharmacist with a total picture of what is happening to the patient, it is preferable to educate the physicians to limit the writing of their drug orders to a single medication order sheet (Fig. 34). Once written, it behooves the responsible party to promptly remove the copy portion of the medication order and transmit it to the pharmacy in order to obviate dispensing delays.

The method most widely employed at present is that in which the nurse, nursing unit manager, or ward secretary transcribes or copies

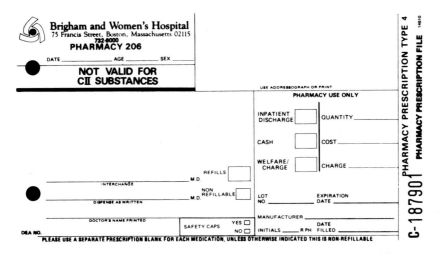

Fig. 35. Prescription form used to order medications other than controlled substances. The reverse side of this form contains the refill record. (See Fig. 36). Controlled substances are dispensed on a similar form but of a different color.

REFILL RECORD

NO.	DATE	QUAN.	INITIALS		EXPIRATION DATE, LOT NO. & MFG.
			BY	R PH	
1					
2					
3					
4					
5					
6					
7					
8					
9					
10					

Fig. 36. Refill record printed on the reverse side of prescription blank.

via a mechanical copying device the physician's written order on to another document (Figs. 39 and 40), sometimes called a drug requisition slip, and sends it to the pharmacy for reviewing and dispensing. This transcribed or copied order is also used by the pharmacist to create his *patient drug profile* and to initiate the medication charge.

If the medication ordered is a non-charge drug, the nurse makes an entry on her records and at the proper time will remove the drug from the ward stock container and administer it to the patient.

PATIENT TRANSFER OR DISCHARGE

The finest drug distribution system will fail if appropriate measures are not taken to record the transfer or discharge of a patient from a nursing unit. If this information is not sent to the pharmacy on a timely basis, the patient's medication may become lost and therefore create a delay in the patient's medication schedule or cause the patient to be charged for drugs never received. To prevent these problems from arising, the pharmacy and nursing services must cooperate with each other. Nursing should notify the pharmacy then remove the medication from the patient's drawer in the unit dose cart, properly identify it with the patient's name and hospital identification number and send it to the patient's new location or return it to the pharmacy, in the case of a discharge, where the necessary credits will be issued. It is also the responsibility of the pharmacy to transfer the patient's drug profile to the new location.

LABELING OF FLOOR STOCK DRUGS

Of further interest to the non-hospital pharmacist members of the profession is the fact that none of the ward stock drugs is labeled with the directions for use. This is so because of the fact that many patients may be receiving the same drug but under a different therapeutic regimen. If one set of directions was affixed to the container under these circumstances, then it is obvious that confusion and error may result. Therefore, packages containing non-charge as well as generally used charge floor stock medications bear a label which shows the name of the ward and the name and strength of the preparation as well as any other pertinent information (Fig. 37).

In contrast, medications being sent to the floor for the specific use of a single patient bear a similar label with the addition of the patient's name (Fig. 38). Once again, the specific directions for use are eliminated because of the fact that the therapeutic regimen may be altered from day to day by the physician in charge. Therefore, the nurse must make frequent checks of the patient's record in order to keep informed of the latest treatment prescribed.

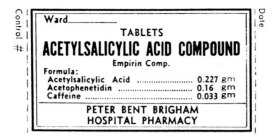

Fig. 37. An example of a non-charge floor stock medication label.

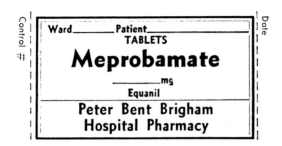

Fig. 38. An example of a charge floor stock medication label.

NURSING POLICY AND PROCEDURE FOR ADMINISTRATION OF A DRUG

Although the hospital pharmacist does not become involved with this aspect of patient care, he should become thoroughly familiar with the procedure used in his particular institution.

There are many different procedures for the administration of drugs by nurses employed in the hospitals of this country; therefore, space will permit only the methodologies employed by one medical center.[1] For other techniques, see Chapter 13.

NURSING MEDICATION ADMINISTRATION REGULATIONS

Purpose

To describe the policy and procedures which guide nursing personnel in the administration of medications, within the limits imposed by Federal and State Law, Professional Nurse Practice Acts and Hospital Policy.

General Regulations for Medication Orders

1. Medications are not to be administered without a written order from the physician.

2. *Verbal Orders*—may be accepted by a registered nurse, from a physician, nurse mid-wife or nurse practitioner, only in an emergency situation and must be countersigned by the physician within 24-hours. *Under no circumstances, including an emergency, may anyone other than a registered nurse accept a verbal order.*

3. *Telephone Orders*—if it should be necessary for a registered nurse to accept a telephone order, the order will be valid only until the following 10:00 AM and the order must be countersigned by the responsible physician as soon as possible, but within 24-hours. *Under no circumstances, including an emergency, may anyone other than a registered nurse accept a telephone order.*

4. A medication may be administered only if a specific dose, route and frequency is ordered.

5. Only those medications which have been dispensed by the Brigham and Women's Hospital Pharmacy may be administered by nursing staff.

6. Medications prepared, but not administered, must be discarded and may not be returned to the drug container. Controlled Substances that have been removed from the narcotic drawer-cabinet and not used must be discarded, witnessed and the narcotic record signed by two (2) professional nurses.

7. Specific regulations for nurses:
   a) The nurse must know the nature of the drug, the desired affect, the average dose, the mathematical preparation of the dose, the toxic symptoms, and the methods of preparation and administration before administering any medication.
   b) The nurse may administer only those medications s/he has prepared (mixed) personally or those premixed by Pharmacy.
   c) The nurse must be familiar with the bulletins and directives relating to medication administration in the Nursing Service Policy Manual and the Nursing Service Procedure Manual.

Regulations for Specific Drugs

Narcotic Medications

1. Narcotic medication (Schedule II drugs) should not be administered if the patient's respiratory rate is below 12 per minute without further orders from the physician. (Exceptions: Patient on a ventilator.)
   a) *Parenteral SC, IM, IV*—narcotic medication and other analgesics may be ordered with a dosage and frequency range as long as the range does not exceed 50 percent of the indicated lower limit. EXAMPLE: Demerol, 60–75 mg, IM every 4–6 hours.

b) *Oral/Rectal*—narcotic medication and other analgesics may be ordered with a dosage and frequency range as long as the range does not exceed 100% of the indicated lower limit.
EXAMPLE:

Percodan $\frac{.}{1}$ to $\frac{..}{11}$ tabs p.o. every 4–6 hours.

2. *Tetanus Antitoxin—Nurses May Not* administer tetanus antitoxin.
3. *Digitalis*—preparations may not be administered if the patient's apical pulse is below 50 without first consulting with the physician, unless other parameters have already been specified by the physician.
4. Registered nurses and licensed practical nurses may administer Rho-GAM (Mass-GAM) according to the procedure found in the Procedure Manual.
5. *Magnesium Sulfate*—must be administered *by a physician* by IV Push. An RN may administer Magnesium Sulfate IV piggyback via pump.
6. Blood pressure must be taken before giving Ergonovine or Methylergonovine. If blood pressure exceed 130/90, consult physician before giving.
7. Orders for Antihypertensives must be accompanied by upper and lower limits of blood pressure to be observed.

Regulations for Various Routes of Administration

1. *Oral Medications*
   a) Only scored tablets may be divided.
   b) Capsules may not be opened in an attempt to alter dose.
2. *Parenteral Medications*—no more than 5ml of any medication may be injected intramuscularly into one (1) site at any time and no more than 2ml of any medication subcutaneously.
3. *Intradermals*—may be performed by an RN who is skilled in the technique.
4. *Rectal Medications*—rectal medications may be administered by retention enema or by suppository.
5. *Intra-arterial Medications*—these are prepared and administered by physicians on the general units. (Exceptions made in specialty units will be specified in writing in the Unit's Policy Manual.)
6. *Instillations*—all genito-urinary irrigants are prepared in the Pharmacy.

Restrictions for Nurses in the Administration of Drugs

The preceding regulations of this bulletin apply to all classifications of nurses (i.e., RN, LPN and student nurse) in conjunction with the following specific instructions:

NOTE: Specific Units in the Hospital, such as the Dialysis Unit, many have policies applicable to that Unit's personnel, based on the staff's specialized training and experience.

1. *Registered Nurses*

   Registered professional nurses may give parenteral medications if they have had adequate instruction and supervision in the method used and have adequate knowledge of the drug.

   They may add medication to IVs in accordance with Intravenous Medication Policy.

2. *Licensed Practical Nurses*

   a) LPNs may administer heparinized saline via heparin lock by IV push. NO other medications may be administered by LPNs by IV push.

   b) LPNs May Hang: IV solutions prepared and labeled by the Pharmacy, IV solutions from the manufacturers to which nothing has been added, hyperalimentation and intralipids piggybacking.

   c) LPNs May Not administer research or investigational drugs.

   d) LPNs May Not administer allergenic extracts.

   e) All restrictions for RNs are also applicable to LPNs.

   Before administering Schedule II drugs, insulin and anticoagulants, the LPN must check the preparared drug and order with a registered nurse.

3. *Professional Nursing Students*

   Students may administer oral, rectal, intramuscular and subcutaneous medication only after qualifying by demonstration to an Instructor. Until that time, a student must check with an instructor or designated alternate relative to the intent and reason for giving the drug; the preparation, action, and anticipated response, the last dose, and the patient's vital signs, if applicable.

MEDICATION PROCEDURE—UNIT DOSE SYSTEM

Purpose: To provide a consistent, safe manner of administering medications to patients.

Equipment: Medication Keys
               Medication Cart
               Medication Kardex
               Ball Point Pen

Procedure:

STEPS	KEY POINTS
A. Preparation	
1. Check Kardex listing and medication cassette drawers to determine that patient's bed location and listing in Kardex correspond.	When a patient is admitted to the Unit or transferred in from another area the Unit Secretary or Nurse will notify the Unit Pharmacy of the room or bed number. Anytime bed numbers are changed within the Unit the Unit Dose Pharmacist must be notified so that the change can be made in the Unit Dose Pharmacy records.
2. Prepare Medication Cart with extra souffle cups, 30 ml medication cups; 90 ml cups—fruit juice, water; straws, alcohol swabs, syringes; etc.	This is helpful when giving medication to a large number of patients. Some "unit of use" packaging is not adequate to serve as a cup, so medication may have to be placed in a cup for administration.
B. Administration	
1. Take Medication Cart and Medication Kardex to patient's bedside and unlock Medication Cart.	There is no need to set up separate tray. Lock releases cassette drawers. Do not unlock the Narcotic drawer unless necessary.
2. Greet patient and explain your purpose.	
3. Check patient's Medication Administration Record information with band. Establish positive patient identification by asking patient to state his/her name.	If a patient does not have on an identification band, inform the Unit Secretary, who should prepare one.
4. Assess patient for special needs pertinent to medication to be administered.	e.g., swallowing, position, state of consciousness, presence of fever, diarrhea, constipation, nausea or vomiting, etc. Some medications require the checking of vital signs, urine or blood tests before administration.

STEPS	KEY POINTS
5. Using the patient's Medication Administration Record, select the unit dose preparation from the patient's cassette drawer to be administered to that patient at that time. Check: a) name of the drug b) dosage of the drug c) route of administration d) date and time drug to be given e) medication order transcription was checked by R.N. f) renewal date if pertinent.	If there is any discrepancy between the unit dose preparation and the medication order in the Medication Administration Record: DO NOT GIVE THE MEDICATION. Check the physician's Order Sheet and/or consult with Unit Dose Pharmacy. Physician's order may be transcribed by Unit Secretary, but must be checked by an R.N. Initials beside order on Medication Administration Record indicate that order was checked. Initials, signature and status should be recorded in upper right column of Record.
6. Take medication and Kardex to the bedside. Verify the patient's identification; the unit dose with the Administration Record, and administer the medication.	Remain with the patient until he/she swallows oral medication. NEVER LEAVE MEDICATION AT THE BEDSIDE except those specified by Pharmacy and Therapeutics Committee.
C. Charting Medication 1. Chart medication *immediately* on the patient's Medication Record in the Kardex, using ball point pen. a) On the appropriate date, sign the time drug was given, injection site if indicated, and your initials.	This is the permanent record. Charting immediately insures accuracy and up-to-date record keeping and decreased errors in medication administration.
b) Sign your name and status beside your initials in the upper right column of the patient's Medication Administration Record.	e.g., J.D.—Jane Doe, R.N.
c) If a medication was not given: 1. See code on the medication record and indicate reason by using the appropriate code; record the time and encircle the two to indicate "not given."	If a drug was given late because of a special test or other reason—record the time the drug was given—not the time scheduled. This may necessitate a change in the schedule.

STEPS	KEY POINTS
2. Make out "Medication Not Given Notice" with patient's name, date, time, bed number, medication and reason not given. Sign form and place in patient's cassette.	This assists Pharmacist in maintaining accurate patient profile.

D. Security of Medication Cart

STEPS	KEY POINTS
1. When medication has been administered LOCK Medication Cart.	It is the responsibility of the nurse administering medications to provide absolute security of the Medication Cart. DO NOT LEAVE THE CART UNATTENDED AND/OR UNLOCKED.
2. Return Kardex to Kardex shelf on cart.	
3. Return cart to designated storage area.	
4. Maintain cleanliness of cart. Discard waste materials. Wipe off cart.	

MEDICATION ADMINISTRATION—GENERAL

Purpose: For uniform administration of oral, parenteral, rectal and vaginal medications.

PROCEDURE	POINTS OF EMPHASIS
1. Check physician's order sheet and medication kardex for physician's order.	
2. Explain medication use and side effects to patient.	
3. Read label on medication.	3. Medications must be checked 3 times: a) When being taken from drawer. b) When preparing medication. c) Before giving medication to patient.
4. After administering, always chart medication given with time and initials on medication kardex. Also, include initials and signature in spaces provided.	

A. *INTRAMUSCULAR AND SUBCUTANEOUS*
Purpose: Injectable medications are given for more rapid absorption of the drug, if the patient is unable to take medication orally, or to avoid inactivation of drug action by gastric enzymes.

PROCEDURE	POINTS OF EMPHASIS
Equipment: Syringe and needle (23/25g for subcutaneous, 21/22g for intramuscular). Two alcohol sponges. Medication as ordered. **Single Dose Vial and Ampules*	
1. Wipe the neck of the ampule or the top of a vial with an alcohol sponge; break off the top of the ampule with a gauze sponge.	
2. Draw up medication into syringe.	2. Leave a 0.2ml bubble of air in syringe after proper dose is drawn up; this bubble will be injected last and block leakage from tissue.
3. Take empty vial or ampule, syringe and alcohol sponge to patient's bedside.	
4. Select site of injection	4. Subcutaneous injections are given in upper anterior arm over the tricep muscle, abdomen for heparin and in the anterior portion of the thigh and rotated with each injection. Intramuscular injections are given in upper outer quadrant of the buttocks or thigh. *Never* given IM injection in the deltoid unless approved by Head Nurse or Supervisor. The maximum amount given by s.c. is 1 cc. and by IM is 3 cc. (except 5 cc. of decadron & 4 cc. for procaine penicillin 2.4 m.u. syringe).
5. Administer medication	5. When giving an injection, make sure that you aspirate the syringe before giving the medication. If blood is aspirated, prepare a new medication.
6. When long term or irritating injections are given, a body chart should be placed on the patient's chart next to medicatition record and the site chart by date and time.	6. Change needles before injecting into patient when irritating medicaitons are being injected, to reduce tissue irritation. Rotating sites helps to reduce tissue irritation and injury.
**Multiple Dose Vial:	
1. Wipe rubber stopper on vial with an alcohol sponge.	1. This will cleanse area to be punctured.

PROCEDURE	POINTS OF EMPHASIS
2. Draw the amount of air equal to the amount of medication to be withdrawn into the syringe. Introduce the needle through the rubber stopper and inject the air. Next, withdraw the correct dose of medication.	2. This is essential so that the liquid in the bottle will not develop either positive or negative pressure.
3. Take medication to patient and administer. Always check patient's identification band and question her regarding allergies prior to administering any medication.	
4. Dispose of used equipment. All needles must be removed from the syringes, using the destrucuclip and plastic syringes must have hub removed also by destructuclip. The remainder of the syringe may be disposed of in a properly labeled syringe disposal box.	4. These steps are necessary to prevent accidents and reuse of contaminated equipment.

B. *OPHTHALMIC PREPARATIONS*

Purpose:　　To dilate or contract pupils, to relieve inflammation and to produce local anesthesia.

Equipment:　Medication in dropper bottle or tube of ophthalmic ointment, as ordered box.
　　　　　　Disposable tissues.

1. Have patient in bed in supine position.	1. Be sure medication is for the EYES and not the EAR.
2. Evert lower eyelid gently, instruct patient to look upward.	
3. Allow number of drops ordered to fall on center of inner surface of lower lid.	3. Do Not allow tips of medicine dropper or tube to touch inner surface of lid or eye. Do Not allow medicine dropper to touch your fingers.
4. If ointment is ordered, apply thin line along inner surface of lower lid, from inner to outer canthus.	
5. Instruct patient to close eyes for a moment.	
6. Wipe off excess with tissue, and discard.	6. Wipe from inner to outer canthus of eye.
7. Replace cover of ointment or medication securely, then replace in medication cart.	
8. Discard waste.	

C. *RECTAL MEDICATIONS*

Purpose:　　Medications are introduced into the rectum for a direct or systemic effect.

Equipment: Suppository
                Lubricant
                Disposable glove

1. Have the patient turn on her/his side and assume a Sim's position.
2. Lubricate index finger of the glove and the end of the medication. Insert medication into the rectum well beyond the internal sphincter.

2. Gentle insertion and withdrawal of the finger minimizes the defecation reflex. By placing the medication beyond the internal sphincter, the possibility of it being readily expelled is reduced.

3. Remove glove, discard in wastebasket.

D. VAGINAL MEDICATIONS

Purpose: To apply medications locally to the cervix and vagina. These are available in creams and suppositories.
Equipment: Medication
                Applicator
                Glove and lubricant

1. Assist the patient in assuming the lithotomy position and place a drape to maintain privacy.
2. Place cream or suppository into the tip of the applicator and separating the labia gently, insert the applicator into the vagina at an angle toward the back, as far as possible.

2. Gentle insertion will reduce the danger of trauma to sensitive vaginal mucosa.

3. Push the plunger to release the medication and gently withdraw the applicator.

3. Always wash the applicator in warm soapy water immediately after use. Instruct the patient to remain in bed for 15–30 minutes to obtain full benefit from the medication.

4. If no applicator is available, the nurse (or patient, when appropriate) should use a clean glove and gently insert suppository in the same manner.

4. The use of lubricant on the glove will eliminate friction during insertion.

5. Inform the patient that the medication will melt at body temperature and a mini pad can be worn to absorb any leakage and prevent staining of underwear.

5. Tampax should *not* be used.

INSPECTION OF NURSING DRUG CABINETS

Once a large supply of drugs is placed in the nursing station, the hospital pharmacist's responsibility is increased. The only way the pharmacist can be sure that the drug supplies on the pavilions are being properly cared for is by personal inspection of the drug cabinets.

Too often, this facet of the pharmacist's responsibility is taken too lightly and may oftentimes be delegated to nursing supervisory personnel who, although well motivated, are not trained to evaluate the state of deterioration of drugs.

In order that the inspection program be successful, it should be carried out by pharmacy and nursing personnel on a regular basis. In addition, there should be developed a regular check list of points to be looked for during each inspection tour.

The following is a check list which may, with modification, be used for the inspection of the drug cabinets on the nursing station of any hospital.

1. Check lock mechanism for security.
2. Check lighting and refrigeration.
3. Check the uniformity of containers.
4. Check the uniformity and completeness of labeling.
5. Check to see that minimal and maximal inventories are being adhered to.
6. Check to see that internal use medications are separated from external use products.
7. Ascertain that all dated pharmaceuticals and related products are still usable.
8. Determine whether non-dated drugs have deteriorated.
9. Check whether research drugs are properly labeled and segregated.
10. Eliminate any samples, non-approved drugs, or non-drug items from the cabinet.
11. Check the storage and rotation of IV solutions.
12. Check emergency or "crash carts" for appropriate drug levels and status of drugs if dated.
13. Check DEA mandated record keeping.
14. Check to see if previous inspection citations have been adequately corrected.
15. Check the general appearance of the drug preparation area.

SELECTED READINGS

Barker, K.N., Harris, J.A., Webster, D.B., Stringer, J.F., Pearson, R.E., Mikeal, R.L., Glotzhober, G.R. and Miller, G.J.: Consultant Evaluation of a Hospital Medication System: Analysis of the Existing System. Am. J. Hosp. Pharm., *41*:2009–2016, 1984.
Ibid: Consultant Evaluation of a Hospital Medication System: Implementation and Evaluation of the New System. Am. J. Hosp. Pharm., *41*:2022–2029, 1984.

REFERENCES

1. Nursing Proc. Manual—1982. Brigham and Women's Hospital, Boston, Mass. 02115.
2. McKenney, J.H. and Wasserman, A.J.: Effect of Advanced Pharmaceutical Services on the Incidence of Adverse Drug Reactions, Am. J. Hosp. Pharm., *36*:1691–1697, (Dec.) 1979.

13

Dispensing to In-Patients

The increased demand for the utilization of hospitals coupled with the growing shortage of professional personnel—nurses, pharmacists, dietitians and social workers—has stimulated thought and research in work simplification through the establishment of criteria which define each and every job performed by this category of personnel.

A great deal of nursing time was consumed by frequent trips to the pharmacy to obtain medications and other ancillary supplies. As a direct result thereof, many administrators have requested the hospital pharmacist and nursing administrative staff to scrutinize present procedures and develop new systems for the distribution and dispensing of drugs.

In the interim, many stop-gap measures were taken simply because they appeared to be the most expedient but which, when viewed in the light of experience and reasoning, were in reality a direct violation of the law.

One such approach was the indiscriminate stocking of drugs on the nursing station in bulk quantities, thereby eliminating the pharmacist's control, for here the physician prescribed, the nurse *dispensed,* and the nurse *administered.* Clearly, in a situation such as this the nurse in performing the dispensing act is infringing upon the professional as well as the legal prerogatives of the pharmacist.

Archambault[1] has stated that drug administration is a nursing act which consists of the removal or withdrawal of a single dose from a drug container and its administration to a patient on the order of a physician or dentist. He has further stipulated that dispensing is a pharmacy act and consists of the pharmacist removing two or more doses from a bulk drug container and placing them in another container for subsequent use.

Pharmacists should be alert to such infringements and should not lend their approval to such procedures. Many hospital administrators would support the pharmacists' stand on this if the matter is brought to his attention with adequate particularity.

Another hasty decision, in some areas, was the installation of vending type machines, only to have the attorneys-general of several states rule that they were illegal. Most of the decisions were based on the fact that state laws provide that registered nurses are not authorized under statute to dispense drugs, but may "administer" them after the prescription has been "dispensed" by a licensed person.

A more rational approach to the subject might be the installation of a messenger service between the pharmacy and the nursing stations, installation of mechanical conveyor systems or pneumatic tube systems or to develop emergency boxes, or the placing of charge floor stock drugs on the pavilion after a limited selection of drugs for this use has been made by the Pharmacy and Therapeutics Committee.

In order to alleviate the nursing burden, some hospital administrators contend that hospital pharmacists must assume responsibility for medications from the time of their selection to the time of their administration. Yet, in designing a system which incorporates this concept, consideration must be given to alleviate the burden placed upon the nursing service for the ordering, preparation and administration of medications.[2]

Many examples are recorded in the literature that illustrate the relationship between a drug distribution system and the nursing system.

One study of nursing activities indicated that approximately 15% of a professional nurse's time is spent in the communication aspects of medication procedures.[3] This is not unusual when compared to other studies which show that: a 22% increase in the amount of time nurses were able to spend at the patient's bedside as a result of changing the drug dispensing system[4]; 5.5 hours per day of nursing time were saved as a result of the installation of a unit dose system[5]; 14.4 hours per day of nursing time for four medical wards were freed by the use of a unit-dose system.[6]

ASPH GUIDELINES FOR HOSPITAL DRUG DISTRIBUTION SYSTEM

Because of the importance of drug distribution systems in the hospital, the American Society of Hospital Pharmacists approved and the American Hospital Association endorsed a *Statement on Hospital Distribution Systems.*[7]

The following guidelines for planning and evaluating hospital drug distribution systems are abstracted from the aforementioned statement:

Traditional methods of distributing drugs in hospitals are now undergoing reevaluation, and considerable thought and activity is being directed toward the development of new and improved drug distribution systems. Some of the newer concepts and ideas in connection with hospital drug distribution systems are centralized or decentralized (single, or unit-dose) dispensing, automated (mechanical and/or electronic) processing of medication orders and inventory control, and automated (mechanical and/or electronic) storage and delivery devices. Several investigators are at work in each of these areas, and the results of their studies may greatly alter current practices and procedures.

Because of the present state of uncertainty regarding the proper scope and optimum design of drug distribution systems for the modern hospital, and as an aid to pharmacists, nurses, physicians, and administrators who are faced with making decisions concerning drug distribution systems during this period of change, the following guidelines for evaluating proposed changes or new ideas or equipment are presented.

Though some of the practices recommended may not be widespread at the present, the adoption of these practices is believed to be a desirable and practical goal. Therefore, it is urged that they be given prime consideration in the design of new drug distribution systems and in modifications of existing ones (particularly where such changes would commit a hospital to a considerable financial investment in a system not including, or not easily altered to include, the recommended practices).

1. Before the initial dose of medication is administered the pharmacist should review the prescriber's original order or a direct copy.
2. Drugs dispensed should be as ready for administration to the patient as the current status of pharmaceutical technology will permit, and must bear adequate identification including (but not limited to); name or names of drug, strength or potency, route(s) of administration, expiration date, control number, and such other special instructions as may be indicated.
3. Facilities and equipment used to store drugs should be so designed that the drugs are accessible only to medical practitioners authorized to prescribe, to pharmacists authorized to dispense, or to nurses authorized to administer such drugs.
4. Facilities and equipment used to store drugs should be designed to facilitate routine inspection of the drug prior to the time of administration.
5. When utilizing automated (mechanical and/or electronic) devices as pharmaceutical tools, it is mandatory that provision be made to provide suitable pharmaceutical services in the event of failure of the device.
6. Such mechanical or electronic drug storage and dispensing devices, as require or encourage the repackaging of drug dosage forms from the manufacturer's original container, should permit and facilitate the use of a new package, which will assure the stability of each drug and meet U.S.P. standards for the packaging and storing of drugs, in addition to meeting all other standards of good pharmacy practice.
7. In considering automated (mechanical and/or electronic) devices as pharmaceutical tools, the distinction between the accuracy required in accounting practices versus that required in dispensing practices should be clearly distinguished.

Subsequently the following ASHP Statement on Unit Dose Drug Distribution was issued.[30]

ASHP STATEMENT ON UNIT DOSE DRUG DISTRIBUTION[a]

The unit dose system of medication distribution is a pharmacy-coordinated method of dispensing and controlling medications in health-care institutions.

---

[a]Approved by the ASHP House of Delegates on June 8, 1981. Revision approved by the ASHP Board of Directors at its meeting of November 13–14, 1980. Originally approved by the Board of Directors on April 19, 1975.

The unit dose system may differ in form depending on the specific needs of the institution. However, the following distinctive elements are basic to all unit dose systems: Medications are contained in single unit packages; they are dispensed in as ready-to-administer form as possible; for most medications not more than a 24-hour supply[a] of doses is delivered to or available at the patient-care area at any time.

Numerous studies concerning unit dose drug distribution systems have been published over the past several decades. These studies indicate categorically that unit dose systems, with respect to other drug distribution methods, are: (1) safer for the patient, (2) more efficient and economical for the institution, and (3) a more effective method of utilizing professional resources.

More specifically, the inherent advantages of unit dose systems over alternative distribution procedures are:

1. A reduction in the incidence of medication errors.
2. A decrease in the total cost of medication-related activities.
3. A more efficient usage of pharmacy and nursing personnel, allowing for more direct patient care involvement by pharmacists and nurses.
4. Improved overall drug control and drug-use monitoring.
5. More accurate patient billings for drugs.
6. The elimination or minimization of drug credits.
7. Greater control by the pharmacist over pharmacy workload patterns and staff scheduling.
8. A reduction in the size of drug inventories located in patient-care areas.
9. Greater adaptability to computerized and automated procedures.

In view of these demonstrated benefits, the American Society of Hospital Pharmacists considers the unit dose system to be an essential part of drug distribution and control in hospitals and other institutional health-care settings in which drug therapy is an integral component of health care delivery.

REFERENCES

1. Sourcebook on unit dose drug distribution systems. Bethesda, MD: American Society of Hospital Pharmacists; 1978.
2. ASHP guidelines on hospital drug distribution and control (with references). Am. J. Hosp. Pharm., 1980; *37*:1097–1103.

Accordingly, this chapter will be devoted to the various means employed by the hospital pharmacist to dispense and distribute various categories of drugs throughout the hospital.

---

[a] In long-term care facilities, a larger supply of medication (e.g., 48 or 72 hours) may be acceptable.

DRUG DISTRIBUTION—FLOOR STOCK SYSTEM

Each pavilion in the hospital, regardless of its size or specialty care, has a supply of drugs stored in the medicine cabinet even though the nursing unit is serviced by a unit dose system. However, the JCAH specifies that the use of floor stock medications should be minimized. In addition, research has shown[2] that the system of drug distribution has an effect upon the incidence of adverse drug reactions. These medications may be classified under two separate headings, each of which serves a specific purpose. Drugs on the nursing station may be divided into *"charge floor stock drugs"* and *"non-charge floor stock drugs."* It is the responsibility of the hospital pharmacist, working in cooperation with the nursing service, to develop ways and means whereby adequate supplies of each are always on hand and, in the appropriate situation, that proper charges are made to the patient's account.

This section will deal with the means whereby floor stock drugs are selected, and leave the methods whereby they are requisitioned by nursing service, distributed by pharmacy personnel and methods of issuing charges to patients, where the situation so warrants, to a later chapter on dispensing and distribution systems in the hospital pharmacy.

Definitions

Charge floor stock drugs may be defined as those medications that are stocked on the nursing station at all times and are charged to the patient's account after they have been administered.

Non-charge floor stock drugs represent that group of medications that are placed at the nursing station for the use of all patients on the pavilion and for which there may be no direct charge to the patient's account. In fact, the cost of this group of drugs is usually calculated in the per diem cost of the hospital room.

Today, there are four systems in general use for dispensing drugs for inpatients. They may be classified as follows: (i) Individual Prescription Order System, (ii) Complete Floor Stock System and (iii) Combinations of (i) and (ii) and the unit dose method.

INDIVIDUAL PRESCRIPTION ORDER SYSTEM

As has been previously stated, this system is generally used by the small and/or private hospital because of the reduced manpower requirements and the desirability for individualized service. Inherent in this system is the possible delay in obtaining the required medication and the increase in cost to the patient. At the same time, there are very definite advantages: (i) all medication orders are directly reviewed by the pharmacist; (ii) provides for the interaction of pharmacist, doctor, nurse and patient and (iii) provides closer control of inventory.

THE "COMPLETE" FLOOR STOCK SYSTEM

Under this system, the nursing station pharmacy carries both "charge" and "non-charge" patient medications. Rarely used or particularly expensive drugs are omitted from floor stock but are dispensed upon the receipt of a prescription or medication order for the individual patient.

Although this system is used most often in governmental and other hospitals in which charges are not made to the patient or when the all inclusive rate is used for charging, it does have applicability to the general hospital.

Obviously, there are both advantages and disadvantages to the complete floor stock system. Advantages include: (i) ready availability of the required drugs; (ii) elimination of drug returns; (iii) reduction in number of drug order transcriptions for the pharmacy and (iv) reduction in the number of pharmacy personnel required. The disadvantages of such a system are: (i) medication errors may increase because the review of medication orders is eliminated; (ii) increased drug inventory on the pavilions; (iii) greater opportunity for pilferage; (iv) increased hazards associated with drug deterioration; (v) lack of proper storage facilities on the ward may require capital outlay to provide them and (vi) greater inroads are made upon the nurses' time.

To be borne in mind by the student is the fact that in some hospitals the complete floor stock system is successfully operated as a decentralized pharmacy under the direct supervision of a pharmacist.

Obviously, when this occurs, many of the disadvantages associated with such a system disappear. In addition, the use of the decentralized pharmacy concept provides for a "home base" for the clinically oriented pharmacist.

In the past, floor stock containers were pre-labeled multiple dose units. Today, the floor stock is in unit-of-use packaging thereby assuring better packaging, control and identity of the medication.

COMBINATION OF INDIVIDUAL DRUG ORDER AND FLOOR STOCK SYSTEMS

Falling into this category are those hospitals which use the individual prescription or medication order system as their primary means of dispensing, but also utilize a limited floor stock. This combination system is probably the most commonly used in hospitals today and is modified to include the use of unit dose medications.

SELECTION OF CHARGE FLOOR STOCK DRUGS

The final decision as to which drugs shall be placed on the pavilions should rest with the Pharmacy and Therapeutics Committee, because this representative group of clinicians possesses a unique and intimate knowledge of the medicinal requirements of the patients within the institution.

This does not mean that the decision as to which drug shall or shall not be admitted to floor stock status should be arbitrarily arrived at. Representatives of nursing service, pharmacy and administration should be consulted for guidance and advice.

Once a floor stock list has been determined, it becomes the responsibility of the hospital pharmacist to make the drugs available, enforce the decision of the Pharmacy and Therapeutics Committee by not permitting deviations, and periodically to re-submit the list to the Pharmacy and Therapeutics Committee for re-evaluation in the light of later experience and therapeutic trends.

In arriving at a list of charge floor stock drugs, the Pharmacy and Therapeutics Committee will be concerned, in all probability, with having available for immediate use drugs of proven efficacy and which the average clinician considers necessary to administer to the patient as soon as a diagnosis is made or, at least, for the immediate symptomatic treatment.

Aside from the storage problem on the pavilion, there should be no valid reason why the decision of the Committee in this respect should not be honored, since each of these agents is chargeable to the patient's account. The only really important criteria to be considered here are the patient's clinical needs. The patient's financial status or ability to pay should have no bearing on his clinical need.

The following represents a typical list of injectable charge floor stock drugs in a large teaching hospital:

Medication and Strength

Parenteral
Ampicillin 1gm
Atropine 0.4mg
Cefoxitin 1gm
Cephalothin 1gm
Diazepam 10mg
Diphenhydramine 50mg
Dexamethasone 4mg
Gentamicin 80mg
Hydralazine 20mg
Hydroxyzine 100mg/2ml
Magnesium sulfate 1gm
Magnesium sulfate 5gm
Pitocin 10U
Prochlorperazine 10mg

    Promethazine 25mg
    Phenobarbital 60mg
    Potassium chloride 40mEq
    Scopolamine 0.43mg
    Terbutaline 1mg
    Trimethobenzamide 200mg
Oral
    Acetaminophen 325mg
    Aspirin 325mg
    Ampicillin 250mg
    Cephalexin 250mg
    Diazepam 2mg
    Diphenhydramine 25mg
    Ergotrate 0.2mg
    Fiorinal
    Hydralazine 10mg
    Chloral Hydrate 500mg
    Methyldopa 250mg
Medication and Strength
    Darvocet N 100
    Flurazepam 15mg
    Flurazepam 30mg
    Lomotil
    Chloral Hydrate 500mg
    Methylergonovine 0.2 mg
    Milk of Magnesia
    Mineral Oil
    MON/MO
    Mylanta
    Phenobarbital 15mg
    Promethazine 25mg
    Prochorperazine 5mg
    Terbutaline 2.5mg
    Terbutaline 5 mg
Refrigerator
    Dulcolax supp
    Prochlorperazine supp 25 mg
    Promethazine supp 25mg
    Methylergonovine amps 0.2mg
    Trimethobenzamide supp 200mg

SELECTION OF NON-CHARGE FLOOR STOCK DRUGS

With regard to the non-charge floor stock drugs a different set of criteria are employed. Here, consideration is usually given to the cost of the preparation, the frequency of use, the quantity used, and the effect upon the hospital budget and reimbursement from third party payors.

In many hospitals, this list is exceptionally small and therefore the patient is billed for numerous single doses of drugs. This, of course, produces bad public relations and the pharmacist should do all in his power to correct the situation.

A list of pharmaceutical and related preparations that are considered to be non-charge floor stock drugs in a university teaching hospital will be found in this Chapter. Each hospital should, of course, arrive at its own list based upon the needs of the staff and the type of patient cared for. Too brief a list will necessarily mean frequent small charges for pharmaceuticals. The sum of several such charges for each dose is usually more than would be charged for a like number of doses issued in one package. This has been a prime cause of adverse public relations for the hospital and should be guarded against whenever possible.

DISPENSING OF CHARGE NON-FLOOR STOCK DRUGS

Perusal of a modern hospital formulary will quickly show the large number of therapeutic agents available to the physician. They also indicate that the ordering, dispensing and accounting of these drugs must consume an inordinate amount of time on the part of nursing service and pharmacy personnel. Therefore, it has become necessary to streamline the paperwork involved through the adoption of semi-automated processes and technics. Having previously discussed the method whereby a physician orders a drug for a patient, this section will deal with the forms of accounting.

One method adopted by the hospital to identify patients is the principle of the charge plate. Here, by use of a plastic or metal card prepared on the patient's admission to the hospital or clinic, much nursing time is conserved. As a matter of fact, all newly-printed hospital forms usually reserve a 1 × 3 inch space in the upper right or left hand corner of the form for the information on the identification plate. Accordingly, all charge stations are equipped for using this time saving device which yields an important by-product—legibility of identity.

Many drug order forms may have such information as name of drug, dosage form and route of administration preprinted on it, thereby again conserving time by requiring only a minimal effort to select the drug, the desired form and route of administration.

Items with an extremely heavy demand have specific cards with all the information preprinted. All that is necessary is the patient's identity which is quickly supplied through the use of the charge plate.

Drug order forms may be prepared on duplicate or triplicate snap out forms which provide a copy for the pharmacy, accounting department and a control copy for the pavilion.

Some hospitals have developed a procedure whereby the hospital pharmacy receives a copy of the nurse's drug administration record or the physician's drug order sheet. Pharmacists then prepare periodic

PHARMACY
207

ORIGINAL TO BE SENT TO PHARMACY

ADDRESSOGRAPH AREA
PATIENT'S NAME John Doe
NUMBER 12-12-12
AREA & FLOOR B-26

IN PATIENT (✓ ONE): [X] PRIVATE; [ ] SEMI-PRIVATE; [ ] WARD PRIVATE; [ ] WARD
OUT PATIENT (✓ ONE): [ ] CLINIC; [ ] EMERGENCY WARD; [ ] PRIVATE AMBULATORY

DATE 1-15-65
REQUESTED BY Dr. Brown

NO SERVICE PERFORMED
WITHOUT PROPERLY FILLED OUT CHARGE REQUISITION

ORIGINAL

REQUEST FOR: (PRINT)	COST	UNITS	CHARGE
2 amps. Drug A	.10	2	.50
1 vial Drug B	1.00	1	1.65
	TOTAL COST	TOTAL UNITS	TOTAL CHARGE
	1.10	3	2.15

FORM 124
CHARGE REQUISITION
PETER BENT BRIGHAM HOSPITAL

Fig. 39. Pharmacy charge floor stock requisition form.

charges to the patient's account and re-stock the pavilions with the items consumed.

One example of a simple snap-out form utilizing the principles of the charge plate system is shown in Figure 39. This form is prepared in duplicate on the ward by the charge nurse or other responsible individual. The original is then forwarded to the pharmacy and the duplicate retained on the ward as a control copy. In addition to dispensing the requested medication, the pharmacist is also required to complete the form by inserting the cost price, the selling price and the number of units dispensed. This information is deemed to be necessary for internal auditing purposes.

A second example of a snap-out form that may utilize the principle of the charge plate is that shown in Figure 40. This form differs from that shown in Figure 40 in that the original portion entitled *Requisition for Medication* is forwarded to the pharmacy and contains on its face complete information relative to the administration of the drug by the nursing service. The second copy is utilized in the billing procedure whereas the third copy is used in the accounting department for internal audit purposes.

THE ENVELOPE SYSTEM

One hospital developed a system whereby an envelope was used to dispense containers of drugs to the nursing station and at the same time was also used as a charge ticket.[9] Under this system the pharmacist fills prelabeled envelopes with the specific drugs and places a predetermined quantity on the nursing unit. When the drug is administered to the patient, the nurse places the patient's name and room number

NEW ENGLAND CENTER HOSPITAL

Requisition for

MEDICATION

Mary Doe

12-12-50

Room 25   Dr. Roe

IN PATIENT USE ☒   HOME USE ONLY ☐ :

IF OFFICE ACC'T. DR.'S NAME:

ORDERED BY DR.: Dr. Roe		ORDER MADE OUT BY: JK					FILLED BY: WH	
	DRUG	DOSE	How Often	Route of Admin.	Quant. Issued	COST	CHARGE	
1.	Drug A	10 mg.	daily	I.M.	1 amp	1.00	1.65	
2.	Drug B	15 mg.	t.i.d.	oral	20 tab.	.30	.50	
3.								
	REQUISITION NO.: 12345				TOTAL	1.30	2.15	

F-51B 1/63

SEND THIS COMPLETE SET TO B.D. PHARMACY

Fig. 40. Combination Requisition for Medication, Charge Slip and Internal Audit developed by the New England Center Hospital.

JEFFERSON MEDICAL COLLEGE HOSPITAL
Philadelphia, Pa.

CHARGE - CREDIT VOUCHER

Date_____

Name

Room— Ward

Admission Number

Sex

Doctor

Complete or Imprint with Address-O-Plate

Explanation of Charge / Credits	√	DEBIT (CHARGE)	CREDIT
		$	

Signature of Person Preparing Voucher

Below this line for Main Office use only.

CODE

1 - Service	7 - Physical Therapy.	11 - 5 Formula & Bracelet	11-11 Hearing & Speech Center	D C Discount Credits
2 - Laboratory	8 - EKG	11 - 6 BMR		T B Transfer of Balance
3 - Drugs	9 - Blood or Plasma	11 - 7 Oxygen	11-12 Guest	P P Part Pay
4 - Operating Rm.	10 - Med.-Surg. Sup.	11 - 8 Nursery	B C Blue Cross	A D P S W
5 - Anesthesia	11 - 3 Telephone	11 - 9 Trfn Lab Svc	B D Bad Debts	Circle Appropriate Letters
6 - X-Ray	11 - 4 Guest Trays	11 - 10 Shock Treat.	B R Board Refunds	

FORM 14

Fig. 41. The multi-purpose Charge-Credit Voucher developed at the Jefferson Medical College Hospital.

on the envelope and places it in her "out" basket. This is later picked up by the messenger service and is delivered to the pharmacy where it is priced and forwarded to the accounting office.

ALLOWANCE OR CREDIT PROCEDURES ON UNUSED CHARGE DRUGS

Much has been written and spoken of the desirability and the moral and legal obligation to extend credit for unused medications consonant with necessary legal and fiscal controls.

Where a credit is to be issued, two things must be done; criteria for issuing credit on pharmaceuticals must be established, and second a proper credit form must be developed.

Many state pharmacy laws prohibit accepting pharmaceuticals for credit return unless the container is an unopened original package. To this should be added the caution that such containers should not have been out of the pharmacist's control for an unreasonable period of time. Most hospital pharmacists accept for credit most unopened ampuls, vials, tubes, and sealed containers of capsules and tablets which are returned from the pavilions. In order to avoid too great a loss to the patient when his therapy is suddenly changed, most hospitals restrict the amount of drug dispensed. A common number of tablets or capsules dispensed to a hospitalized patient is 20.

In some hospitals, a multi-purpose Charge-Credit Slip is utilized for extending credit to the patient's account for returned medications (Fig. 41). On the other hand, some institutions prefer to separate the functions of the two procedures and utilize two separate slips. One specif-

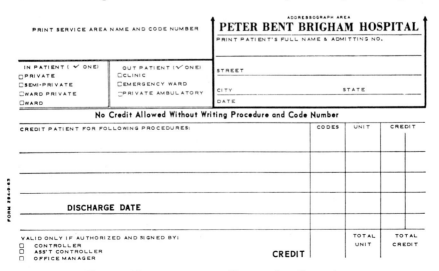

Fig. 42.   The separate or specific type of credit voucher.

PETER BENT BRIGHAM HOSPITAL

PHARMACY REQUISITION FOR FLOOR STOCK

AREA .... CODE .... DATA ....

Drugs listed below are to be considered floor stock and supplied Monday—Wednesday—Friday. All other drugs must be ordered as charge drugs.

MEDICINE CLOSET

Amt.	AMPULS	Price
	Adrenalin 1 ml 1:1000	
	Aminophylline 10 ml 250 mg	
	Atropine Sulfate 20 ml 0.4 mg/ml	
	Digitoxin 1 ml 0.2 mg	
	Digoxin 2 ml 0.25 mg/ml	
	Lidocaine HCl 50 ml 1%	
	Lidocaine HCl 50 ml 2%	
	Lidocaine HCl 1% with Epinephrine 1:1000 50 ml	
	Phenolsulfonphthalein (P.S.P.) 1 ml 6 mg/ml	
	Saline for Injection 30 ml	
	Scopolamine H. Br 1 ml 0.65 mg	
	Sodium Dehydrocholate (Decholin) 5 ml 1 gm/5 ml	
	Sulfobromophthaelin Sod. (B.S.P.) 3 ml 50 mg/ml	
	Water for Injection 30 ml	

Amt.	CAPSULES & TABLETS	Price
	Acetylsalicylic Acid (Aspirin) 0.3 gm	
	Acetylsalicylic Acid Buffered	
	Acetylsalicylic Acid Compound	
	Ammonium Chloride E.C. 0.5 gm	
	Amobarbital Sodium 0.2 gm	
	Atropine Sulfate T.T. 0.65 mg	
	Bisacodyl (Dulcolax) 5 mg	
	Bishydroxycoumarin (Dicoumarol) 25 mg	
	Cascara Sagrada Ext. 0.3 gm	
	Chloral Hydrate 0.5 gm	
	Digitalis 0.1 gm	
	Digitoxin 0.1 mg	
	Digoxin 0.25 mg	
	Ferrous Gluconate 300 mg	
	Ferrous Sulfate 0.3 gm	
	Nitroglycerin H.T. 0.3 mg	
	Nitroglycerin H.T. 0.6 mg	
	Pentobarbital 50 mg	
	Phenobarbital 15 mg	
	Placebos	
	Polyvitamins	
	Potassium Chloride E.C. 1 gm	
	Propoxyphene HCl (Darvon) 32 mg	
	Propoxyphene HCl Darvon Compound–65 mg	
	Quinidine HCl 0.2 gm	
	Secobarbital 50 mg	
	Sodium Bicarbonate 0.6 gm	

Amt.	SOLUTIONS—INTERNAL		Price
	Ammonium Chloride Syr.	8 oz	
	Belladonna Tr.	2 oz	
	Benzoin Comp. Tr.	4 oz	
	Cascara Fldext Aromatic	4 oz	
	Castor Oil	8 oz	
	Chloral Hydrate 1 gm/5 ml	8 oz	
	Glyceryl Guaiacolate- (Robitussin)	4 oz	
	Kaolin-Pectin Mixture	8 oz	
	Opium Tr. Camphorated	4 oz	
	Peppermint Spirit	2 oz	
	Potassium Chloride Elixir	8 oz	
	Potassium Iodide Sat. Sol.	2 oz	
	Potassium Triple Ion Elixir	8 oz	
	Terpin Hydrate Elixir	4 oz	
	Terpin Hydrate & Codeine Elixir	8 oz	
	Vanilla Flavor	4 oz	

Amt.	POWDERS		Price
	Dextrose (D-Glucose)	100 gm Units	
	Sodium Bicarbonate	16 oz	
	Talcum—Individual Units*		
	Thymol Iodide (Aristol)*	2 oz	
	*Store in Utility Room		

Amt.	MISCELLANEOUS	Price
	Amyl Nitrite	
	Aromatic Ammonia	

REFRIGERATOR

Amt.	SUPPOSITORIES		Price
	Acetylsalicylic Acid	0.6 gm	
	Aminophylline	500 mg	
	Bisacodyl (Dulcolax)	10 mg	

Amt.	LIQUID		Price
	Hydrogen Peroxide 3 Vol.	16 oz	
	Magnesia, Milk of	32 oz	
	Petrolatum, Liquid	32 oz	

Fig. 43. (Continued on opposite page)

UTILITY ROOM

Amt.	SOLUTIONS—EXTERNAL		Price
	Alcoholic Sponge Lotion	32 oz	
	Alkaline Aromatic Solution (Mouth Wash)	32 oz	
	Amphyl–2%	Gal	
	Back Rub Lotion	Ind	
	Benzalkonium Chloride 1:750	gal	
	Benzalkonium Chloride 1:1000	gal	
	Benzalkonium Chloride 1:20,000	gal	
	Benzalkonium Chloride Tr.	16 oz	
	Benzoin Tr.	4 oz	
	Calamine Lotion	8 oz	
	Chlorinated Soda—5%	32 oz	
	Collodion Flexible	4 oz	
	Creo-Napol 1:50	Gal	
	Denatured Alcohol for Lamps	8 oz	
	Deodorizing Spray	16 oz	
	Ether—Not For Anesthesia	8 oz	
	Ether—Alcohol Mixture	8 oz	
	Glycerin	8 oz	
	Hand Lotion	8 oz	
	Hexachlorophene Deterg.	32 oz	
	Hexachlorophene Liquid Soap	32 oz	
	Iodine Aqueous—2%	8 oz	
	Iodine Tr.—2%	8 oz	
	Instrument Sterilizing Solution	32 oz	
	Isopropyl Alcohol—50%	32 oz	
	Magnesium Sulfate—Glycerin Solution	16 oz	
	P.C.G. Solution	8 oz	
	Thermometer Germicide Solution	32 oz	

Amt.	OINTMENTS & CREAMS		Price
	A & D Ointment	1 oz	
	Lanolin	1 oz	
	Lanolin—Stearin Cream	4 oz	
	Petrolatum	1 oz	
	Surgical Lubricant—Single use unit		
	Zinc Oxide Ointment	1 oz	

Amt.	REAGENTS		Price
	Acetone	8 oz	
	Acetic Acid—50%	4 oz	
	Benzidine Reagent	4 oz	
	Schiller's Solution	8 oz	
	Sulfuric Acid—50%	2 oz	
	Sulfuric Acid—0.5%	2 oz	
	Toluene	8 oz	
	Topfer's Reagent	4 oz	
	Wright's Stain	8 oz	

THIS SPACE FOR PHARMACY
OFFICE USE ONLY

Filled by . . . .

Checked by: . . . .

Price Total for sheet . . . $ . . . .

Previous Total $ . . . .

Current Total $ . . . .

Form 16-Drug

Fig. 43 *(Continued).* Pharmacy requisition for non-charge floor stock supplies.

ically for the charge and the other for extending credit. See Figure 42 for this type of form.

DISPENSING AND DISTRIBUTION OF NON-CHARGE FLOOR STOCK DRUGS

This category of drugs and related products being predetermined and stable is amenable to a variety of unique methods whereby the drugs are conveyed from the pharmacy to the nursing station.

Basic to all the distribution systems is the preparation of a printed list which indicates the name and strength of the product, the size of the unit, and its location on the nursing station. Figure 43 represents one such form which encompasses non-charge floor stock drugs as well as various lotions, germicides, mouthwashes and sterilizing solutions.

DRUG BASKET METHOD

One method formerly used by hospitals for stocking non-charge floor stock drugs and related products on the nursing station is the "drug basket method." Under this system, the night nurse checks the medicine closet, utility room and drug refrigerator inventory of supplies against a master list provided by the pharmacy through the nursing service. The nurse places a check mark on the number required for each drug on the requisition for floor stock supplies (Fig. 43). Where there is an empty container, she places it in the drug basket. Once the procedure is completed, the drug basket containing the empty containers and requisition for floor stock supplies, is then sent to the pharmacy.

Immediately upon opening in the morning the pharmacy staff commences to fill each container and dispense the requested ampuls and vials as ordered. Once the basket is complete, it is delivered to the floor via a messenger service or, in the newer institutions, via a dumb-waiter or basket ejector delivery system.

MOBILE DISPENSING UNIT

A mobile dispensing system, previously described, for the hospital pharmacy[8] utilizes a specially constructed stainless steel truck measuring 60 inches high, 48 inches wide and 25½ inches deep. The main body of the truck is mounted on six 8-inch balloon tires, the center wheels being stationary while the remaining four are swivel-type. The main compartment is provided with two locking sliding doors, a handle for steering and pushing, a heavy duty steel and rubber protective bumper and a 2-inch rim on the top to permit carrying empty containers being returned to the pharmacy.

The interior of the unit consists of four shelves which allow for the transport of all size containers.

Under this system, two mobile units are put into operation in order to permit one unit to be in use while the other is being serviced. The frequency of delivery and the hours during which the mobile unit will visit the pavilion can be selected in cooperation with the Nursing Service.

By using this system, it will not be necessary for the night nurse to check the pharmacy inventory or have empty containers transported to the pharmacy. Instead, the pharmacist or the pharmacy aide manning the mobile unit will inventory the pavilion drug cabinets and check off the items and quantity of supplies left. The carbon copy of the *Requisition for Floor Stock Supplies* is left on the pavilion as a record of the delivery, and the original is returned to the pharmacy where it will serve the following three purposes.

1. to re-stock the mobile unit
2. to determine rate of use or consumption
3. to serve as a charge document for the internal allocation of costs.

Although it would appear that this method primarily conserves nursing personnel time, it has a number of advantages which are beneficial to the pharmacy, particularly if the truck is manned by a pharmacist.

For example, the drugs and the nursing station drug cabinets will always be under the supervision of professional personnel. The pharmacist is brought out of the pharmacy and made available for on the spot consultations by clinical and nursing staffs, and through the routine checking of the medicine closet, deteriorated, out-dated and non-approved drugs and drug samples may be quickly removed.

PATIENT SERVERS CONCEPT

A decentralized system of unit dose distribution of patients' medications to each individual hospital room was incorporated into the construction of two new floors of a hospital. Essentially, locked medication drawers are located in "patient servers" which are specially designed supply closets built into the hall wall at the entrance to each

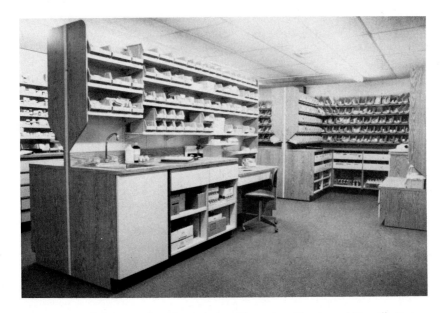

Fig. 44. View of pharmacy featuring unit dose dispensing. (Courtesy of Lionville Systems, Inc., Lionville, Pa.)

patient's room. The patient servers are designed to allow access to the medication drawer and the drawer containing the patient's chart from the hall or from within the patient's room. This allows the nurse access to the patient's medication and chart without leaving the room, while the pharmacy technician may gain access to the medication drawer without entering the room. The drawer containing the patient's chart may also be reached from the hall without entering the room.[28]

It has been stated that the use of "patient servers" can be costly for a pharmacy department and state that a medication cart system is more cost-effective from the standpoint of remodeling costs, and personnel time involved (primarily in exchange of medication drawers, and duplication of floor stock supplies).[28]

UNIT DOSE DISPENSING—GENERAL

Unit-dose medications have been defined[10] as—

"those medications which are ordered, packaged, handled, administered and charged in multiples of single dose units containing a predetermined amount of drug or supply sufficient for one regular dose, application or use."

The concept of unit-dose dispensing is not a new innovation to pharmacy and medicine. For many years, pharmaceutical manufacturers have prepared and sold prefilled, single-dose disposable syringes of medications and single-unit foil or cellophane wrapped capsules and tablets. Because the concept is broad, one might even consider the individual ampul or single-dose vial as the precursor to unit-dose dispensing.

Although unit-dose dispensing is a pharmacy responsibility, it cannot be instituted in the hospital without the cooperation of the nursing, administrative and medical staffs. Thus, it is recommended that a planning committee be created and charged with the responsibility of developing the approach to the utilization of a unit-dose system in the hospital. Despite the motivation of the committee membership, experience dictates that the hospital pharmacist should take the time to thoroughly educate them in the concepts of unit-dose dispensing. This may be accomplished via literature reprints, film strips and visitations to institutions that have implemented a unit-dose system. Throughout the educational and developmental period, liaison must be maintained with the medical, nursing and administrative staffs by the hospital pharmacist.

The following are some advantages attributed to a unit dose system:

(1) Patients receive improved pharmaceutical service 24 hours a day and are charged for only those doses which are administered to them.

(2) All doses of medication required at the nursing station are prepared by the pharmacy thus allowing the nurse more time for direct patient care.
(3) Allows the pharmacists to interpret or check a copy of the physician's original order thus reducing medication errors.
(4) Eliminates excessive duplication of orders and paper work at the nursing station and pharmacy.
(5) Eliminates credits.
(6) Transfers intravenous preparation and drug reconstitution procedures to the pharmacy.
(7) Promotes more efficient utilization of professional and non-professional personnel.
(8) Reduces revenue losses.
(9) Conserves space in nursing units by eliminating bulky floor stock.
(10) Eliminates pilferage and drug waste.
(11) Extends pharmacy coverage and control throughout the hospital from the time the physician writes the order to the time the patient receives the unit-dose.
(12) Communication of medication orders and delivery systems are improved.
(13) The pharmacists can get out of the pharmacy and onto the wards where they can perform their intended function as drug consultants and help provide the team effort that is needed for better patient care.

The method whereby drugs are obtained from the pharmacy to the nursing station for administration to the patient is by means of the doctor's order written on a Doctor's Order Sheet in the patient's medical record. It is from this source that the nurse prepares the medication for administration to the patient (See Chapter 12).

The student will understand the importance of the doctor's drug order and its relationship to the unit dose system (or any other drug distribution system) from the following excerpt from the ASHP Technical Assistance Bulletin of Hospital Drug Distribution and Control.[31]

ASHP TECHNICAL ASSISTANCE BULLETIN ON HOSPITAL DRUG DISTRIBUTION AND CONTROL (UNIT DOSE SECTION)

Medication distribution is the responsibility of the pharmacy. The pharmacist, with the assistance of the pharmacy and therapeutics committee and the department of nursing, must develop comprehensive policies and procedures that provide for the safe distribution of all medications and related supplies to inpatients and outpatients.

For reasons of safety and economy, the preferred method to distribute drugs in institutions is the *unit dose system.* Though the unit dose system may differ in form depending on the specific needs, resources, and characteristics of each institution, four elements are common to all: (1) medications are contained in, and administered from, single-unit or unit-dose packages; (2) medications are dispensed in ready-to-administer form, to the extent possible; (3) for most medications, not more than a 24-hour supply of doses is provided to or available at the patient care area at any time, and (4) a patient medication profile is concurrently maintained in the pharmacy for each patient. Floor stocks of drugs are minimized and limited to drugs for emergency use and routinely used "safe" items such as mouthwash and antiseptic solutions.

(1) *Physician's Drug Order: Writing the Order.* Medications should be given (with certain specified exceptions) only on the *written* order of a qualified physician or other authorized prescriber. Allowable exceptions to this rule (i.e., telephoned or verbal orders) should be put in written form immediately and the prescriber should countersign the nurse's or pharmacist's signed record of these orders within 48 (preferably 24) hours. Only a pharmacist or registered nurse should accept such orders. Provision should be made to place physician's orders in the patient's chart, and a method for sending this information to the pharmacy should be developed.

Prescribers should specify the date and time medication orders are written.

Medication orders should be written legibly in ink and should include:

- Patient's name and location (unless clearly indicated on the order sheet).
- Name (generic) of medication.
- Dosage expressed in the metric system, except in instances where dosage must be expressed otherwise (i.e., units, etc.).
- Frequency of administration.
- Route of administration.
- Signature of the physician.
- Date and hour the order was written.

Any abbreviations used in medication orders should be agreed to and jointly adopted by the medical, nursing, pharmacy, and medical records staff of the institution.

Any questions arising from a medication order, including the interpretation of an illegible order, should be referred to the ordering physician by the pharmacist. It is desirable for the pharmacist to make (appropriate) entries in the patient's medical chart pertinent to the patient's drug therapy. Also, a duplicate record of the entry can be maintained in the pharmacy profile.

In computerized patient data systems, each prescriber should be assigned a unique identifier; this number should be included in all medication orders. Unauthorized personnel should not be able to gain assess to the system.

(2) *Physician's Drug Order: Medication Order Sheets.* The pharmacist (except in emergency situations) must receive the physician's original order or a direct copy of the order before the drug is dispensed. This permits the pharmacist to resolve questions or problems with drug order

before the drug is dispensed and administered. It also eliminates errors which may arise when drug orders are transcribed onto another form for use by the pharmacy. Several methods by which the pharmacy may receive physician's original orders or direct copies are:

1. Self-copying order forms. The physician's order form is designed to make a direct copy (carbon or NCR) which is sent to the pharmacy. This method provides the pharmacist with a duplicate copy of the order and does not require special equipment. There are two basic formats:
   a. Orders for medications included among treatment orders. Use of this form allows the physician to continue writing his orders on the chart as he has been accustomed in the past, leaving all other details to hospital personnel.
   b. Medication orders separated from other treatment orders on the order form. The separation of drug orders makes it easier for the pharmacist to review the order sheet.
2. Electromechanical. Copying machines or similar devices may be used to produce an exact copy of the physician's order. Provision should be made to transmit physicians' orders to the pharmacy in the event of mechanical failure.
3. Computerized. Computer systems, in which the physician enters orders into a computer which then stores and prints out the order in the pharmacy or elsewhere, are used in some institutions. Any such system should provide for the pharmacist's verification of any drug orders entered into the system by anyone other than an authorized prescriber.

(3) *Physician's Drug Order: Time Limits and Changes.* Medication orders should be reviewed automatically when the patient goes to the delivery room, operating room, or a different service. In addition, a method to protect patients from indefinite, open-ended drug orders must be provided. This may be accomplished through one or more of the following: (1) routine monitoring of patients' drug therapy by a pharmacist; (2) drug class-specific, automatic stop-order policies covering those drug orders not specifying a number of doses or duration of therapy; (3) automatic cancellation of all drug orders after a predetermined (by the pharmacy and therapeutics committee) time interval unless rewritten by the prescriber. Whatever the method used, it must proect the patient, as well as provide for a timely notification to the prescriber that the order will be stopped *before* such action takes place.

(4) *Physician's Drug Order: Receipt of Order and Drug Profiles.* A pharmacist must review and interpret every medication order, and resolve any problems or uncertainties with it, before the drug is entered into the dispensing system. This means that he must be satisfied that each questionable medication order is in fact, acceptable. This may occur through study of the patient's medical record, research of the professional literature or discussion with the prescriber or other medical, nursing, or pharmacy staff. Procedures to handle a drug order the pharmacist still believes is unacceptable (e.g., very high dose or a use

beyond that contained in the package insert) should be prepared (and reviewed by the hospital's legal counsel). In general, the physician must be able to support the use of the drug in these situations. It is generally advisable for the pharmacist to document actions (e.g., verbal notice to the physician that a less toxic drug was available and should be used) relative to a questionable medication order on the pharmacy's patient medication profile form or other pharmacy document (not in the medical record).

Once the order has been approved, it is entered into the *patient's medication profile.* A medication profile must be maintained in the pharmacy for all inpatients and those outpatients routinely receiving care at the institution. (Note: equivalent records also should be available at the patient care unit.) This essential item, which is continuously updated, may be a written copy or computer-maintained. It serves two purposes. First, it enables the pharmacist to become familiar with the patient's total drug regimen, enabling him to detect quickly potential interactions, unintended dosage changes, drug duplications and over-lapping therapies, and drugs contraindicated because of patient allergies or other reasons. Second, it is required in unit dose systems in order for the individual medication doses to be scheduled, prepared, distributed, and administered on a timely basis. The profile information must be reviewed by the pharmacist *before* dispensing the patient's drug(s). (It also may be useful in retrospective review of drug use.)

Patient profile information should include:

- Patient's full name, date hospitalized, age, sex, weight, hospital I.D. number, and provisional diagnosis or reason for admission (the format for this informaiton will vary from one hospital to another)
- Laboratory test results.
- Other medical data relevant to the patient's drug therapy (e.g., information from drug history interviews).
- Sensitivities, allergies, and other significant contraindications.
- Drug products dispensed, dates of original order, strengths, dosage forms, quantities, dosage frequency or directions, and automatic stop dates.
- Intravenous therapy data (this information may be kept on a separate profile form but there should be a method for the pharmacist to review both concomitantly).
- Blood products administered.
- Pharmacist's or technician's initials.
- Number of doses or amounts dispensed.
- Items relevant or related to the patient's drug therapy (e.g., blood products) not provided by the pharmacy.

(5) *Physician's Drug Order Records.* Appropriate records of each medication order and its processing in the pharmacy must be maintained. Such records must be retained in accordance with applicable state laws and regulations. Any changes or clarifications in the order should be

written in the chart. The signature(s) or initials of the person(s) verifying the transcription of medication orders into the medication profile should be noted. A way should be provided to determine, for all doses dispensed, who prepared the dose, its date of dispensing, the source of the drug, and the person who checked it. Other information, such as the time of receipt of the order and management data (number of orders per patient day, and the like) should be kept as desired. Medication profiles also may be useful for retrospective drug use review studies.

(6) *Physician's Drug Order: Special Orders.* Special orders (i.e., "stat" and emergency orders, and those for nonformulary drugs, investigational drugs, restricted-use drugs or controlled substances) should be processed according to specific written procedures meeting all applicable regulations and requirements.

(7) *Physician's Drug Order: Other Considerations.* The pharmacy, nursing, and medical staffs, through the pharmacy and therapeutics committee, should develop a schedule of standard drug administration times. The nurse should notify the pharmacist whenever it is necessary to deviate from the standard medication schedule.

A mechanism to continually inform the pharmacy of patient admissions, discharges, and transfers should be established.

The unit-dose dispensing concept may be introduced into the hospital in either of two ways—the choice depending upon the individual hospital and its pharmacist. The first method is the **centralized unit-dose drug distribution system,** often abbreviated as CUDD, and the **decentralized unit-dose drug distribution system,** often abbreviated as DUDD. Some pharmacists have developed a plan whereby they use a combination of the two methods.

The initiation of a unit-dose dispensing system in the hospital is not an easy task and requires a great deal of planning both within the pharmacy and with the nursing service. The hospital pharmacist should enter into such a program a step at a time. He should commence by distributing as many injectables as possible in individual disposable syringes; he may commence the distribution of tablets and capsules in strip-packages; certain lotions, creams and ointments are already available on the drug market in single dose aluminum foil or plastic containers and thus lend themselves to the concept of unit-dose dispensing.

The adoption of a unit-dose dispensing system in the hospital can save personnel time both in the pharmacy and on the nursing service; provide contamination free positive identification of the medication up to the time of administration; eliminate labeling errors; permit far more accurate medication charges; and prevent the loss of partially used medications.

Personnel time can be saved in the pharmacy because under the unit-dose system it no longer becomes necessary for the pharmacy to repackage and label the product in smaller dispensing units. Since this step is eliminated, so, too, is the cumbersome procedure for the preparation of adequate records for the purpose of recalling all available containers of a specific product should the occasion arise

Unit-dose dispensing of medications can be accomplished in many ways. One means is through the use of strip-packaging and vial and syringe filling equipment in the hospital. (See Chapter 20 Pre-Packaging in the Hospital.) Figure 45 shows a solid oral packaging machine for convenient economical, and reliable institutional use. Vials of 15, 30 and 60 ml may be filled by the use of a programmable dispensing pump (Fig. 47) along with a manual bench capper as shown in Figure 48. An example of one product in a 30-ml vial with the cap properly applied is shown in Figure 49. Injectable drugs may also be prepared for the unit dose system within the hospital. Disposable glass syringes in 0.5, 1, 2.5, and 10-ml sizes are commercially available and can be filled in the hospital using a syringe filling stand and transfer needle. Once filled, the syringes are placed in a plastic tray and labeled. Before commencing such a program, the student should become familiar with

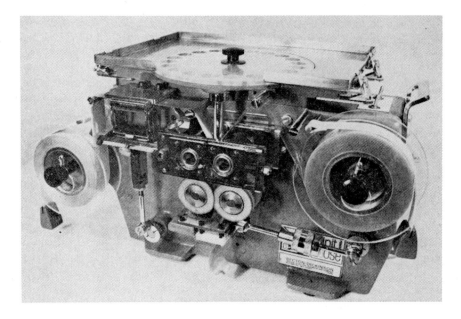

Fig. 45.   Una-Strip Packer, Model SA Oral Solid Packaging Machine. (Courtesy of Becton, Dickinson and Co., Rutherford, New Jersey.)

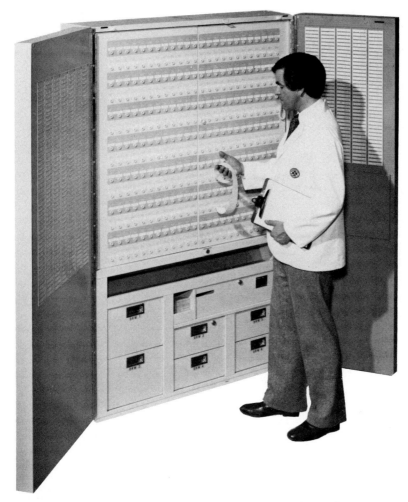

Fig. 46. The DocuMed® Pharmacy Night Cabinet. (Courtesy of Lionville Systems Inc., Lionville, Pa.)

the American Society of Hospital Pharmacists' *Guidelines for Single Unit Packages of Drugs.* See Chapter 20, page 421.

A second method may be to purchase the packaging service from an outside contractor or by the joint purchase and sharing of equipment with a neighboring hospital.

The third method is to purchase all drugs in unit dose packages. For example, Philips Roxane Laboratories distribute unit of use galenicals, magmas and suspensions whereas Wyeth Laboratories, via the "Wyeth System," makes available a combination of single packaged and labeled tablets and capsules and pre-filled, single unit disposable sterile car-

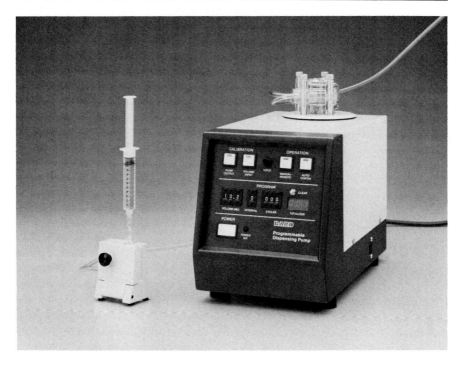

Fig. 47.   Programmable dispensing pump. (Courtesy of Bard MedSystems, Divison C.R. Bard Inc., Murray Hill, N.J.)

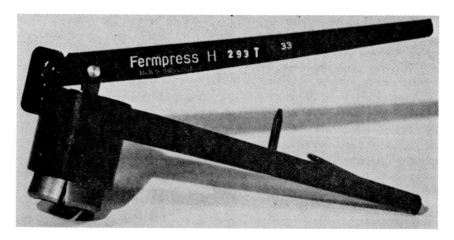

Fig. 48.   Fermpress hand capper. Applies unit dose three-piece aluminum closures to 15-, 30- and 60-ml glass vials. (Courtesy Becton, Dickinson and Co., Rutherford, New Jersey.)

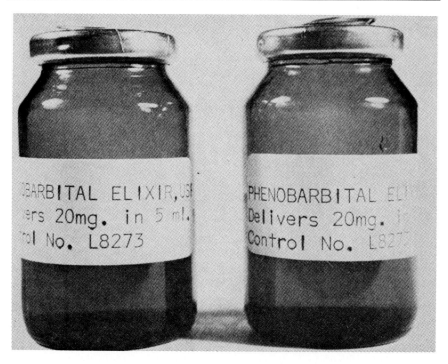

Fig. 49. An example of a 30-ml vial with closure properly applied and labeled. (Courtesy of Becton, Dickinson and Co., Rutherford, New Jersey.)

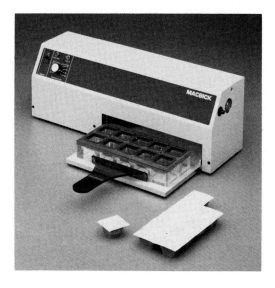

Fig. 50. Unit dose heat sealer. (Courtesy of Bard MedSystems, Division of C.R. Bard Inc., Murray Hill, N.J.)

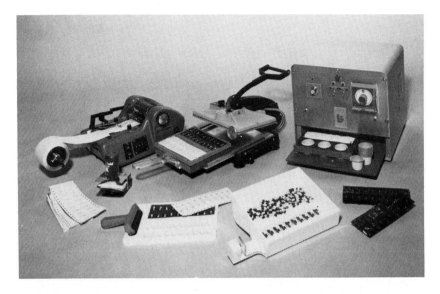

Fig. 51. A full range of unit dose packaging equipment. (Courtesy of Lionville Systems Inc., Lionville, Pa.)

tridge-needle units (Tubex®)[a] and a specially designed medication dispensing cabinet. Other manufacturers produce solid orals in unit dose packages and produce injectables in ready-to-use plastic syringes.

It should be noted at this point that the Wyeth medication dispensing cabinet differs completely from the dispensing machine type of unit which is a component of the Brewer System. Where the Brewer unit required various "control plates" to cause it to operate, the Wyeth unit requires none. Where the Brewer unit could imprint labels and drug charge information, the Wyeth unit does not. These differences are stated here merely for the purpose of impressing upon the student that one is not similar to the other in either design or concept. Each performs a special type of function or service.

One interesting feature of the Wyeth system is its adaptability to utilize three different packagings of oral unit doses—a soft-pack strip pack consisting of a roll of single dose medications which can be dispensed from a re-usable reel-type of dispenser, the Redipak® strip pack, the same cellophane roll of single dose medications described above except that here the outer casing is a disposable cardboard box, and finally, the commonly used strip pack.

The medication dispensing cabinet is available in two styles; a large stationary unit for use at the nursing station or a smaller mobile unit (see Figs. 53, 54, 55) which may be used as a complete medication cart.

---

[a]Tubex® Wyeth Laboratories.

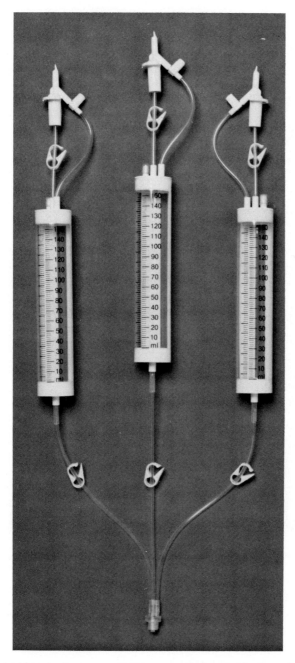

Fig. 52. The Multi-Meter System, a precision metered-chamber fluid transfer system designed for the preparation of TPN and other specialty IV fluids. (Courtesy of Burron Medical Inc., Bethlehem, Pa.)

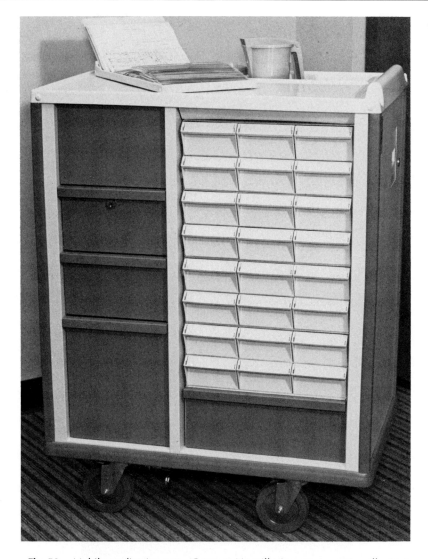

Fig. 53. Mobile medication cart. (Courtesy Lionville Systems Inc., Lionville, Pa.)

By introducing a full-line single unit package of drugs, the hospital pharmacist has the advantage of what has been described as a "pre-system" phase-in from which accrue the following:[11]

(i)   "acquaint nurses with the various new containers from which they will be administering medication;

(ii)   assist in planning for and stocking of various inventory levels;

(iii) provide the many benefits of single unit packaging itself even though a unit dose system is not operational."

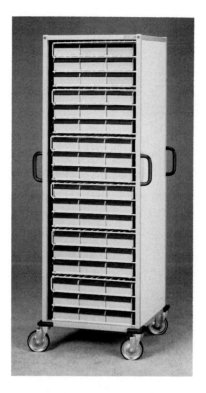

Fig. 54. The vertical transfer system cart. (Courtesy of Bard MedSystem, Division of C.R. Bard Inc., Murray Hill, N.J.)

UNIT DOSE DISPENSING PROCEDURE

The characteristic features of centralized unit-dose dispensing are that all in-patient drugs are dispensed in unit-doses and all the drugs are stored in a central area pharmacy and dispensed at the time the dose is due to be given to the patient. To operate the system effectively, electronic data processing equipment is not required, however delivery systems such as medication carts and dumbwaiters are needed to get the unit-doses to the patients; also suction tube systems (called pneumatic tubes) or other means are required to send a copy of the physician's original medication order to the pharmacy for direct interpretation and filling.

The *decentralized* unit-dose system, unlike the centralized system, operates through small satellite pharmacies located on each floor of the hospital. The main pharmacy in this system becomes a procurement, storage, manufacturing and packaging center serving all the satellites. The delivery system is accomplished by the use of medication carts. This type of system can be used for a hospital with separate buildings or old delivery systems.

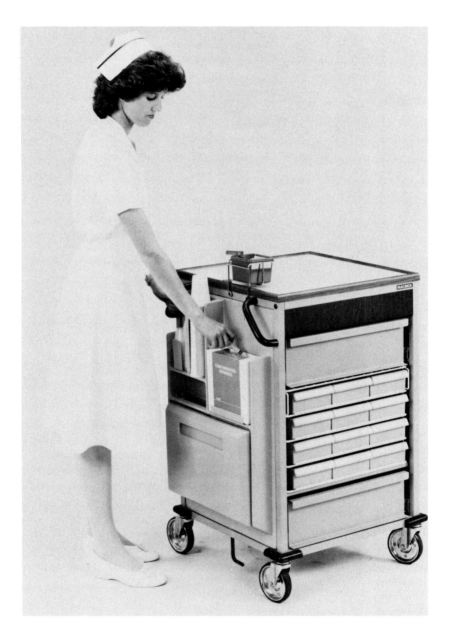

Fig. 55.   Nursing cart for use in unit dose dispensing systems. (Courtsey of Bard Med-
Systems, Division C.R. Bard, Inc., Murray Hill, N.J.)

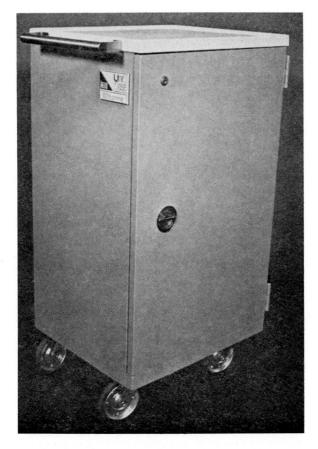

Fig. 56. B-D Nursing Cart with door. (Courtesy of Becton, Dickinson and Co., Rutherford, New Jersey.)

Although each hospital introduces variations, the following is a step-by-step outline of the procedure entailed in a decentralized unit-dose system:

1. Upon admission to the hospital, the patient is entered into the system. Diagnosis, allergies and other pertinent data are entered on to the Patient Profile card.
2. Direct copies of medication orders are sent to the pharmacist.
3. The medications ordered are entered on to the Patient Profile card.
4. Pharmacist checks medication order for allergies, drug-interactions, drug-laboratory test effects and rationale of therapy.
5. Dosage scheduled is coordinated with the nursing station.
6. Pharmacy technician picks medication orders, placing drugs in bins of a transfer cart per dosage schedule (Fig. 54).
7. Medication cart is filled for particular dosage schedule delivery (Figs. 55 and 56).

8. Pharmacist checks cart prior to release.
9. The nurse administers the medication and makes appropriate entry on her medication record.
10. Upon return to the pharmacy, the cart is rechecked.
11. Throughout the entire sequence, the pharmacist is available for consultation by the doctors and nurses. In addition he is maintaining a surveillance for discontinued orders.

UNIT DOSES NOT ADMINISTERED

Accountability of dispensed medications is important to the hospital pharmacist working in a unit-dose distribution system. By learning about and following up on those medications not administered and returned in the patient bins of the drug cart or cassette, the pharmacist utilizes the unit-dose system to its utmost for the purpose of preventing medication errors.[29]

To help facilitate finding out why a drug was not given, many hospitals with unit-dose systems have devleoped communication forms for use by nurses to inform pharmacists. They are usually placed in the bin with the returned medication and sent to the pharmacy.[29] These forms contain the patient identification, drug identity and dose, reason for the drug not being given, a statement to the effect that the prescribing physician has been so notified and a new time for administration if such is warranted.

OTHER CONCEPTS IN DISPENSING

Of late, much has been written about placing a pharmacist on the nursing station to assume all responsibility concerning the ordering, stocking and preparation of drugs for administration as well as to be readily available for consultation by the clinical and nursing staffs. If funds and a sufficient number of pharmacists were available, all would agree that this would be a desirable step forward in ensuring drug safety through a marked reduction in medication errors.

This would be possible because the pharmacist is sufficiently trained and legally licensed to deal with all aspects of drug selection and handling with the exception of administering it to the patient. On the pavilion, the pharmacist may help the physician in the selection of the most therapeutically beneficial drug, assist the nurse by interpreting the physician's order as well as the preparation of each dose for administration, and the ordering, storage, charging and control of all drugs and related products on the nursing station.

Because the funds and personnel are not presently available, some pharmacists[12,13] have experimented with a centralized unit-dose system. Under this method, the department of pharmacy prepares a single dose of medication ready for administration to the patient and delivers it to the pavilion a few minutes before it is to be administered by the nurse.

Both of these studies indicated that nursing time could be saved, that the incidence of error was in all probability reduced and that the system gained "nurse acceptance" in a relatively short time.

Researchers at the University of Arkansas Medical Center worked on an extremely interesting study whereby they developed a centralized unit-dose system for general hospital use.[14,17]

As described, the methodology requires that a copy of the physician's order be forwarded to an IBM Keypunch operator who interprets the order via a code system onto the cards which are then processed through a sorter, reproducer and card-type converter.

Another of these sophisticated electronic data systems permits the physician to write his order and insert the written sheet into a machine, which then transmits a view of the order on to a videoscope in the pharmacy. Here it is checked for accuracy by the pharmacist and if correct, he may activate the dispensing portion of the machine by pressing a button which automatically activates a computer and an entire series of events takes place. The drug is dispensed, the nurse is alerted to administer the medication, a charge is entered upon the patient's account and upon the administration of the drug by the nurse, another press of a button enters the fact upon the patient's hospital record. The computer can also notify the doctor if the drug is not in inventory, is not prescribed according to the dose or route of administration recommended in the hospital formulary and will alert the nurse if she has failed to administer the drug within a predetermined period of time.

It should be clear that the use of electronic data processing equipment in conjunction with the dispensing of unit-dose medications can provide a broad spectrum of useful statistical data governing drugs and their use. Obviously then, such equipment must already be in use in the hospital in order to make the undertaking of a comprehensive automated dispensing program a feasible venture.

One method which does not make use of mechanical or electronic dispensing devices for the distribution of patient-charge drugs is employed at the Massachusetts General Hospital in Boston and is entitled MOSAICS—an abbreviation for **Medication Order Supply and Individual Charge System.**[18] This system places all of the drugs in current use at the hospital in the nurses' drug cabinet.

The Mosaic system is stated to reflect a simple but basic change, namely, that in the past the patient was admitted first and the drug was then requisitioned. Under the Mosaics plan, the drug is already on the floor awaiting the patient. The modus operandi is relatively simple in that a pharmacist visits the patient floor on a regular schedule, re-stocks the unit and makes a charge to the patient or patients consuming the drugs. The information necessary for the charging procedure comes from the Doctor's Order Sheet, Nursing Kardex or Medication Charting Sheets.

The architects of the Mosaic system have demonstrated that by placing the pharmacist on the patient pavilion, it was possible for him to serve as a drug advisor and consultant to the medical and nursing staffs. In addition, he was in a better position to perform the pharmaceutical functions of checking upon the storage, administration, expiration data, contamination and degradation of drugs and biologicals.

SELF-MEDICATION PROGRAMS

The large number of effective therapeutic agents which are now available has created a serious problem in the proper treatment of patients. Because of the specificity of pharmacological response of many of these drugs, it is often necessary to employ several in order to obtain the desired clinical reponse. Frequently, this has led to confusion, improper administration of the drug on the part of the patient and poor therapeutic results.

In an informal survey conducted by the Nursing Service and the Department of Pharmacy of a metropolitan teaching hospital, it was learned that approximately 50% of the ambulatory patients receiving medications were not aware of the reasons for taking the drugs and that nearly 40% exhibited errors in the way they were taking their medications. Upon closer scrutiny of this figure, it was clearly demonstrated that an extremely high percentage of the errors were made when the signa of the prescription indicated "As directed" and the patient received more than one prescription.

Since the above observations were being similarly made in other hospitals throughout the country, many physicians, pharmacists and nurses have become interested in the development of a program for the education of patients relative to the *what, why* and *when* of the drugs which have been prescribed for their use.

One way whereby such a program may be initiated is to place patients, who are capable of cooperating, on a self-medication program while they are in the hospital. After the initial stage of alarm caused by proposing such a radical departure from standard hospital procedure has given way to sound reasoning, many will agree that this concept is really no different from that of progressive patient care or that of the ill patient at home who, of necessity, must resort to self adminstration of prescribed medications.

There are many advantages that would accrue from a satisfactorily developed program, the most important being the education of the patient whereby medication would be taken as intended by the physician when the patient was discharged from the hospital and secondly, while an inpatient, much nursing time could be conserved and devoted to other forms of patient care.

In response to a question as to whether or not physicians may order a medication to be left at the patient's bedside to be taken at the patient's discretion, Kenneth B. Babcock, M.D., former Director of the **Joint Commission on Accreditation of Hospitals** replied[19]—

"The answer is an emphatic 'No.' No medication should ever be left at the patient's bedside to be taken at his or her discretion. Every dose of any medication should be administered by a qualified person and recorded on the chart. This is important not only from the standpoint of the welfare of the patient, but also from a legal aspect."

Based on this opinion, the hospital pharmacist is advised to proceed with caution in the recommendation of such a program for use in the hospital. However, if such a program is, for one reason or another approved for use in a particular hospital, the hospital pharmacist should make every effort to assist in the design of a procedure that would ensure maximal safety for the patient yet protect the hospital and its staff from medicolegal implication.

Since Dr. Babcock's 1964 statement, there have been a number of hospitals and hospital pharmacists who have experimented with self-medication programs.[20,21,22] Some of the projects have been conducted at a physical rehabilitation hospital,[23,24] in an extended care facility,[25] on a geriatric ward of a large New York City hospital and on a cardiology unit of a medical center.[26]

Some hospitals permit self-administration of medicine after the first 24-hours of hospitalization. This is achieved only if the medication is properly labeled and dispensed by the hospital pharmacy. Schedule II, III, and IV as well as investigational use drugs should not be allowed to be self-administered. The self-medication order requires the written order to specific as to the medication, dose and frequency of administration. The nursing staff should record the patient's reported frequency, route of administration and dose of self-administered medication.

Barker and associates[32] studied the effect of an automated bedside dispensing machine (McLaughlin Dispensing System) on medication errors. The "system" consisted of a bedside locked medication cabinet that was electronically programmed to allow the nurse access to doses due at a particular time. The control system was the decentralized unit dose system. This limited study revealed that the error rate was significantly lower for the automated dispensing system than for the system using unit-doses dispensed from a satellite pharmacy. The authors suggest that automated dispensing systems may be useful in reducing errors in administration and time and dose omissions.

A review of the literature reveals that most investigators conducting these studies believe them to be successful. Thus Joint Commission on Accreditation of Hospitals standards allow for self-medication programs.

SELECTED READINGS

Zilz, David A.: Budget and Financial Implication in Implementing and Maintaining Unit Dose Drug Distribution Systems. Hosp. Pharm., 7:12:405, (Dec.) 1972.

Garrison, Thomas J.: Designing a Unit Dose Medication System. Hosp. Pharm., 7:12:413 (Dec.) 1972.

Grousse, W.L.: Computer System for Unit Dose Drug Distribution. Am. J. Hosp. Pharm., 35:711–714, (June) 1978.

Barker, K.N., Harris, J.A., Webster, D.B., Stringrt, J.F., Pearson, R.E., Mikeal, R.L., Glotzhober, G.R. and Miller, G.J.: Consultant Evaluation of a Hospital Medication System: Analysis of the Existing System. Am. J. Hosp. Pharm., 41:2009–2016, 1984.

Ibid: Consultant Evaluation of a Hospital Medication System: Synthesis of a New System. Am. J. Hosp. Pharm., 41:2016–2021, 1984.

Ibid: Consultant Evaluation of a Hospital Medication System: Implementation and Evaluation of the New System. Am. J. Hosp. Pharm., 41:2022–2029, 1984.

REFERENCES

1. Archambault, George F.L.: The Law of Hospital Pharmacy. Am. J. Hosp. Pharm., 15:7:593, 1958.
2. Connors, Edward J.: The Hospital Administrator's Responsibility for Drug Distribution, Hospitals. J.A.H.A., 42:23:46, (Dec.) 1968.
3. Hsieh, R.: Evaluation of Formal Communication Systems in a Hospital. Health Serv. Res., 1:222, Winter, 1966.
4. ———: Hospital Medication Errors. J.A.M.A., 195:31, (Jan.) 1966.
5. Freund, R.G.: How the Centralized Unit-Dose Concept Works in a Community Hospital. J.A.H.A., 40:152, (Sept.) 1966.
6. Tester, W.: A Study of Patient Care Involving a Unit-Dose System, College of Pharmacy, University Hospital, University of Iowa, Iowa City, Iowa, 1967.
7. Statement on Hospital Drug Distribution Systems. Am. J. Hosp. Pharm., 21:11:535, 1964.
8. Hassan, William E., Jr.: Mobile Dispensing for the Hospital Pharmacy. Am. J. Hosp. Pharm., 17:8:490, 1960.
9. Bjerke, P. and Missan, L.C.: An Envelope System for Floor Medications. Hospital, J.A.H.A., 34:63, (Aug.) 1960.
10. Unit Dose Medication Dispensing, Wyeth Laboratories, Philadelphia, Pa.
11. ———: A Brief Review of the Physical, Mechanical, and Packaging Requirements in Unit-Dose Distribution Systems—Part II, Phillips Roxane Laboratories, Columbus, Ohio, 1971.
12. Schwartau, N. and Sturdavant, M.: A System of Packaging and Dispensing Drugs in Single Doses. Am. J. Hosp. Pharm., 18:9:542, 1961.
13. McConnell, W., Barker, K., and Garrity, L.: Centralized Unit-Dose Dispensing. Am. J. Hosp. Pharm., 18:9:531, 1961.
14. Barker, Kenneth N. and Heller, William M.: The Development of a Centralized Unit-Dose Dispensing System, Part I, Description of the U.A.M.C. Experimental System. Am. J. Hosp. Pharm., 20:11:568, 1963.
15. ———: Ibid., 20:12, 612, 1963.
16. ———: Part III, An Editing Center for Physicians' Medication Orders. Am. J. Hosp. Pharm., 21:2:66, 1964.
17. Heller, William M., Sheldon, Eleanor C. and Barker, Kenneth N.: The Development of a Centralized Unit-Dose Dispensing System for U.A.M.C. Part IV, The Roles and

Responsibilities of the Pharmacist and Nurse Under the Experimental System. Am. J. Hosp. Pharm., *21*:8:230, 1964.

18. Tucci, Ralph G. and Webb, John W.: Mosaics, Medication Order Supply and Individual Charge System. Am. J. Hosp. Pharm., *21*:8:307, 1964.

19. Babcock, Kenneth B.: Accreditation Problems, Hospitals, J.A.H.A., *38*:41, (July) 1964.

20. Gordon, H.L., Keller, C.J. and Lentini, V.: Self-Medication Programs in Public Hospitals I. A Survey of Practices in Veterans Administration Hospitals. Hosp. Comm. Psych., *17*:355, (Dec.) 1966.

21. Pope, H.L.: Self-Medication Programs in Public Hospitals II. A Prelude to Discharge. Hosp. Comm. Psych., *17*:357 (Dec.) 1966.

22. Henderson, J.H.: Self-Medication in a Psychiatric Hospital. Lancet, *I*:1055, (May) 1967.

23. Reibel, E.M.: Study to Determine the Feasibility of a Self-Medication Program for Patients at a Rehabilitation Center. Nurs. Res., *18*:65, (Jan.–Feb.) 1969.

24. Johnson, E.W., Roberts, C.J. and Godwin, H.N.: Self-Medication for a Rehabilitation Ward. Arch. Phys. Med. Rehab., *51*:300, (May) 1970.

25. Libow, L.S. and Mehle, B.: Self-Administration of Medications in Hospital or Extended Care Facilities. J. Amer. Geriat. Soc., 18:81, (Jan.) 1970.

26. Buchanan, E.C., Brooks, M.R., and Greenwood, R.B.: A Self-Medication Program for Cardiology Patients. Am. J. Hosp. Pharm., *29*:11:928, (Nov.) 1972.

27. Austin, L H.: Using a Computer to Run a Modern Hospital Pharmacy. Hosp. Pharm., *14*:74–80, (Feb.) 1979.

28. Lovett, L.T.: Locked Medication Drawer at the Patient's Room—Experience in One Hospital. Hosp. Pharm., *14*:584–593, (Oct.) 1979.

29. Bannon, J.A.: Drug Not Given Notice. Hosp. Pharm., *14*:140–142, (Mar.) 1979.

30. ASHP Statement on Unit Dose Drug Distribution. Am. J. Hosp. Pharm., *38*:1214, (Aug.) 1981.

31. ASHP Technical Assistance Bulletin on Hospital Drug Distribution and Control. Am. J. Hosp. Pharm., *37*:1097–1103, (Aug.) 1980.

32. Barker, K.N., Pearson, R.E., Hepler, C.D., Smith, W.E., and Pappas, C.A.: Effect of an Automated Bedside Dispensing Machine on Medication Errors. Am. J. Hosp. Pharm., *4*:1:1352–1358, 1984.

14

Dispensing to Ambulatory Patients

"Ambulatory" refers to patients not occupying beds in hospitals or other inpatient settings, and to care given in physicians' offices, clinics, health centers, and other places where ambulatory patients usually go for health care. Today hospitals break down their ambulatory patient load into three categories—emergency, referral or tertiary care and primary care. The term **emergency care** is self explanatory and **tertiary care** means care beyond that of primary care. Stated simply, primary health care is what most people use most of the time for most of their health problems. Primary care is **majority** care. It describes a range of services adequate for meeting the great majority of daily personal health needs. This majority includes the need for preventive health maintenance and for the evaluation and management on a continuing basis of general discomfort, early complaints, symptoms, problems, and chronic intractable aspects of disease.

Most primary care is used by patients who are ambulatory, and most, but not all, ambulatory care is primary care. Primary care does not include service that is intensive, or very specialized, or both. These characteristics describe other levels of comprehensive health care.

In an organizational sense, primary health care describes a locus which should serve the patient as an entry point into a comprehensive health care system. Once entry is made—and initial care needed at the time of entry given—the primary care locus or program should be responsible for assuring continuity of all the care the patient may subsequently need.

The growth of ambulatory care clinics may be attributed to the following:

(a) The need of the hospital to supplement its in-patient teaching program.
(b) The demand by the community, lay as well as professional, for comprehensive diagnostic and treatment centers.
(c) The new philosophy of hospitals—to take a more active role in the community health programs.

(d)   The need of the hospital and physician to exercise greater control over patients receiving investigational use drugs.

(e)   The lack of a sufficient number of physicians in some areas, thereby causing the population to travel to the medical center for comprehensive care.

(f)   The fact that the emergency service of a hospital is always available, whereas a physician, in some rural areas, may not always be available.

Because of this volume and the prospect of growing larger within the next 20 years, many community pharmacists have been quick to cite the economic hardship this trend may create in the community. Although this is an important factor to be considered, it would appear that the crux of the problem is the lack of understanding by the community practitioner of the purpose and scope of a complete or comprehensive ambulatory service.

With the aim of alleviating this situation, the American Pharmaceutical Association and the American Society of Hospital Pharmacists established a Commission to study out-patient hospital pharmacy service and related hospital-community-pharmacy problems.

REPORT OF THE COMMISISON ON PHARMACEUTICAL SERVICES TO AMBULANT PATIENTS BY HOSPITALS AND RELATED FACILITIES

The two groups recognized that the goal of such a commission would not be realized without the cooperative effort of the medical and hospital associations. Thus an invitation to participate was extended to the American Medical Association and to the American Hospital Association.

The Commission, on October 22, 1964, modified its original name of Commission on Out-Patient Dispensing to read, **Commission on Pharmaceutical Services to Ambulant Patients by Hospitals and Related Facilities.**

One of the objectives adopted by the Commission was—"To obtain accurate data and reliable information regarding pharmaceutical services to out-patients by hospitals and other facilities."

Upon the completion of its studies, the Commission published a report entitled *The Challenge to Pharmacy in Times of Change.* This scholarly publication should be read by every student and practitioner of pharmacy.

Because of the depth of the study and the limited nature of this textbook, it is necessary to concentrate only on the following portion of the Commission's summary.[1]

2. **Hospital out-patient pharmaceutical service:** As a general rule, hospitals do not solicit private out-patient prescription patronage. The hospital out-patient department is in a very favorable position to attract private patients because of the convenience factor, but the location of the pharmacy in the hospital, a limited stock of health supplies, and the limitations of the formulary system, are often deterrents to maximum out-patient services. The hospital pharmacist is burdened with the care of hospital patients and has little time to develop a personal consumer loyalty with private patients. The community pharmacist, on the other hand, can develop a personal relationship through a high level of professional and individualized service that will permit him to compete favorably with the convenience advantage that a hospital or a medical center-based pharmacy service offers the patient. The patient has the same right to select his pharmacist as he does his physician or other health practitioner, and none of the parties involved should adopt procedures that circumvent this right.

Since the Commission Report, the profession has made great strides in recognizing the need to advance ambulatory pharmaceutical service to the level necessary to meet the need of the new healthcare delivery systems which are preponderantly ambulatory oriented. The ASHP in recognition of this need promulgated the following Statement[2] and Guidelines[3] for ambulatory care pharmaceutical services.

ASHP STATEMENT ON THE PROVISION OF PHARMACEUTICAL SERVICES IN AMBULATORY CARE SETTINGS[a]

The concern for increasing access to health care services and containing health care costs has led to increased demands for ambulatory patient care services in organized health care settings. Ambulatory care encompasses the provision of health care services and education to patients who are able to seek medical attention, yet do not require admission to an institution for health care needs. To meet these needs, organized settings for delivery of ambulatory health care are being created within institutional structures as well as in satellite clinics and noninstitutional ambulatory health care systems, including Group Medical Practices and Health Maintenance Organizations.

This expansion of health care into ambulatory settings has been accompanied by an evolution of patient-oriented pharmaceutical services that extend beyond traditional preparation and dispensing of medications. Many of the activities outlined in the American Society of Hospital Pharmacists' Statement on Clinical Functions in Institutional Pharmacy Practice[1] have been adapted to a variety of ambulatory care

---

[a]Developed by the ASHP Council on Clinical Pharmacy and Therapeutics. Approved by the ASHP Board of Directors on March 20, 1980, and by the ASHP House of Delegates on April 21, 1980.

settings. The scope of these activities may vary with practice site, but commonly include:

1. Obtaining and documenting patient medication histories.
2. Monitoring the safety and efficacy of drug therapy through the maintenance of medication profiles.
3. Providing drug information to prescribers and other health care practitioners.
4. Assisting prescribers in the proper selection and adjustment of drug therapy through application of pharmacokinetic and other principles.
5. Utilizing assessment skills in the management of acute and chronic diseases and providing appropriate referrals to other health care providers.
6. Detecting and reporting adverse drug reactions, interactions, and noncompliant patient behavior.
7. Educating and counseling patients and the general public in the proper use of medications.
8. Participating in drug-use reviews, patient care audits, and clinical drug investigations.
9. Participating in the education of health care providers.
10. Supervising the storage, preparation, dispensing, and administration of medications in the patient care area.
11. Developing systems for the delivery of pharmacy services in the institutional setting and the community.
12. Developing and utilizing systems for fiscal management and reimbursement.

Directors of pharmacy services in institutions and pharmacists in noninstitutional settings have the responsibility to develop and maintain comprehensive pharmaceutical services commensurate with the individual needs of each health care setting and to evaluate and document the health care benefits of such services. The American Society of Hospital Pharmacists recognizes and supports the development and implementation of comprehensive ambulatory pharmaceutical services in organized health care settings.

REFERENCE

1. ASHP statement on clinical functions in institutional pharmacy practice. Am. J. Hosp. Pharm., 1978; *35*:813.

ASHP GUIDELINES: MINIMUM STANDARD FOR AMBULATORY-CARE PHARMACEUTICAL SERVICES[a]

Services to ambulatory patients are an important part of many institutional pharmacy programs. The need for such services probably will increase substantially in the 1980s.

[a]Approved by the ASHP Board of Directors, November 19, 1981.

The Society has identified 12 activities in which institutional pharmacists will be involved in the ambulatory-care setting.[1] However, providing all these services in all institutions at all times is not feasible. At a minimum, ambulatory patients require certain critical pharmaceutical services. The essential elements of any ambulatory-care pharmaceutical service program are as follows:

1. The ambulatory-care pharmacy program must be directed by a qualified pharmacist.
2. The appropriateness of the choice of drug and its dosage, route of administration, and amount must be verified by the pharmacist. This will require the maintenance of medication profiles for patients routinely treated at the institution to prevent duplicate drug therapies and the use of contraindicated drugs.
3. All medications dispensed to patients will be completely and correctly labeled and packaged in accordance with all applicable regulations and accepted standards of practice.
4. Upon dispensing a new (to the patient) medication, the pharmacist will ensure that the patient or his representative receives and understands all information required for proper use of the drug.[2]
5. All drugs in ambulatory-care service areas will be properly controlled.[3]

The American Society of Hospital Pharmacists believes that patients in all ambulatory-care facilities should expect these five pharmaceutical services, without exception.

REFERENCES

1. ASHP statement on the provision of pharmaceutical services in ambulatory care settings. Am. J. Hosp. Pharm., 1980; *37*:1095.
2. ASHP statement on pharmacist-conducted patient counseling. Am. J. Hosp. Pharm., 1976; *33*:644.
3. ASHP guidelines on hospital drug distribution and control (with references). Am. J. Hosp. Pharm., 1980; *37*:1097–103.

Ambulatory-care pharmacy practice has reached the stage whereby its practitioners have become specialized in this branch of pharmaceutical services. As a result thereof, specialized postgraduate programs have evolved to train residents. The following is the ASHP Supplemental Standard and Learning Objectives for Residency Training in Ambulatory-Care Pharmacy Practice.[4]

ASHP SUPPLEMENTAL STANDARD AND LEARNING OBJECTIVES FOR RESIDENCY TRAINING IN AMBULATORY CARE PHARMACY PRACTICE

Preamble[a]

Definition. A specialized residency in ambulatory-care pharmacy practice is defined as a postgraduate program of organized education and training that meets the requirements set forth and approved by the American Society of Hospital Pharmacists. The ASHP Accreditation Standard for Specialized Residency Training,[1] together with this supplement, are the basic criteria used to evaluate ambulatory-care pharmacy residency training programs in institutions applying for accreditation by the American Society of Hospital Pharmacists.

A specialized residency in ambulatory-care pharmacy practice must be organized and conducted to develop expert skills and competency in this area of practice, differentiated in scope, depth, and proficiency from those expected of institutional pharmacy residents. Objectives of such training should include extensive experience in providing comprehensive clinical pharmacy services to ambulant patients, as well as the management of drug-distribution systems in ambulatory-care facilities.

Qualifications of the Training Site. The parent facility for an accredited residency in ambulatory-care pharmacy practice shall meet the requirements set forth in Standard I in the body of the ASHP Accreditation Standard for Specialized Pharmacy Residency Training.[1] Facilities may include, but are not limited to, institutional ambulatory-care settings, satellite clinics, and noninstitutional ambulatory health-care systems, including group medical practices and health-maintenance organizations.

Qualifications of the Pharmacy Service. The pharmacy service in which an accredited ambulatory-care practice residency is based must meet the requirements set forth in Standard II of the ASHP Accreditation Standard for Specialized Pharmacy Residency Training.[1] In addition, the pharmacy service must provide a comprehensive program of ambulatory-care services, far surpassing that required in the ASHP Minimum Standard for the Provision of Ambulatory-Care Pharmaceutical Services.[2] The following specific requirements are established for the ambulatory-care service program:

1. *Medical records.* All patient-related records must be accessible before, during, and after the provision of pharmaceutical services.
2. *Drug information resources.* Each facility shall maintain a centralized

---

       body of pharmaceutical and medical literature, containing current primary, secondary, and tertiary literature sources.

3. *Scope of service.* The ASHP Statement on the Provision of Pharmaceutical Services in Ambulatory Care Settings[3] sets forth the fundamental scope of services that should be provided by such a program. Although provision of non-prescription drugs and health-related devices and appliances is included within the intent of this requirement, the sale of sundries and general merchandise is specifically excluded.

4. *Preceptors serving as independent proprietors.* In those instances in which the preceptor may also serve as sole proprietor of an independent (noninstitutional) ambulatory health-care setting, particular attention should be focused on section II-B of the Accreditation Standard for Specialized Pharmacy Residency Training.[1] Administative and business concerns of the preceptor in such a setting should not be allowed to detract from the objectives of the residency program.

5. *Review of quality.* There shall be an ongoing quality-assurance program to evaluate the pharmacy services being provided.

Qualification of the Preceptor. The preceptor of an accredited ambulatory-care pharmacy practice residency must meet the requirements set forth in Standard III of the ASHP Accreditation Standard for Specialized Pharmacy Residency Training.[1] The area of specialization of the preceptor shall be ambulatory-care pharmacy practice. Additionally, the preceptor shall demonstrate proficiency as a clinical pharmacist within this area of practice.

Qualifications of the Applicant. In addition to meeting the requirements set forth in Standard IV of the ASHP Accreditation Standard for Specialized Pharmacy Residency Training,[1] the applicant should have completed formal academic instruction in the following subject areas or their equivalents: pathophysiology, physical assessment, communication techniques, and drug-literature evaluation.

The following learning objectives shall be approved by the Commission on Credentialing following review annually by a committee appointed from the Special Interest Group on Ambulatory-Care Pharmacy Practice of the American Society of Hospital Pharmacists.

Learning Objectives and Areas of Emphasis

I.   **Learning Objectives.** A resident who completes an accredited residency program in ambulatory-care pharmacy practice shall be able to:

    A.   Develop an appreciation for the organization and operation of an ambulatory-care pharmacy service, including physical accommodations, reference sources, computer applications, professional and supportive personnel, budgeting, relationships with other health-care departments, patient flow, assumed or designated responsibilities, and documentation of services.

B. Obtain and document, in the patient's medical record, medication histories, medication profiles, and other pertinent information that may directly affect the intended therapeutic plan.

C. Manage a patient's drug therapy by:
    1. Advising prescribers in designing a drug-therapy treatment plan,
    2. Using established therapeutic protocols, or
    3. Independently prescribing or adjusting drug therapy in instances where supportive legislation allows.

D. Monitor the safety and efficacy of drug therapy through the use of physical-assessment skills, interpretation of laboratory data, patient interview, and medical-record review.

E. Provide drug information to prescribers and other health-care practitioners.

F. Refer the patient, when necessary, to other appropriate health-care providers.

G. Supervise the storage, preparation, and dispensing of medications and the provision of surgical and ostomy supplies.

H. Participate in, or recommend alternative methods of, administering medications to ambulatory-care patients in either the medically supervised or home health-care setting.

I. Identify and initiate strategies to correct noncompliant patient behavior.

J. Establish functional systems for detecting, reporting, and managing adverse drug reactions, interactions, allergies, and other untoward drug-related effects.

K. Educate and counsel patients,[4] the general public, and health-care providers in the proper use of medications and drug-delivery systems.

L. Establish criteria for safe and effective drug use and coordinate drug-use reviews and patient-care audits.

M. Organize an ongoing educational program directed toward the professional advancement of all health-care staff members.

N. Develop and defend a proposal for obtaining reimbursement for patient-care activities.

O. Establish a quality-assurance program directed toward continuous assessment of the patient-care pharmaceutical services being provided.

P. Participate in the management of medical emergencies.

II. **Areas of Emphasis.** The resident's training program shall be directed toward solving specific clinical problems. It must occur in a multidisciplinary setting, in which each member of the health-care team has a defined patient-care responsibility. The program should also focus on drug-literature analysis and associated communication skills. It must be organized in a way that makes possible the attainment of the learning objectives. Exposure to a widely varied patient population is expected. To meet these criteria, experiences should be provided in, but not necessarily restricted to, many of the following areas:

A. Acute illnesses
    1. Upper-respiratory infections
    2. Headaches
    3. Diarrhea
    4. Otitis media

      5. Skin allergies
      6. Acne
      7. Local fungal infections
      8. Hay fever
      9. Viral gastroenteritis
    10. Streptococcal pharyngitis
    11. Parasitic infections
    12. Venereal disease
    13. Urinary-tract infections

B. Chronic illnesses
      1. Diabetes mellitus
      2. Hypertension
      3. Seizure disorders
      4. Parkinsonism
      5. Rheumatoid arthritis
      6. Tuberculosis
      7. Chronic obstructive pulmonary disease
      8. Asthma
      9. Angina pectoris
    10. Congestive heart failure
    11. Thrombosis
    12. Neoplastic disease
    13. Renal failure/transplantation
    14. Peptic ulcer disease
    15. Ulcerative colitis
    16. Thyroid disorders
    17. Gout
    18. Anemias
    19. Glaucoma
    20. Intractable pain

C. Preventive care
      1. Nutrition
      2. Hygiene
      3. Exercise programs
      4. Alcohol-abuse rehabilitation program
      5. Smoking-cessation program
      6. Weight-reduction program
      7. Stress-reduction program

D. Self care (nonprescription-medication use)

E. Emergency care
      1. Cardiopulmonary resuscitation
      2. Acute burn therapy
      3. Shock
      4. Trauma

F. Family planning
      1. Contraception
      2. Pregnancy testing
      3. Teratogenicity
      4. Maternogenicity

G. Devices
      1. Nutrition-delivery systems
      2. Drug-delivery systems
      3. Prosthetic devices
      4. Home health-care supplies

  5. Ostomy supplies
  6. Oxygen systems
  7. Surgical appliances
  8. Durable medical equipment
H. Communication skills
   The resident shall have numerous assignments throughout the year aimed at developing written and verbal communication skills. The residency preceptor shall be specifically responsible for setting goals for the resident's growth and development in these areas, monitoring the resident's progress, and counseling the resident on a regular basis concerning communication abilities.

Extramural Experiences

When appropriate, rotations or visitations to other health-care settings should be scheduled to augment the resident's training. Extramural rotations may be conducted either as full-time training activities (e.g., a one-month block), or on a regularly scheduled part-time basis. Examples of such experiences might include providing nursing-home or long-term care facility consultations, or participation in regularly scheduled home health-care visits to patients requiring drug therapy or device monitoring. If extramural rotations are scheduled for the purpose of pursuing one or more of the fundamental learning objectives, there must be a pharmacist preceptor who has defined responsibilities for monitoring the progress and evaluating the accomplishments of the resident. A detailed set of objectives for extramural rotations must be prepared in advance. Extramural rotations must represent not more than 25% of the resident's experience. The qualifications of the extramural training site are subject to review and approval by the American Society of Hospital Pharmacists.

Research Projects

The residency training schedule shall make provision for the resident's participation in a self-directed or collaborative research project. The purpose of such activities is to teach the application of the scientific method. The resident should submit a final report of the project, which should be of publishable quality.

REFERENCES

1. American Society of Hospital Pharmacists. ASHP accrediation standard for specialized pharmacy residency training (with guide to interpretation). Am. J. Hosp. Pharm. 1980; *37*:1229–32.
2. American Society of Hospital Pharmacists. ASHP minimum standard for ambulatory-care pharmaceutical services. Am. J. Hosp. Pharm. 1982; *39*:316.
3. American Society of Hospital Pharmacists. ASHP statement on the provision of

pharmaceutical services in ambulatory care settings. Am J Hosp. Pharm. 1980; *37*:1096.

4. American Society of Hospital Pharmacists. ASHP guidelines on pharmacist-conducted patient counseling. Am. J. Hosp. Pharm. 1976; *33*:644–5.

LOCATION OF OUT-PATIENT DISPENSING AREA

There is no set rule as to the best area to locate an out-patient dispensing pharmacy. This is evidenced by the fact that in today's practice three equally suitable provisions are made for this area:

(a)   A separate out-patient pharmacy is available.
(b)   A combined in-patient and out-patient unit with service provided from the same "window."
(c)   A combined in-patient and out-patient unit with service provided from separate "windows."

A separate out-patient pharmacy is usually established whenever the out-patient department and the pharmacy are geographically widely separated. Although this arrangement has the advantage of being a separate and distinct unit with a specialized function, it possesses the disadvantages of requiring a separate staff as well as consuming a great deal of time, on the part of other pharmacy department personnel, in transporting supplies and drugs to the area.

The above disadvantages are obviously eliminated whenever both in-patient and out-patient facilities are combined. An additional advantage to this arrangement is that the director of the pharmacy service is able to exert a greater degree of control and supervision.

TYPES OF PRESCRIPTIONS RECEIVED

Depending upon the location and kind of hospital, the prescriptions received in the out-patient department pharmacy will generally include those of private patients (where permitted by the state board of registration in pharmacy), indigent patients, non-indigent patients, employees, and patients being discharged from the hospital. It is a known fact that in any large metropolitan teaching hospital, the largest volume of prescriptions comes from the indigent or partially indigent group of patients. It is also established that every patient who visits the clinics does not have his prescription filled in the hospital. Indeed, hospitals with 500 or more beds fill approximately 1 prescription per 3 out-patient visits, whereas the 100 to 199-bed hospitals average about 1¼ prescriptions for each visit.[5]

Because many of these indigent patients are supported by some type of welfare program, their prescriptions require special identification, and the billing for such must be in accord with the requirements of the particular agency. In some states, a special pricing for the drugs dis-

PRESCRIPTION CHECK

№ 5007

Name _____

Address _____   —Pharmacy Portion

PRICE $

PETER BENT BRIGHAM HOSPITAL
721 Huntington Avenue
Boston 15, Mass.

—Patient's Portion

PETER BENT BRIGHAM HOSPITAL
DEPARTMENT OF PHARMACY
Boston 15, Mass.

To avoid errors please present this check when calling for your prescription

№ 5007

Fig. 57.   Prescription Call Check used in the out-patient dispensing pharmacy as a means of matching the correct patient and prescription.

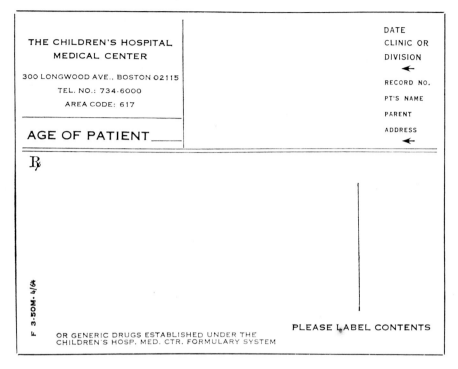

THE CHILDREN'S HOSPITAL
MEDICAL CENTER

300 LONGWOOD AVE., BOSTON 02115

TEL. NO.: 734-6000

AREA CODE: 617

AGE OF PATIENT____

DATE

CLINIC OR

DIVISION

RECORD NO.

PT'S NAME

PARENT

ADDRESS

℞

F 3-50M- 4/64

OR GENERIC DRUGS ESTABLISHED UNDER THE
CHILDREN'S HOSP. MED. CTR. FORMULARY SYSTEM

PLEASE LABEL CONTENTS

Fig. 58. A prescription blank developed by The Children's Hospital Medical Center in Boston. Note the emphasis on the patient's age.

pensed is in effect. See Chapter 19 for an example and discussion of one such system.

DISPENSING ROUTINE

The dispensing pattern involved in providing clinic patients as well as those patients being discharged with "take home drugs" is identical with that carried on by a community pharmacy.

In both instances, a prescription is written by the physician and the patient takes it to the pharmacy where it is compounded by a pharmacist. If there is to be a waiting period, the pharmacist will make use of a prescription call check which numerically identifies the patient, and the finished prescriptions (Fig. 57). Once in the hands of the pharmacist, the prescription and label are numbered by a numbering machine; the directions and other pertinent information are placed on the label; ancillary labels are affixed; the proper medication is then placed in the container; a check for accuracy is then conducted; and finally the prepared prescription is wrapped and dispensed.

For internal audit purposes, hospital prescriptions are separated into out-patient and in-patient discharges and therefore may utilize two different colored blanks.

Figure 58 represents one type of hospital prescription. It is rather ingenious combination of prescription call check, prescription and label in a single form was that of the Philadelphia General Hospital now closed. This form (Fig. 59) has many advantages in that it combines

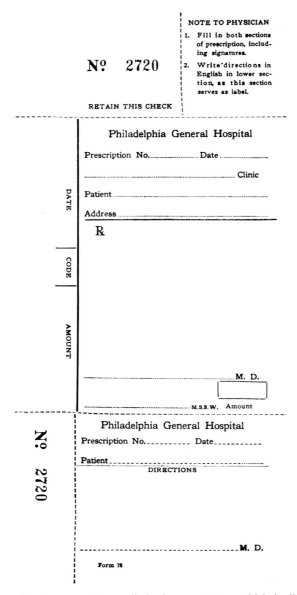

Fig. 59.   A combination prescription call check, prescription and label, all in one form.

three forms into one; it saves the pharmacist's time in handing out a call check and typing a label; and finally, it is probably more economical. It would seem that its only disadvantages are that the prescription on file does not carry the directions for use and that the directions for use written by the physician on the label portion of the form, more often than not, will be illegible to the patient.

Many other types of prescription forms are in current use in the hospitals of the nation. Some consist of multiple pages attached to a pre-punched card ready for use in a computer system; others consist of a prescription blank the back of which is affixed with coded magnetic tape thereby rendering the prescription suitable for use in automatic billing and electronic data-retrieval systems.

PRESCRIPTIONS INVOLVING RESEARCH PROJECTS

The department of pharmacy in a teaching hospital is often called upon either to assist in or to conduct a special research program designed to ascertain the prescribing habits of the staff physicians, the correlation between diagnosis and drug prescribed, as well as cost studies which involve the cost of drugs to both hospital and patient.

Such studies usually involve designing a special prescription blank, an example of which is shown in Figure 60. This two part carbonized prescription form is designed to provide, in addition to the usual information obtained on a prescription, special data required for the particular study. The days of therapy and cost information are provided by the pharmacist compounding the prescription, and the information concerning the diagnosis is obtained by research personnel from the medical record.

The prescription number, patient number, date, age, sex, drug prescribed, quantity prescribed, directions for use, physician's code, days of therapy, cost data and diagnosis are then transferred to a punched tape. The tape is then processed and fed into a computer for a final analysis of the information thus gathered.

I.R.S. RULING ON OUT-PATIENT DISPENSING

Revenue received by a non-profit pharmacy for filling prescriptions for in-patients or out-patients is not considered "unrelated business taxable income" and is not subject to federal income tax, the Internal Revenus Service has ruled.

But, if a hospital pharmacy is open to the general public and prescriptions are filled for patients walking in from the street or if sales of non-prescription items are made under the same conditions, this revenue is subject to taxation. One of the rulings permits prescription sales without taxation by a hospital which fills occasional prescriptions

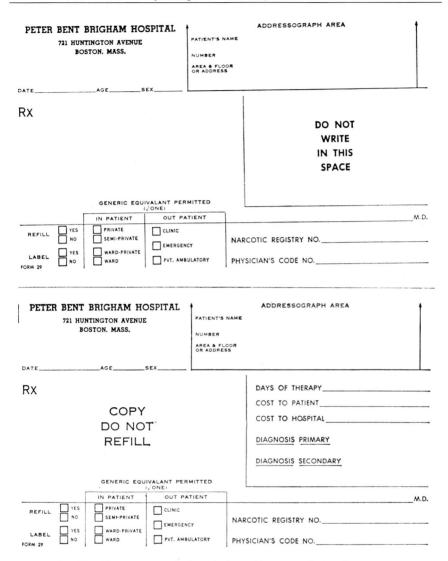

Fig. 60. Two-part prescription blank used in a prescription data survey.

written by staff physicians who practice in consultation rooms provided by the hospital. IRS has ruled that these were merely "casual" sales, made as a courtesy to staff physicians.

In ruling that out-patients may have prescriptions filled in hospital pharmacies without subjecting the income received by the institution to federal taxations, IRS also included refills for former patients or prescriptions originally written when the patients were received hospital treatment. It also extended the non-taxable income rule to treatment received in home care and extended care facilities operated by or supervised by a hospital.[6]

Revenue Rule 68-374 provides as follows:

"Section 513 of the Code defines the term 'unrelated trade or business' as any trade or business the conduct of whch is not substantially related (aside from the need of such organization for income or funds or the use it makes of the profit derived) to the exercise or performance by such organization of its exempt functions.

To the extent relevant here, section 513 (a)(2) of the Code further states that the term 'unrelated trade or business' does not include any trade or business which is carried on by an organization described in section 501 (c)(3) primarily for the convenience of its patients."

Section 512 of the Code defines the term 'unrelated business taxable income' as the income computed in this section derived by organizations from any unrelated trade or business regularly carried on.

Section 1.513(c)(1) of the Income Tax Regulations states that "in determining whether trade or business from which a particular amount of gross income derives is 'regularly carried on' within the meaning of section 512, regard must be had to the frequency and continuity with which the activities productive of the income are conducted and the manner in which they are pursued."

Section 1.513-1(c)(2)(ii) of the regulations states that "in determining whether or not intermittently conducted activities are regularly carried on, the manner of conduct of the activities must be compared with the manner in which commercial activities are normally pursued by non-exempt organizations. In general, exempt organization businesses which are engaged in discontinuously or periodically will not be considered regularly carried on if they are conducted without the competitive and promotional efforts typical of commercial endeavors."

Section 1.513-1(c)(2)(ii) of the regulations further states that "where an organization sells certain types of goods or services to a particular class of persons in pursuance of its exempt functions 'primarily for the convenience' of such persons within the meaning of section 513(a)(2), casual sales in the course of such activity which do not qualify as related to the exempt function involved or as described in section 513(a)(2) will not be treated as regular. On the other hand, where the non-qualifying sales are not merely casual, but are systematically and consistently promoted and carried on by the organization they meet the section 512 requirement of regularity."

Dispensing to Emergency Patients

After receiving treatment in the Emergency Ward of a hospital, the patient may receive a prescription. If the prescription is presented to a hospital pharmacist, he follows the methodology described earlier in this chapter (see page 312).

Mar and associates[7] have developed a system which uses a special cabinet containing medication bins which store selected and limited quantities of medications packaged in single-unit containers. Additionally, intravenous solutions, irrigating solutions, eye tray medications, drugs for cardiopulmonary resuscitation and refrigerated drugs are kept in areas of ready access. The system provides for punched cards containing information of the drug. These cards are stored with the medication and are used for billing and re-ordering purposes. A 24-hour supply of medications that may be dispensed after pharmacy hours are packaged in prelabeled, zipper-locked plastic bags.

SELECTED READINGS

Mehl, Bernard and Kissner, Edward A.: Ambulatory Pharmaceutical Services in a Changing Urban Communnity. Am. J. Hosp. Pharm., *29*:5:407, (May) 1972.

Johnson, Richard E., Myers, John E. and Egan, Douglas M.: A Resource Planning Model for Outpatient Pharmacy Operations, Am. J. Hosp. Pharm., *29*:5:411 (May) 1972.

Klienman, Kurt: Outpatient Pharmacy—New Design Encourages Comprehensive Pharmaceutical Service. Am. J. Hosp. Pharm., *29*:5:419, (May) 1972.

Madden, E.E., Vaughn, C.M. and Trahan, G.J.: Outpatient Pharmacy Prescription Automation. Am. J. Hosp. Pharm., *26*:151–159, (Mar.) 1979.

Vemuri, Sriram: Simulated Analysis of Patient Waiting Time in an Out-patient Pharmacy. Am. J. Hosp. Pharm., *41*:1127–1130, 1984.

REFERENCES

1. Brodie, Donald C.: *The Challenge to Pharmacy in Times of Change,* A.Ph.A. and A.S.H.P., Washington, D.C., 1966.
2. ASHP Statement on the Provision of Pharmaceutical Services in Ambulatory Care Settings. Am. J. Hosp. Pharm., *37*:1096, (Aug.) 1980.
3. ASHP Guidelines: Minimum Standards for Ambulatory-Care Pharmaceutical Services. Am. J. Hosp. Pharm., *39*:316, (Feb.) 1982.
4. ASHP Supplemental Standard and Learning Objectives for Residency Training in Ambulatory-Care Pharmacy Practice. Am. J. Hosp. Pharm., *39*:1967–1969, (Nov.) 1982.
5. Francke, Don E., Latiolais, Clifton J., Francke, Gloria N. and Ho, Norman, F.C.: *Mirror to Hospital Pharmacy,* Washington, D.C., p. 120.
6. Internal Revenue Bulletin No. 1968-29, July 15, 1968.
7. Mar, D.D., Hanan, Z.I. and LaFontaine, R.: Improved Emergency Room Medication Distribution. Am. J. Hosp. Pharm., *35*:70–73, (June) 1978.

15

Distributing Ancillary Supplies

A trend in hospital pharmacy is the assumption of responsibility for the purchase, stocking and distribution of the various ancillary medical, surgical and laboratory supplies. The range of inventory for this type of goods is extremely broad and may consist of costly surgical instruments, catheters, sutures, needles, syringes, sphygmomanometers, and laboratory ware.

Whether or not this is a desirable trend depends upon the individual pharmacist and the hospital administration. Certainly the assignment of this added special type of responsibility to the pharmacist is a clear indication of the administration's respect for his multiple talents. In addition, a few years of experience in handling these supplies will better qualify him to assume responsibility for the central sterile supply room or for the purchasing division if the occasion should ever arise.

Certainly, in the small hospital such an assignment is highly desirable for it may mean the difference between hiring a pharmacist or not hiring one on the basis of insufficient pharmaceutical duties.

QUALIFICATIONS OF THE PHARMACIST

There should be no doubt about the fact that the pharmacist is certainly capable of undertaking such a task for he, in all probability, will have had greater training than the lay person who might be assigned the task. In addition, he will have a greater understanding relative to the use to which these items are to be put to and therefore may be able to act in an advisory capacity relative to the selection of one item over another. Furthermore, because of his experience in the handling and accounting of pharmaceuticals, the hospital will be assured of proper control.

PURCHASING

Because of the nature of ancillary supplies, they are usually purchased from sources other than a pharmaceutical house or drug wholesaler. Therefore, the pharmacist must acquaint himself with the various agencies, distributors and general wholesaler. Due to the extremely keen competition in this area, the pharmacist is cautioned to take the time to ascertain the integrity and reliability of the vendor, as well as his ability and desire to be cooperative and render special services when called upon in an emergency situation.

Since many distributors have the agency for the same product, it is wise to purchase as many items via the bid process with the right to bid being open to all, but the specifications and other service demands associated with the shipping, billing, etc. being set at a level that only the most reliable vendors can meet.

The purchasing of the supplies should not be mixed with the purchasing of pharmaceuticals and separate records and inventories should be maintained. Depending upon the scope of the ancillary supply inventory, some items may be extremely slow in turn-over; therefore unless a separate physical inventory is maintained and recorded, it is possible to warp the true operation of the drug portion of the pharmacy by reducing the number of times of turn-over of the true pharmacy inventory.

Pharmacists who take on the responsibility for the procurement, inventorying and distribution of ancillary supplies should give serious consideration to having the hospital join a successful group purchasing program. By so doing, the institution can derive many benefits which include lower prices due to volume purchasing; in some instances centralized storage and on-call delivery thus minimizing the utilization of hospital space; elimination of sales personnel thereby conserving the pharmacist's time; specifications and bids are centrally prepared thus resulting in uniform products in use throughout the service area and on-going monitoring of price fluctuations.

For those products that are not available from a group purchasing organization or a local wholesaler, the pharmacist should give consideration to the following when dealing with a purveyor:[1]

1. Manufacturers, upon request, must be able to provide data relating to analytical control, sterility testing, descriptions of test procedures for raw materials and finished product or any other information which would confirm the safety and quality of the product.
2. The company should not have a history of recurring product recalls.
3. Whenever applicable, packaging and labeling must conform to FDA requirements.
4. Delivery of items such as sutures and sterile fluids and catheters should be confined to a single lot number.
5. The expiration date should be sufficiently advanced to permit appropriate use and turn-over.
6. Vendor should accept and credit any unopened packages after the expiration date.
7. Supplier should ship all merchandise freight prepaid, provide inside delivery with a packing slip which indicates back ordered items and their anticipated delivery.

8. Vendor must warrant title to all products supplied by him; warrant them free from defects; fit for any rational use of the product; indemnify and hold harmless the purchaser against any and all legal actions (including attorney fees) arising from claims by third parties relating to the product.

Once the responsibility of handling these items is assigned to the pharmacist, it is suggested that the procedure for the purchase of drugs discussed in Chapter 9 be followed.

DISTRIBUTION

Ancillary supplies are of such a nature that the laboratories, pavilions and special service areas can predict their rate of use and consequently order them from the pharmacy on a weekly or bi-weekly basis.

The day on which these orders are placed inarbitrary, but it is recommended that a specific day be selected in addition to a time deadline. This is necessary if the suppliers are to be ready for pick-up and distribution by the hospital messenger service.

There are two methods whereby the pavilions, laboratories and special service areas may be informed as to exactly what is carried in inventory. They are via a pre-printed requistion form which lists all the supplies or by issuing a catalogue.

If the total number of items stocked is not too great, then a pre-printed requisition form is ideal and the most practical.

One the other hand, the best way to inform those who must requisition the supplies for their area is by means of a published catalogue should be cross-indexed to facilitate its use and should show the unit size of the package to be dispensed. This will save a great deal of time for the dispensing personnel as well as for the pricing clerk.

In hospitals where a catalogue has been published, a special requisition form must also be put into use. This form must, of necessity, be quite simple and yet capable of being used for any type of supply. A sample of such a form is shown in Figure 61.

When preparing this requisition, the department head usually prepares it in duplicate in order that he may retain a copy of the original order as a receiving slip to make sure that all supplies ordered have been received.

Because some items will at one time or another be out of inventory, it is advisable to use an OUT OF STOCK NOTICE to so inform the requisitioning department. A sample of this form is shown in Figure 62. This form is initiated in duplicate by the pharmacist filling the requisition. The original is retained in the pharmacy and the duplicate is sent to the requisitioning department. When the supplies are again in inventory, it is a simple matter to forward the item to the laboratory or ward without their issuing a new request.

PETER BENT BRIGHAM HOSPITAL
REQUISITION TO PHARMACY FOR WARD AND LABORATORY SUPPLIES ONLY

For use in ....Ward A... Date...1/4/80.......

Requisitions for Ward and Laboratory Supplies must be in the Pharmacy by 10:30 A.M. daily. Supplies may be picked up any time between 3:30 P.M. and 5:00 P.M. There will be only one order daily. No requisitions will be filled on Sundays and holidays. Please watch your stock supplies, and see that you are well supplied.

WANTED		DESCRIPTION OF ITEM	✓	COST
Amount	Size			
1	100	Sugar Testing Tablets		
12	1"	Adhesive Tape		
12	---	Oral Thermometers		
1	2oz.	Benzidine Test Reagent		

Requested by ...Jane Doe, Head Nurse........................

Approved by ...Mary Doe, Supervisor...................   Received by ....Helen Doe, Ward Clerk..................

Form 16A - Drugs

Fig. 61. A requisition to the pharmacy for ward and laboratory supplies. This form is prepared on the ward or in the laboratory and sent to the pharmacy. The pharmacist checks off each item dispensed, prices it, and forwards the completed requisiton form to the pharmacy accounting section.

Form 191   **PETER BENT BRIGHAM HOSPITAL**

PHARMACY

DATE   1-5-80

DEPT.   Operating Room

NAME ON ORIGINAL REQ. Jane Doe

We are temporarily out of the following:

Quantity	ITEMS
1 doz.	Sutures # 123
	☐ Charged ☒ Not charged

When these items are available, your order will be completed.

PLEASE DO NOT REORDER

Fig. 62. Out of Stock Notice.

APPLICATION OF ECONOMIC ORDER QUANTITY MODEL

If the pharmacist assumes the managerial responsibility for the dispensing of ancillary supplies, then he must utilize modern techniques to maintain control over the investment in inventory. One such method is the utilization of the economic order quantity model (see Chapter 9).

A number of economic order quantity models have been devised to assist one in the control of inventory locked dollars. Basically, these mathematical models determined the opimum inventory level by calculating the optimum order quantity and re-order points. In addition, such additional information as *procurement cost, average holding cost per unit, average investment per unit,* and *optimum turn-over rate,* should be considered.

A model for this purpose has been presented and described in Chapter 9 *Purchasing and Inventory Control.* The same model has application for the control of any type of inventory be it drugs or ancillary supplies.

SELECTED READINGS

Caufman, M.: Utilizing the Computer for a Hospital Bid Program. Hosp. Pharm., *19*:1:13, (Jan.) 1984.
Sok, J.E.: Pharmacy Inventory Management (PIM) Strategy. Topics in Hosp. Pharm. Mgt., *4*:4:33, (Feb.) 1985.
Smith, J.E.: Expanding Hospital Pharmacy Services to Meet Developing Markets. Topics in Hosp. Pharm. Mgt., *4*:4:67, (Feb.) 1985.

REFERENCES

1. *Pharmacy Policy and Procedure Manual 1981,* Dept. Pharmacy Service, Brigham & Women's Hospital, Boston, Mass. 02115.

16

Dispensing of Controlled Substances

The Federal Harrison Narcotic Act was originally passed in 1914 and was designed to protect the health of the American people and to serve as a source of tax revenue to the Government. Regulation No. 5 of the Harrison Narcotic Act and subsequent treasury department decisions concerned themselves with the practical application of this law.

In 1965, the Federal Food, Drug and Cosmetic Act was amended by the passage of the Drug Abuse Control Amendments of 1965. Thus, the combination of the Federal Harrison Narcotic Act and the Drug Abuse Control Amendments of 1965 formed the basis for the control of the majority of special drugs within the hospital environment. In 1970, the Congress enacted the Comprehensive Drug Abuse Prevention and Control Act, which in effect, combined the Federal Harrison Narcotic Act and Drug Abuse Control Amendments of 1965 and imposed stricter controls over a large number of stimulant and depressant drugs. Thus, the new law required the profession of pharmacy to devise new ways to control a large segment of the medications dispensed.

COMPREHENSIVE DRUG ABUSE PREVENTION AND CONTROL ACT OF 1970

The above act, also known as Public Law 91-513, and as the Controlled Substances Act, has as its purpose to "amend the Public Health Service Act and other laws to provide increased research into, and prevention of, drug abuse and drug dependence; to provide for treatment and rehabilitation of drug abusers and drug dependent persons; and to strengthen existing law enforcement authority in the field of drug abuse."[1]

The Act is divided into four "titles" dealing with the following subjects:

Title I   — Rehabilitation Programs Relating to Drug Abuse
Title II — Control and Enforcement
Title III — Importation and Exportation; Amendments and Repeal of Revenue Laws
Title IV — Report on Advisory Councils

Title I, Rehabilitation Programs Relating to Drug Abuse amends Part D of the Community Mental Health Centers Act to include under its provisions persons with drug abuse and drug dependence problems. In addition, it provides for increased budgetary allocations for drug abuse education programs; funding for special projects for narcotic addicts and drug dependent persons; broader treatment authority in public health service hospitals; and research under the Public Health Service Act in drug use, abuse and addiction.

Title II, dealing with control and enforcement is also known as the Controlled Substances Act. In passing this Act, the Congress made the following findings and declarations:

1. Drugs included under this title have a legitimate and useful medical purpose and are necessary to maintain the health and general welfare of the American people.
2. Illegal importation, manufacture, distribution, possession and improper use of controlled substances have a detrimental effect on the health and welfare of the American people.
3. The manufacture, local distribution, and possession of controlled substances have a direct effect upon interstate commerce.
4. Local distribution and possession of controlled substances contribute to the interstate traffic in such substances.
5. It is not a practical matter to attempt to differentiate between controlled substances manufactured and distributed interstate and controlled substances manufactured and distributed intrastate.
6. Federal control of both types of traffic is essential.
7. The United States must establish effective control over domestic and international traffic in controlled substances to be in compliance with the Single Convention of Narcotic Drugs of 1961 to which it was a party.

In order to understand the contents of Title II completely, it is necessary first to be familiar with the definitions contained within the text:

Addict: any individual who habitually uses any narcotic drug so as to endanger the public morals, health, safety or welfare, or who is so far addicted to the use of narcotic drugs as to have lost the power or self-control with reference to his addiction.

Administer: the direct application of a controlled substance to the body of a patient or research subject by a practitioner or his agent or by the patient or research subject at the direction and in the presence of the practitioner.

Agent: an authorized person who acts on behalf of or at the direction of a manufacturer, distributor or dispenser; exceptions being common contract carriers and warehouse men.

Control: the addition of a drug or other substance, or immediate precursor, to a schedule under Part B of this title, whether by transfer from another schedule or otherwise.

Controlled Substances: a drug or other substance, or immediate precursor, included in Schedule I, II, III, IV or V of Part B of this title. The term does not include distilled spirits, wine, malt beverages or tobacco, as those terms are defined or used in subtitle E of the Internal Revenue Code of 1954.

Counterfeit Substance: a controlled substance whose container or label has, without authorization, the identification of a producer other than the actual producer.

Deliver or Delivery: the actual, constructive, or attempted transfer of a controlled substance, whether or not there exists an agency relationship.

Depressant or Stimulant Substance:

(A)   a drug which contain any quantity of (1) barbituric acid or any of the salts of barbituric acid; or (2) any derivative of barbituric acid which has been designated by the Secretary as habit-forming under section 502 (d) of the Federal Food, Drug, and Cosmetic Act [21 U.S.C. 352(d)]; or

(B)   a drug which contains any quantity of (1) amphetamine or any of its optical isomers; (2) any salt of amphetamine or any salt of an optical isomer of amphetamine; or (3) any substance which the Attorney General, after investigation, has found to be, and by regulation designated as, habit-forming because of its stimulant effect on the central nervous system; or

(C)   lysergic acid diethylamide; or

(D)   any drug which contains any quantity of a substance which the Attorney General, after investigation, has found to have, and by regulation designated as having, a potential for abuse because of its depressant or stimulant effect on the central nervous system or its hallucinogenic effect.

Dispense: to deliver a controlled substance to an ultimate user or research subject by, or pursuant to the legal order of a practitioner, including the prescribing and administering of a controlled substance and the packaging, labeling, or compounding necessary to prepare the substance for such delivery.

Dispenser: a practitioner who so delivers a controlled substance to an ultimate user or research project.

Distribute: to deliver (other than by administering or dispensing) a controlled substance.

Distributor: a person who so delivers a controlled substance.

Drug: the same as that provided by section 201 (g) (1) of the Federal Food, Drug, and Cosmetic Act.

Immediate Precursor: a substance which

(A)   the Attorney General has found to be and by regulation designated as being the principal compound used, or produced primarily for use, in the manufacture of a controlled substance;

(B)   which is an immediate chemical intermediary used or likely to be used in the manufacture of such controlled substances; and

(C)   the control of which is necessary to prevent, curtail, or limit the manufacture of such controlled substances.

Manufacture: the production, preparation, propagation, compounding, or processing of a drug or other substance, either directly or by extraction from substances of natural origin, or independently by means of chemical synthesis or by a combination of extraction and chemical synthesis, and includes any packaging or repackaging of such substance or labeling or relabeling of its container; except that such term does not include the preparation, compounding, packaging, or labeling of a drug or other substance in conformity with applicable state or local law by a practitioner as an incident to his administration or dspensing of such drug or substance in the course of his professional practice. The term "manufacturer" means a person who manufactures a drug or other substance.

Manufacturer: a person who manufacturers a drug or other substance.

"Marihuana": all parts of the plant *Cannabis sativa L.,* whether growing or

not; the seeds thereof; the resin extracted from any part of such plant; and every compound, manufacture, salt, derivative, mixture, or preparation of such plant, its seeds or resin. Such term does not include the mature stalks of such plant, any other compound, manufacture, salt, derivative, mixture, or preparation of such mature stalks (except the resin extracted therefrom), fiber, oil, or cake, or the sterilized seed of such plant which is incapable of germination.

Narcotic Drug: means any of the following, whether produced directly or indirectly by extraction from substances of vegetable origin, or independently by means of chemical synthesis, or by a combination of extraction and chemical synthesis.

(A) opium, coca leaves and opiates.

(B) a compound, manufacture, salt, derivative, or preparation of opium, coca leaves or opiates.

(C) a substance (any compound, manufacture, salt, derivative, or preparation thereof) which is chemically identical with any substance referred to in (A) or (B) above. Excluded are decocainized coca leaves or extracts of coca leaves which do not contain cocaine or ecgonine.

Opiate: any drug or other substance possessing an addiction-forming or addiction-sustaining liability similar to morphine or being converted into a drug having such capabilities.

Opium Poppy: the plant (excluding the seeds) of the species *Papaver somniferum L.*

Practitioner: a physician, dentist, veterinarian, scientific investigator, pharmacy, hospital, or other person licensed, registered or otherwise permitted, by the United States or the jurisdiction in which he practices or does research, to distribute, dispense, conduct research with respect to, administer, or use in teaching or chemical analysis, a controlled substance in the course of professional practice or research.

Production: includes the manufacture, planting, cultivation, growing or harvesting of a controlled substance.

Ultimate User: a person who has lawfully obtained and who possesses, a controlled substance for his own use or for the use of a member of his household or for an animal owned by him or a member of his household.

AUTHORITY TO CONTROL

Part B of Title II authorizes the Attorney General to apply the provisions of this title to the controlled substances listed within Section 202 of this title and (a) add to such a schedule or transfer between such schedules any drug or other substance if he finds that such material has a potential for abuse, and (b) remove any drug or other substance from the schedules if he finds that the drug or other substance does not meet the requirements for inclusion in any schedule. In making these decisions, the Attorney General is required to give consideration to the following factors:

1. The drug's or other substances' actual or relative potential for abuse.
2. Scientific evidence of its pharmacological effect, if known.
3. The state of current scientific knowledge regarding the drug or other substance.
4. Its history and current pattern of abuse.

5. What, if any, risk there is to the public.
6. Its psychic or physiologic dependence liability.
7. Whether the substance is an immediate precursor of a substance already under this title.

The Attorney General may disregard the requirements of this title and control any drug or substance if control of such is required by United States obligations under international treaties, conventions or protocols. He may also, without regard to the findings required by this title, place an immediate precursor in the same schedule in which the controlled substance of which it is an immediate precursor is placed or in any other schedule with a higher numerical designation. Excepted is the drug dextromethorphan although the exclusionary wording allows for its control at some future time if such becomes necessary.

SCHEDULES FOR CONTROLLED SUBSTANCES

The key section of Public Law 91-513 is Section 202(a) for within it is created the five schedules of controlled substances, known as Schedules I, II, III, IV and V. The listings within each schedule must be updated and republished one year after the date of enactment and annually thereafter.

Except where control is required by a United States obligation, a drug or other substance may not be placed in any schedule unless the findings required for each schedule are made with respect to such drug or other substance. The findings required for each of the schedules are as follows:

(1) SCHEDULE I
  (A) The drug or other substance has a high potential for abuse.
  (B) The drug or other substance has no currently accepted medical use in treatment in the United States.
  (C) There is a lack of accepted safety for use of the drug or other substance under medical supervision.
(2) SCHEDULE II
  (A) The drug or other substance has a high potential for abuse.
  (B) The drug or other substance has recurrently accepted medical use in treatment in the United States or a currently accepted medical use with severe restrictions.
  (C) Abuse of the drug or other substances may lead to severe psychological or physical dependence.
(3) SCHEDULE III
  (A) The drug or other substance has a potential for abuse less than the drugs or other substances in schedules I and II.
  (B) The drug or other substance has a currently accepted medical use in treatment in the United States.
  (C) Abuse of the drug or other substance may lead to moderate or low physical dependence or high psychological dependence.

(4) SCHEDULE IV
    (A) The drug or other substance has a low potential for abuse relative to the drugs or other substances in schedule III.
    (B) The drug or other substance has a currently accepted medical use in treatment in the United States.
    (C) Abuse of the drug or other substance may lead to limited physical dependence or psychological dependence relative to the drugs or other substances in schedule III.

(5) SCHEDULE V
    (A) The drug or other substance has a low potential for abuse relative to the drugs or other substances in schedule IV.
    (B) The drug or other substance has a currently accepted medical use in the United States.
    (C) Abuse of the drug or other substance may lead to limited physical dependence or psychological dependence relative to the drugs or other substances in schedule IV.

(c) Schedules I, II, III, IV, and V shall, unless and until amended pursuant to section 201, consist of the following drugs or other substances, by whatever official name, common or usual name, chemical name, or brand name designated.

REGISTRATION REQUIREMENTS

Part C of this title describes the registration of manufacturers, distributors and dispensers of controlled substances. Generally, it authorizes the Attorney General to promulgate rules and regulations and to charge reasonable fees relating to the registration and control of the manufacture, distribution, and dispensation of controlled substances.

Every person falling into one or more of the above cited areas must obtain annually a registration issued by the Attorney General. Exempted from registering are the following:

1. An agent or employee of any registered manufacturer, distributor, or dispenser of any controlled substance if he is acting within the usual scope of the business or employment.
2. A common or contract carrier or warehouseman, or an employee thereof, whose possession of the controlled substance is in the usual scope of his business or employment.
3. An ultimate user who possesses such substance for his own use or for the use of a member of his household or for an animal owned by him or a member of his household.

Since the new law went into effect, the Internal Revenue Service and the Food and Drug Administration are no longer issuing a registration authorizing a person or firm to handle controlled substances. Registration with the Bureau of Narcotics and Dangerous Drugs (BNDD), now DEA, became effective with the new law. (*See* footnote, p. 330)

The registration fees are as follows:

Manufacturer (includes repackers and relabelers) $50
Distributor (wholesalers) 25
Importer or Import Broker/Forwarder 25
Exporter or Export Broker/Forwarder 25
Foreign Firm (manufacturing for importation into the U.S.A.)... 25
Retail Pharmacy 5
Hospital and Clinic 5
Practitioner 5
Researcher 5
Analytical Laboratory 5
Teaching Institution 5

The Attorney General may, in accord with the rules and regulations promulgated by him, inspect the establishment of a registrant or applicant for registration.

Registration may be granted to the applicant if the Attorney General determines that such registration is in the public interest. The following are some of the factors that are considered in determining the public interest:

1. Maintenance of effective control against diversion of the controlled substances into other than legal channels;
2. Compliance with applicable state and municipal law;
3. Prior conviction record of the applicant;
4. Past experience in the distribution of controlled substances;
5. Such other factors as may be relevant to and consistent with the public health and safety.

REGISTRATION EXEMPTION FOR HOSPITAL HOUSE STAFF

When the Federal Controlled Substances Act became effective on May 1, 1971 every physician was required to register with the Bureau of Narcotics and Dangerous Drugs, now DEA, in order to prescribe, dispense and administer controlled substances. This policy applied to interns, residents, and foreign-trained physicians working in hospitals. The only exception allowed was where a person administered or dispensed controlled drugs as the employee of the registrant, such as a nurse or intern working with in-patients in a registered hospital.

The problem this policy caused soon became apparent in that interns, residents and foreign-trained physicians had to obtain BNDD, now DEA, registrations even though their occasion to use the registration was limited to the times they prescribed controlled substances in the emergency or ambulatory clinics. To alleviate this situation, an alternative procedure was developed which allowed the temporary or provisionally licensed doctor to prescribe controlled substances without an individual registration with DEA.

Under the new policy, the intern, resident or foreign-trained physician does not have to register individually but may use the hospital's registration number for writing prescriptions, provided that the hospital complies with the following:

First, the hospital has the responsibility for verifying that the intern, resident or foreign-trained physician may lawfully write prescription while working in the hospital.

Second, the hospital must assign a code system which designates individual physicians using the hospital's registration number. This code serves as the intern's, resident's or foreign-trained physician's individual number in lieu of the DEA[a] registration number.

Third, the hospital must assure that the individual physician uses the full number assigned to him and not merely the code number which the hospital added to its registration number to identify him. In addition, the physician should have his name stamped, or typed, or hand-printed on the hospital's prescription form.

Fourth, upon the request of an outside pharmacy, law enforcement agency, or other registered person seeking to verify the authority of the prescribing individual practitioner, the hospital will determine whether or not the prescription is written by one of its staff by checking the name and code number of the physician as requested against a current list of internal code numbers and the corresponding individual practitioners.

SEPARATE REGISTRATION FOR INDEPENDENT ACTIVITIES

The following eight groups of activities are deemed to be independent of each other:

1. Manufacturing (including repackaging and relabeling) controlled substances.
2. Distributing controlled substances.
3. Dispensing (including prescribing and administering) narcotic and non-narcotic, and conducting research with non-narcotic, and conducting instructional activities with narcotic and non-narcotic controlled substances listed in schedules II through V.
4. Conducting research with narcotic controlled substances listed in schedules II through V.
5. Conducting research and instructional activities with controlled substances listed in schedule I.
6. Conducting chemical analysis with controlled substances in any schedule.
7. Importing controlled substances.
8. Exporting controlled substances listed in schedules I through IV.

---

[a]A new agency, the Drug Enforcement Administration, was created under Reorganization Plan No. 2 of 1973 which assumed the functions of various enforcement arms of the Department of Justice, including the Bureau of Narcotics and Dangerous Drugs (BNDD), and the investigative functions of the Bureau of Customs. Effective date was July 1, 1973.

Every person who engages in more than one group of independent activities must obtain a separate registration for each group of activities, with the following exceptions. Any person, when registered to engage in the group of activities described hereinafter shall be authorized to engage in the coincident activities, provided that, unless specifically exempted, he complies with all requirements and duties prescribed by law for persons registered to engage in such coincident activities: For example—

1. A person registered to manufacture or import any controlled substance or basic class of controlled substance shall be authorized to distribute that substance or class which he is not registered to manufacture or import.
2. A person registered to manufacture any controlled substance listed in schedules II through V shall be authorized to conduct chemical analysis and preclinical research (including quality control analysis) with narcotic and non-narcotic controlled substances listed in those schedules in which he is authorized to manufacture.
3. A person registered to conduct research with a basic class of controlled substances listed in schedule I shall be authorized to manufacture such class if and to the extent that such manufacture is set forth in the research protocol filed with the application for registration.
4. A person registered to conduct chemical analysis with controlled substances shall be authorized to manufacture and import such substances for analytical or instructional purposes, to distribute such substances to other persons registered to conduct chemical analysis or instructional activities and to persons exempted from registration pursuant to Section 301.26, to export such substances to persons in other countries performing chemical analysis or enforcing laws relating to controlled substances or drugs in those countries, and to conduct instructional activities with controlled substances.
5. A person registered to conduct research with narcotic controlled substances listed in schedules II through V shall be authorized to conduct research with non-narcotic controlled substances listed in schedules II through V.

One or more controlled substances listed in schedules II through V may be included in a single registration to engage in any independent activity. Only one basic class of controlled substance listed in schedule I, and no controlled substances listed in other schedules, may be included in a single registration, except that a registration to conduct chemical analysis with basic classes of controlled substances listed in schedule I may include more than one basic class and also controlled substances listed in any other schedule.

SEPARATE REGISTRATIONS FOR SEPARATE LOCATIONS

A separate registration is required for each principal place of business or professional practice at one physical location where controlled substances are manufacturered, distributed, or dispensed by a person. An office used by a practitioner (who is registered at another location) where controlled substances are prescribed but neither administered nor otherwise dispensed as a regular part of the professional practice of the practitioner at such office and where no supplies of controlled substances are maintained shall be deemed not to be places where controlled substances are manufactured, distributed or dispensed by a person.

EXEMPTION OF AGENTS AND EMPLOYEES

The requirement of registration is waived for any agent or employee of a person who is registered to engage in any group of independent activities, if such agent or employee is acting in the usual course of his business or employment. An individual practitioner who is an agent or an employee of another practitioner registered to dispense controlled substances may, when acting in the usual course of his employment, administer and dispense (other than by issuance of prescription) controlled substances if and to the extent that such individual practitioner is authorized or permitted to do so by the jurisdiction in which he practices, under the registration of the employer or principal practitioner in lieu of being registered himself. For example, a pharmacist employed by a hospital need not be registered individually to fill a prescription for controlled substances if the hospital pharmacy is so registered.

TIME FOR APPLICATION FOR REGISTRATION

Any person who is required to be registered and who is not so registered may apply for registration at any time. No person required to be registered may engage in any activity for which registration is required until the application for registration is granted and a Certificate of Registration is issued to him.

EXPIRATION OF REGISTRATION

Any person who is registered may apply to be re-registered not more than 60 days before the expiration date of his registration.

At the time any person is first registered, he will be assigned to one of twelve groups, which shall correspond to the months of the year. The expiration date of the registrations of all persons within any group will be the last day of the month designated for that group. In assigning any person to a group, the DEA may select a group the expiration date of which is less than 1 year from the date such person was registered. If the person is assigned to a group which has an expiration date less than 3 months from the date on which the person is registered, the registration will not expire until 1 year from that expiration date; in all other cases, the registration will expire on the expiration date first following the date on which the person is registered.

APPLICATION FORMS

Individuals seeking registration under the Act are required to file special forms. A person applying for registration:

1. To manufacture or distribute controlled substances shall apply on DEA Form 225.
2. To dispense narcotic or non-narcotic, or to deduct research with non-narcotic, or to conduct instructional activities with narcotic or non-narcotic controlled substances listed in schedule II through V, shall apply on DEA Form 224.
3. To conduct research with narcotic controlled substances listed in schedules II through V, shall apply on DEA Form 225.
4. To conduct research with a controlled substance listed in schedule I, shall apply on DEA Form 225, with two copies of a research protocol describing the research project attached to the Form.
5. To conduct instructional activities with a controlled substance listed in schedule I, shall apply as a researcher on DEA Form 225 with two copies of a statement describing the nature, extent and duration of such instructional activities attached to the Form.
6. To conduct chemical analysis with controlled substances listed in any schedule, shall apply on DEA Form 225.
7. To import or export controlled substances listed in any schedule, shall apply on DEA Form 225.

Applications for registration must include all of the information called for in the form, unless the item is not applicable, in which case this fact must be indicated. In addition, each application, attachment, or other document filed as part of an application, shall be signed by the applicant, if an individual; by a partner of the applicant, if partnership; or by an officer of the applicant, if a corporation, corporate division, association, trust or other entity. Another person may be authorized to sign for the applicant, if proof of authority (e.g. general power of attorney) accompanies the application.

MODIFICATION IN REGISTRATION

Any registrant may request a modification of his registration by submitting a letter of request to the Registration Branch, Drug Enforcement Agency, Central Station, Washington, D.C. 20005. Each letter of request for modification must be signed and dated by the same person who signed the most recent application for registration or reregistration.

INVENTORY REQUIREMENTS

Every registrant, other than an individual practitioner, must on the day he is first registered and every two years thereafterr, make a complete and accurate record of all stocks of controlled substances under his control. The record must indicate the date on which the inventory was taken and whether taken at the close or opening of business; be signed by the person responsible for the taking of the inventory; and be maintained at the location appearing on the registration for a period of two years.

The term "individual practitioner" means a physician, dentist, veterinarian, or other individual licensed, registered, or otherwise permitted by the United States or the jurisdiction in which he practices, to dispense a controlled substance in the course of professional practice, but does not include a pharmacist, a pharmacy, or an institutional practitioner.

Under the law, a registered individual practitioner is not required to keep records with respect to narcotic controlled substances listed in schedules II through V which he prescribes or administers in the lawful course of his professional practice. However, he must keep records with respect to such substances that he dispenses other than by prescribing or administering. A registered individual practitioner is not required to keep records with respect to non-narcotic controlled substances listed in schedules II through V which he dispenses in any manner unless he regularly charges his patients, either separately or together with charges for other professional services, for such substances so dispensed (e.g. when he substitutes his services for those of a pharmacist).

In addition to the above, Section 307 (a) through (3) requires that, after inventory, every registrant shall maintain, on a current basis, a complete and accurate record of each substance manufactured, received, sold, delivered or otherwise disposed of by him. A perpetual inventory is not required.

Furthermore, records to be kept must be in conformity with the regulations of the Attorney General; they must be maintained separately from all other records of the registrant; the records of the non-narcotic controlled substances must be in such form that information required by the Attorney General is readily retrievable from the ordinary business records of the registrant; and all records pertaining to this law must be maintained for a period of two years.

PRESCRIPTIONS

In studying the contents of Section 309 which follows, the reader is urged to make constant reference to the Federal Food, Drug, and Cosmetic Act Section 503(b).

Section 309 provides the following requirements:

1. Except when dispensed directly by a practitioner, other than a pharmacist, to an ultimate user, no controlled substance in Schedule II, which is a prescription drug as determined under the Federal Food, Drug, and Cosmetic Act, may be dispensed without prescription of a practitioner.
2. Drugs may be dispensed on an oral prescription in an emergency situation.
3. Prescriptions shall be retained in conformity with the requirements of this law.
4. No prescription for a controlled substance in Schedule II may be refilled.
5. Controlled substances in Schedule III or IV may not be dispensed without a written or oral prescription in conformity with Section 503 (b) of the Federal Food, Drug, and Cosmetic Act.
6. Such prescriptions may not be filled or refilled more than 6 months after the date thereof or be refilled more than 5 times after the date of the prescription unless renewed by the practitioner.
7. No controlled substance in Schedule V which is a drug may be distributed or dispensed other than for a medical purpose.

Prescriptions filled with controlled substances in Schedule II must be written in ink or indelible pencil and must be signed by the practitioner issuing them.

No prescription for a controlled substance in Schedule II may be refilled and such prescriptions, as well as prescriptions for narcotic substances in Schedules III, IV and V, must be kept in a separate file.

Prescriptions for controlled substances in Schedule II or IV may be issued either orally or in writing and may be refilled if so authorized. These prescriptions may not be filled or refilled more than 6 months after the date issued, or be refilled more than 5 times after the date issued. After 5 refills or after 6 months the practitioner may renew any such prescription. A renewal should be recorded on a new prescription blank and a new prescription number should be assigned to that prescription.

OFFENSES AND PENALTIES

Part D concerns itself with a listing of prohibited acts, most of which are familiar to the pharmacist. Examples include:

1. Dispensing controlled drugs without first becoming registered.
2. Removing, altering or obliterating a symbol or label required by this title.
3. Refusing or failing to make, keep or furnish any record, report, notification, declaration, order or order forms, statement, invoice or information required under this title.
4. Refusing an entry into any premises or inspection authorized by this title.

Finally, the section provides for various penalties to be assessed for the various violations and range from fines, imprisonment or both depending upon the seriousness of the violation.

LABELING AND PACKAGING REQUIREMENTS

Labeling and packaging requirements under this law are cited in Section 305 (a), (b), (c) and (d). Generally, they require that containers of controlled substances must meet the labeling requirements of the Federal Food, Drug, and Cosmetic Act or the regulations to be promulgated by the Attorney General.

Each controlled substance manufactured after December 1, 1971 must have on its label a symbol designating to which schedule it belongs. The symbol will be a letter C with the Roman numeral I, II, III, IV or V. This symbol will appear in the upper right hand portion of the label. Manufacturers and other registrants will be given adequate time, to be specified by regulations, in order to comply with the symbol requirements.

MODEL SET OF HOSPITAL CONTROLLED SUBSTANCES REGULATIONS

The Controlled Substance regulations here set forth comply with Title II of the 'Comprehensive Drug Abuse Prevention and Control Act of 1970' and subsequent amendments or proclamations concerned with the implementation of the Federal Law. The law is administered by the Drug Enforcement Agency. This regulation deals specifically with Schedule II substances which include drugs formerly known as Class A narcotics, amphetamines, methamphetamines, and any subsequent additions.

Definitions:

1. "Order": The direction for the drug, strength and frequency of administration as written on the Doctor's Order Sheet of the patient's Medical Record.
2. "Prescription": The direction for the drug, strength, quantity, and frequency of administration as written on a prescription blank by a doctor for dispensing by the Pharmacy.
3. "Administer": The word "administer" is employed when a nurse or other properly qualified individual gives medication to a patient, pursuant to the order of a qualified practitioner.
4. "Dispense": The word "dispense" is employed when a pharmacist gives medication to a nurse or other properly qualified individual in accord with the directions of a properly written prescription.
5. "Doctor": This term is herein employed to indicate an individual who has qualified for and has received a number from the Drug Enforcement Agency.

6. *Controlled Drugs Requisition* (Fig. 63) is used by the head nurse to order drugs from the Pharmacy.
7. *Daily Controlled Drugs Administration Form* (Fig. 64) serves three purposes: a 24-hour administration record for all Schedule II substances administered, allows space for inventory count for each nursing shift, and a section which serves as a record of losses and as a basis for review of errors.
8. *Monthly Controlled Drugs Inventory* (Fig. 65) serves as a monthly dispensing record for each nursing unit and receipt for Schedule II substances dispensed directly from Pharmacy.

Registration

A.   *HOSPITAL*
The hospital is registered with the Drug Enforcement Agency.
B.   *DOCTORS*
Doctors (Practitioners), in order to prescribe narcotics for or order administered (dispensed) to their patients in the hospital, must be licensed to practice under the laws of the state and must be duly registered with the DEA.
C.   *INTERNS and RESIDENTS*
Interns and Residents who are attending patients in the hospital or hospital clinics must obtain a license to practice medicine in this State. According to the *Federal Register,* Vol. 36, No. 140, p. 13390, registration requirements were waived to allow interns and residents to dispense and prescribe controlled substances under the registration of the hospital by which they are employed, provided that:
   a.   Such dispensing or prescribing is done in the usual course of professional practice.
   b.   Such individual practitioner is authorized or permitted to do so by the jurisdiction in which he is practicing.
   c.   The hospital which employs him has determined that the individual practitioner is so permitted to dispense or prescribe drugs by the jurisdiction.
   d.   Such individual practitioner is acting only within the scope of his duties within the hospital.
   e.   The hospital authorizes the intern, resident, or foreign physician to dispense or prescribe under the hospital registration and designates a specific internal code number for each intern, resident, or foreign physician so authorized. The code number shall consist of numbers or letters, or a combination thereof and shall be a suffix to the hospital's DEA registration number. Example: AM1901176-WH2.
A Hospital House Staff Identification card may be obtsined from the Medical Staff Registrar and the DEA number will be issued by the Pharmacy upon request.

Hospital Control Procedures

A.   *RESPONSIBILITY for CONTROLLED SUBSTANCES in the HOSPITAL*
The administrative head of the hospital is responsible for the proper safeguarding and the handling of controlled substances within the hospital. Responsibility for the purchase, storage, accountability and proper dispensing of bulk controlled substances within the hospital is delegated to the Pharmacist-in-Chief. Likewise, the Head Nurse of a nursing unit

is responsible for the proper storage and use of the nursing unit's controlled substances.

B.   *PREPARATION of ORDERS*
All controlled substances orders and records must be typed or written in ink or indelible pencil and signed in ink or indelible pencil.

C.   *ORDERING WARD STOCK CONTROLLED SUBSTANCES from the PHARMACY*
   1.   A requisition for ward stock controlled substances is completed by placing a check mark opposite the name, strength, form of the controlled substance desired. The completed form is then sent to the pharmacy along with the empty containers and the nurse's inventory sheet. Figure 63 is an example of this type of form.
   2.   Before any new controlled substances are issued to a ward, the previous supply must be fully accounted for. Therefore, each request for a new supply must be accompanied by the Daily Controlled Drugs Administration Form shown in Figure 64. Whenever a new supply of drug is issued, it is accompanied by one of these forms. This form serves three purposes: a 24-hour administration record for all Sched-

---

Ward _____ Code _____ Date _____

Each floor is entitled to 2 containers of each of the following tablets and 2 units of the injectables. Empty bottles **except** tubex, along with narcotic or barbiturate accounting sheets must be returned to the pharmacy. All other narcotics and barbiturates must be ordered for and charged to the patient. These special narcotic and barbiturate orders must be accompanied by a prescription.

No. of Tabs-Caps mls.	(√)	Check item needed	Price
25		Codeine Sulfate Tablets 15 mg	
25		Codeine Sulfate Tablets 30 mg	
10		Codeine Sulfate 30 mg Tubex	
10		Codeine Sulfate 60 mg Tubex	
10		Hydromorphone (Dilaudid) 2 mg Tubex	
10		Hydromorphone (Dilaudid) 4 mg Tubex	
10		Meperidine HCl 50 mg Tubex	
10		Meperidine HCl 75 mg Tubex	
10		Meperidine HCl 100 mg Tubex	
25		Meperidine HCl Tablets 50 mg	
10		Morphine Sulfate 8 mg Tubex	
10		Morphine Sulfate 10 mg Tubex	
10		Morphine Sulfate 15 mg Tubex	
10		Methadon HCl Ampul 10 mg /1 ml	
15		Methadon HCl Tablets 5 mg	
15		Percodan Tablets	
25		Chloral Hydrate Capsules 500 mg	
1		Pentobarbital Injection 50 mg /ml 20 ml	
25		Pentobarbital Capsules 50 mg	
25		Phenobarbital Tablets 15 mg	
25		Secobarbital Capsules 50 mg	

FORM 107 REV.

Fig. 63.   Requisition form for ward stock controlled substances.

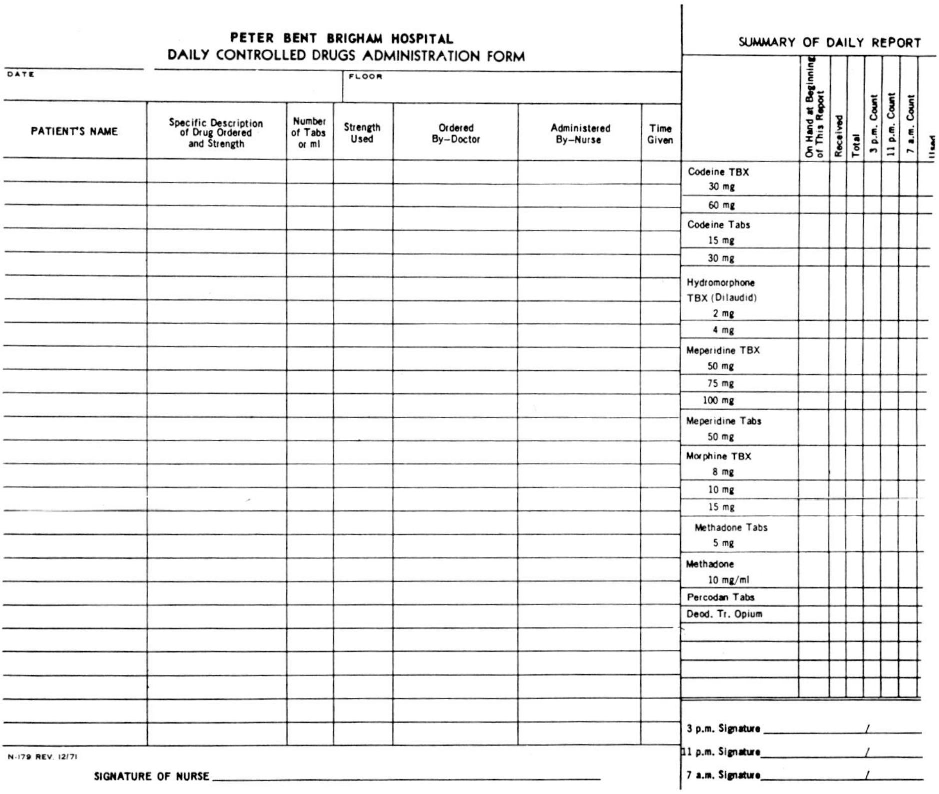

PETER BENT BRIGHAM HOSPITAL
DAILY CONTROLLED DRUGS ADMINISTRATION FORM

DATE ______ FLOOR ______

PATIENT'S NAME	Specific Description of Drug Ordered and Strength	Number of Tabs or ml	Strength Used	Ordered By–Doctor	Administered By–Nurse	Time Given

N-179 REV. 12/71

SIGNATURE OF NURSE ______

SUMMARY OF DAILY REPORT

	On Hand at Beginning of This Report	Received	Total	3 p.m. Count	11 p.m. Count	7 a.m. Count	Used
Codeine TBX 30 mg							
60 mg							
Codeine Tabs 15 mg							
30 mg							
Hydromorphone TBX (Dilaudid) 2 mg							
4 mg							
Meperidine TBX 50 mg							
75 mg							
100 mg							
Meperidine Tabs 50 mg							
Morphine TBX 8 mg							
10 mg							
15 mg							
Methadone Tabs 5 mg							
Methadone 10 mg/ml							
Percodan Tabs							
Deod. Tr. Opium							

3 p.m. Signature ______ / ______
11 p.m. Signature ______ / ______
7 a.m. Signature ______ / ______

Fig. 64. Daily Controlled Drugs Administration Form.

ule II substances administered, allows space for inventory count for each nursing shift, and a section which serves as a record of losses and as a basis for review of errors.

3. Whenever a dose of a drug is lost or wasted on the ward, the nurse in charge must prepare a report to cover the incident. This is accomplished by using a special report form shown in Figure 66. This report is prepared in duplicate and sent to the pharmacy along with the nurse's account sheet and a request for a new supply of drug. The original is filed in the pharmacy and the duplicate is forwarded to the Nursing Office.

D. *DOCTOR'S ORDERS for ADMINISTRATION of CONTROLLED DRUGS*

The doctor's orders for the administration of ward stock controlled drugs must be written on the doctor's order sheet of the patient's chart. However, if the desired controlled drug is not on ward stock a complete controlled drug prescription must be written on a hospital prescription blank. The signed prescription must be sent to the pharmacy. A notation must then be made on the patient's chart by the doctor or nurse indicating that the doctor's signature for the order is in the pharmacy.

A *controlled drug order* must be *written* by a *licensed physician or a registered intern or resident.*

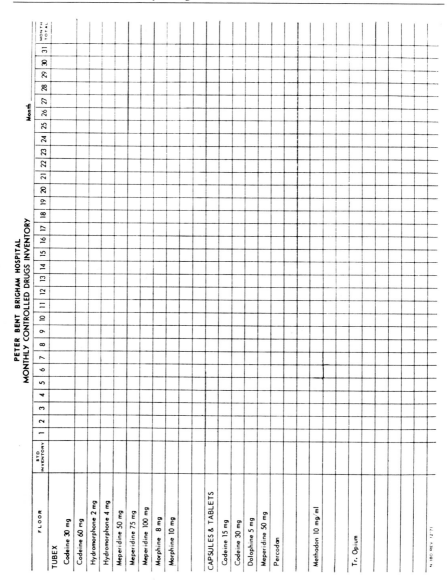

Fig. 65.   Monthly Controlled Drugs Inventory Form.

E.   *INFORMATION WHICH MUST APPEAR on the DAILY CONTROLLED DRUGS ADMINISTRATION SHEET*
The full information required on the Daily Controlled Drugs Administration Sheet (Fig. 64) is as follows:
1.   Date
2.   Amount given
3.   Patient's full name
4.   Patient's hospital number

REQUEST FOR REPLACEMENT
OF CONTROLLED SUBSTANCE LOSS OR WASTE ON WARDS

Date _____

Send Original and One Copy
TO PHARMACY

ml.
Name of Drug _____ Quantity _____ Tab.

Bottle No. _____   Narcotic Sheet No. _____

Explicit statement of what happened:

_____
Signature of Nurse Making Report

Attested by Head Nurse or
        Nursing Supervisor _____

Reviewed by Pharmacist _____

This report must be prepared in duplicate and sent to the Pharmacy. The signed report is brought to the Pharmacy along with a requisition for a new supply of the lost narcotic. The report will be signed by the Pharmacist on duty. The reports will be retained in the pharmacy.
Form 248

Fig. 66. Controlled Substance Loss or Waste Form.

5.   Name of doctor ordering

6.   Signature of nurse administering

The following information is requested for auditing purposes and is not required by Federal law:

1.   Number of tablets or ml administered

3.   Filing out inventory column (to be retained for Pharmacy).

F.   *DOCTOR'S SIGNATURE*

The doctor's full name or initials are required on the doctor's order sheet. The doctor's full name is required on a controlled drug prescription.

In each of the above, the signature must be by the doctor's own hand.

G.   *PRO RE NATA (p.r.n.) or SI OPUS SIT (s.o.s.) ORDERS*

A p.r.n. or s.o.s. order for controlled drugs must be discouraged except under special circumstances.

H.   *TELEPHONE ORDERS*

A doctor may order a controlled drug by telephone in case of necessity. The nurse will write the order on the doctor's order sheet, stating that it is a telephone order and will sign the doctor's name and her own initials. The controlled drug may then be administered at once. The order must then be *signed by the doctor* with either his signature or his initials within 24 hours.

I.   VERBAL ORDERS

A verbal order may be given by a doctor in an *extreme emergency* where time does not permit writing the order. The nurse must write the order on the doctor's order sheet. The doctor must sign the order with either his signature or his initials within 24 hours.

J.   *ORDERING NON-WARD STOCK CONTROLLED DRUGS from PHAR-MACY*

Drugs which are not stocked on the nursing stations may be ordered from the Pharmacy on written prescription only.

The amount of drugs sent to the nursing unit is the amount covered on the prescription by the doctor's signature. If more is needed a new signed prescription must be obtained. The prescription must have the following information:

1.   Patient's full name

2.   Patient's address or hospital number

3.   Date

4.   Name and strength of drug prescribed

5.   Total amount of drug to be dispensed

6.   Registration number of the licensed physician

The prescription must be written in ink or indelible pencil. It shall not bear erasures, or alterations of any kind.

A doctor may not write a prescription for controlled drugs for his own use.

K.   *PRESCRIBING CONTROLLED DRUGS in the OUT-PATIENT DEPART-MENT*

Prescriptions for Schedule II and other controlled substances drugs may be dispensed from Pharmacy and must include the following information.

a.   Patient's full name

b.   Patient's address or hospital number

c.   Date

d.   Name and strength of drug prescribed.

e.   Quantity of drug to be dispensed

f.   DEA number and signature of physician

g.   Frequency and route of administration

The prescription must be written in ink or indelible pencil and shall not bear cross outs or erasures. Discharge prescriptions for Schedule II drugs must be picked up by a registered nurse.

L. *DISPENSING CONTROLLED DRUGS for HOME USE when PHARMACY IS CLOSED*

Occasionally patients who require drugs for use at home are discharged from the hospital or released from the Emergency Ward during hours when the Pharmacy is closed. Whenever possible, a prescription signed by a member of the staff who has a License to practice medicine and a DEA number should be obtained.

A staff physician whose DEA number is issued to an outside office should use his own prescription blank. If this is not available, then he must insert his office address on the hospital prescription blank. This will permit the patient or his relative to purchase the drugs at an outside pharmacy. If no physician is available, or during hours when the local pharmacies are closed, the following procedure is allowed, but only as an EMERGENCY MEASURE:

The attending doctor will calculate the smallest amount of the drug necessary to treat the patient until the Pharmacy opens. He will write a prescription for this amount and the nurse may dispense the medication from her stock supply. The prescription will be presented to the pharmacy the following morning for replacement of stock.

M. *PROCEDURE in CASE of WASTE, DESTRUCTION, CONTAMINATION ETC.*

1. *Aliquot Part of Narcotic Solutions Used for Dose:*
   The nurse shall use the proper number of tablets or ampuls from nursing stock. She shall record the number of tablets or ampuls used and the dose given in the proper columns on Daily Controlled Drugs Administration Form (Fig. 64). She shall, in arriving at the proper aliquot part, expel into the sink that portion of the solution that is not used.

2. *Prepared Dose Refused by Patient or Cancelled by Doctor:*
   When a dose has been prepared for a patient but not used, due to a refusal by the patient or because of cancellation by the doctor, the nurse shall expel the solution into the sink and record why the drug was not administered. Examples: "Discarded," "Refused by patient" or "order cancelled by Dr. _____ ." The head nurse of the unit shall countersign the statement.

3. *Accidental Destruction and Contamination of Drugs:*
   When a solution, ampul, tablet etc., is accidentally destroyed or contaminated on a Nursing Unit, the person responsible shall indicate the loss on Figure 66.

MISCELLANEOUS REGULATIONS

1. Ward supplies of narcotics are to be used only for patients on the ward. They may not be given to patients to take home (except as an emergency measure as noted above) and are not for the treatment of employees.

2. Narcotic prescriptions may not be refilled.

3. A nurse, though the agent of a hospital or doctor, as such, may be partially or wholly responsible for the violation of any of the

regulations described above or any others under the Federal Narcotic Act as amended, but not included here.

4. Federal regulations do not allow a shortage from a vial of injectable narcotic.
5. A physician may not prescribe narcotics for his own personal use.

CONTROL OF NARCOTICS BY NURSES

Once the narcotics for the pavilion have been dispensed from the pharmacy, the nursing service assumes the responsibility for the administration, control and auditing of the inventory.

The auditing of the narcotic inventory takes place with each change of nursing shift. At this time, both the nurse coming on duty and the nurse going off duty take a physical count of the narcotics then on the nursing station. If the tally is correct both sign the audit record (Fig. 67). If the tally is incorrect, then a check of the medications ordered for the day by the physicians is in order so that the omission of recording is immediately corrected. On the other hand, if the error cannot be explained, then a narcotic loss report must be executed and forwarded to the department of pharmacy.

NARCOTICS DELIVERY TO NURSING STATION

The delivery of narcotics from the pharmacy to the nursing station may be assigned to any reliable person in the hospital's employ. It is usually entrusted to a member of the messenger staff since it is presumed that sufficient control records are maintained so that any narcotics that are delivered for illegal use would be immediately detected and appropriate measures taken for their recovery.

EIGHT HOUR NURSE AUDIT RECORD

DATE	7 A. M.		3 P. M.		11 P. M.	
	SIGNATURE ON-COMING NURSE	INITIALS OFF-GOING NURSE	SIGNATURE ON-COMING NURSE	INITIALS OFF-GOING NURSE	SIGNATURE ON-COMING NURSE	INITIALS OFF-GOING NURSE

RETURNED TO THE PHARMACY BY _____

DATE _____

Fig. 67

Charges to Patients for Narcotics

Charging for narcotics depends upon the policy of the individual hospital. Many hospitals make a charge for each dose received while others make a flat charge to cover all narcotics and hypnotics. In general, hospitals include narcotics along with other floor stock drugs for which no specific charge is made to the patient. Where there is a split policy in operation, the general plan is not to charge the patient for routinely used narcotics but to make a charge for those that must be obtained on special order.

Narcotics which commonly fall into the routinely used category are Codeine Phosphate Injection, Codeine Sulfate Tablets and Morphine Sulphate Injection.

One factor affecting the decision as to which narcotic drug should be included in the per diem charge is its cost. Accordingly, large teaching hospitals with a sterile products manufacturing section produce, at reasonably low cost, a large variety of injectable narcotic preparations and therefore make these available to the patient at no charge.

Smaller hospitals, which purchase their narcotics in ampul form, find it necessary to charge for each dose administered.

PROTOCOL FOR REPORTING DRUG ABUSE OR DIVERSION

Because of the possibility of drug abuse or diversion of controlled substances in the hospital, the Director of Pharmacy Services in collaboration with the Director of Personnel and the Director of Security should develop a protocol for use when drug abuse or diversion is detected. By so doing, confusion is avoided when an incident occurs. The following is a sample protocol that could be modified to meet the needs of a specific institution.

I. *Drugs included in this Protocol*
    All drugs in Schedules 2, 3, 4, and 5 of the Controlled Substances Act of 1970. These drugs are listed in the Current Practice Manual, 1-16-1.

II. *Persons affected by this Protocol*
    Employees, patients, and visitors, of The Peter Bent Brigham Hospital.

III. *Explanation of Outside Agencies*
    A. D.E.A.—Federal Drug Enforcement Administration.
    B. D.I.U.—Diversion Investigation Unit of the State Police
    C. Board of Pharmacy—Massachusetts State Board of Pharmacy
    D. Local Police—Self explanatory

IV. *Events covered by this Protocol which should be reported to Outside Agencies*
    A. Diversion—Any unexplained loss or theft of controlled substances.
    B. Abuse—Any problems such as unusual behavior which are suspected to be caused by the use of controlled substances.

V. *Procedure for reporting suspected diversion or abuse within the hospital*
    A. An employee who has knowledge of drug diversion or abuse by a fellow employee, patient, or visitor has an obligation to report such information.
    B. Any incident involving drug diversion or abuse shall be reported by the person involved or the person observing the incident.

C.   Reporting should be done in the following manner:

DIVERSION

Report in writing on Controlled Substances Incident Report Form to the Pharmacy:

1. Known loss or theft.
2. Discrepancy found in inventory or audit.
3. Observation of container seals and caps which have been tampered.
4. Any other incident in which diversion is suspected.

ABUSE

1. The first occurrence of an unusual behavior by an employee should be observed and reported to the supervisor for evaluation.
2. If in the judgment of the supervisor the employee is incapable of performing normal work functions, it should be suggested that the employee go to the Employee Health Clinic.
3. If the employee refuses, the employee should be sent off duty by the supervisor, and the event should be reported to the Personnel Department.
4. If the employee is seen in the Employee Health Clinic and it is determined that the problem is due to the employee's use of controlled substances without prescription of a physician or in a manner differing from that indicated by the prescription, this should be reported in writing by the Employee Health Clinic to both the Pharmacy and the Personnel Department. If the employee refuses to provide a blood sample, the employee should be sent off duty by the supervisor and the event should be reported to the Personnel Department.
5. If abuse is suspected of a patient or visitor, this should be reported to the Hospital Security Department who will send a copy of the report to the Pharmacy.

VI.   *Investigation of incidents within the hospital*

A.   The number of hospital personnel involved in investigating a possible abuse or diversion should be limited.
B.   Reports received by the Pharmacy will be investigated to determine if diversion is involved. This investigation will include:
    1. Verification of records which should reflect the drug, dose, by whom prescribed, by whom administered, time of administration, and to whom administered.
    2. A check of the 8-hour Nursing Service Audits.
    3. If necessary an assessment will be made with nursing and medical assistance of the patient response to the medication.
C.   Investigation of potential employee abuse will be conducted by the department involved with the consultation of the Employee Health Clinic and the Personnel Department. The Hospital Security Department will assist in any investigation as requested.
D.   Investigation of potential abuse by patients and visitors will be conducted by the Hospital Security Department.
E.   Factual information gained during the investigation should be co-signed by the individuals gathering the information.
F.   The rights of individuals will be respected and police methods will be avoided by hospital personnel.
G.   If it is determined in the internal investigation that diversion or abuse

is not involved, the incident report will be filed in the Pharmacy, or in some cases of abuse it will be filed in the Personnel Department, and observed for the possible development of a pattern.
    H.   If diversion is suspected by the Pharmacy or abuse reported by the Employee Health Clinic or the Personnel Department, then the outside agencies will be contacted.

VII.   *Procedure for making reports to outside agencies*
    A.   The Pharmacy is responsible for making reports.
    B.   Pharmacy to notify Hospital Security Department before making report.
    C.   **For reporting diversion:**
       1. Pharmacy will call D.E.A. and describe event.
       2. Call will be followed with a certified letter describing event.
       3. D.E.A. will send copies of Report Form #106.
       4. Pharmacy will call local police, describe the event, and advise police that D.E.A. has also been contacted.
       5. Call will be followed with a certified letter describing the event.
       6. Upon receipt of Form #106 Pharmacy will complete copies and send to—
          a. D.E.A. (Pharmacy will send two (2) copies and D.E.A. will forward one (1) to D.I.U.)
          b. Board of Pharmacy
          c. Local police
    D.   **For reporting abuse:**
       1. Pharmacy will call D.E.A., D.I.U., and local police describing event.
       2. Pharmacy will follow calls with certified letters to each agency describing the event.

VIII. *Ground for dismissal of hospital employees*
    A.   Felony conviction on a drug charge.
    B.   An established drug dependency.
       1. This will first result in a suspension.
       2. If the condition is cured, the employee will be reinstated to a low risk area.
       3. If the condition is not cured, dismissal will take place.

IX.   *Educational Program*
The Personnel Department will conduct periodic educational programs to assist personnel in carrying out their responsibilities which are described in this Protocol. Assistance in conducting these programs will be obtained from the Pharmacy, Nursing Service, the Hospital Security Department, and the D.E.A.

Mailing of Controlled Substances

The Drug Enforcement Administration has published the mailing requirements for controlled substances as set forth in the U.S. Postal Services (Domestic) regulations TL-34, 3-7-75, Issue 97. The DEA-Postal Service regulations are reprinted for your information:

124.5 Controlled Substances, Narcotics (18 U.S.C. 1716)

.51 Definitions

.511 Controlled Substances
A controlled substance is any narcotic, hallucinogenic, stimulant or depressant

drug in Schedules I through V of the Controlled Substances Act (Public Law 91-513), 21 U.S.C. 801, et. seq., and the regulations thereunder, 21 C.F.R. 1300, et. seq.

.512 Narcotic Drugs

Narcotic drugs, as defined in the Controlled Substances Act, include opium, cocaine and opiates (synthetic narcotics) and the derivatives thereof.

.52 Declarations as to Injurious Nature

Controlled substances are, by reason of their addictive nature or capacity for abuse, hereby declared to be Articles, Compositions, or materials which may kill or injure another within the intent and meaning of 18 U.S.C. 1716.

.53 Nonmailable Generally

Except under the conditions specified in 124.5 controlled substances are non-mailable matter and shall not be conveyed in the mails or delivered from any post office or station thereof nor by any letter carrier.

.54 Mailing Requirements

.541 Authorized Mailings

Controlled substances may be transmitted in the mails between persons registered with the Drug Enforcement Administration or between persons who are exempted from registration such as military, law enforcement, and civil defense personnel in the performance of their official duties. Prescription medicines containing non-narcotic controlled substances may be mailed from a registered practitioner or dispenser to an ultimate user. Prescription medicines containing narcotic drugs may be mailed only by Veterans Administration medical facilities to certain veterans. Parcels containing controlled substances must be prepared and packed for mailing in accordance with the requirements of 124.542.

.542 Preparation and Packing

a. The inner container of any parcel containing controlled substances must be marked and sealed in accordance with the applicable provisions of the Controlled Substances Act, 21 U.S.C. 801, and the regulations promulgated thereunder, 21 C.F.R. 1300 et seq.

b. The inner container of prescription medicines containing controlled substances must, in addition to the marking and sealing requirements set forth in *a*, be labeled to show the name and address of the practitioner, or the name and address of the pharmacy or other person dispensing the prescription if other than the practitioner, and the prescription number.

c. Every parcel containing controlled substances shall be placed in a plain outer container or securely overwrapped in plain paper.

d. No markings of any kind which would indicate the nature of the contents shall be placed on the outside of any parcel containing controlled substances.

.543 Use of Registered Mail Required

Parcels containing controlled substances, including those sent to DEA Regional Offices for disposal (see 21 CFR 1307.2) generally must be sent by registered mail, return requested. The Drug Enforcement Administration number or exemption status of the sender shall be set forth in the sender's address Section of Form 3877, as applicable. This information shall appear in the following format:

DEA REGISTRATION No. 654321

or

DEA Exempt—Police

.544 Regular Mail Permitted
The following may be sent by regular mail without regard to the provision of 124.543:

   a. Prescription medicines containing non-narcotic controlled substances listed in Schedule II in amounts not exceeding 100 dosage units.
   b. Prescription medicine containing non-narcotic controlled substances listed in Schedules III, IV, and V in amounts not exceeding a 100-day supply or 300 dosage units whichever is less.
   c. Physician's sample of medicines containing non-narcotic controlled substances in amounts not exceeding the limitations; set forth in 124.544 *a* or *b*.

.55 Exempt Shipments

Small quantities of unknown matter suspected of containing controlled substances may be sent by regular mail without regard to the other provisions of 124.5 only when addressed to a Federal, state or local law enforcement agency for law enforcement purposes. Such mailings must comply with 124.542 (c) and (d).

.56 Violations

Violations of this section shall be referred to the Inspection Service.

OTHER SYSTEMS

Although the system herein described for the distribution of floor stock narcotics has been used by many hospital pharmacists and has been found to be dependable and satisfactory, some hospital pharmacists have developed modifications for which they claim the advantage of saving personnel time and the reduction of the possibility of error.[1,2]

In addition, the pharmaceutical industry has developed new concepts in the packaging of narcotics for distribution in the hospital. One of these systems provides narcotic injectables in a single-dose ampul which is packaged in a space-saving, see-through dispenser of ten, which in turn is packaged in a carton of two floor-stock dispenser trays.

Narcotic tablets are being packaged in strip packs thereby permitting the pharmacist and the nurse to easily identify each individual tablet up to the time of its consumption as well as to "measure count" for inventory purposes.[3–6]

SPECIAL USES

The ASHP Technical Assistance Bulletin on Institutional Use of Controlled Substances[7] provides two sections (VIII and IX) that are of importance to the Hospital pharmacist. They are as follows:

VIII. RESEARCH, LABORATORY PROCEDURES AND INSTRUCTIONAL USES

(A) *Registration.*

(1) *General.* Persons engaged in research, laboratory procedures or instructional uses with controlled substances are required to register under the Controlled Substances Act. A person already registered to dispense controlled substances in Schedules II through V is authorized by virtue of such registration to use controlled substances in research and related activities including preclinical and clinical investigations of drugs, laboratory procedures and for instructional use without separate registration, provided they are otherwise permitted to do so under applicable federal and state laws. Methadone research or dispensing is not authorized for persons registered to dispense controlled substances unless the general requirements discussed in Section IX of these Guidelines are complied with.

(2) *Use of Schedule I Drugs.* The conduct of research with controlled substances listed in Schedule I requires separate registration. Registration for Schedule I research requires submission of a research protocol with the application describing each research project. Research will be authorized only with those substances listed in an approved research protocol.

(3) *Separate Locations.* If research or related activities are conducted with controlled substances in more than one general physical location, a separate registration is required for each location.

(B) *Records and Reports.*

(1) *General Requirement.* Each person registered or authorized to conduct research or related activities with controlled substances is required to keep records. A registered person using a controlled substance in research conducted at a registered establishment need not maintain separate records if the establishment maintains records in compliance with an IND. The registered person must notify DEA of the name, address and registration number of the establishment maintaining the investigational use records. Notice to DEA is given in the form of an attachment to the application for registration or re-registration.

(2) *Inventory.* The inventory requirements of a person registered to dispense or authorized to conduct research or related activities with controlled substances include an accounting for each controlled substance in finished form and controlled substances awaiting disposal,

held for quality control purposes or maintained for extemporaneous compoundings or similar purposes.

(3) *Receipt and Dispensing.* Receipt and dispensing records must be kept by the registrant. If the registrant is a hospital, the required records should be kept by the pharmacist in the same manner as records for other controlled substances.

(C) *Security.* In a registered institution the pharmacist should be the custodian of all controlled substances. Controlled substances may be dispensed only to or for authorized investigators, laboratory personnel or instructors. The pharmacist should be responsible for the security of controlled substances used in research and related activities.

IX. METHADONE

(A) *Registration and Approval.*

(1) *General.* The use of methadone in an institution is controlled jointly under FDA and DEA regulations. The FDA methadone regulations (21 CFR 310.305) provide for approved uses of methadone in a hospital and in a methadone treatment program. A hospital may be approved to dispense methadone for detoxification and temporary maintenance of inpatients or for analgesia in severe pain for both inpatients and outpatients. If a hospital desires to establish a methadone treatment program for detoxification and maintenance of drug-dependent persons, separate approval is required. In either case, the hospital must be registered with DEA to dispense Schedule II controlled substances in addition to receiving approval under the FDA methadone regulations.

(2) *Hospital Use of Methadone.* In order for a hospital pharmacy to lawfully receive or dispense methadone for its approved hospital uses, the hospital must submit form FD 2636, "Hospital Request for Methadone for Analgesia in Severe Pain and for Detoxification and Temporary Maintenance Treatment." The application must be approved by the responsible state authority and the FDA. The form requires detailed information about the hospital, including the name of the pharmacist responsible for receiving and securing supplies of methadone.

(3) *Methadone Treatment Programs.* To obtain approval to establish a methadone treatment program, the sponsor must submit Form FD 2632, "Application for Approval of Use of Methadone in a Treatment Program." The application must receive the approval of the responsible state authority and the FDA with the concurrence of DEA. In order to assure that each participating physician in a methadone treatment program is aware of his professional and administrative responsibilities, the FDA requires that form FD 2633, "Medical Responsibility Statement for use of Methadone in a Treatment Program," be completed by each physician licensed to dispense or administer methadone in an approved

program. These statements must accompany the program application. All patients in the program are required to give their consent for treatment by signing Form FD 2635, "Consent for Methadone Treatment."

(B) *Records and Reports.*

(1) *Hospital Use of Methadone.* All records must be kept in compliance with the DEA requirements for Schedule I and II controlled substances. Hospitals must also maintain accurate records traceable to specific patients and they must include dates, quantity and batch or code marks of the drug dispensed. Methadone records must be retained for a three-year period instead of the two-year period required for other controlled substances. The hospital does not have to submit a detailed annual report. The hospital is required to report to FDA annually the name and address of all physicians who prescribed methadone for outpatient use during the previous year.

(2) *Methadone Treatment Program.* All records must be kept in compliance with the DEA requirements for Schedule I and II controlled substances. The FDA methadone regulations require also that there be accurate records traceable to specific patients and they must include dates, quantity and batch or code marks of the drug dispensed. The record retention period for methadone records is three years. The methadone treatment program is required to file an annual report with the responsible state authority and the FDA. The content of the annual report is detailed in FD Form 2634, "Annual Report for Treatment Program Using Methadone."

(C) *Security.* The FDA regulations require that the security for methadone treatment programs must be in compliance with DEA guidelines prior to final FDA approval.

SELECTED READINGS

Regulations No. 5, I.R.S. Publication No. 428 (6-29), Superintendent of Documents, U.S. Government Printing Office, Washington D.C. 20402.

Hibbard, F.J., Bair, J.N., and Sylvester, K.L.: Pharmacy-Based Controlled Substances Distribution for a University Campus. Am. J. Hosp. Pharm., *40*:74–77, 1983.

ASHP Technical Assistance Bulletin and Hospital Drug Distribution and Control. Am. J. Hosp. Pharm., *37*:1097–1103, (Aug.) 1980.

REFERENCES

1. Davis, Neil M.: A Case Study in Narcotic Control, Hospitals. J.A.H.A., *36*:56, 1962.
2. Eckel, Fred M. and Latiolais, Clifton J.: An Effective Narcotic Control System Using Electronic Data Processing. Am. J. Hosp. Pharm., *22*:9:519, 1965.
3. Mabol, Philip D.: Evaluation of a New Ready-to-Dispense System for Oral Narcotics. Am. J. Hosp. Pharm., *24*:10:543, 1967.
4. Zellers, Darryl D. and Derewiczs, Henry J.: Twenty-Four Hour Narcotic Disposition Recording System. Am. J. Hosp. Pharm., *24*:10:550, 1967.

5. Wirth, Bradford P.: A Computerized System for Restricted Drug Control and Inventory. Am. J. Hosp. Pharm., *24*:10:556, 1967.
6. Austin, Leonard H.: A Simplified Narcotic Distribution System. Am. J. Hosp. Pharm., *24*:10:561, 1967.
7. ASHP Technical Assistance Bulletin on Institutional Use of Controlled Substances. Am. J. Hosp. Pharm., *31*:582–588, (June) 1978.

17|

Tax-Free Alcohol—Its Procurement and Control

Because the hospital is a prime user of tax-free alcohol which is commonly purchased, stored, dispensed and accounted for by the hospital pharmacist, it seems proper to devote a separate chapter to the technical procedures involved in the above processes.

The hospital pharmacist should obtain from the U.S. Government Printing Office the latest document[1] governing the distribution and use of tax-free alcohol. In addition, the local assistant regional commissioner will make available the appropriate "Industry Circular," a publication of the Office of the Commissioner of Internal Revenue, Alcohol and Tobacco Tax Division.

Although this chapter will deal with the various aspects of Section D, Part 22, Code of Federal Regulations, the reader is cautioned to make reference to the Federal publication and where questions arise to consult freely with the assistant regional commissioner.

In the following discussion, the various sections of Part 22 will be listed along with their subtitles. Where the section should be of particular interest to the hospital pharmacist, its content will be quoted and, where necessary, elaborated upon. Samples of all the forms discussed in the various sections may be obtained from the Assistant Regional Commissioner (Alcohol and Tobacco Tax) for study along with the appropriate section. These regulations are effective June, 1985.

FEDERAL REGULATIONS

Subpart—Definitions

§ 22.11 Meaning of terms.

When used in this part and in forms prescribed under this part, the following terms have the meanings given in this section. Words in the plural form include the singular, and vice versa, and words importing the masculine gender include the feminine. The terms "includes" and "including" do not exclude things not enumerated which are in the same general class.

354

Alcohol. Spirits having a proof of 190° or more when withdrawn from bond, including all subsequent dilutions and mixtures thereof, from whatever source or by whatever process produced.

Area supervisor. The supervisory officer of the Bureau of Alcohol, Tobacco and Firearms area office.

ATF officer. An officer or employee of the Bureau of Alcohol, Tobacco and Firearms (ATF) authorized to perform any function relating to the administration or enforcement of this part.

CFR. The Code of Federal Regulations.

Clinic. When used in this part the term includes veterinary clinics.

Delegate. Any officer, employee, or agency of the Department of the Treasury authorized by the Secretary of the Treasury directly, or indirectly by one of more redelegations of authority, to perform the function mentioned or described in the context.

Director. The Director, Bureau of Alcohol, Tobacco and Firearms, the Department of the Treasury, Washington, D.C.

Executed under penalties of perjury. Signed with the prescribed declaration under the penalties of perjury as provided on or with respect to the claim, form, or other document or, where no form of declaration is prescribed, with the declaration "I declare under the penalities of perjury that this _____(insert type of document, such as statement, report, certificate, application, claim, or other document), including the documents submitted in support thereof, has been examined by me and, to the best of my knowledge and belief, is true, correct, and complete."

Fiduciary. A guardian, trustee, executor, administrator, receiver, conservator, or any person acting in any fiduciary capacity for any person.

Gallon or wine gallon. The liquid measure equivalent to the volume of 231 cubic inches.

Hospital. When used in this part the term includes veterinary hospitals.

Initial order. The first order of tax-free alcohol placed by a permittee or Governmental agency with a distilled spirits plant or vendor, and, the first order placed following the issuance of an amended or corrected permit.

Liter or litre. A metric unit of capacity equal to 1,000 cubic centimeters of alcohol, and equivalent to 33.814 fluid ounces. A liter is divided into 1,000 milliliters (ml). The symbol for milliliter or milliliters is "ml".

Permit. The document issued under 26 U.S.C. 5271(a), authorizing a person to withdraw tax-free alcohol from the premises of a distilled spirits plant and use such alcohol under specified conditions.

Permittee. Any person holding a permit, on Form 5150.9, issued under this part to withdraw and use tax-free alcohol.

Person. An individual, trust, estate, partnership, association, company, or corporation.

Proof. The ethyl alcohol content of a liquid at 60° Fahrenheit, stated as twice the percent of ethyl alcohol by volume.

Proof gallon. A gallon at 60° Fahrenheit which contains 50 percent of volume of ethyl alcohol having a specific gravity of 0.7939 at 60° Fahrenheit referred to water at 60° Fahrenheit as unity, or the alcoholic equivalent thereof.

Region. A Bureau of Alcohol, Tobacco and Firearms Region.

Regional director (compliance). The principal ATF regional official responsible for administering regulations in this part.

Restoration. Restoring to the original state of recovered tax-free alcohol, including redistillation of the recovered alcohol to 190° or more of proof and the removal of foreign materials by redistillation, filtration, or other suitable means.

Secretary. The Secretary of the Treasury or his delegate.

Spirits or distilled spirits. The substance known as ethyl alcohol, ethanol, or spirits of wine, having a proof of 190° or more when withdrawn from bond, including all subsequent dilution and mixtures thereof, from whatever source or by whatever process produced.

This chapter. Title 27, Code of Federal Regulations, Chapter I (27 CFR Chapter I).

U.S.C. The United States Code.

Subpart C—Administrative Provisions

Authorities

§ 22.21 Forms prescribed.

(a) The Director is authorized to prescribe all forms required by this part, including bonds, applications, notices, claims, reports, and records. All of the information called for in each form shall be furnished as indicated by the headings on the form and the instructions on or pertaining to the form. In addition, information called for in each form shall be furnished as required by this part.

(b) ATF Publication 1322.1, Public Use Forms, is a numerical listing of forms issued by the Bureau of Alcohol, Tobacco and Firearms. This publication is available from the Superintendent of Documents, U.S. Government Printing Office, Washington, DC 20402.

(c) Requests for forms should be mailed to the ATF Distribution Center, 3800 South Four Mile Run Drive, Arlington, Virginia 22206.

§ 22.22 Alternative methods of procedures; and emergency variations from requirements.

(a) *Alternate methods of procedures.*—(1) *Application.* A permittee, after receiving approval from the Director, may use an alternate method or procedure (including alternate construction or equipment) in lieu of a method or procedure prescribed by this part. A permittee wishing to use an alternate method of procedure may apply to the regional director (compliance). The permittee shall describe the proposed alternate method or procedure and shall set forth the reasons for its use.
(Sec. 201, Pub. L. 85-859, 72 Stat. 1375, as amended (26 U.S.C. 5311))

Liability for Tax

§ 22.31 Persons liable for tax.

All tax-free alcohol removed, sold, transported, or used in violation of law or regulations in this part, is subject to all provisions of law relating to taxable alcohol, including the requirement for payment of tax on the alcohol. The person removing, selling, transporting, or using tax-free alcohol in violation of law or regulations pertaining to tax-free alcohol shall be required to pay the lest distilled spirits tax on the alcohol.
(Sec. 201, Pub. L. 85-859, 72 Stat. 1314, as amended (26 U.S.C. 5001))

Destruction of Marks and Brands

§ 22.33 Time of destruction of marks and brands.

(a) Any person who empties a package containing tax-free alcohol shall immediately destroy or obliterate the marks, brand, and labels required by this chapter to be placed on packages of tax-free alcohol.
(b) A person may not destroy or obliterate the marks, brands or labels until the package or drum has been emptied.
(Sec. 201, Pub. L. 85–859, 72 Stat. 1358, as amended (26 U.S.C. 5206))

Document Requirements

§ 22.35 Execution under penalties of perjury.

(a) When any form of document prescribed by this part is required to be executed under penalties of perjury, the permittee or other authorized person shall:
(1) Insert the declaration "I declare under the penalties of perjury that I have examined this _____(insert the type of document such as claim, application, statement, report, certificate), including all sup-

porting documents, and to the best of my knowledge and belief, it is true, correct, and complete''; and

(2) Sign the document.

(b) When the required document already bears a perjury declaration, the permittee or other authorized person shall sign the document. (Act of August 16, 1954, 68A Stat. 745 (26 U.S.C. 6056))

§ 22.36 Filing of qualifying documents.

All documents returned to a permittee or other person as evidence of compliance with requirements of this part, or as authorization, shall except as otherwise provided, be kept readily available for inspection by an ATF officer during business hours.

Subpart D—Qualification

Application for Permit, Form 5150.22

§ 22.41 Application for industrial alcohol user permit.

(a) *Users.* Each person desiring to withdraw and use tax-free alcohol shall, before commencing business, file an application on Form 5150.22 for, and obtain a permit, Form 5150.9, except permittees who were previously qualified to withdraw and use tax-free alcohol on the effective date of this regulation.

(b) *Filing.* All applications and necessary supporting documents, as required by this subpart, shall be filed with the regional director (compliance). All data, written statements, affidavits, and other documents submitted in support of the application are considered a part of the application.

(1) Applications filed as provided in this section, shall be accompanied by evidence establishing the authority of the officer or other person to execute the application.

(2) A State, political subdivision thereof, or the District of Columbia, may specify in the application that it desires a single permit authorizing the withdrawal and use of tax-free alcohol in a number of institutions under its control. In this instance, the applicable, Form 5150.22, or an attachment, shall clearly show the method of distributing and accounting for the tax-free alcohol to be withdrawn.

§ 22.42 Data for application, Form 5150.22.

(a) Unless waived under § 22.43, each application on Form 5150.22 shall include as applicable, the following information:

(1) Serial number and purpose for which filed.

(2) Name and principal business address.

(3) Based on the bona fide requirements of the applicant, the esti-

mated quantity of tax-free alcohol in proof gallons, which will be procured during a 12-month period (one calendar year).

(4) Location, or locations where tax-free alcohol is to be used, if different from the business address.

(5) Statement showing the specific manner in which, or purpose for which, tax-free alcohol will be withdrawn and used.

(6) Statement that tax-free alcohol will be stored in accordance with the requirements of this part.

§ 22.44 Disapproval of application.

The regional director (compliance) may, in accordance with Part 200 of this chapter, disapprove an application for the permit to withdraw and use tax-free alcohol, if on examination of the application (or inquiry), the regional director (compliance) has reason to believe that:

(a) The applicant is not authorized by law and regulations to withdraw and use alcohol free of tax;

(b) The applicant (including, in the case of a corporation, any officer, director, or principal stockholder, and, in the case of a partnership, a partner) is, by reason of their business experience, financial standing, or trade connections, not likely to maintain operations in compliance with 26 U.S.C. Chapter 51, or regulations issued under this part;

(c) The applicant has failed to disclose any material information required, or has made any false statement as to any material fact, in connection with their application; or

(d) The premises at which the applicant proposes to conduct the business are not adequate to protect the revenue.

§ 22.45 Organizational documents.

The supporting information required by § 22.42(a)(7) includes, as applicable:

(a) *Corporate documents.* (1) Certified true copy of the certificate of incorporation, or certified true copy of certificate authorizing the corporation to operate in the State where the premises are located (if other than that in which incorporated).

(2) Certified list of names and addresses of officers and directors, along with a statement designating which corporate officers, if applicable, are directly responsible for the tax-free alcohol activities of the business.

(3) Statement showing the number of shares of each class of stock or other evidence of ownership, authorized and outstanding, the par value thereof, and the voting rights of the respective owners or holders.

(b) *Articles of partnership.* True copy of the articles of partnership or association, if any, or certificate of partnership or association where required to be filed by any State, county, or municipality.

(c) *Statement of interest.* (1) Names and addresses of persons owning

10% or more of each of the classes of stock in the corporation, or legal entity, and the nature and amount of the stockholding or other interest of each, whether such interest appears in the name of the interested party or in the name of another for him or her. If a corporation is wholly owned or controlled by another corporation, persons owning 10% or more of each of the classes of stock of the parent corporation are considered to be the persons interested in the business of the subsidiary, and the names and addresses of such persons shall be submitted to the regional director (compliance) if specifically requested.

(2) In the case of an individual owner or partnership, name and address of every person interested in the business, whether such interest appears in the name of the interested party or in the name of another for the interested person.

Industrial Alcohol User Permit, ATF F 5150.9

§ 22.48 Conditions of permits.

Permits to withdraw and use tax-free alcohol will designate the acts which are permitted, and include any limitations imposed on the performance of these acts. All of the provisions of this part relating to the use or recovery of tax-free alcohol are considered to be included in the provisions and conditions of the permit, the same as if set out in the permit.

§ 22.49 Duration of permits.

Permits to withdraw and use tax-free alcohol are continuing unless automatically terminated by the terms thereof, suspended or revoked as provided in § 22.51, or voluntarily surrendered. The provisions of § 22.58 are considered part of the terms and conditions of all permits.

§ 22.50 Correction of permits.

If an error on a permit is discovered, the permittee shall immediately return the permit to the regional director (compliance) for correction.

§ 22.51 Suspension of revocation of permits.

The regional director (compliance) may institute proceedings under Part 200 of this chapter to suspend or revoke a permit whenever there is reason to believe that the permittee—

(a) Has not in good faith complied with the provisions of 26 U.S.C. Chapter 51, or regulations issued under that chapter;

(b) Has violated the conditions of that permit;

(c) Has made any false statements as to any material fact in the application for the permit;

(d) Has failed to disclose any material information required to be furnished;

(e) Has violated or conspired to violate any law of the United States relating to intoxicating liquor or has been convicted of an offense under Title 26, U.S.C., punishable as a felony or of any conspiracy to commit such offense;

(f) Is, by reason of its operations, no longer warranted in procuring and using tax-free alcohol authorized by the permit; or

(g) Has not engaged in any of the operations authorized by the permit for a period exceeding two years.

§ 22.52 Rules of practice in permit proceedings.

The regulations of Part 200 of this chapter apply to the procedure and practice in connection with the disapproval of any application for a permit and in connection with suspension or revocation of a permit.

§ 22.53 Power of attorney.

An applicant or permittee shall execute and file with the regional director (compliance) a Form 1534, in accordance with the instructions on the form, for each person authorized to sign or to act in its behalf. Form 1534 is not required for persons whose authority is furnished in accordance with § 22.42(a)(10).

§ 22.54 Photocopying of permits.

A permittee may make photocopies of its permit exclusively for the purpose of furnishing proof of authorization to withdraw tax-free alcohol from a distilled spirits plant.

§ 22.55 Posting of permits.

Permits issued under this part will be kept posted and available for inspection on the permit premises.

Changes After Original Qualification

§ 22.57 Changes affecting applications and permits.

(a) *General.*—(1) *Changes affecting application.* When there is a change relating to any of the information contained in, or considered a part of the application on Form 5150.22 for a permit, the permittee shall, within 30 days (except as otherwise provided in this subpart) file a written notice with the regional director (compliance) to amend the application.

(2) *Changes affecting waivers.* When any waiver under § 22.43 is terminated by a change to the application, the permittee shall include the current information as to the item previously waived with the written notice required in paragraph (a)(1) of this section.

(3) *Changes affecting permit.* When the terms of a permit are affected by a change, the written notice required by paragraph (a)(1) of this

section (except as otherwise provided in this subpart) will serve as an application to amend the permit.

(4) *Form of notice.* All written notices to amend an application on Form 5150.22 with—

(i) Identify the permittee;

(ii) Contain the permit identification number;

(iii) Explain the nature of the change and contain any required supporting documents;

(iv) Identify the serial number of the applicable application, Form 5150.22; and

(v) Be consecutively numbered and signed by the permittee or any person authorized to sign on behalf of the permittee.

(b) *Amended application.* The regional director (compliance) may require a permittee to file an amended application on Form 5150.22 when the number of changes to the previous application are determined to be excessive, or when a permittee has not timely filed the written notice prescribed in paragraph (a)(1) of this section. If items on the amended application remain unchanged, they will be marked "No change since Form 5120.22, Serial No. _____ ."

(c) *Changes in officers, directors and stockholders*—(1) *Officers.* In the case of a change in the officers listed under the provisions of § 22.45(a)(2), the notice required by paragraph (a)(1) of this section shall only apply (unless otherwise required, in writing, by the regional director (compliance)) to those offices the incumbents of which are responsible for the operations covered by the permit.

(2) *Directors.* In the case of a change in the directors listed under the provisions of § 22.45(a)(2), the notice required by paragraph (a)(1) of this section shall reflect the changes.

(3) *Stockholders.* In lieu of reporting all changes, within 30 days, to the list of stockholders furnished under the provisions of § 22.45(c)(1), a permittee may, upon filing written notice to the regional director (compliance) and establishing a reporting date, file an annual notice of changes. The notice of changes in stockholders does not apply if the sale or transfer of capital stock results in a change in ownership or control which is required to be reported under § 22.58.

(Approved by the Office of Management and Budget under control number 1512-0335)

§ 22.58 Automatic termination of permits.

(a) *Permit not transferable.* Permits issued under this part are not transferable. In the event of the lease, sale, or other transfer of such a permit, or of the operations authorized by the permit, the permit shall, except as provided for in this section, automatically terminate.

(b) *Corporations.* (1) If actual or legal control of any corporation holding a permit issued under this part changes, directly or indirectly, whether by reason of a change in stock ownership or control (in the permittee corporation or any other corporation), by operation of law, or in any other manner, the permittee shall within 10 days of the change, give written notice to the regional director (compliance). The written notice shall be accompanied by (or within 30 days of the change) an application and supporting documents on Form 5150.22 for a new permit. If an application on Form 5150.22 for a new permit is not filed within 30 days of the change, the outstanding permit will automatically terminate.

(2) If an application on Form 5150.22 for a new permit is filed within the 30-day period prescribed in paragraph (b)(1) of this section, the outstanding permit will remain in effect until final action is taken on the application. When final action is taken, the outstanding permit will automatically terminate and the permittee shall forward it to the regional director (compliance) for cancellation.

§ 22.61 Change in name of permittee.

(a) *Permit.* When the only change is a change in the individual, firm, or corporation name, a permittee may not conduct operations under the new name until a written notice, accompanied by necessary supporting documents, to amend the application and permit has been filed and an amended permit has been issued by the regional director (compliance).

(b) *Bond.* If required to file a bond, the permittee shall furnish a consent of surety on Form 1533 or a new bond to cover the change in name.

(Approved by the Office of Management and Budget under control number 1512-0335)

§ 22.62 Change in trade name.

Where there is to be a change in, or addition of, a trade name, the permittee may not conduct operations under the new trade name until a written notice has been filed and an amended permit has been issued by the regional director (compliance). A new bond or consent of surety is not required for changes in trade names.

(Approved by the Office of Management and Budget under control number 1512-0335)

§ 22.63 Change in location.

(a) *Permit.* When there is to be a change in location within the same region, a permittee may not conduct operations at the new location until a written notice, accompanied by necessary supporting information, to amend the application and permit has been filed and an amended permit has been issued by the regional director (compliance).

(b) *Bond.* If required to file a bond, the permittee shall furnish a consent of surety on Form 1533 or a new bond to cover the new location. (Approved by the Office of Management and Budget under control number 1512-0335)

§ 22.64 Return of permits.

Following the termination, surrender or revocation of a permit, or the issuance of a new or amended permit, caused by a change, the permittee shall (a) obtain and destroy all photocopies of the previous permit from its suppliers and (b) return the original of the permit or obsolete permit to the regional director (compliance) for cancellation.

Registry of Stills

§ 22.66 Registry of stills.

Part 196 of this chapter applies to stills located on the premises of a permittee. The listing of a still on Form 5150.22 and the issuance of a permit constitute registration of that still in lieu of filing Form 26.

Permanent Discontinuance of Use of Tax-Free Alcohol

§ 22.68 Notice of permanent discontinuance.

(a) *Notice.* A permittee who permanently discontinues the use of tax-free alcohol shall file a written notice with the regional director (compliance) to cover the discontinuance. The notice will be accompanied by the permit, and contain—

(1) A request to cancel the permit.

(2) A statement of the disposition made, as provided in § 22.154, of all tax-free and recovered alcohol, and

(3) The date of discontinuance.

(b) *Bonds.* The bond of a permittee may not be canceled until all tax-free and recovered alcohol has been properly disposed of in accordance with the provisions of this part.

(Approved by the Office of Management and Budget under control number 1512-0335)

Subpart E—Bonds and Consents of Surety

§ 22.71 Bond.

(a) Any bond previously approved, under this chapter, on Form 1448 (5150.25) which fulfills the penal sum requirements of paragraph (b) of this section shall remain valid and will be regulated by the same provisions of this subpart as it refers to bonds on Form 5150.25.

(b) Each person who intends to withdraw more than 1,500 proof gallons of tax-free alcohol per annum shall file a bond, Form 5150.25, before issuance of the permit. The penal sum of the bond will be as follows:

Minimum annual withdrawals	Bond penal sum
0 to 1,500 proof gallons	No bond required.
Over 1,500 but not over 3,000 proof gallons.	$2,000 plus $100 for each additional 100 proof gallons up to a maximum of $3,000 (2,500 proof gallons).
Over 3,000 but not over 6,000 proof gallons.	$3,000 plus $200 for each additional 100 proof gallons up to a maximum of $7,500 (5,250 proof gallons).
Over 6,000 proof gallons	$7,500 plus $250 for each additional 100 proof gallons up to a maximum penal sum of $15,000 (9,000 proof gallons).

(c) The following are some examples:

If your annual withdrawals are	Your penal sum is
1,250 proof gallons	No bond required.
2,800 proof gallons	$3,000 ($2,000 plus $1,000 ($100 × 10 units), last 300 proof gallons does not require additional bond coverage).
8,250 proof gallons	$13,000 ($7,500 plus $5,500 ($250 × 22 units), the remaining 50 proof gallons does not increase the bond since it is not an "additional" 100 proof gallon unit).

§ 22.72 Evaluation of bond penal sum.

(a) *Permittee's evaluation.* Each permittee shall, for the period from January 1 through the following December 31, make an annual evaluation of its previous and future needs for tax-free alcohol. Based on the results of this evaluation:

(1) The permittee shall file a new bond in increased penal sum, if the existing bond no longer meets the penal sum requirements of § 22.71, or

(2) The permittee may file a new bond in decreased penal sum, if the existing bond exceeds the penal sum requirements of § 22.71.

(b) *Authority of regional director (compliance).* The regional director (compliance) may, at any time, require a permittee to file a new bond in a larger penal sum, or require a satisfactory explanation why a new bond should not be filed.

(Chapter 390, Pub. L. 80-280, 61 Stat. 648 (6 U.S.C. 6, 7))

Subpart F—Premises and Equipment

§ 22.91 Premises.

All persons qualified to withdraw and use tax-free alcohol shall have premises suitable for the business being conducted and adequate for the protection of the revenue. Storage facilities shall be provided on the premises for tax-free alcohol received or recovered. The storage facilities may consist of a combination of storerooms, compartments, or stationary storage tanks.

§ 22.92 Storage facilities.

(a) Storerooms or compartments shall be so constructed and secured as to prevent unauthorized access and will be equipped for locking. These storage facilities shall be of sufficient capacity to hold the maximum quantity of tax-free alcohol which will be on hand at one time.

(b) Each stationary storage tank used to hold tax-free alcohol shall be equipped for locking in such a manner as to control access to the spirits. All stationary storage tanks shall be equipped with an accurate means of measuring the spirits.

§ 22.102 Prohibited uses.

(a) *Usage.* Under no circumstances may tax-free alcohol withdrawn under this part be used for beverage purposes, food products, or in any preparation used in preparing beverage or food products.

(b) *Selling.* Persons qualified under this part are prohibited from selling tax-free alcohol, using tax-free alcohol in the manufacture of any product for sale, or selling any products resulting from the use of tax-free alcohol. A separate charge may be made by a hospital, sanitarium or clinic for medicines compounded with tax-free alcohol and dispensed to patients for use on the premises, as provided in § § 22.105 and 22.106. Hospitals may not furnish tax-free alcohol for use of physicians in their private practice.

(c) *Removal from premises.* Persons qualified under this part may not remove tax-free alcohol or products resulting from the use of tax-free alcohol from the permit premises unless specifically authorized by the terms of their permit, or permission is obtained from the regional director (compliance), except that:

(1) Products made through the use of tax-free alcohol which contain no alcohol may be removed to other premises for the sole purpose of further research; or

(2) Under the provisions of § § 22.105 and 22.106, clinics operated for charity and not for profit may compound bona fide medicines with tax-free alcohol, and dispense the medicine from the premises for use by its patients outside of the clinic, if the furnishing of the medicine is not conditioned upon payment.

(d) *Liability for tax.* Permittees who use tax-free alcohol in any manner prohibited by this section become liable for the tax on the alcohol. Any permittee who sells tax-free alcohol also becomes liable for special (occupational) tax as a liquor dealer.

(Sec. 201, Pub. L. 85-859, 72 Stat. 1314, as amended, 1343, as amended, 1362, as amended (26 U.S.C. 5001, 5121, 5214))

§ 22.103 States and the District of Columbia.

Except as otherwise provided in this section, tax-free alcohol withdrawn by a State or political subdivision of a State, or the District of Columbia shall be used solely for mechanical and scientific purposes, and except on approval of the regional director (compliance), the use of tax-free alcohol or the use of any resulting product will be confined to the premises under the control of the State or political subdivision of a State, or the District of Columbia. Tax-free alcohol withdrawn for use in hospitals, clinics, and other establishments specified in § § 22.104 through 22,108, operated by a State, political subdivision of a State, or the District of Columbia, shall be used in the manner prescribed for those establishments.

(Sec. 201, Pub. L. 85-859, 72 Stat. 1362, as amended (26 U.S.C. 5214))

§ 22.104 Educational organizations, colleges of learning, and scientific universities.

(a) *Educational organizations.* Educational organizations authorized to withdraw and use tax-free alcohol under § 22.101 are those organizations which normally maintain a regular faculty and curriculum and which normally have a regularly enrolled body of students in attendance at the place where their educational activities are regularly carried on and which are exempt from Federal income tax under 26 U.S.C. 501(a).

(b) *Colleges of learning.* Colleges of learning, for the purposes of this subpart, have a recognized curriculum and confer degrees after specified periods of attendance at classes or research work.

(c) *Scientific universities.* Scientific universities include any university incorporated or organized under any Federal or State law which provides training in the sciences.

(d) *Uses.* Tax-free alcohol withdrawn by educational organizations, scientific universities, and colleges of learning shall be used only for scientific, medicinal, and mechanical purposes. Use of tax-free alcohol and resulting products are limited by the provisions of § 22.102.

(Sec. 201, Pub. L. 85-859, 72 Stat. 1362, as amended (26 U.S.C. 5214))

§ 22.105 Hospitals, blood banks, and sanitariums.

(a) Tax-free alcohol withdrawn for use by hospitals, blood banks, and sanitariums shall be used exclusively for medicinal, mechanical (analysis or test) and scientific purposes and in the treatment of patients. The use of tax-free alcohol and of products resulting from the use of tax-free alcohol shall be confined to the permit premises, except as provided in this section and § 22.102. Medicines compounded with tax-free alcohol on the premises of a hospital or sanitarium, for use of patients on the premises, may not be sold, but a separate charge may be made for the medicine.

(b) A hospital, operating a clinic on premises, may withdraw tax-free alcohol for use in the clinic, if the clinic is operated for charity and not for profit. Medicines compounded with tax-free alcohol may be dispensed to patients at a clinic for use outside of the clinic, if the furnishing of the medicine is not conditioned upon payment.

(c) A hospital or sanitarium, operating a pathological or other laboratory on premises, may withdraw tax-free alcohol for authorized use in the laboratory.
(Sec. 201, Pub. L. 85-859, 72 Stat. 1362, as amended (26 U.S.C. 5214))

§ 22.106 Clinics.

Tax-free alcohol withdrawn by clinics operated for charity and not for profit shall be used only for medicinal, scientific, and mechanical purposes and in the treatment of patients. Medicine compounded with tax-free alcohol may be dispensed to patients for use off the premises, if the furnishing of the medicine is not conditioned upon payment. A separate charge may be made for medicine compounded on the clinical premises with tax-free alcohol for use of patients on the premises. Except as provided in this section and in § 22.102, the use of tax-free alcohol shall be confined strictly to the premises of the clinic.
(Sec. 201. Pub. L. 85-859, 72 Stat. 1362, as amended (26 U.S.C. 5214))

§ 22.107 Pathological laboratories.

(a) Pathological laboratories, not operated by a hospital or sanitarium, may withdraw and use tax-free alcohol if exclusively engaged in making analyses or tests for hospitals or sanitariums. If a pathological laboratory does not exclusively conduct analyses or tests for hospitals or sanitariums, it does not qualify for the permit issued under this part.

(b) A pathological laboratory which uses tax-free alcohol for any other purpose, except as provided in this section, shall become liable for the tax on the alcohol.

(c) Except as provided in § 22.102, the use of tax-free alcohol and of products resulting from the use of tax-free alcohol shall be confined strictly to the permit premises.
(Sec. 201, Pub. L. 85-859, 72 Stat. 1314, as amended. 1362, as amended (26 U.S.C. 5001, 5214))

§ 22.108 Other laboratories.

Laboratories, other than pathological laboratories specified in § 22.107, may withdraw and use tax-free alcohol exclusively in scientific research. The use of tax-free alcohol or of products resulting from the use of tax-free alcohol shall be confined strictly to the laboratory premises, except as provided in § 22.102.
(Sec. 201, Pub. L. 85-859, 72 Stast. 1362, as amended (26 U.S.C. 5214))

Subpart H—Withdrawal and Receipt of Tax-Free Alcohol

§ 22.111 Withdrawals under permit.

(a) *General.* The permit, Form 5150.9, issued under Subpart D of this part, authorizes a person to withdraw tax-free alcohol from the bonded premises of a distilled spirits plant or, under the provisions of 26 U.S.C. 5688(a)(2)(B), receive alcohol from the General Services Administration.

(b) *Photocopying of permit, Form 5150.9.* (1) As provided in § 22.54, a permittee may make photocopies of its permit, or amended permit, for the exclusive purpose of furnishing proof of authorization to withdraw tax-free alcohol.

(2) A permittee need only furnish the photocopy of its permit, or amended permit, to a distilled spirits plant for the "initial order" from that distilled spirits plant.

(3) When a permittee makes photocopies of its permit, Form 5150.9, each copy shall be signed, dated, and contain the word "COPY" across the face.

(4) A permittee is responsible for obtaining and, as applicable, destroying all photocopies of its permit from distilled spirits plants when (i) an amended or corrected permit is issued which supersedes the copy on file, (ii) the permit is canceled by reason of requalification as a new permittee, (iii) the permit is revoked or suspended, or (iv) upon permanent discontinuance of use of tax-free alcohol.

(c) *Withdrawals under permit.* (1) When a permittee places an initial order for tax-free alcohol it shall forward a signed copy of the permit, for retention by the distilled spirits plant, along with the purchase request.

(2) When the permittee places a subsequent order for tax-free alcohol, the purchase request, in addition to any other information, shall contain the permit identification number and date of issue along with a statement that the permittee possesses a valid permit to withdraw tax-free alcohol, a copy of which is on file.

(3) Shipments shall not be made by a proprietor of a distilled spirits

plant until it is in possession of a signed copy of a valid permit, Form 5150.9.

(Sec. 201, Pub. L. 85-859, 72 Stat. 1395, as amended (26 U.S.C. 5555))

§ 22.112 Regulation of withdrawals.

(a) Each permittee shall regulate its withdrawals of tax-free alcohol to ensure that (1) the quantity on hand and unaccounted for does not exceed the capacity of the storage facilities, and (2) the cumulative quantity withdrawn or received in any calendar year does not exceed the quantity authorized by the permit, Form 5150.9. Recovered alcohol and alcohol received from the General Services Administration shall be taken into account in determining the total quantity of alcohol on hand.

(b) For the purpose of this section, tax-free alcohol and recovered alcohol shall be considered as unaccounted for if lost under circumstances where a claim for allowance is required by this part and the claim has not been allowed, or if used or disposed of in any manner not provided for in this part.

§ 22.113 Receipt of tax-free alcohol.

(a) When tax-free alcohol is received, it shall be placed in the storage facilities prescribed by § 22.91 and kept there under lock until withdrawn for use. Unless required by city or State fire code regulations or authorized by the regional director (compliance) or the terms of the permit, the permittee may not remove tax-free alcohol from the original packages or containers in which received until the alcohol is withdrawn for use. If the tax-free alcohol is transferred to "safety" containers in accordance with fire code regulations, the containers to which they are transferred shall be appropriately marked to identify the package from which transferred, the quantity transferred, the date of transfer, and the name and address of the vendor.

(b) When tax-free alcohol is received, the permittee shall ascertain and account for any losses in transit in accordance with Subpart I of this part. The permittee shall note any loss or deficiency in the shipment on the record of receipt.

(c) Records of receipt shall consist of the consignors invoice or bill. Records of receipt may be filed in accordance with the permittee's own filing system as long as it does not cause inconvenience to ATF officers desiring to examine the records. The filing system shall systematically and accurately account for the receipt of all tax-free alcohol.

§ 22.114 Alcohol received from the General Services Administration.

Any nonprofit charitable institution holding a permit on Form 5150.9, and receiving alcohol from the General Services Administration under the provisions of 26 U.S.C. 5688(a)(2)(B), shall include any quantity of alcohol received in computing the quantity of tax-free alcohol that may be procured under its permit during the calendar year. The alcohol, on receipt, shall be placed in the storage facilities prescribed in § 22.91 and kept there under lock until withdrawn for use.

Subpart I—Losses

§ 22.121 Liability and responsibility of carriers.

(a) A person or carrier transporting tax-free alcohol to a consignee or returning the alcohol to the consignor is responsible for the safe delivery and is accountable for any tax-free alcohol not delivered.

(b) A person or carrier transporting tax-free alcohol in violation of any law or regulation pertaining thereto, is subject to all provisions of law relating to alcohol subject to and the payment of tax thereon, and shall be required to pay the tax.

(Sec. 201, Pub. L. 85-859, 72 Stat. 1314, as amended [26 U.S.C. 5001)]

§ 22.122 Losses in transit.

(a) *Reporting losses.* Upon discovering any loss of tax-free alcohol while in transit, the carrier shall immediately inform the consignee, in writing, of the facts and circumstances relating to the loss. In the case of theft, the carrier shall also immediately notify the consignee's regional director (compliance) of the facts and circumstances relating to the loss.

(b) *Recording losses.* At the time the shipment or report of loss is received, the consignee shall determine the quantity of tax-free alcohol lost. The consignee shall note the quantity lost on the receiving document and attach all relevant information to the record of receipt, prescribed in § 22.113. For the purpose of maintaining the records prescribed in Subpart M of this part, receipts on tax-free alcohol shall only include the quantity actually received.

(c) *Claims.* A claim for allowances of losses of tax-free alcohol shall, as prescribed in § 22.125, be filed:

(1) If the quantity lost in transit exceeds 1 percent of the total quantity shipped and is more than 5 proof gallons, the consignee shall file a claim for allowance of the entire quantity lost; or

(2) If the loss was due to theft or other unlawful removal, the consignee shall file a claim for allowances of the entire quantity lost, regardless of the quantity or percentage involved.

(Reporting approved by the Office of Management and Budget under control number 1512-0335; recordkeeping approved by the Office of Management and Budget under control number 1512-0334.)

§ 22.123 Losses on premises.

(a) *Recording of losses.* A permittee shall determine and record, in the records prescribed by Subpart M of this part, the quantity of tax-free or recovered alcohol lost on premises—

(1) At the end of each semi-annual period when the inventory required by § 22.162 is taken, or

(2) Immediately upon the discovery of any loss due to casualty, theft or other unusual causes.

(b) *Claims.* A claim for allowances of losses of tax-free alcohol shall be filed as prescribed in § 22.125, in the following circumstances—

(1) if the quantity lost during any semi-annual inventory period exceeds 1 percent of the quantity to be accounted for during that period, and is more than 10 proof gallons, or

(2) if the loss was due to theft or unlawful use or removal, the permittee shall file a claim for allowances of losses regardless of the quantity involved.

(Approved by the Office of Management and Budget under control number 1512-0334)

§ 22.124 Incomplete shipments.

(a) Subject to the provisions of this part and Part 19 of this chapter, when containers of tax-free alcohol have sustained losses in transit other than by theft, and the shipment will not be delivered to the consignee, the carrier may return the shipment to the distilled spirits plant.

(b) When tax-free alcohol is returned to the distilled spirits plant, in accordance with this section, the carrier shall inform the proprietor, in writing, of the facts and circumstances relating to the loss. In the case of theft, the carrier shall also immediately notify the shipper's regional director (compliance) of the facts and circumstances relating to the loss.

(c) Subject to the limitations for loss prescribed in § 22.122, the proprietor of the distilled spirits plant shall file a claim for allowance of the entire quantity lost, in the same manner provided in that section. The claim shall include the applicable date required by § 22.125.

§ 22.125 Claims.

(a) Claims for allowances of losses of tax-free or recovered alcohol shall be filed, on Form 2635 (5620.8), with the regional director (compliance) within 30 days from the date the loss is ascertained, and shall contain the following information:

(1) Name, address, and permit number of claimant;

(2) Identification and location of the container(s) from which the tax-free or recovered alcohol was lost, and the quantity lost from each container;

(3) Total quantity of tax-free or recovered alcohol covered by the claim and the aggregate quantity involved;

(4) Date of loss or discovery, the cause or nature of loss, and all relevant facts, including facts establishing whether the loss occurred as a result of negligence, connivance, collusion, or fraud on the part of any person, employee or agent participating in or responsible for the loss; and

(5) Name of carrier where a loss in transit in involved.

(b) The carriers statement regarding a loss in transit, prescribed by § 22.122 or 22.124, shall accompany the claim.

(c) The regional director (compliance) may require additional evidence to be submitted in support of the claim.

See Figure 69 for ATF Form 1451 which is used to report the annual use of tax-free alcohol.

CONTINUING WITHDRAWAL PERMITS

On November 23, 1982, the Department of the Treasury Bureau of Alcohol, Tobacco and Firearms issued Industry Circular No. 82-13 entitled Continuing Withdrawal Permits for Tax-Free Alcohol Users. The Circular, addressed to Tax-Free Alcohol Users and Distilled Spirits Plant Proprietors (DSP) states:

Purpose. The purpose of this circular is to advise industry members of the new regulations regarding the elimination of the requirement for tax-free alcohol users to annually make application for and receive a new withdrawal permit.

The final rule, T.D. ATF-103, amended regulations in 27 CFR Parts 211 and 213. The specific changes which affect tax-free alcohol users and DSP proprietors are as follows:

(a) Tax-Free Alcohol Users—Withdrawal permits issued on Form 1450 (5150.13) to tax-free alcohol users which are annotated to expire on April 30, 1983, will continue in effect indefinitely. It is not necessary to submit an application for renewal of the May 1, 1983–April 30, 1984 withdrawal permit, or for any succeeding withdrawal permit. (Section 213.111 of 27 CFR is removed).

(b) Shipments by DSP Proprietors—DSP proprietors are authorized to make shipments after April 30, 1983, of tax-free alcohol to users whose permits expire on April 30, 1983. This authorization is based on the fact that all the above mentioned withdrawal permits will be "valid" after the expiration date, indefinitely, in the same manner as "limited" withdrawal permits.

ATF believes this amendment will significantly reduce administrative burdens on both industry and the Government.

Inquiries. Inquiries concerning this circular should refer to it by number and be addressed to: Assistant Director, (Regulatory Enforcement),

FORM **2600** (REV. 7-60)	U. S. TREASURY DEPARTMENT · INTERNAL REVENUE SERVICE **APPLICATION FOR PERMIT TO** **USE ALCOHOL FREE OF TAX**	1. INDUSTRIAL USE PERMIT *(If amendment of industrial use permit)* TF –

This form shall be executed in duplicate and filed with the assistant regional commissioner of the region in which the premises are situated.

Applications on this form which are not executed in accordance with instructions and regulations or which do not contain all the information required by the regulations will be returned to the applicant or permittee for correction.

TO	**ASSISTANT REGIONAL COMMISSIONER (ALCOHOL AND TOBACCO TAX)** *(City and State)*	2. DATE OF APPLICATION

Application is hereby made for an industrial use permit to use alcohol free of tax, as described herein.

3. APPLICATION MADE BY *(If individual owner, give full name and address; if partnership, give full name and address of each person interested in enterprise; if corporation, give name of corporation, State under laws of which incorporated and address of principal office)*

4. TRADE NAME AND OFFICE WHERE REGISTERED	5. MAXIMUM NO. PROOF GALLONS WHICH WILL BE ON HAND, IN TRANSIT, AND UNACCOUNTED FOR AT ANY ONE TIME1/

6. SERIAL NUMBER	7. PURPOSE FOR WHICH FILED *("For original industrial use permit," "For amendment of industrial use permit to authorize (state privilege desired)," etc.)*

8. PERMIT IS FOR ☐ USE OF ALCOHOL FREE OF TAX ☐ RECOVERY OF TAX-FREE ALCOHOL	9. *(If application is made by central authority, as a State, municipality, university, etc., for use of alcohol by an agency, institution, department, etc., thereof, the name of such agency, etc., shall be stated)*

10. PREMISES ON WHICH ALCOHOL WILL BE USED *(Number, street, city or town, zone, State)*

11. ALCOHOL TO BE USED IN THE FOLLOWING MANNER *(The specific use which will be made of the alcohol and resulting products (if any), that is, the purpose or purposes for which the alcohol will be used, shall be stated explicitly, and not in general terms. For example, when the alcohol is to be used at a hospital, the specific purposes for which the alcohol will be used shall be stated, such as clinical use, treatment of patients, compounding medicines for use of patients in the hospital, preserving specimens of anatomy, etc. If alcohol so used is recovered, state that fact)2/*

12. SIZE AND COMPLETE DESCRIPTION OF THE ALCOHOL STORAGE FACILITIES

CONDITIONS

The applicant fully understands that any permit that may be issued pursuant to this application will be subject to the following conditions:

1. That this application contains no misrepresentation of fact; that he and all persons employed by him in any connection with such permit privileges, and all persons employed by him while on the permit premises, will in good faith observe and conform to all the terms and conditions of said permit, the laws of the United States relating to the manufacture, taxation, and control of and traffic in, intoxicating liquors, and all regulations issued pursuant to such laws which are now, or may hereafter be, in force; and he

will pay the tax, together with penalties and interest, on all alcohol diverted while being transported to him, and on all alcohol withdrawn, transported, used, or disposed of by him in violation of laws and regulations now or hereafter in force; and that he and all persons interested in the business to be conducted under said permit are duly qualified, under the law and regulations pertaining thereto, to receive the permit privileges herein applied for.

2. That all data, written statements, evidence, affidavits, and other documents, submitted in support of this application, or upon hearing thereon, shall be deemed to be included in the provisions and conditions of this application and any permit issued pursuant thereto the same as if set out at length therein.

I declare under the penalties of perjury that this application has been examined by me and to the best of my knowledge and belief is a true, correct, and complete application.

13. SIGNATURE OF APPLICANT 3/	14. BY *(Name and capacity)*

FORM **2600** (REV. 7-60)

Fig. 68

DEPARTMENT OF THE TREASURY – BUREAU OF ALCOHOL, TOBACCO AND FIREARMS
REPORT OF TAX-FREE ALCOHOL USER
(Prepare in duplicate – See instructions on reverse)

1. INDUSTRIAL USE PERMIT No. TF-

2. NAME OF PERMITTEE

3. ADDRESS (Number, Street, City, State, ZIP Code)

4. REPORT FOR CALENDAR YEAR 19_____

MONTH a	ON HAND BEGINNING OF MONTH (Proof gallons) b	RECEIVED (Proof gallons) c	RECOVERED (Proof gallons) d	USED (Proof gallons) e	ON HAND END OF MONTH* (Proof gallons) f	GAINS (Proof gallons) g	LOSSES (Proof gallons) h	RECAPITULATION (Proof gallons)
Jan.								(1) ON HAND BEGINNING OF YEAR
Feb.								(2) TOTAL RECEIVED
Mar.								(3) TOTAL RECOVERED
April								(4) GAINS
May								(5) TO BE ACCOUNTED FOR (Total lines (1) through (4))
June								
July								(6) TOTAL USED
Aug.								(7)
Sept.								(8)
Oct.								(9) LOSSES
Nov.								(10) ON HAND END OF YEAR
Dec.								(11) ACCOUNTED FOR (Total lines (6) through (10))
5. CUMULATIVE TOTALS								

*IMPORTANT: Regulations require actual physical inventory of tax-free alcohol to be taken at the end of each month (See 27 CFR 213.172)

FOR USE OF REGIONAL REGULATORY ADMINISTRATOR	Under penalties of perjury, I declare that I have examined this report (including any accompanying explanations, statements and schedules) and, to the best of my knowledge and belief, it is true, correct, and complete and includes all transactions required by law or regulations to be reported.	
AUDITED BY: (Initials)	6. DATE	7. SIGNATURE
DATE:		8. TITLE

ATF Form 1451 (5150.28) (7-79) EDITION OF 12-77 MAY BE USED

Fig. 69

Bureau of Alcohol, Tobacco and Firearms, 1200 Pennsylvania Avenue, NW, Washington, DC 20226.

DISPENSING ALCOHOLIC LIQUORS TO PATIENTS

In the summer of 1965, the Internal Revenue Service division of Alcohol and Tobacco Tax issued **Industry Memorandum No. NA 65-7** to hospitals and similar institutions. The purpose of the memorandum was to advise hospitals and institutions regarding liability for special tax which may be incurred by dispensing alcoholic liquors to patients.

Memorandum No. NA 65-7 provides that:

Internal Revenue laws impose special taxes on persons engaging or carrying on the business or occupation of selling, or offering for sale, any alcoholic liquors for use as a beverage whether or not such liquors are fit for such use. Regulations issued pursuant to Internal Revenue law provide that hospitals and similar institutions furnishing liquor to patients are not required to pay special tax, provided that no specific or additional charge is made for the liquor so furnished. This regulation is found at section 194.187 of the Federal Liquor Dealer regulations. The words "no specific or additional charge" are interpreted as applying, for example, to those cases where a hospital or institution makes a fixed charge for treatment, subsistence, medicine, etc., and the over-all fee or charge remains the same regardless of whether alcoholic liquors are furnished to the patient.

A hospital or similar institution incurs liability for special tax as a retail liquor dealer whenever it furnishes an alcoholic liquor to a patient, whether pursuant to a prescription or otherwise, under conditions constituting a sale. These conditions would include any manner of accounting for a specific or additional charge made to a patient for alcoholic liquor furnished him. Totaling of charges for various items under a general headline, such as "Drugs and Dressings," would not give relief from special tax liability, if a charge for alcoholic liquors is one of the items included in the total.

Any hospital or similar institution which dispenses alcoholic liquors under conditions constituting a sale will be required to pay special tax as a retail liquor dealer. Special tax is paid by filing a tax return on Form 11 with the District Director of Revenue in the District in which the hospital is located. The special tax rate for a retail liquor dealer is $54.00 for each fiscal year beginning July 1.

ALCOHOL RECORDS AND AUTOMATIC DATA PROCESSING

Industry Circular No. 65-5 was issued to advise users of tax-free alcohol, among others, of the provisions of **Revenue Procedure 64-35, I.R.B. 1964-37, 21.**

The revenue procedure requires that the methodology built into a computer's accounting program "must include a method of producing from the punched cards or tapes visible and legible records which will provide the necessary details required by the regulation covering the respective operations, or such details must be available in supplemental records."

In addition, the revenue procedure suggests that the Assistant Regional Commissioner, Alcohol and Tobacco Tax, be notified in advance of the actual installation of an automatic data processing system in order to assure the adequacy of the system as it relates to the required records.

SELECTED READINGS

All of the following publications can be obtained from the Superintendent of Documents, U.S. Government Printing Office, Washington, D.C., 20402.

Distribution and Use of Denatured Alcohol and Rum, Part 211 of Title 26, Code of Federal Regulations, I.R.S. Publication No. 443.

Formulas for Denatured Alcohol and Rum, Part 212, Title 26, Code of Federal Regulations, I.R.S. Publication No. 368.

Distribution and Use of Tax-Free Alcohol, Part 213, Title 27, Code of Federal Regulations, ATF 5100.9 (12-77).

Drawback on Distilled Spirits Used in Manufacturing Nonbeverage Products, Part 197, Title 26, Code of Federal Regulations, I.R.S. Publication No. 206.

Rules of Practice in Permit Proceedings, Part 200, Title 26, Code of Federal Regulations, I.R.S. Publication No. 289.

REFERENCES

1. Distribution and Use of Denatured Alcohol and Rum, and Tax-Free Alcohol; Final Rule Part II Department of the Treasury Bureau of Alcohol, Tobacco and Firearms, Federal Register, March 6, 1985.
2. Kaul, A.F., Vogenberg, R., and Harsfield, J.C.: Simplified Method of Calculating and Recording the Use of Tax-Free Alcohol. Am. J. Hosp. Pharm., *39*:1525–1528, 1982.

18

Dispensing During Off-Hours

At one time, the major criticism of the small hospital was the lack of clinical ancillary services on a 168 hour per week basis. Over the years, the clinical laboratories, radiology, blood bank and the emergency service have successfully coped with the demand. The one area which has not kept pace has been the pharmaceutical service. Many reasons have been offered for this dilemma, the major ones being the shortage of trained personnel and the prohibitive cost. The percentage of hospital pharmacies providing around-the-clock service has increased from 6% in 1975 to 12% in 1978.[1] and to 19.3% in 1982.[2] The 1982 figures showed 24-hour service in 2.8% of the hospitals with less than 200 beds, 25.4% in hospitals with between 200 to 399 beds, and 70.3% in hospitals with 400 or more beds.[2]

Much has been published relative to the various means whereby a hospital may provide 24-hour a day pharmacy coverage[3,4] and the following represents a brief review of them.

USE OF NURSING SUPERVISORS

The first and probably the commonest method employed today is to permit the evening and night nursing supervisor to enter the pharmacy and provide a limited type of service. Although this method is the most widely used, it is dangerous and in some areas an illegal practice. Those who advocate such a practice are prone to cite the argument that there exists a correlation between the nurse selecting a medicine from the drug cabinet on the pavilion and selecting the same item from the pharmacy. The fallacy of this view is the fact that medications which have been forwarded to the nursing station have already had the benefit of special packaging, handling and labeling by professionally competent and legally qualified individuals.

Therefore, if this is the only means available to the small hospital, it should be practiced with caution. Nursing personnel serving in this category should be specifically prohibited from compounding a mixture and restricted to dispensing from the selection of pre-labeled and pre-packaged items.

378

EMERGENCY BOXES AND NIGHT DRUG CABINETS

The literature is replete with data concerning emergency boxes and night drug cabinets. Since these two items serve a different purpose, we shall discuss them separately.

The *emergency box,* although an integral part of the twenty-four-hour a day pharmacy coverage, is necessary to expedite treatment in situations where time is of the essence. Therefore, the emergency, or as it is often called the "STAT" box, must be large enough to contain the necessary supplies and yet sufficiently compact to facilitate handling them. The box should be kept in a readily accessible place, known to all ward personnel, and should be ready for use at all times. In order to accomplish this goal, the pharmacy should have reserve boxes prepared so that the units may be handled on an exchange basis and thereby reduce the period of time a ward may be without a ready-to-use emergency box.

If it is the hospital's policy to make a charge for the supplies used from the emergency box, then the nurse should prepare a charge ticket and submit it to the pharmacy along with the "used" box.

Some of the larger teaching hospitals have expanded on the emergency box concept and have developed the "emergency cart" or "resuscitation cart." These mobile units have on them the same basic supplies contained in the emergency box plus facilities for the administration of oxygen, the application of suction, and a cardiac pacemaker.

For the convenience of those desiring to establish an emergency box, a list of the pharmaceuticals and ancillary supplies which should be in it is given in Chapter 4, p. 114. However, where the services of a Pharmacy and Therapeutics Committee are available, the pharmacist should consult with the Committee prior to the adoption of a specific list of supplies.

Once an emergency box system is put into effect, the hospital pharmacist is reminded that it should not be forgotten. Many of the drugs which may be placed in the unit may deteriorate if not used within a reasonable period of time, and therefore are useless in an emergency. Therefore, a system of checking all emergency boxes must be initiated and pursued on a regular basis.

One such system requires the hospital pharmacist to check each emergency box on a monthly basis in order to remove outdated and deteriorated medications. This system requires placing an inventory and product control card in the box (Fig. 70). First, it serves as an inventory of the emergency box; second, it shows when the unit was last checked; and third, it provides the nursing personnel with adequate directions for replenishing any item which may have been used.

The *night drug supply cabinet* is basically an adjunct to the charge floor stock medications already on the pavilion. These units also range

EMERGENCY BOX INVENTORY & CONTROL CARD

Inventory	Product	Monthly Control Check											
		J	F	M	A	M	J	J	A	S	O	N	D
6 ampuls	Aminophyllin 250 mg I.V.	√	√	√	√								
4 ampuls	Calcium Gluconate 10 ml I.V.	√	√	√	√								
6 ampuls	Digitoxin 0.2 mg I.M.	√	√	√	√								

Fig. 70.

from a simple cabinet with drawers to large elaborate installations which include narcotic vaults and refrigerated compartments.[5]

The large cabinets are usually constructed in a wall of the pharmacy so that the unit may be serviced from within the pharmacy yet is accessible from the corridor side to authorized nursing personnel.

The night drug supply cabinet should be stocked with pre-packaged and labeled containers of the drug listed in the hospital formulary which the Pharmacy and Therapeutics Committee deems advisable. In addition, many hospitals also store certain medical and surgical supplies such as Foley catheters, oxidized cellulose and elastic hosiery.

The nursing supervisor opening the unit is required to leave a properly identified charge ticket listing the item removed and to whom it was administered. The next morning, pharmacy personnel restock the unit and forward the charge tickets to the accounting office.

Although the cost of purchase and installation of a night service cabinet may seem high to those who have inquired about such a unit, it would seem to be reasonably safe to state that the control of inventory which such a unit provides will more than offset its initial purchase and installation. Any plans for the construction of a new pharmacy or the renovation of existing quarters should include such a unit.

USE OF PHYSICIANS

Next to the use of registered pharmacists, a safe administrative and legal practice would be to prohibit nursing personnel from entering the pharmacy after hours and require that the physician enter the pharmacy and obtain any special medication not provided through the floor stocks, night cabinets or emergency box.

The major drawbacks to this method are first that the physician might waste a great deal of time searching for a product in unfamiliar surroundings and second, in these days of physician shortages, it is an unfair burden to place upon their already heavily taxed work hours.

This system does, however, possess one major advantage in that rather than enter the pharmacy, the physician may be influenced to use a drug which will accomplish the same purpose, yet is more readily available.

PHARMACIST-ON-CALL

Like all professional personnel, the hospital pharmacist understands the necessity of providing twenty-four-hour coverage and, therefore, will not hesitate to accept his share of an on-call assignment. In order to encourage this type of coverage, many administrators have developed bonus or extra pay plans to compensate the pharmacist.

Where the hospital employs a number of pharmacists, the institution of a rotational plan of on-calls will not burden any single individual.

In communities where more than one hospital is in operation, it is recommended that the pharmacists join forces in providing twenty-four hour on-call service. Under such a system, one pharmacist will be assigned to on-call duty for any one period of time and he, therefore, will answer the needs of both institutions. This type of cooperation will spread out the frequency of on-call duty and, at the same time, acquaint a second person with the routine of each hospital in case of an emergency or sick leave and vacation coverage.

PURCHASED SERVICE

Hospitals employing only one staff pharmacist have found a practical solution to the dilemma by contracting with the local community pharmacy for night, holiday and vacation relief for the staff pharmacist.

This method is a safe and legal one which, while protecting the drug needs of the hospital and patient, establishes good will in the community and perhaps a better understanding of the efforts of the hospital to safe-guard the health needs of the area on a round-the-clock basis.

Where there is more than one pharmacy in the community, care should be taken to avoid any claims of favoritism or politics. One method by which this may be accomplished is to develop a set of specifications and requirements concerning the desired service and request the local establishments to submit their bids. Obviously, the specifications should be so prepared that only the retail pharmacies with adequate staff, inventory, and delivery service can qualify to bid.

In recent years, much has been done to make drugs available on the pavilions in order to cope with every emergency. Some of these methods include the use of mechanical dispensing units, self-medication programs and centralized unit dose dispensing system available around the clock.

EXTENDING PHARMACY SERVICE HOURS

Emergency after-hour pharmacy services in hospitals have been replaced by around the clock coverage by staff pharmacists. In those smaller hospitals that are currently struggling to provide safe medications during off-hours, efforts should be made to convince hospital administration to financially support the broader pharmaceutical coverage. One survey[2] reveals that hospital pharmacists utilized the following reasons to convince management to support the extension of services:

1. Provided continuity for the IV admixture program.
2. Provided continuity for the unit dose program.
3. Provided medication to the night shift that is least experienced and newest to the hospital; reluctance or refusal by, and the time constraints on the night nursing supervisor allowed more involvement with nursing rather than pharmacy problems.
4. Provided continuity with the drug information service.
5. Provided continuity for the drug monitoring system.
6. Helped to prevent serious medication error(s) at night.

The ASHP Technical Assistance Bulletin on Hospital Drug Distribution and Control provides the following statements with regard to emergency medical supplies and the provision of pharmaceutical service after hours:[6]

Emergency Medication Supplies. A policy to supply emergency drugs when the pharmacist is off the premises or when there is insufficient time to get to the pharmacy should exist. Emergency drugs should be limited in number to include only those whose prompt use and immediate availability are generally regarded by physicians as essential in the proper treatment of sudden and unforeseen patient emergencies. The emergency drug supply should not be a source for normal "stat" or "p.r.n." drug orders. The medications included should be primarily for the treatment of cardiac arrest, circulatory collapse, allergic reactions, convulsions, and bronchospasm. The pharmacy and therapeutics committee should specify the drugs and supplies to be included in emergency stocks.

Emergency drug supplies should be inspected by pharmacy personnel on a routine basis to determine if contents have become outdated and are maintained at adequate levels. Emergency kits should have a seal which visually indicates when they have been opened. The expiration date of the kit should be clearly indicated.

Pharmacy Service When the Pharmacy is Closed. Hospitals provide services to patients 24 hours a day. Pharmaceutical services are an integral part of the total care provided by the hospital, and the services of a pharmacist should be available at all times. Where around-the-clock operation of the pharmacy is not feasible, a pharmacist should be available on an "on-call" basis. The use of "night cabinets" and drug dispensing by nonpharmacists should be minimized, and eliminated wherever possible. (See Chapter 14, Fig. 46.)

Drugs must not be dispensed to outpatients or hospital staff by anyone other than a pharmacist while the pharmacy is open. If it is necessary for nurses to obtain drugs when the pharmacy is closed and the pharmacist is unavailable, written procedures covering this practice should be developed. They generally should provide for a limited supply of the drugs most commonly needed in these situations; the drugs should be in proper single-dose packages and a log should be kept of all doses removed. This log must contain the date and time the drugs were removed, a complete description of the drug product(s), name of the (authorized) nurse involved, and the patient's name.

Drugs should not be dispensed to emergency room patients by non-pharmacist personnel if the pharmacy is open. When no pharmacist is available, emergency room patients should receive drugs packaged, to the extent possible, in single unit packages; no more than a day's supply of doses should be dispensed. The use of an emergency room "formulary" is recommended.

SELECTED READINGS

Ross, A.J.: Extended Hours of Service. Pharm. J., *221*:526–527, (Dec.) 1978.
Upton, J.H.: Justifying 24-Hour Pharmaceutical Services. Am. J. Hosp. Pharm., *39*:2072–2078, (Dec.) 1982.

REFERENCES

1. Stolar, M.H.: National Survey of Hospital Pharmacy Services—1978. Am. J. Hosp. Pharm., *36*:316:316–325, (Mar.) 1979.
2. Kessler, H. and Davis, N.M.: Survey of 24-Hour, 7-Day/Week Hospital Pharmacy Service. Hosp. Pharm., *19*:5:327, (May) 1984.
3. Hassan, William E. Jr.: Six Ways to Provide Pharmacy Coverage After Normal Hours, Hospitals. J.A.H.A., *32*:54, May 16, 1958.
4. Jeffrey, Louis P.: Around the Clock Pharmacy Service. Am. J. Hosp. Pharm., *15*:12:1064, 1958.
5. Thompson, Richard F. and Feely, William J.: A Pharmacy Night Cabinet. Hospital Pharmacy, *6*:10:21, (Oct.) 1971.
6. ASHP Technical Assistance Bulletin on Hospital Drug Distribution and Control. Am. J. Hosp. Pharm., *37*:1097–1103, (Aug.) 1980.

19

Hospital Reimbursement

Because of the remarkable change in the manner in which the health care industry is reimbursed, it is important for the institutional practitioner to be aware of these reimbursement systems and their evolution. Irrespective of the reimbursement methodology of the third party payors or the jurisdiction in which the hospital is located, there is an impact on the daily operation of the department of pharmacy services.

BLUE CROSS PLAN

Established in the 1930s, the concept of the Blue Cross plan today boasts a membership of upwards of 60 million people. The importance of this plan is further emphasized when one learns that in some hospitals nearly 75% of all admissions are covered by a Blue Cross plan.

Under this type of coverage the hospital is paid, in addition to a portion of the room and board charge, an amount for ancillary services which is determined by a "reimbursement formula" or published charges, whichever is the lower.[a] In arriving at the actual dollar rate of reimbursement, the Blue Cross auditors exclude the cost of teaching, research and capital expenditures.

Since the reimbursement rate for ancillaries includes the cost of drugs, the pharmacist should be aware of the fact that the drug portion of this reimbursement is arrived at by determining the average drug cost per patient day.

The average drug cost per patient day is calculated by dividing the actual cost of drugs issued by the hospital for the fiscal year by the total number of patient days for the same period. The average cost per patient day is also ascertained for all other ancillary services rendered by the hospital.

A state-approved reimbursement formula is then applied to the average cost per patient day figures which then results in a dollar rate which will be paid to the hospital for every Blue Cross patient day of service rendered to the plan's subscribers.

With the advent of the DRG prospective payment system, Blue Cross,

---

[a]Varies with plan.

as Medicare intermediary, reimburses hospitals for all Medicare patients on that basis.

Many Blue Cross plans have developed and operate a wholly owned HMO subsidiary as a defensive measure to prevent an erosion of Plan membership to competing alternative health care delivery systems.

COMMERCIAL INSURANCE PLANS

Present-day insurance plans are of the deductible and co-insurance type. The deductible portion of the policy is primarily intended to eliminate small nuisance claims. However, many individuals who have a Blue Cross plan paid for by their employer purchase a commercial policy with the deductible portion being the maximum allowed by the Blue Cross plan. One of the reasons advanced for this is the lower cost to the subscriber and yet it provides him with extremely broad hospitalization insurance.

Because the deductible and co-insurance type of policy often provides for a specific maximum aggregate benefit, insurance carriers imposed the co-insurance factor as a control on the quantity and type of medical care to be received by the policyholder. Under such plans, the insurance carrier will pay a stated percentage of the medical expense and the policyholder undertakes to pay the balance.

Under the commercial insurance plans, the insured, if he has no other type of coverage, pays the deductible amount of his policy and the co-insurance amount, the balance being covered by the insurance company.

From the above brief comparison of the Blue Cross plan with that of a commercial type health insurance plan, it should be clear that the Blue Cross subscriber utilizing the hospital pays for his drugs and other ancillary services on the basis of actual cost to the hospital, whereas the patient without any form of coverage or with commercial health insurance may pay the hospital's published charges.

MEDICARE COST-PER-CASE MANAGEMENT CONCEPT

The 1982 Medicare Amendments made drastic changes in hospital payment policies. These changes (1) replaced routine per diem cost limits with total operating cost-per-case limits; (2) authorized "incentive payments" to hospitals that hold costs below a Medicare cost-per-case target; and (3) mandated the development of a prospective payment proposal for consideration by the Congress in 1983.

Historically, the Medicare program was created in 1965 to improve access to needed health services by the elderly. It provided for a comprehensive benefit package for patients with modest cost-sharing; physician payment based on usual, customary and reasonable fees; and

hospital payment based on "reasonable costs." It was these incentives
that caused increased utilization and intensity of services that has
nearly bankrupted the system.

The new revisions limit average Medicare reimbursable total operating cost-per-case. For each hospital, two limits are set: a target cost-
per-case and a Section 223 maximum allowable cost-per-case. The
lower of these two limits is applied, although costs in excess of the
target cost-per-case are partially reimbursable while 100% of the costs
in excess of the Section 223 limit must be absorbed by the hospital.[18]

The cost-per-case target is calculated by applying an allowable rate
of increase to the hospital's actual historical cost-per-case. The limit
applies to total operating costs, including both routine and ancillary
services but excluding capital and teaching costs. The allowable rate
of increase is determined by the HCFA market basket index plus one
percent. Hospitals able to contain their average cost-per-case to a level
below their target ae permitted to retain 50% of the savings.[18]

MEDICARE PROSPECTIVE PRICING CONCEPT

On March 24, 1983, Congress approved a Medicare prospective pricing plan as part of the Social Security Amendments of 1983. Unlike
the system of the Tax Equity and Fiscal Responsibility Act cost-per-
case limits, the approach to Medicare prospective pricing (1) sets pricing for each Diagnosis Related Group (DRG) rather than establish a case
mix adjusted cost-per-case limit for the hospital; (2) severs the traditional relationship between Medicare revenues and costs; and (3) places
the hospital "at risk" for differences between average costs within DRGs
and the DRG prices.[19]

Because of the "at-risk" factor, hospitals must be managed within
the limits of available revenues and therefore must control the length
of stay, use of ancillary services and the mix of patients admitted within
each DRG.

Basis of Payment

The discharge will be the unit of payment in the Medicare prospective
pricing system. Over a 4-year period, a system of prospective pricing
will be phased in that establishes separate urban and rural national
DRG price schedules, adjusted for variations in wage levels. During the
phase-in period, the payment for each Medicare discharge will be computed by blending a hospital-specific cost-per-case amount, the regional
urban or rural price for the DRG to which the patient is assigned (adjusted for variations in wage levels), and the national urban or rural
price for the DRG to which the patient is assigned (adjusted for variations in wage levels).

- In the first year, the payment for each Medicare patient will be equal to:
— 75% of the hospital-specific cost-per-case amount; PLUS
— 25% of the regional average price for the patient's DRG.
- In the second year, the payment for each Medicare patient will be equal to:
— 50% of the hospital-specific cost-per-case amount; PLUS
— 37.5% of the regional average price for the patient's DRG; PLUS
— 12.5% of the national average price for the patient's DRG.
- In the third year, the payment for each Medicare patient will be equal to:
— 25% of the hospital-specific cost-per-case amount; PLUS
— 37.5% of the regional average price for the patient's DRG; PLUS
— 37.5% of the national average price for the patient's DRG.

In the fourth year, payments will be based on the urban or rural national average price for each DRG, adjusted for differences in area wages.[19]

The American Hospital Association has succinctly summarized this legislation as follows:[19]

Hospitals and Services Covered. All hospitals except long-term, children's, psychiatric and rehabilitation hospitals. Distinct part psychiatric and rehabilitation units of general hospitals are also exempt, and hospitals designated as sole community providers are given special treatment. Outpatient services and services provided in exempt distinct part units of general hospitals will be paid for on the basis of retrospectively determined costs.

Effective Dates. Prospective payment replaces the TEFRA cost-per-case limits in hospital fiscal years beginning on or after October 1, 1983.

Unit of Payment. When the prospective pricing system is fully phased in separate prices will be established for each of the Medicare Diagnosis Related Groups (DRGs). During the phase-in period payments will be calculated on a per-discharge basis.

Method of Computing Payments. During a three year phase-in period, the payment for each hospital discharge will be a blend of a hospital cost-per-case amount, a regional average price for the DRG to which a patient is assigned, and the national average price for the patient's DRG. Separate DRG prices will be computed for urban and rural hospitals. The regional and national prices will be adjusted for the wage level in the hospital's area. Beginning in the fourth year, prices will be set on the basis of the national average price for urban or rural hospitals.

Price Adjustment Factor. During the first two years of prospective pricing a base year cost-per-case will be rolled forward by the rate of increase in the hospital market basket, plus one percent for technology. Adjustments will be made to ensure that total Medicare expenditures are no greater under prospective payment than under the TEFRA cost-per-case limits. In subsequent years, the price adjustment factor will be determined by the Secretary in consultation with an independent commission.

Payments for "Outliers" and "Atypical Cases". "Atypical" or "outlier" cases include patients whose length of stay exceeds the average for the DRG by either a fixed number of days or a fixed number of standard deviations and, if approved by HCFA, patients whose costs are a "fixed multiple" of the average cost in the DRG to which the patient is assigned. Payments for "outlier" cases will be based on the "marginal costs" of the days beyond the cut-off level.

Payment of Exempt Providers. Hospitals exempt from the prospective payment system, including distinct part rehabilitation and psychiatric units of general hospitals will be reimbursed on the basis of retrospectively determined costs, subject to the cost-per-case limit on the allowable rate of increase established by TEFRA. The "section 223" limit will not apply to these hospitals.

Treatment of Capital Costs. During the first three years of the program, capital expenses will be reimbursed on the basis of retrospectively determined costs. Separate identification of capital costs incurred after the date of enactment may be required. Capital costs will be incorporated into the prospective prices beginning in year four.

Treatment of Education Costs. The direct expenses of approved education programs will be reimbursed on the basis of retrospectively determined costs.

Treatment of Indirect Medical Education Costs. The indirect costs of medical education will be reimbursed on the basis of an "indirect medical education allowance" equal to 12.12% of direct operating costs for each increment of 0.1 in the ratio of full time equivalent interns and residents to beds.

Appeals. Hospitals may appeal the incorrect application of the prospective pricing methodology and errors in calculation. The adequacy of the prices established by the correct application of the methodology may not be appealed.

DRUG UTILIZATION REVIEW (DUR)

Hoffman[20] has described a strategy aimed to reduce drug expenditures with a drug utilization review (DUR) program. The importance of this type of program is underscored by the spiraling rise in health care expenditures and the influence of costly new drug technology. The program described consists of a utilization review of high cost drugs for which a lower cost alternative exists. The following is a condensation of the essential elements of the Hoffman strategy:

1 Establish drug usage criteria through literature review and consultations.
2. Obtain medical staff approval and endorsement.

3. Inservice the pharmacy staff on the approved drug usage criteria.
4. Employ a DUR pharmacist who will, on a daily basis, compare the prescribed drug use to the approved criteria and contact the prescriber when the usage appears to be inappropriate.

Hoffman[20] also presents a job description for a DUR pharmacist. Some of the representative duties include but are not limited to:

1. Implements DUR programs as needed in conjunction with the pharmacy and medical staff.
2. Conducts regular educational programs for medical, nursing and pharmacy staffs regarding drug utilization.
3. Monitor drug expenses and utilization on a regular basis.
4. Maintains and updates DUR literature file.
5. Assists in the maintenance of the hospital drug formulary.

PRICING OF DRUGS

Much has been published concerning the pricing of prescriptions in the retail pharmacy.[1-3] In addition, various pricing schedules have been developed and made available to the community pharmacist.[4]

On the other hand, the problem of pricing policy has remained local in nature. That is, some state hospital pharmacy groups have undertaken pricing surveys and have published the data obtained.[5] This type of information, although of local comparative value, does nothing in the way of establishing a workable nation-wide hospital pharmacy prescription pricing formula from which each hospital may develop its own schedule of prescription prices.

At the present time, too many hospital pharmacists establish prescription prices blindly. That is to say, their prices are simply based on a percentage mark-up over cost. The percentage selected is usually that of a neighboring hospital or what is thought to be prevalent in the local community pharmacies.

In hospitals with low direct and indirect costs, the arbitrarily selected percentage mark-up figure may be high enough to permit a profitable operation. If, on the other hand, the direct and indirect costs are high, an operating loss seems a reasonable certainty.

Therefore, it behooves the hospital pharmacist to work closely with the comptroller in order to establish the departmental direct and indirect cost. Once ascertained, this figure when divided by the number of prescriptions filled will result in a unit prescription portion of the operational expense. From this, it should not be too difficult for the pharmacist to visualize the end of the spectrum in which he is operating. In this calculation, "the number of prescriptions filled" has been used as the denominator. For general purposes, "prescription" here is intended to mean out-patient prescription, take-home drug prescription and in-patient drug order since irrespective of how the medication is administered or where it is consumed, the *dispensing* aspect remains the same.

To this point, discussion has been aimed at developing an equitable price for drugs to be charged to all categories of patients and yet to be in a position to fully protect the hospital's financial interests in any transaction involving the sale of drugs to patients who do not have any form of insurance, as well as those who are covered by a commercial carrier whose policy provides for the payment of posted charges. There-fore, nothing has been mentioned of those patients whose hospital and medical needs are paid for by third party payors, other than Blue Cross, Medicare and commercial insurance companies. These third party pay-ors may be welfare agencies, industrial accident groups, or various governmental bureaus providing aid to the blind, to families of de-pendent children, to crippled children or for vocational rehabilitation.

Patients admitted to the hospital under the sponsorship of these agen-cies are accepted for a specified all-inclusive per diem rate, generally the Medicaid rate. Therefore, any difference between the hospital's posted charges and the per diem rate is considered to be an allowance by the hospital.

However, when the patients of some of these agencies are seen in the hospital clinics and receive a prescription, an entirely different pricing policy may be put into effect. This special pricing schedule is usually prepared by the agency and becomes a part of the agency's contract with the hospital.

PER DIEM DRUG CHARGE

The itemized pharmacy charges for 250 patients were studied to determine the average daily charges for drugs and pharmaceutical serv-ices. A comparison of the actual charges and the projected per diem rate indicated that the per diem rate would produce the same revenue as the itemized charging method. The per diem system enabled the hospital to reduce administrative and accounting costs while contin-uing to provide quality pharmaceutical service.[17]

Other hospitals have explored various methods of combining the per diem drug charge with fees for special clinical services. Yet others have advocated flat fees based on the medication record; a mark-up plus a dose fee and a combined product and service per diem fee. These concepts may be explored further by reading the articles cited under **Selected Readings** at the end of this chapter.

PROFESSIONAL FEE CONCEPT

The fee concept has been defined[6] as follows.

"...the exclusive use of a professional fee to meet all operating expenses, including overhead and compensation, but not the actual cost of drug and container."

Many hospital pharmacists have developed a professional fee system to be used in their hospitals.[7-10] These individuals report that the concept has found acceptance with both the public and medical staff.

One hospital pharmacist[11] states:

"This system incorporates two basic elements in the charge; the cost of the medication and an added fee that will recover the expense of operating the pharmacy and the share of the total hospital expense assumed by the pharmacy. These two elements are combined into one charge to the patient."

The professional fee concept should not be confused with the traditional retail theory of "mark-up" or "margin." These two terms generally imply that a per cent of the wholesale cost or selling price is used as the basis for recovering all direct and indirect expenses.

Many pharmacists are of the opinion that, as a professional member of the health team, the pharmacist should make a charge for his services which is separate and distinct from the cost of the medication and its container. It is further argued that the fee concept is more equitable to and better understood by the patient since he is accustomed to paying professional fees to doctors, dentists or lawyers.

The House of Delegates of the American Society of Hospital Pharmacists adopted the following resolution.[12]

Whereas the professional fee concept is recognized as a project consistent with the objectives, basic truths and goals of the ASHP statement on Goals for Hospital Pharmacy, now therefore be it
RESOLVED that the Society urge the adoption of the professional fee concept by hospital pharmacists, and be it further
RESOLVED that the Society assist hospital pharmacists in adopting the professional fee concept by providing information in the American Journal of Hospital Pharmacy, at continung education programs, and through related sources.

In order to make use of the fee concept in the pricing of prescriptions, the hospital pharmacist should become acquainted with all aspects of his direct and indirect operating costs so that he may arrive at a "fee" which in fact will meet all operating expenses. The thought has been advanced, in some circles, that a professional fee should be the same for all pharmacists in any one locality. Although this concept of standardizing the professional fee rates highly when one considers the public relations aspect, it is not advisable according to sound business and legal principles.

Reimbursement for pharmaceutical services under Title XIX (Medicaid) programs is now based upon "actual acquisition costs of the drug plus a fixed fee." The "fixed fee" is the terminology used by the Federal government for "professional fee."

At the present time, there rages within the profession a controversy relative to the definition of the term "acquisition cost." The issue seems to center around the role to be given to free goods, special discounts and direct purchasing credits in ascertaining the actual acquisition cost.

BREAK-EVEN POINT PRICING

A useful tool in the overall analysis of cost-volume-profit relationships is the break-even point which is defined as that level at which there is neither profit or loss.

Foulke[13] states that the existence of a break-even point is not a matter of theory but is a practical analytical factor which is useful in the comparison of net sales, expenses and operating profits within a budget; to ascertain the necessary increase in net sales to justify expansion of plant or personnel and to determine the effect upon net profits by any changes in personnel or material costs.

The application of the break-even principle has been applied to the pricing of drugs both in the in-patient and out-patient pharmacies.[14]

To adapt the break-even point to the pricing of drugs requires that the pharmacist be in a position to ascertain the fixed and indirect expenses of his department, and then be in a position to charge to the dispensing unit its fair share of these expenses.

In general, the costs of a department of pharmacy should include its proportionate cost of the hospital's administration, maintenance and housekeeping, depreciation of plant and equipment, and labor. These figures may be obtained from the hospital's comptroller since they are usually required of him in the preparation of the hospital's annual report to the Department of Public Health's Division of Hospitals. If these figures are not available, then the pharmacist may, with the co-operation of the comptroller, determine them.

For example, the pharmacy's share of the maintenance and house-keeping costs may be determined by calculating the total cost of these services to the hospital and dividing this figure by the total number of square feet of floor space utilizing these services. The resulting figure is the maintenance and housekeeping costs per square foot. By taking the total number of square feet in the pharmacy dispensing unit and multiplying by the maintenance-housekeeping cost per square foot, the pharmacy dispensing unit thereby is charged with its fair share. The actual cost of these services divided by the number of prescriptions filled on an average day results in the cost of these services per prescription.

1. Total cost of maintenance and housekeeping to the
   hospital $100,000
2. Total of number square feet in the hospital 100,000
3. Maintenance-Housekeeping costs per square foot $1.00
4. Pharmacy dispensing unit in square feet 25
5. Maintenance-Housekeeping costs per sq. ft. of dispensing
   unit (#3 multiplied by #4)............................ $25.00
6. Number of prescriptions filled daily 100
7. Maintenance-Housekeeping cost per prescription .... $.25

Other indirect overhead costs such as the unit's share of administration, heat, light, water (these are not usually metered to each department) may be similarly obtained by arriving at a common denominator such as square feet or space; total number of personnel employed or number of quota hours assigned to the department.

Depreciation of equipment and direct costs, such as the pharmacist's time, cost of container and label, laundry, etc., are readily calculable.

Once the direct and indirect operational costs are determined, to them is added the cost of the container and the cost of the drug. The total of these factors represents the break-even point.

COMPUTERIZED PRICING AND INVENTORY CONTROL

A computerized on-line pharmacy pricing and inventory control system has been developed and is in use in a 940-bed hospital. The program requires input of only four pieces of information: (1) patient number; (2) drug identification number; (3) dose factor; and (4) total number of doses dispensed.

In the pricing formula, the charge to the patient is calculated by adding the product of the total cost of medication and the mark-up factor to the product of the dose fee and the total number of doses received.

The system is stated to have the following advantages: (1) the patient or third party payor can be given an itemized bill for all pharmaceutical charges; (2) the system accounts for all medication costs whether or not they are charged to the patient; (3) the revenue for the department can be projected and adjusted accurately; (4) the charges are fair and equitable; (5) the patient is charged for medication administered only; and (6) the system produces accurate statistical reports for both the pharmacy and financial departments. A major disadvantage is stated to be the number of man-hours needed for the pricing function.[16]

PUBLIC LAW 89-97 (MEDICARE)

This legislation provides three programs for health insurance and medical care under the Social Security Act.

The basic responsibility for administration of the insurance program is vested in the Secretary of Health and Human Services. Within this authority, the administrative and operational responsibility will be in the Social Security Administration, with responsibility for certain professional aspects in the Public Health Service.

The Social Security Administration will make use of state agencies and organizations to assist in the administration of the program.

In view of the fact that drugs will be an integral part of the care rendered under these programs, it is essential that the hospital pharmacist familiarize himself with the basic requirements of each in order that he may develop proper charge procedures for the drugs dispensed to the enrollees.

I. TITLE XVIII (A)—COMPULSORY HOSPITAL PROGRAM

The first of these programs, the "compulsory hospital program," became effective July 1, 1966, and provides the following basic benefits to about 19 million persons aged 65 or older:

1. *In-patient hospital services*—For up to 90 days in semi-private accommodations during an illness. The patient pays the first $400 of the costs. If he stays in the hospital for more than a 60-day period, he also pays $100 for each day between 61st and 90th days. Psychiatric hospital in-patient services are limited to 190 days during a lifetime.
2. *Posthospital extended care services*—For up to 100 days, beginning January 1, 1967. The patient pays $18 for each day over 20 days.
3. *Posthospital home health services*—Nurses' or technicians' services for up to 100 home visits after discharge from a hospital or extended care facility.
4. *Out-patient hospital diagnostic services*—Patient pays $75 deductible and 20% of any charges in excess of $75 during a 20-day period.

Life-time reserve—Limited to 60 days during which the patient is required to pay for services rendered up to $200 per day.

The "in-patient hospital services" benefits includes drugs and biologicals ordinarily furnished by the hospital for the care and treatment of in-patients. "Posthospital extended care services" include drugs and biologicals ordinarily furnished by the nursing home. Drugs and biologicals are presently excluded from coverage in the "posthospital home health services."

The terms "drugs and biologicals" are specifically limited by the law to drugs included (or approved for inclusion) in *The United States Pharmacopeia, The National Formulary, The United States Homeopathic Pharmacopeia, New Drugs,* or *Accepted Dental Remedies,* and drugs approved by the Pharmacy and Therapeutics Committees of the furnishing hospitals.

This program will be financed by increased social security payments. Payments for benefits will be made directly by the Federal Government to the providers of services who have entered into an agreement with the Secretary of Health and Human Services or by selected private insurance carriers who will act as intermediaries.

II. TITLE XVIII (B)—VOLUNTARY INSURANCE PROGRAM

The second of the programs, the "voluntary insurance program," became effective on July 1, 1966, and provides medical insurance for persons 65 or over who elected to enroll under it at a cost of $3 each. It was financed from premiums paid by the enrollees and by funds appropriated by the Federal Government. The services provided under this program are:

1. Home health services for up to one hundred visits during a calendar year.
2. Medical and other health services including:
   a. Physicians' and surgeons' services, whether furnished in the hospital, office, or home.
   b. Diagnostic x rays and laboratory tests, electrocardiograms, and other diagnostic tests.
   c. Surgical dressings and splints; casts and other devices for reduction of fractures and dislocations; braces and artificial limbs; prosthetic devices; rental of durable medical equipment such as iron lungs, oxygen tents, hospital beds, and wheelchairs used in patients' homes.
   d. Ambulance services.

Payment for these services will be made by the Federal Government directly to the provider of such services or by private insurance carriers based upon a co-payment factor. Drugs and biologicals are specifically excluded from "home health services." They are only covered in the "medical and other health services" if they cannot be self-administered and if they are furnished either as an incident to a physician's professional service or as a hospital service incident to a physician's service rendered to outpatients.

III. TITLE XIX—MEDICAID

Basically, Title XIX is an extended Kerr-Mills type of program. As written, it will have the following effects:

1. Serve to foster the present "vendor payment" type of system by increasing the amount of Federal matching funds under a formula based on state per capita income (ranges from 55 to 83%).

2. Consolidate all state programs under one state administrator.
3. Broaden the scope of state programs to include more people and more services for many of these people by providing at least the following services to those eligible:
   a. In-patient hospital services
   b. Out-patient hospital services
   c. Other laboratory and x-ray services
   d. Skilled nursing home service
   e. Physician's services

Under this program the supply of drugs is optional, but it is felt that most states will elect to supply them.

Title XIX is potentially larger than the other two Medicare programs since it authorizes and encourages government-assisted medical care to *all* persons receiving public assistance and to many other persons in need of medical aid regardless of age. It has been estimated that this program could encompass as many as 35 million people.

CONDITIONS OF PARTICIPATION

The rules governing the aspects of the Medicare program are known as the *Conditions of Participation for Hospitals.* These were issued by the Social Security Administration after extensive consultation with the Health Insurance Benefits Advisory Council—commonly referred to as HIBAC.

Accordingly, it is from this document[15] that the following information governing the participation of hospitals and allied health agencies is obtained.

General Hospitals

Since the Joint Commission on Accreditation of Hospitals has adopted a requirement for utilization review, any hospital accredited by this group would generally be conclusively presumed to meet all the conditions for participation in the program.

The regulations also provide that accreditation by the American Osteopathic Association, or any other national accrediting body, may also be accepted if it is reasonable to do so, as evidence that a hospital meets some or all of the conditions of participation.

Further stipulations require the hospital to be licensed, certified or approved by the state (local law equivalents to licensing meet this requirement) and it must substantially comply with regulations pertaining to medical records, medical staff by-laws, pharmacy and therapeutics committees to mention a few.

Further requirements necessary to the health and safety of patients may be imposed by the Government; however, these health and safety requirements cannot be more strict than the comparable conditions enforced by the Joint Commission on Accreditation of Hospitals.

The regulations also permit the state to establish stricter requirements if such are specified under its Federal-State medical assistance programs. These stricter requirement may be enforced by the sovereign state even if they are not used in its own programs.

Psychiatric and Tuberculosis Hospitals

In order to avoid paying for care that is merely custodial in nature, the conditions of participation require that the institution:
(1) be accredited by the Joint Commission on Accreditation of Hospitals:
(2) maintain clinical records which are adequate to ascertain the degree ad intensity of treatment furnished to the insured; and
(3) meet staffing requirements commensurate with those needed for carrying out an active treatment program.

The regulations also dictate that a distinct part of the institution may participate as a psychiatric or tuberculosis hospital, if it meets the above conditions, even though the institution of which it is a part does not. Also, if the distinct part of the institution meets requirements equivalent to accreditation requirements, it may qualify under the program even though the institution is not accredited.

Conditions of Participation for an Extended Care Facility

An extended care facility is liberally defined as a skilled nursing home or a distinct part of an institution, such as a ward or wing of a hospital.

An institution which is primarily for the care and treatment of mental diseases or tuberculosis is excluded from the definition of an extended care facility.

In general, extended care facilities will be required to have an agreement with a hospital for the transfer of patients and interchange of medical records. This requirement may be waived where an extended care facility has attempted, in good faith, to arrange a transfer agreement but failed and the State agency finds that the facility's participation in the hospital insurance program is in the public's interest and essential to assuring necessary care to the insured inhabitants of the community.

It should be emphasized that the requirement for a transfer agreement does not mean that a patient would have to be transferred between a hospital and extended care facility which have such an arrangement between them. A transfer agreement with any hospital would qualify the facility so that the patient's extended care would be paid for if he was admitted upon transfer from some other hospital.

Since the extended care facility is expected to render high-quality convalescent and rehabilitative care, it must meet the following requirements. They include:
(1) around-the-clock nursing services with at least one registered nurse employed full time;
(2) the availability of a physician to cope with emergencies;
(3) utilization review;
(4) proper methods for handling drugs; and
(5) the maintenance of adequate medical policies, governing the nursing care and related services.

Conditions of Participation for a Home Health Agency

Visiting nurse organizations, hospital-operated home-care services as well as agencies specifically established to provide a broad spectrum of home health services are examples of home health agencies which may qualify under the program. A private organization providing home care on a profit basis may qualify if it is licensed, where State law requires it, and if it meets specified standards.

In general, a home health agency in order to partipate will have to be:
(1) publicly owned; or
(2) a nonprofit organization exempt from Federal taxation; or
(3) licensed and meet staffing requirements and other conditions and standards prescribed by regulation.

It should be recognized that not all institutions desiring to participate will be certified for this purpose. Therefore, it will be possible for an insured person to encounter a medical emergency and find that he is admitted to a hospital not participating in the hospital insurance program. In these situations, the law permits the payment of benefits for emergency hospital diagnostic services or in-patient care until it is no longer necessary from a medical point of view to care for the patient in a non-participating institution provided that the hospital agrees not to charge the patient amounts (except the deductibles and co-insurance) in addition to the program's payments for covered services.

Conditions of Participation for Hospitals:
VIII Pharmacy or Drug Room

Drugs and biologicals furnished to hospital patients for their use while in-patients will be paid for under the health insurance program provided that the conditions of participation applicable to the pharmacy or drug room are complied with.

The following are conditions of participation as they apply to the hospital pharmacy.

STANDARD A—PHARMACY SUPERVISION

There is a pharmacy directed by a registered pharmacist or a drug room under competent supervision.

Factor 1. The pharmacist is trained in the administration of hospital pharmacy.
Factor 2. The pharmacist is responsible to the administration of the hospital for developing, supervising, and coordinating all the activities of the pharmacy department.
Factor 3. If there is a drug room with no pharmacist, prescriptions are compounded by a qualified pharmacist elsewhere, and only storing and distributing are done in the drug room. A consulting pharmacist assists in drawing up the correct procedures, rules, and regulations for the distribution of drugs, and visits the hospital on a regularly scheduled basis in the course of his duties. Whenever possible, the pharmacist, in dispensing drugs, works from the prescriber's original order or a direct copy.

STANDARD B—PHYSICAL FACILITIES

Facilities are provided for the storage, safeguarding, preparation, and dispensing of drugs.

Factor 1. Drugs are issued to floor units in accordance with approved policies and procedures.
Factor 2. Drug cabinets on the nursing units are routinely checked by the pharmacist. All floor stocks are properly controlled.
Factor 3. There is adequate space for all pharmacy operations and the storage of drugs at a satisfactory location provided with proper lighting, ventilation, and temperature controls.
Factor 4. If there is a pharmacy, equipment is provided for the compounding and dispensing of drugs.
Factor 5. Special locked storage space is provided to meet the legal requirements for storage of narcotics, alcohol, and other prescribed drugs.

STANDARD C—PERSONNEL

Personnel competent in their respective duties are provided in keeping with the size and activity of the department.

Factor 1. The pharmacist is assisted by an adequate number of additional registered pharmacists and such other personnel as the activities of the pharmacy may require to insure quality pharmaceutical services.
Factor 2. The pharmacy, depending upon the size and scope of its operations, is staffed by the following categories of personnel:
(i) Chief pharmacist; (ii) One or more assistant chief pharmacists; (iii) Staff pharmacists; (iv) Pharmacy residents (where a program has been activated); (v) Non-professionally trained pharmacy helpers; (vi) Clerical help.
Factor 3. Provision is made for emergency pharmaceutical services.
Factor 4. If the hospital does not have a staff pharmacist, a consulting pharmacist has overall responsibility for control and distribution of drugs and a designated individual(s) has responsibility for day-to-day operation of the pharmacy.

STANDARD D—RECORDS

Records are kept of the transactions of the pharmacy (or drug room) and correlated with other hospital records where indicated. Such special records are kept as are required by law.

Factor 1. The pharmacy establishes and maintains, in cooperation with the accounting department, a satisfactory system of records and bookkeeping in accordance with the policies of the hospital for:
(i) Maintaining adequate control over the requsitioning and dispensing of all drugs and pharmaceutical supplies; (ii) Charging patients for drugs and pharmaceutical supplies.

Factor 2. A record of the stock on hand and of the dispensing of all narcotic drugs is maintained in such a manner that the disposition of any particular item may be readily traced.

Factor 3. Records for prescription drugs dispensed to each patient (in-patients and out-patients) are maintained in the pharmacy or drug room containing the full name of the patient and the prescribing physician, the prescription number, the name and strength of the drug, the date of issue, the expiration date for all time-dated medications, the lot and control number of the drug, the name of the manufacturer (or trademark) and (unless the physician directs otherwise) the name of the medicaiton dispensed.

Factor 4. The label of each out-patient's individual prescription medication container bears the lot and control number of the drug, the name and the manufacturer (or trademark) and (unless the physician directs otherwise) the name of the medication dispensed.

STANDARD E—CONTROL OF TOXIC OR DANGEROUS DRUGS

Policies are established to control the administration of toxic or dangerous drugs with specific reference to the duration of the order and the dosage.

Factor 1. The medical staff has established a written policy that all toxic or dangerous medications, not specifically prescribed as to time or number of doses, will be automatically stopped after a reasonable time limit set by the staff.

Factor 2. The classificaiton ordinarily thought of as toxic or dangerous drugs are narcotics, sedatives, anticoagulants, antibiotics, oxytocics and cortisone.

STANDARD F—COMMITTEE

There is a committee of the medical staff to confer with the pharmacist in the formulation of policies.

Factor 1. A Pharmacy and Therapeutics Committee (or equivalent committee), composed of physicians and pharmacists, is established in the hospital and serves as the liaison between the medical staff and the pharmacist.

Factor 2. The committee assists in the formulation of broad professional policies regarding the evaluation, appraisal, selection, procurement, storage, distribution, use, and safety procedures, and all other matters relating to drugs.

Factor 3. The committee performs the following specific functions: (i) Serves as an advisory group to the hospital medical staff and the pharmacist on matters pertaining to the choice of drugs; (ii) Develops and reviews periodically a formulary or drug list accepted for use in the hospital; (iii) Establishes standards concerning the use and control of experimental drugs and research in the use of recognized drugs; (iv) Evaluates clinical data concerning new drugs or preparations requested for use in the hospital; (v) Makes recommendations concerning drugs to be stocked on the nursing unit floors and by other services; (vi) Prevents unnecessary duplication in stocking the same basic drug and its preparation.

Factor 4. The committee meets at least quarterly and reports to the executive committee and the medical staff.

STANDARD G—DRUGS TO BE DISPENSED

Drugs dispensed are included (or approved for inclusion) in the *United States Pharmacopoeia, National Formulary, United States Homeopathic Pharmacopeia, New Drugs,* or *Accepted Dental Remedies* (except for any drugs unfavorably evaluated therein), or are approved for use by the Pharmacy and Therapeutics Committee (or equivalent committee) of the hospital staff.

Factor 1. The pharmacist, with the advice and guidance of the Pharmacy and Therapeutics Committee, is responsible for specifications as to quality, quantity, and source of supply of all drugs.

Factor 2. There is available a formulary or list of drugs accepted for use in the hospital which is developed and amended at regular intervals by the Pharmacy and Therapeutics Committee (or equivalent committee) with the cooperation of the pharmacist (consulting or otherwise) and the administration.

Factor 3. The pharmacy or drug room is adequately supplied with preparations so approved.

ASHP GUIDELINES FOR IMPLEMENTING AND OBTAINING REIMBURSEMENT FOR CLINICAL PHARMACEUTICAL SERVICES[21]*

During the past 10 years, pharmacies in institutions and other organized settings have been evolving from a product-centered structure to a more service-oriented practice. This trend will continue as drug therapy becomes more complex and sophisticated. Many innovative pharmaceutical services have been described in recent literature. Examples of these services are formalized patient education sessions and pharmacokinetic consultations. Many pharmacists are planning on initiating these and other new programs in their institutions. However, until these activities become the "norm," they may have to meet certain

---

*Approved by the ASHP Board of Directors, November 13–14, 1980. Originally developed by the ASHP Task Force on Payment for Pharmacy Services; reviewed and approved by the ASHP Council on Clinical Pharmacy and Therapeutics.

administrative requirements. These are: (1) obtaining approval from the institution's administration for the provision of the service on a routine basis (along with the resources required); (2) delineating the costs of the service and an appropriate patient charging mechanism; and (3) obtaining reimbursement and payment for the provider.[a]

The ASHP Task Force on Payment for Pharmacy Services has concluded that, generally, there are no policies of Blue Cross plans, private insurance companies, or other third-party carriers that prohibit their reimbursing and paying providers for clinical pharmacy services. However, their support is predicated upon acceptance and endorsement of the service by the involved administrative and medical staffs (and, in the case of those covered by private insurance plans, by their desire to have the service as a covered benefit of their plan).

This document presents a set of general guidelines for use in obtaining administrative support and subsequent reimbursement and payment for a new pharmaceutical service. Often, many steps of the process may be omitted. For example, it should not be necessary to conduct a preliminary trial of a widely accepted, though not universally adopted, service (such as use of patient medication profiles). Likewise, it may not be necessary to generate cost or other data if they are available in the literature or elsewhere. The context in which these guidelines are written is that of a pharmacy director working in a hospital—they are adaptable to other situations as well (such as a pharmacist providing services as part of a medical group practice).

Guidelines

1. Prepare, for the provider's administration, a written proposal for a short-term (e.g., three-month) implementation project for the proposed service. This document should include the following elements:
   a. A clear, concise description of the service.
   b. The rationale for the service. Include published references if available.
   c. Written support for the service by the pharmacy and therapeutics committee and other appropriate parties (e.g., infections committee, department of nursing).
   d. The expected benefits of the service to patients and the institution in terms of costs and quality of care as measured by indices such as: (i) decrease in length of stay; (ii) decrease in the incidence of therapeutic failures; (iii) decrease in drug expenditures.
   e. Estimated start-up and operating expenses and revenue[b] of the service, plus its personnel, equipment, and material requirements.
2. Obtain formal approval of the implementation project from administration.

---

[a]The term "provider" refers to an individual practitioner (e.g., pharmacist) or organization (e.g., hospital or group practice).

[b]Depending upon the acceptance of the service within the health-care system and in cooperation with the provider's fiscal offices, a determination should be made if payment for the service can or should be received.

3. Initiate the project, keeping complete records of all expenses, outputs (i.e., the number of patient consults or whatever quantitative measure is appropriate), and man-hours devoted to it. This information will be needed in developing charges for the service and for obtaining reimbursement and payment.

4. Upon its completion, prepare a report of the implementation project for administration. This report should contain fiscal and workload data, including total pharmacy cost per patient or service unit and a suggested charge based on these data. Information on acceptance of the program by patients and staff should be included, as should whatever measures of its effectiveness (see 1.d.) are possible. This report should also project the manpower and financial resources needed to perform the service as a regular pharmacy function.

5. Obtain formal approval from administration to implement the service provider-wide.

6. Assist the institution's administration and financial manager in developing the information needed to include the costs of the service in its reimbursement agreements with third-party carriers. In obtaining this reimbursement, certain administrative requirements (such as formal approval of the service by the pharmacy and therapeutics committee) may have to be met.

7. It may be useful to prepare annual updates on the impact of the service (reporting, for example, annual cost savings or decreased readmissions over a baseline period). Annual assessments of the financial and manpower requirements of the service also will be useful in preparing pharmacy budgets.

These guidelines pertain to reimbursement and payment to institutions or other organized providers for the costs of pharmaceutical services. There may be circumstances under which pharmacists wish to obtain direct reimbursement or payment, as independent practitioners, for their services. The procedures outlined in this document, generally, are applicable to these situations as well. It should be noted, however, that such direct remuneration may be extremely difficult to obtain and may, in fact, possess certain disadvantages (such as substantial paperwork requirements).

USE OF CHARGE CARDS

Most hospitals are reimbursed for prescription drugs—both in-patient and out-patient—by third-party payors or a direct billing basis. Lately, some institutions have begun to accept charge-card systems such as **Master Card** and **Visa** to cover not only out-patient prescription drug charges, but for all other services rendered by the hospital.

A number of companies have been formed to act as prescription program administrators for insurance companies, private firms, government agencies, HMO's and other organizations who offer their employees a prescription reimbursement program. These programs represent a fringe benefit to the employees. Also, it is to the advantage of the sponsoring firm to avoid the cost of establishing and monitoring a reimbursement program and to have someone else perform this function. The procedure followed is that the outside contractor enters into an agreement with a firm to supply identification cards and reimbursement services for all that firm's employees. The employee then has the prescription filled at a pharmacy and uses the identification card to pay for the prescription (generally a co-payment is involved).

The pharmacist, in order to obtain reimbursement, collects all such evidence of prescription activity and submits it to the contractor for reimbursement in the aggregate via a prescription claim form. The contractor then processes each prescription claim on a computer, verifying product identification, costs, eligibility, and completeness of data and reimburses the pharmacy for all valid claims. The contractor then bills the contracting firm, or its insurance carrier, for its services plus the cost of the prescription.

SELECTED READINGS

Smith, W.E. and Weiblen, J.W.: Charging for Hospital Pharmaceutical Services: Product Cost, Per Diem Fees and Fees for Clinical Services. Am. J. Hosp. Pharm., *36*:355–359, (Mar.) 1979.

Fish, K.H., Jr.: Charging for Hospital Pharmaceutical Services: Computerized System Using a Markup and a Dose Fee. Am. J. Hosp. Pharm., *36*:360–363, (Mar.) 1979.

Dirks, I. and Pang, F.J.: Charging for Hospital Pharmaceutical Services: Combined Product-Service Per Diem Fees. Am. J. Hosp. Pharm., *36*:363–365, (Mar.) 1979.

Wyatt, B.K.: Charging for Hospital Pharmaceutical Services: Flat Fee Based on the Medication Record. Am. J. Hosp. Pharm., *36*:365–367, (Mar.) 1979.

Iglehart, J.K.: Health Policy Report: Medicare Begins Prospective Payment of Hospitals. N. Engl. J. Med., *308*:23:1428, (June 9) 1983.

Huffman, Jr. D.C. and Kilgore, S.M.: Changing Concepts in Hospital Reimbursement. Current Concepts in Hosp. Pharm. Mgt., *6*:3;13, (Fall) 1984.

Curtis, F.R.: Looking Beyond DRGs: Opportunity for Hospital Pharmacy. Am. J. Hosp. Pharm., *41*:721–723, 1984.

REFERENCES

1. *Systematic Prescription Pricing Digest.* Syracuse, Bristol Laboratories, Inc.
2. *The Lilly Digest.* Indianapolis, Eli Lilly & Co.
3. *The American College of Apothecaries Operational Survey.* Philadelphia, American College of Apothecaries.
4. *The Universal Prescription Costing and Pricing Calculator.* Rutherford, N.J., Becton, Dickinson & Co.
5. Narinian, George: Pharmaceutical Pricing in Hospitals. Hosp. Mgt., *90*:2:83, 1960.
6. Hartlieb, Charles J., Flack, Herbert L., and Abrams, Robert E.: A Rational Method of Prescription Pricing—The Professional Fee Concept. J.A.Ph.A. Pract. Ed., *21*:11:696, 1960.
7. Latiolais, Clifton J.: Experiences with the Professional Fee System in Hospital Pharmacy Practice at Ohio State University Hospital. Am. J. Hosp. Pharm., *23*:9:511, 1966.
8. Butler, John L. and Parker, Paul F.: Experience with the Professional Fee System in Hospital Pharmacy Practice at the University of Kentucky Medical Center. Am. J. Hosp. Pharm., *23*:9:516, 1966.
9. Rourke, Sr. Mary Vera: Experiences with the Professional Fee System in Hospital Pharmacy Practice at Mercy Hospital (Buffalo). Am. J. Hosp. Pharm., *23*:9:520, 1966.

10. Ulan, Martin S.: Experiences with the Professional Fee System in Hospital Pharmacy Practice at the Hackensack Hospital. Am. J. Hosp. Pharm., *23*:9:522, 1966.
11. Kashino, Minoru: Experiences with the Professional Fee System in Hospital Pharmacy Practice at the Palo Alto-Stanford Hospital Center. Am. J. Hosp. Pharm., *23*:9:518, 1966.
12. Provost, George P.: An Opportunity for Hospital Pharmacy. Am. J. Hosp. Pharm., *23*:9:487, 1966.
13. Foulke, R.A.: *Practical Financial Statement Analysis,* 5th ed. New York, McGraw-Hill Book Co., 1961.
14. Provost, George P. and Hiller, William M.: How Break-Even Pricing of Drugs Works. The Modern Hospital, *94*:122, 1960.
15. Health Insurance for the Aged, Conditions of Participation for Hospitals, Publication HIM-1 (2–66), Social Security Administration, U.S. Department of Health, Education and Welfare, Washington, D.C.
16. Fish, K.H.: Charging for Hospital Pharmaceutical Services: Computerized System Using a Markup and a Dose Fee. Am. J. Hosp. Pharm., *36*:360–363, (Mar.) 1979.
17. Dirks, I. and Pang, F.J.: Charging for Hospital Pharmaceutical Services: Combined Product-Service Per Diem Fees. Am. J. Hosp. Pharm., *36*:363–365, (Mar.) 1979.
18. Anon. Medicare Payment: Cost-Per-Case Management Special Report No. 1, August 1982. American Hospital Association, Office of Public Policy Analysis, Chicago, Ill. 60611.
19. Anon. Medicare Payment: Cost-Per-Case Management Special Report No. 3, April, 1983. American Hospital Association, Office of Public Policy Analysis, Chicago, Ill. 60611.
20. Hoffmann, R.P.: A Strategy to Reduce Drug Expenditures with a Drug Utilization Review Program. Hosp. Pharm., *19*:1:7–12, 1984.
21. ASHP Guidelines for Implementing and Obtaining Reimbursement for Clinical Pharmaceutical Services. Am. J. Hosp. Pharm., *38*:386, (Mar.) 1981.

20|

Prepackaging in the Hospital

Prepackaging of drugs is not a new concept to the profession of pharmacy. It has been in practice since the apothecary of old grew his own herbs and drugs and harvested and packaged them for sale. Many retail pharmacies purchase various over-the-counter tablets and syrups in bulk quantities and prepackage the material in smaller-sized containers.

In the hospital pharmacy, the concept of prepackaging is utilized in both the large and the small hospital for it is, oftentimes, the means of coping with the periods of peak demand for pharmaceutical service. In the small hospital, the pharmacist may prepackage only those items which he considers require too much time if filled only when called for. In some hospital pharmacies, items which fall into this category are narcotics, barbiturates oily products, heavy syrups or magmas.

Most large hospitals have found it economical to prepackage all ward stock items as well as the often prescribed tablets, capsules, syrups, ointments and creams used both by the in-patients as well as the out-patient clinics. Because of the scope of ths phase of a large hospital pharmacy operation, it often requires a separate work force, special equipment, and detailed control procedures to ensure against the possibility of errors.

PREPACKAGING POLICY—ITS DETERMINATION

The decision as to what product and how much of it should be prepackaged is one which can be made only after a comprehensive study of the local situation. No rule of thumb can be reasonably stated which would be applicable in a majority of the instances.

Some of the factors which must be considered are:

a. Demand for the product.
   Is it a year 'round demand or is it a seasonal demand?
   Is the demand one which originates from the clinics or the pavilions?
   Can this product be purchased in quantities to meet the demand, yet have it packaged in small units by the manufacturer at a price lower than the hospital cost to prepackage the same item in a similar container?

406

b. What size units should be packaged? How many of each size?

c. What type of containers and closures must be used in order to maintain therapeutic integrity?

d. What special labeling will be required?

e. Can the item be machine packaged or must hand counting be resorted to?

f. What is the stability of the product?
   Is it dated?

g. What will the unit cost of prepackaging amount to? Who should pay it?

Those experienced with the problem are convinced that almost every item in the pharmacy can be prepackaged. This includes preparations considered to be free ward stock as well as the items prescribed as charge drugs.

The size of each container of drug can best be ascertained by consulting the nursing service as well as the Pharmacy and Therapeutics Committee. The nursing service can be most helpful in providing data concerning the quantities and rate of use of such items as ward stock hypnotics, sedatives, antitussives, antiseptics, mouth washes, back rub lotions, etc. On the other hand, the Pharmacy and Therapeutics Committee can establish a quota regarding the number of capsules and tablets or volume of liquid preparations which may be sent to the pavilions. The figure is usually included in the published formulary as the quantity to prescribe and is arrived at by a decision not to permit more than a specific number of days of therapy on any one drug order. In a majority of hospitals, 20 to 25 capsules or tablets are considered as adequate for hospitalized patients and are therefore the commonly prepackaged sizes.

Insofar as prepackaging for the out-patient clinic is concerned, the most important factor to be considered is the cycle for obtaining subsequent appointments. If it is accepted hospital policy to schedule patients for appointments every 30 or 45 or 60 days, then the quantity of drug, if the therapy warrants it, should be sufficient to last until the date of the subsequent appointment. Failure to do this will result in burdening the patient by forcing him to return to the hospital for an unscheduled appointment for the purpose of obtaining authorization for a refill. Thus quantities of 50, 75 and 100 unit doses may be prepackaged for clinic dispensing.

As has been previously stated, no set rule can be provided which will be of universal value in determining the total volume of material to be prepackaged. Some hospital pharmacists have developed a routine whereby items are prepackaged in a volume estimated to last for a period of 60 days, whereas others vary from as little as 30 days to as much as 120 days. In this regard, a word of caution must be interjected—

namely, an extremely large volume of prepackaging of a single item may be quite risky should the use fall off or be jeopardized by reports of adverse reactions resulting from its use. The prepackaged items may not be returned to the manufacturer for credit and may become a total loss to the hospital.

PREPACKAGING OPERATION

In the small hospital, the prepackaging operation is usually accomplished by the staff pharmacist with the assistance of a part-time helper. This is a practical approach to the problem when the volume is not great for it permits the pharmacist to remain busy throughout the work week. Under these circumstances, no special area need be set aside nor is there the need for any special counting equipment other than manual tablet counters or moderately sensitive scales for weighing.

Hospitals requiring large scale prepackaging operations have found it feasible to establish a separate unit for this facet of the total operation. Here, a separate lay work force is marshalled under the supervision of a pharmacist, and the monumental task is undertaken with the assistance of automatic filling machines for liquid preparations, automatic tablet and capsule counters and automatic labeling machines.

In between these two extremes lies the majority of the hospitals. That is, the volume is too great for a total hand operation, yet too small for a separate automated division within the department proper. Here, the pharmacy staff usually rotates the responsibility for maintaining a supply of prepackaged goods. Oftentimes, the pharmacist may have available the assistance of lay personnel already on the pharmacy payroll, other staff pharmacists during off-peak hours, or members of the volunteer staff in the hospital.

The prepackaging of drugs in this type of operation usually makes use of some semi-automatic packaging aids such as the various types of automatic and electronic tablet and capsule counters, automatic filling and capping machines, pipetting machines, and semi-automatic labeling equipment. Figure 71 demonstrates one such piece of equipment—the King "Dispensa" electronic tablet and capsule counter.

Although the above-mentioned equipment is intended for use in the larger hospital, there is on the market a number of units intended for use in the small hospital. This is particulary true with the various tablet counters.

TYPES OF CONTAINERS

The literature is amply documented[1,2] with the pros and cons associated with the choice of container for dispensing pharmaceuticals. This controversy was made possible by the advent of the plastic con-

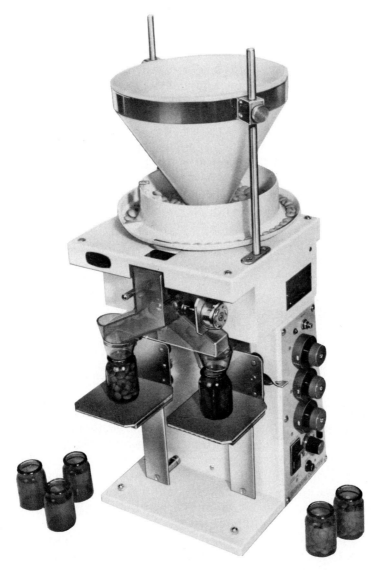

Fig. 71. The King "Dispensa." (Courtesy of Modular Packaging Systems, Inc., E. Hanover, N.J.)

tainer, the plasticized paper or cardboard package, and the strip package. Those opposed to the use of these modern packaging aids often cite the requirements of the *United States Pharmacopeia* and *National Formulary* which direct that the official preparations be packaged, stored and preserved in air-tight, light-resistant containers.

The general claim is usually based upon the observation that some plastic containers do not meet the standards of moisture vapor transmission set for well-closed containers, that volatile oils and certain dyes migrate through the walls of polyethylene containers, and that "plastic containers" do not withstand heat sterilization.

A sophisticated study of the literature will quickly dispel many of these observations for, in fact, high density polyethylene containers do protect against migration of volatile oils, do measure up to high standards in the moisture vapor transmission tests, and can be subjected to heat sterilization.

Although plastic materials do all these things, it is the considered opinion of many that they still do not fully meet the requirements of the official compendia.

Despite these generally divergent views, the ASHP Technical Assistance Bulletin on Single Unit and Unit Dose Packages of Drugs provides the following information:[3]

ASHP TECHNICAL ASSISTANCE BULLETIN ON SINGLE UNIT AND UNIT DOSE PACKAGES OF DRUGS[a]

Drug packages must fulfill four basic functions: (1) identify their contents completely and precisely; (2) protect their contents from deleterious environmental effects (e.g., photodecomposition); (3) protect their contents from deterioration due to handling (e.g., breakage, contamination); (4) permit their contents to be used quickly, easily, and safely. Modern drug-distribution systems use single unit packages to a great extent and, in fact, such packages are central to the operation of unit dose systems, intravenous admixture services, and other important aspects of pharmacy practice. These guidelines have been prepared to assist pharmaceutical manufacturers and pharmacists in the development and production of single unit and unit dose packages, the use of which has been shown to have substantial benefits.

A *single unit* package is one which contains one discrete pharmaceutical dosage form, i.e., one tablet, one 2-ml volume of liquid, one 2-g mass of ointment, etc. A *unit dose* package is one which contains that particular dose of the drug ordered for the patient. A single unit package is also a *unit dose* or *single dose* package if it contains the particular dose of the drug ordered for the patient. A unit dose package could, for example, contain two tablets of a drug product.

---

[a]Approved by the ASHP Board of Directors, November 14–15, 1984. Revised by the ASHP Council on Clinical Affairs. Supersedes the previous version, which was approved on March 31–April 1, 1977.

General Considerations

Packaging Materials. Packaging materials (and the package itself) must possess the physical characteristics required to protect the contents from (as required) light, moisture, temperature, air, and handling. The material should not deteriorate during the shelf life of the contents. Packages should be of lightweight, nonbulky materials that do not produce toxic fumes when incinerated. Materials that may be recycled or are biodegradable, or both, are to be preferred over those that are not. Packaging materials should not absorb, adsorb, or otherwise deleteriously affect their contents. Information should be available to practitioners indicating the stability and compatibility of drugs with various packaging materials.

Shape and Form. Packages should be constructed so that they do not deteriorate with normal handling. They should be easy to open and use, and their use should require little or no special training or experience. Unless the package contains a drug to be added to a parenteral fluid or otherwise used in compounding a finished dosage form, it should allow the contents to be administered directly to the patient (or IPPB apparatus or fluid administration set) without any need for repackaging into another container or device (except for ampuls).

Label Copy. Current federal labeling requirements must be adhered to, with attention also given to the items below. The desired copy and format are as follows:

Nonproprietary Name
(and propietary name, if to be shown)
Dosage Form (if special or other than oral)
Strength
Strength of Dose and Total Contents
Delivered
(e.g., no of tablets and their total dose)
Special Notes (e.g., refrigerate)
Expiration Date
Control Number

1. *Nonproprietary and Proprietary Name(s).* The nonproprietary name and the strength should be the most prominent part of the package label. It is not necessary to include the proprietary name, if any, on the package. The name of the manufacturer or distributor should appear on the package. In addition, the name of the manufacturer of the finished dosage form should be included in the product labeling. The style of type should be chosen to provide maximum legibility, contrast, and permanence.
2. *Dosage Form.* Special characteristics of the dosage form should be a part of the label, e.g., extended release. Packages should be labeled as to the route of administration if other than oral, e.g., topical use. In a package containing an injection, the acceptable injectable route(s) of administra-

tion should be stated on both outer and inner packages, i.e., both on the syringe unit and carton (if any).

3. *Strength.* Strength should be stated in accordance with terminology in the *American Hospital Formulary Service.* The metric system should be used, with dosage forms formulated to provide the rounded-off figures in the USP table of approximate equivalents and expressed in the smallest whole number.

   Micrograms should be used through 999, then milligrams through 999, then grams. Thus, 300 mg, *not* 5 gr, nor 325 mg, nor 0.3 g; 60 mg, *not* 1 gr. nor 0.06 g, nor 64.5 mg, nor 65 mg; 400 µg, *not* 1/150 gr, nor 0.4 mg, nor 0.0004 g; ml (milliliters) should be used instead of cc (cubic centimeters).

4. *Strength of Dose and Total Contents Delivered.* The total contents *and* total dose of the package should be indicated. Thus, a unit dose package containing a 600-mg dose as two 300-mg tablets should be labeled: "600 mg (as two 300-mg tablets)." Likewise, a 500-mg dose of a drug in a liquid containing 100 mg/ml should be labeled: "Delivers 500 mg (as 5 ml of 100 mg/ml)."

5. *Special Notes.* Special notes such as conditions of storage (e.g., refrigerate), preparation (e.g., shake well, moisten), and administration (e.g., not to be chewed) that are not obvious from the dosage form designation are to be included on the label.

6. *Expiration Date.* The expiration date should be prominently visible on the package. If the contents must be reconstituted prior to use, the shelf life of the final product should be indicated. Unless stability data warrant otherwise, all expiration dates should fall during January and July to simplify product recall procedures.

7. *Control Number (Lot Number).* The control number should appear on the package.

Product Identification Codes. The use of product identification codes, appearing directly on the dosage form, is encouraged.

Evidence of Entry. The package should be so designed that it is evident, when the package is still intact, that it has never been entered or opened.

Specific Considerations

Oral Solids.
1. *Blister Package.* A blister package should
   a. Have an opaque and nonreflective backing (flat upper surface of package) for printing,
   b. Have a blister (dome or bubble) of a transparent material that is, preferably, flat bottomed,
   c. Be easily peelable, and
   d. If it contains a controlled substance, be numbered sequentially for accountability purposes.
2. *Pouch Package.* A pouch package should
   a. Have one side opaque and nonreflective for printing,
   b. Be easily deliverable, i.e., large tablets in large pouches, small tablets in small pouches,

c. Tear from any point or from multiple locations, and

d. If it contains a controlled substance, be numbered sequentially for accountability purposes.

3. The packages should be such that contents can be delivered directly to the patient's mouth or hand.

Oral Liquids.

1. The packages should be filled to deliver the labeled contents. It is recognized that overfilling will be necessary, depending on the shape of the container, the container material, and the formulation of the dosage form.

2. The label should state the contents as follows: Delivers _____mg (or g or µg) in _____ml.

3. If reconstitution is required, the amount of vehicle to be added should be indicated. These directions may take the form of "fill to mark on container" in lieu of stating a specific volume.

4. Syringe-type containers for oral administration should not accept a needle and should be labeled "For Oral Use Only."

5. Containers should be designed to permit administration of the contents directly from the package.

Injectables.

1. The device shall be appropriately calibrated in mililiters and scaled from the tip to the fill line. Calibrated space may be built into the device to permit addition of other drugs. The label should state the contents as follows: Delivers _____mg (or g in µg) in _____ml.

2. An appropriate-size needle may be an integral part of the device. The needle sheath should not be the plunger. The plunger should be mechanically stable in the barrel of the syringe.

3. The device should be of such a design that it is patient-ready and assembly instructions are not necessary.

4. The sheath protecting the needle should be a nonpenetrable, preferably rigid material, to protect personnel from injury. The size of the needle should be indicated.

5. The device shall be of such a design that easy and visible aspiration is possible. It should be as compact as possible and to such a size that it can be easily handled.

Pareteral Solutions and Additives

1. The approximate pH and osmolarity of parenteral solutions should be stated on the label. The amount of overfill also should be noted. Electrolyte solutions should be labeled in both meq (or millimole) and mg concentrations. Solutions commonly labeled in terms of percent concentrations, e.g., dextrose, should also be labeled in w/v terms.

2. Parenteral fluid container labels should be readable when hanging and when upright or in the normal manipulative position.

3. Drugs to be mixed with parenteral infusion solutions should be packaged into convenient sizes that minimize the need for solution transfers and other manipulations.

4. Partially filled piggyback-type containers should
   a. Be recappable with a tamperproof closure,
   b. Have a hanger,
   c. Have volume markings,

    d. Be designed to minimize the potential for contamination during use, and

    e. Contain a partial vacuum for ease of reconstitution.

  5. If an administration set is included with the container, it should be compatible with all large-volume parenteral delivery systems.

Other Dosage Forms—Ophthalmics, Suppositories, Ointments, etc. Dosage forms other than those specifically discussed above should be adequately labeled to indicate their use and route of administration and should adhere to the above and other required package labeling and design criteria.

    The following excerpts from ASHP Technical Assistance Bulletin on Hospital Drug Distribution and Control[10] are useful to the student:

ASHP TECHNICAL ASSISTANCE BULLETIN ON HOSPITAL DRUG DISTRIBUTION AND CONTROL

    (10) *Medication Containers, Labeling and Dispensing: Inpatient Medications.* Drug products should be as ready for administration to the patient as the current status of pharmaceutical technology permits. Inpatient medication containers and packages should conform to applicable USP requirments and the ASHP guidelines.

    Inpatient self-care and "discharge" medications should be labeled as outpatient prescriptions (see below).

    (11) *Medication Containers, Labeling and Dispensing: Outpatient Medications.* Outpatient medications must be labeled in accordance with state board of pharmacy and federal regulations. As noted, medications given to patients as "discharge medication" must be labeled in the pharmacy (not by nursing personnel) as outpatient prescriptions.

    The source of the medication and initials of the dispenser should be noted on the prescription form at the time of dispensing. If feasible, the lot number also should be recorded.

    An identifying check system to ensure proper identification of outpatients should be established.

    Outpatient prescriptions should be packaged in accordance with the provisions of the Poison Prevention Packaging Act of 1970 and any regulations thereunder. They must also meet any applicable requirements of the USP.

    Any special instructions to or procedures required of the patient relative to the drug's preparation, storage, and administration should be either a part of the label or accompany the medication container received by the patient. Counseling of the patient sufficient to ensure understanding and compliance (to the extent possible) with his medication regimen must be conducted. Nonprescription drugs, if used in the institution, should be labeled as any other medication.

LABELING

The ASHP Technical Assistance Bulletin on Hospital Drug Distribution and Control states the following:[10]

(9) *Medication Containers, Labeling and Dispensing: Stock Containers.* The pharmacist is responsible for labeling medication containers. Medication labels should be typed or machine-printed. Labeling with pen or pencil and the use of adhesive tape or china marking pencils should be prohibited. A label should not be superimposed on another label. The label should be legible and free from erasures and strikeovers. It should be firmly affixed to the container. The labels for stock containers should be protected from chemical action or abrasion and bear the name, address, and telephone number of the hospital. Medication containers and labels should not be altered by anyone other than pharmacy personnel. Prescription labels should not be distributed outside the pharmacy. Accessory labels and statements (shake well, may not be refilled, and the like) should be used as required. Any container to be used outside the institution should bear its name, address, and phone number.

Important labeling considerations are:

1. The metric system should be given prominence on all labels when both metric and apothecary measurement units are given.
2. The names of all therapeutically active ingredients should be indicated in compound mixtures.
3. Labels for medications should indicate the amount of drug or drugs in each dosage unit (e.g., per 5 ml., per capsule).
4. Drugs and chemicals in forms intended for dilution or reconstitution should carry appropriate directions.
5. The expiration date of the contents, as well as proper storage conditions, should be clearly indicated.
6. The acceptable route(s) of administration should be indicated for parenteral medications.
7. Labels for large-volume sterile solutions should permit visual inspection of the container contents.
8. Numbers, letters, coined names, unofficial synonyms, and abbreviations should not be used to identify medications, with the exception of approved letter or number codes for investigational drugs (or drugs being used in blinded clinical studies).
9. Containers presenting difficulty in labeling, such as small tubes, should be labeled with no less than the prescription serial number, name of drug, strength, and name of the patient. The container should then be placed in a larger carton bearing a label with all necessary information.
10. The label should conform to all applicable federal, state, and local laws and regulations.

11. Medication labels of stock containers and repackaged or prepackaged drugs should carry codes to identify the source and lot number of medication.

12. Nonproprietary name(s) should be given prominence over proprietary names.

13. Amount dispensed (e.g., number of tablets) should be indicated.

The labeling of the various prepackaged drugs must be considered as one of the most important steps in the entire operation, yet, unfortunately, too many hospital pharmacists take this step for granted. Consider the following implications which may result from improperly labeled units.

1. If the preparation of the label to be applied to a particular batch of prepackaged drug is wrong, then every container in the lot, whether it be 50 units or 500 units, is also improperly labeled. This could lead to innumerable incidents on the pavilions and thereby cast reflections upon the accuracy of the pharmacy staff.

2. Insufficient information on the label may cause the nurse or physician or even the patient to make unnecessary and time-consuming telephone calls to the pharmacy.

3. Improperly or inaccurately labeled containers are an indication that the safety controls and checks are not functioning adequately.

4. In case of a drug recall by the manufacturer, it may be difficult to remove the affected containers from circulation due to the insufficient data on the label.

5. Labels which are ambiguous may lead to medication errors or may mislead the prescriber as to its contents.

One hospital pharmacist[4] utilizes a $\frac{1}{4} \times 2$-inch pressure sensitive label upon which is printed the following information:

Proprietary name	Pharmaceutical classification
Generic name	Description of the product
Strength	Control number

The finished label in this instance is quite informative and in itself has a number of built-in checks against improper package contents and the possible administration of the wrong medication to a patient. Figure 72 is an example of this type of label.

Labeling a medication container with the generic name of the product is considered to be proper. However, the use of a brand or proprietary name other than the one which actually describes the contents is never proper; as a matter of fact it may be considered to be fraudulent. It is also considered to be improper if the proprietary name is used in such a manner as to imply that the contents are the same, although every one concerned knows that they are of a different make.

The format in Figure 73 has been recommended for the labeling of

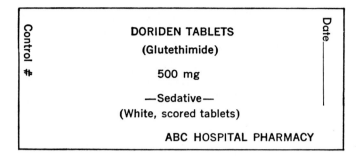

Fig. 72

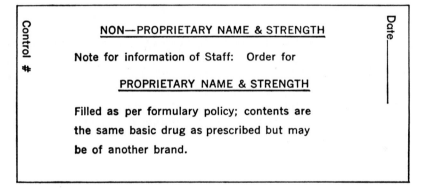

Fig. 73

medication containers in the hospital in order to overcome the above situations.

Because many drugs which are prepackaged in the hospital bear an expiration date, it is advisable to include this on an ancillary label. Although some hospital pharmacists feel that this is not needed because of the rapid consumption of drugs in the hospital and the fact that the proper control record will provide this information, it is suggested that the hospital prepackaging operation should comply with the rules set for manufacturers or other prepackagers of drugs.

In this regard, it is of interest to note that the regulations governing the location of expiration dates on labels of drug packages appeared in the *Federal Register of July 16, 1958* and reads as follows:

"3.507 *Location of Expiration Date in Drug Labeling.* Drugs which require an expiration date should show the expiration date on the immediate container. When the immediate container is packaged in an individual carton, the expiration date should also be placed on the carton. When single dose containers are packed in single cartons, the expiration date may properly appear on the carton only. . . ."

For the benefit of the student or those who wish to, for the first time, establish a prepackaging program, the following is a program of labeling which when pursued will provide the safety and control needed in a successful operation.

Step One.—Using a marking or printing machine, prepare the proper number of self-adhering labels bearing the following information:

    a. Date of prepackaging by month and year.
       e.g. 8/79.
    b. On the next line insert the name of the manufacturer.
    c. On the third line insert the control number assigned by the man-
       ufacturer.
    d. If the item is a dated product, place the expiration date on the far
       right of the first line, *e.g.* 8/79 (on left), 9/80 (on right).

Thus the completed tag will appear as shown in Figure 74.

This tag is then affixed to the container and is not to be removed by nursing or pharmacy personnel. Whenever dry goods are packaged, the label is placed on the inside of the cap of the capsule or tablet vial thus reducing the temptation to remove it.

Step Two.—Again using a marking or printing machine prepare the proper number of self-adhering labels bearing the following information:

    a. Date of prepackaging by month and year.
    b. Name and strength of the drug.
    c. Unit cost—coded if desirable.
    d. Unit selling price.
    e. Number of capsules on far right of the first line.

Thus, the finished tag appears as shown in Figure 75 and is affixed to the outside of the container.

Step Three.—Affix any ancillary labels which are required, *e.g.* for the Eye; for the Nose; Refrigerate, etc.

Step Four.—When the unit is dispensed, the tag described in Step Two is removed from the container and affixed to the prescription or to the medication order slip.

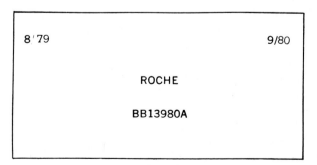

8'79   9/80

ROCHE

BB13980A

Fig. 74

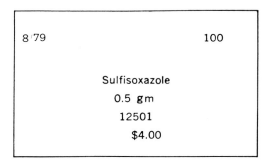

8/79   100

Sulfisoxazole

0.5 gm

12501

$4.00

Fig. 75

Many pharmacists have expressed the opinion that this final step is unnecessary and is burdensome; however it serves the purpose of affording the checking pharmacist another visible means (in addition to the characterstic color or shape of the dispensed product) of ascertaining accuracy.

Recently a national survey[11] was conducted to determine the policies of hospital pharmacies regarding expiration dates for repackaged pharmaceuticals. The results were that less than one third of the responding institutions followed the current FDA recommendations for dating oral solids repackaged from bulk. Almost one quarter used the manufacturer's date. Only 5.6% of the hospitals used more conservative dating. Similar percentages were found for the dating of oral liquids. One third of the hospitals used 30 to 90 days to date repackaged injectables.

The Control Record

Besides accurate and comprehensive labeling practices, it is essential that the pharmacist maintain a written control record. Many different varieties of records may be kept; that is, sheets, cards, books, etc. What is important is the information which appears on these records.

Miller[5] recommends the use of a control card upon which is transcribed the following information:

a. Item packaged
b. Manufacturer's control number
c. Total number of units
d. Size of each unit
e. Identity of the prepacker
f. Identity of the checker
g. Type of container and closure

Figure 76 is an example of one type of prepackaging record. Of interest here is the fact that a separate sheet is used for each product prepackaged and should be retained for a period of one year after the last entry.

HOSPITAL PHARMACY

PRE-PACKAGING CONTROL RECORD

PRODUCT: _____
STRENGTH: _____

FORM
(Check One)

Capsule _____   Elixir _____   Solution _____
Tablet _____   Syrup _____   Ointment _____
Powder _____   Tincture _____   Other _____

MFG.	MFG. LOT #	DATE OF PURCHASE	HOSPITAL PRE-PACK LOT #	UNIT OF PRE-PACK	DATE OF PRE-PACK	NUMBER PRE-PACKED	PACK'D BY	LABELED BY	CHECK'D BY

MISCELLANEOUS COMMENTS

Fig. 76

Strip Packaging

In discussing the various methods of drug distribution in the hospital (Chap. 13), reference was made to the commercial availability of many drug products in strip packages. The pharmaceutical industry has made many drugs available to the hospital pharmacy in prepackaged strips of 5 tablets or capsules, rolls of 25 and rolls of 100. Each strip of 5 is then placed in a bulk dispensing carton, whereas the rolled strips are packaged in cardboard reel-type dispensing packages.

In spite of industry's good intentions, there still remains a large number of drugs, in common hospital use, that are not strip packaged. Thus, some hospital pharmacists have, in cooperation with industrial packagers, sought to develop a practical yet inexpensive means of strip packaging within the hospital. One such study at the University of Kentucky Medical Center[6] has resulted in the development of both a machine and a program.

In describing the project, the authors state that the operational principles of the machine are basic:

Two strips of packaging material are fed through the machine from reels mounted on each side. As this packaging material is pulled into the meshing crimp rollers: (1) the packaging material is labeled where the pocket is to be formed; (2) the tablet or capsule is placed in position to be entrapped in the pocket; (3) the two strips of packaging material are sealed around the tablet or capsule to form the pocket and are then pulled from the heated crimp rollers. Thus, the three phases of the packaging operation are completed.

The packaging machine is known as the Una-Strip Packer.

Prior to undertaking such a program, the hospital pharmacist should undertake studies to ascertain the volume of drugs which must be prepackaged. He must develop a satisfactory label to comply with all legal requirements, and finally he must select the proper packaging material to protect the product against air, moisture, and light.

A comparison of five hospitals to determine labor savings if single unit packaged medications replaced those now prepared and dispensed from bulk containers revealed the following figures:[7]

(a) Estimated labor cost per dose in the pharmacy for existing methods averaged 1.61 cents while the unit dose average was 1.33 cents. For nurses, the figures were 14.6 cents and 14 cents respectively. This represents a cost of 16.2 cents per dose for existing methods as opposed to 14.3 cents for unit dose.

(b) There was a direct labor savings of two cents per unit with single-dose dispensing over existing bulk-methods, versus an average cost increase of one cent per single-unit of medications over conventional bulk containers.

Because many hospital pharmacists operating in a large medical center prefer for reasons of availability and economy to repackage oral solids and liquids in single unit and unit dose packages, it is important that certain precautions be undertaken to assure the integrity of the final package. In a collaborative effort the American Society of Hospital Pharmacists and the American Society of Consultant Pharmacists developed a set of guidelines for repackaging oral medications in single unit and unit dose packages. The following is a verbatim, presentation of these **Guidelines.**[8]

ASHP TECHNICAL ASSISTANCE BULLETIN ON REPACKAGING ORAL SOLIDS AND LIQUIDS IN SINGLE UNIT AND UNIT DOSE PACKAGES[a]

To maximize the benefits of a unit dose drug distribution system, all drugs must be packaged in single unit or unit dose packages.[b] However, not all drugs are commercially available in single unit (or unit dose) packages. Therefore, the institutional pharmacist must often repackage drugs obtained in bulk containers (e.g., bottles of 500 tablets) into single unit packages so that they may be used in a unit dose system.

---

[a]Revised by the ASHP Board of Directors, November 16–17, 1978. This document was developed originally by a joint working group of the American Society of Hospital Pharmacists and the American Society of Consultant Pharmacists and representatives of the drug packaging industry. The original document subsequently was approved officially by the boards of directors of ASHP and ASCP. The Food and Drug Administration reviewed the original document and commended ASHP and ASCP for developing the Guidelines.

[b]A *single unit* package is one which contains one discrete pharmaceutical dosage form, e.g., one tablet, one 5-ml volume of liquid, etc. A *unit dose* package is one which contains the particular dose of drug ordered for the patient. A *single unit* package is a *unit dose* (or *single dose*) package if it contains that particular dose of drug ordered for the patient.

Certain precautions must be taken if the quality of drugs repackaged by the pharmacist is to be maintained. The guidelines presented herein will assist the pharmacist in developing procedures for repackaging drugs in a safe and acceptable manner.

1. The packaging operation should be isolated, to the extent possible, from other pharmacy activities.
2. Only one drug product at a time should be repackaged in a specific work area. No drug products other than the one being repackaged should be present in the immediate packaging area. Also, no labels other than those for the product being packaged should be present in the area.
3. Upon completion of the packaging run, all unused stocks of drugs and all finished packages should be removed from the packaging area. The packaging machinery and related equipment should then be completely emptied, cleaned and inspected before commencing the next packaging operation.
4. All unused labels (if separate labels are utilized) should be removed from the immediate packaging area. The operator should verify that none remain in the packaging machine(s). If labels are prepared as part of the packaging operation, the label plate (or analogous part of the printing apparatus) should be removed or adjusted to "blank" upon completion of the run. This will help assure that the correct label is printed during any subsequent run. There should be a procedure to reconcile the number of packages produced with the number of labels used (if any) and/or destroyed (if any) and the number of units or volume of drug set forth to be packaged.
5. Before beginning a packaging run, an organoleptic evaluation (color, odor, appearance and markings) of the drug product being repackaged should be made. The bulk container should also be examined for evidence of water damage, contamination or other deleterious effects.
6. All packaging equipment and systems should be operated and used in accordance with the manufacturer's or other established instructions. There should be valid justification and authorization by the supervisor for any deviation from those instructions on the part of the operator.
7. The pharmacist should obtain data on the characteristics of all packaging materials used. This information should include data on the chemical composition, light transmission, moisture permeability, size, thickness (alone or in laminate), recommended sealing temperature and storage requirements.
8. Unit dose packages and labels should, to the extent possible, comply with the American Society of Hospital Pharmacists' "Guidelines for Single Unit and Unit Dose Packages of Drugs."[1]
9. Whenever feasible, a responsible individual, other than the packaging operator, should verify that: (a) the packaging system (drug, materials, machines) is set up correctly and (b) all procedures have been performed properly. Ultimate responsibility for all packaging operations rests with the pharmacist.
10. Control records of all packaging runs must be kept. These records should include the following information: (1) complete description of the product, i.e., name, strength, dosage form, route of administration, etc.; (2) the product's manufacturer or supplier; (3) control number; (4) the pharmacy's control number if different from the manufacturer's; (5) expiration dates of the original container and the repackaged product; (6) number

of units packaged and the date(s) they were packaged; (7) initials of the operator and checker (if any); (8) a sample of the label and, if feasible, a sample of the finished package which should not be discarded until after the expiration date and which should be examined periodically for signs of deterioration; (9) description (including lot number) of the packaging materials and equipment used.

11. It is the responsibility of the pharmacist, taking into account the nature of the drug repackaged, the characteristics of the package, and the storage conditions to which the drug may be subjected, to determine the expiration date to be placed on the package. This date must not be beyond that of the original package.[a]

12. All drugs should be packaged and stored in a temperature- and humidity-controlled environment to minimize degradation caused by heat and moisture. A relative humidity of 75% at 23° C should not be exceeded. Packing materials should be stored in accordance with the manufacturer's instructions and any applicable regulations.

13. Written procedures (both general and product-specific) governing repackaging operations should be prepared and updated as required. Any deviation from these procedures should be noted and explained on the control record. Operators must understand the procedures (and operation of all packaging equipment) before commencing the run.

14. Applicable FDA and USP requirments concerning the type of package required for specific drug products must be followed.

15. Drugs and chemicals with high vapor pressures should be stored separately from other products in order to minimize cross contamination.

REFERENCES

1. American Society of Hospital Pharmacists. ASHP guidelines for single unit and unit dose packages of drugs. Am. J. Hosp. Pharm., 1977; *34*:613–4.
2. Stolar, M.H.: Expiration dates of repackaged drug products. Am. J. Hosp. Pharm., 1979; *36*:170. Editorial.

QUALITY CONTROL GUIDELINES FOR SINGLE PACKAGING OF PARENTERALS

The primary manufacturer of a product is liable for the quality and safety of his product until such time as another party assumes the responsibility from him. In the hospital pharmacy, the manufacturer may be relieved of his responsibility for the product whenever the hospital pharmacist undertakes to repackage it. Thus, to repackage and store these products without an adequate quality control program may result in a lawsuit for the hospital.

A good quality control program should concern itself with the details involved in container selection in order to eliminate stability and compatibility programs arising from a reaction with capping material or even the plunger tip. Contamination of the parenteral solution must be

[a]For specific recommendations on expiration-date policy, see reference 2.

guarded against from such sources as personnel, environment, and containers. Vials and syringes should be checked for accuracy of calibration in order that the amount of overfill be ascertained.

The filling process should be performed under a laminar airflow hood and detailed records should be maintained.[9]

SELECTED READINGS

Turco, S.J.: Chairman's Overview—National Coordinating Committee on Large Volume Parenterals. Infusion, *2*:4–7, (Jan.–Feb.) 1979.
———: Recommendations for the Labeling of Large Volume Parenterals. Infusion, *1*:2:50, (Nov.–Dec.) 1977.

REFERENCES

1. Archambault, G.F.: Plastics and the U.S.P. Requirements for Tight, Light-Resistant Containers. Am. J. Hosp. Pharm., *15*:877, 1958.
2. ———: Standards for Prescription Containers. Am. J. Hosp. Pharm., *20*:538, 1952.
3. ASHP Technical Assistance Bulletin on Single Unit and Unit Dose Packages of Drugs. Am. J. Hosp. Pharm., *42*:378–379, 1985.
4. Benya, Theodore J.: Labeling Pre-packaged Medication. Am. J. Hosp. Pharm., *19*:1:20, 1962.
5. Webb, John W.: Methods of Promoting Safety and Control in Hospital Pharmacy. Am. J. Hosp. Pharm., *15*:11:977, 1958.
6. Samuels, Tom M. and Guthrie, Don L.: Unit Dose Packaging—a New Machine for Strip Packaging Tablets and Capsules. Am. J. Hosp. Pharm., *23*:1:4, 1966.
7. Blasingame, W.G., Drevno, Harold, Godley, Leo F., Kratz, Richard L., Vona, Joseph P., and Minott, Paul: Some Time and Motion Considerations with Single-Unit Packaged Drugs in Five Hospitals. Am. J. Hosp. Pharm., *26*:6:310, (June) 1969.
8. ASHP Guidelines fo Repackaging Oral Solids and Liquids in Single Unit and Unit Dose Packages. Am. J. Hosp. Pharm., *40*:451–452, (Mar.) 1983.
9. Patel, J.A., Curtis, E.G., and Phillips, G.L.: Quality Control Guidelines for Single Unit Packaging of Parenterals in the Hospital Pharmacy. Am. J. Hosp. Pharm., *29*:11:947, (Nov.) 1972.
10. ASHP Technical Assistance Bulletin on Hospital Drug Distribution and Control. Am. J. Hosp. Pharm., *37*:1097–1103, (Aug.) 1980.
11. Chaney, R.F. and Summerfield, M.: Survey of Expiration Dating Policies for Repackaged Pharmaceuticals. Am. J. Hosp. Pharm., *41*:1150–1152, 1984.

21|

Manufacturing—
Bulk and Sterile

Statistical data on manufacturing or bulk compounding in hospitals[1] revealed that approximately 41% of 1853 hospital pharmacies operate a manufacturing program. The survey further demonstrated that 78% of the sample group prepared galenical pharmaceuticals; 74%, products not commercially available; 42%, sterile solutions for topical use; 33%, sterile pharmaceuticals such as collyria, ointments etc.; and 30%, small volume injectable solutions.

In addition, the same survey[2] showed that hospital pharmacists were also active in the preparation of sterile products such as surgical irrigating fluids, large volume injectable solutions, and special sterile products for investigational use.

This volume of hospital manufacturing may surprise the neophyte pharmacist particularly when viewed in the light of the magnitude of the American pharmaceutical industry. Obviously, there must be some explanation to this paradox. Those knowledgeable in the ways of the profession have advanced a number of reasons the more important of which are *(a)* that there exists a close relationship between doctors and pharmacists in hospitals, *(b)* that commercially available products are not often suited for the treatment of certain unusual illnesses which the physician with a hospital practice is expected to cope with, and *(c)* that, because of the physician-pharmacist relationship in the hospital, doctors feel at ease in requesting the pharmacist to prepare a special pharmaceutical form either for clinical or experimental use.

Also worthy of consideration here is the fact that hospital pharmacists engaged in this type of practice often encourage and promulgate its expansion and growth because they are of the consensus that such an activity promotes economy within the hospital, complements the operation of the formulary system, increases the prestige of the hospital pharmacist, and provides the research clinician with the opportunity to develop new pharmaceutical formulations.

Those responsible for the education and training of future hospital pharmacists consider a manufacturing or bulk compounding program to be an extremely useful endeavor which draws together the classroom concepts of courses in product development, physical chemistry, instrumental methods of analysis, and preservation and stabilization of pharmaceutical products.

A manufacturing program within the department of pharmacy is also of interest to trustees and administrators because of its ability to reduce the cost of pharmaceuticals to patients and is, therefore, encouraged by them, whenever the pharmacist shows the desire and the ability to undertake such an endeavor.

For the purposes of this chapter, a manufacturing program for the hospital pharmacy shall be deemed to encompass both bulk compounding of pharmaceuticals and the preparation of sterile products. The same meticulous standards and principles should apply to the preparation of both classes of products.

Control

The word "control" is defined[3] as

"To test or verify (a statement or experiment) by counter or parallel evidence or experiment."
"To exercise directing, guiding or restraining power over."

The ASHP Technical Assistance Bulletin on Hospital Drug Distribution and Control makes the following provision:[17]

ASHP TECHNICAL ASSISTANCE BULLETIN ON HOSPITAL DRUG DISTRIBUTION AND CONTROL

In-house Manufacturing, Bulk Compounding, Packaging and Labeling. As with commercially marketed drug products, those produced by the pharmacy must be accurate in identity, strength, purity, and quality. Therefore, there must be adequate process and finished-product controls for all manufacturing/bulk compounding and packaging operations. Written master formulas and batch records (including product test results) must be maintained. All technical personnel must be adequately trained and supervised.

Packaging and labeling operations must have controls sufficient to prevent product/package/label mixups. A lot number to identify each finished product with its production and control history must be assigned to each batch.

The Good Manufacturing Practices of the Food and Drug Administration is a useful model for developing a comprehensive control system.

The pharmacist is encouraged to prepare those drug dosage forms, strengths, and packagings which are needed for optimal drug therapy, but which are commercially unavailable. Adequate attention must be given to the stability, palatability, packaging, and labeling requirements of these products.

Klemme[4] has suggested that hospital pharmacists should consider control of their manufacturing program from two vantage points—"quality control" to govern the quality, purity and strength of the manufactured product and "budgetary control" to regulate the economic aspects of the program. All too often, the hospital pharmacist devotes a great deal of thought and effort to the quality control aspect of the manufacturing program only to learn that he has a technically and professionally sound program but at the same time one which is in economic distress.

Accordingly, the principles of budgetary and quality control will be discussed under separate sections within this chapter.

BUDGETARY CONTROL

In order to develop adequate budgetary control over the manufacturing program, the hospital pharmacist is required to give lengthy consideration to his *inventory* and *consumption rate* for the *finished product, raw materials requirement, manufacturing capacity, available personnel* and *operating costs.*

Manufacturing Requirements

Probably the most difficult task lies in prognosticating, with reasonable accuracy, the consumption rate for each item to be included in a manufacturing program. This can be done by reviewing the records of the previous year or two and comparing this figure with the staff's present prescribing pattern. Since the figure to be arrived at is, at best, an educated guess, the pharmacist should not become too alarmed if, at the end of the first quarter, he realizes that he has overestimated or underestimated his requirements. Whichever the case may be, corrective measures may be put into effect for the second quarter, namely, increase the rate or volume of production or reduce the batch quantity or frequency of manufacture or eliminate one batch of the product which is considered to be above desirable inventory limits.

Material Requirements

Once the hospital pharmacist has determined what products he intends to manufacture and in what volume and quantity, he must next arrange for the procurement of the necessary supplies. These supplies should include, in addition to raw materials, such items as containers, labels and ancillary materials such as filter paper, filter pads, boxes, and special labels.

The first step in this direction is to take each formula and determine the quantity of chemical or other material which will be required to produce the annual supply. This is done by taking the quantities of raw materials from the working formula and packaging specifications of each item and multiplying these quantities by the number of times the formula must be produced to satisfy the estimated annual requirement.

The second step is to enter these quantities on a *summary sheet* because the same drug, chemical or container may be required by many different formulas.

By totaling the quantities under each item on the summary sheet, the pharmacist will now have available to him his annual supplies and material needs to undertake the contemplated manufacturing program.

Since the budget period of the hospital is on a yearly basis, the purchasing agent or the purchasing pharmacist will divide the material and supply requirements into four quarters. This will allow the purchasing group ample time to utilize the basic principles of good purchasing technics and at the same time ensure against over inventory and shortage of materials in the pharmacy.

Manufacturing Capacity

Two important considerations in any bulk compounding program are first whether or not the pharmacist has available to him the kind of equipment necessary to produce the formulas selected and secondly, whether or not the machinery is capable of producing the desired quantity.

Because time is the costliest factor in any manufacturing program, it behooves the pharmacist to utilize the maximum capacity of his equipment. In addition, the selection of equipment should be made on the basis of the multiple or variety of uses to which a single piece of equipment can be put. This will prevent costly equipment from accumulating idle time.

Manufacturing Equipment and Its Sources

The kind and size of manufacturing equipment required in the hospital pharmacy will vary from institution to institution. Primary consideration must be given to the scope of the manufacturing program, the quantities to be produced during any production run as well as to the length of time that will be required to consume the product, the availability of personnel and the availability of physical facilities.

Modern technology has developed equipment to meet every production need. The available machinery can handle amounts that are considered to be of "practical volume or quantity" for a small or medium sized hospital. In addition, the larger hospitals have available to them automatic and semi-automatic heavy duty production equipment which is capable of handling large volume in a minimum of time.

In *Remington's Practice of Pharmacy,*[5] the student will find pictures and a brief description of the various pieces of equipment which may be useful in the formulation of pharmaceutical preparations.

As a means of assisting the pharmacist desirous of mechanizing his bulk compounding department, many producers of pharmaceutical manufacturing and packaging equipment have prepared excellent descriptive brochures and catalogues which are of value in assisting the pharmacist in selecting the most versatile equipment for his particular use and needs.

Manufacturing Staff

Next to equipment, personnel represent the most important consideration in a bulk compounding program. Too many personnel will raise the cost of a manufactured product to the point where it would be more economical to purchase it from a commercial supplier and too little help may mean the inability to maintain an adequate production schedule and potential errors—neither of which may be condoned.

Accordingly, production time must be determined for each formula in order that proper planning and scheduling be effected.

The manufacturing section of the pharmacy must be supervised by a technically competent, legally qualified pharmacist. In addition he must be supported with ancillary personnel who can be trained to carry on such non-technical pursuits as bottling, filtering, labeling, etc. Under no circumstances should a bulk compounding program be undertaken without the services of a pharmacist under the pretense that this is justified by the reduction in labor cost and that reasonably intelligent lay help can be trained to perform specific tasks with accuracy and dependability.

Operating Costs

A review of the literature pertaining to manufacturing programs in hospital pharmacies and central sterile supply rooms leads one to believe that many so-called "profitable ventures" are classified as such mainly because of an understated operating cost. In these instances, the operating cost was shown to consist of the direct costs only—direct labor and cost of materials.

Correctly used, operating costs should include both direct and indirect costs.[6] The terminology "overhead costs" is usually used interchangeably with "indirect costs" and, for the purpose of this section, is intended to include such items as the cost of supervisory personnel, space rental, insurance, equipment depreciation, maintenance, housekeeping, etc. In some hospitals, those items not directly connected with the pharmacy operation are included in a figure obtainable from the comptroller's office known as the *"overhead per square foot"* figure.

By whatever means obtainable, the indirect costs should be compared with the direct costs for the purpose of calculating a ratio of overhead dollars to direct labor dollars which may later be applied in ascertaining the true dost of the product.

An example of the above principle is best demonstrated as follows:
  a. Assume that the ratio of indirect costs to direct costs in hospital X is 100%.
  b. Further assume that 5 gallons of product "A" require $4.25 in materials and $5.50 in direct costs. Therefore,

              Direct Cost
                   Materials .... $ 4.25
                   Labor 5.50
              Indirect Cost............   9.75
                   TOTAL COST ......$19.50 for 5 gallons

It is of importance to call the student's attention at this point to the fact that if the quantity of product "A" in the above example were doubled, only the cost of materials could double. The direct and indirect costs *do not* increase in direct proportion because it requires little more time to manufacture 10 gallons than it does to manufacture 5 gallons. The packaging segment of the operation is where the direct labor cost will be in direct proportion to the batch size.

Since the increase in batch size will, to a point, reduce the unit cost, the student is cautioned that the cost curve does not decrease geometrically with the increase in batch size. Also, it is unwise to manufacture in a volume which will not be consumed within a reasonable period of time for this will now introduce problems in storage, long term product preservation, and reduced inventory turn-over.

QUALITY CONTROL

The term "quality control" should not be confused with the term "statistical quality control" which involves the application of statistics for the control of sizes, weights and other physical characteristics of articles undergoing mass production. Statistical quality control plays an important role in large scale pharmaceutical production plants but has little value in the control aspect of hospital pharmacy manufacturing programs.

What is more important to hospitals, their staff and patients is a quality control that will ensure the integrity of the label. This can best be accomplished by developing a series of cross checks and laboratory analyses.

It should be clearly understood that no two hospitals develop control systems which are identical in every respect,[7,8] and therefore no system can here be recommended which will serve every purpose. Accordingly, it becomes the responsibility of the hospital pharmacist to make whatever modifications he deems necessary to ensure a product which will meet high pharmaceutical standards.

The FDA has published good manufacturing practices regulations which went into effect on March 28, 1979. Because one lawyer specializing in pharmacy law has stated[16] the concern that pharmacists may be required to comply with these regulations, they are presented here in order to permit the hospital pharmacist to compare his recent quality control program with the specific considerations which ordinarily form the basis of a quality control program utilized by the pharmaceutical industry.

GOOD MANUFACTURING PRACTICE REGULATIONS

Title 21, Code of Federal Regulations sections 211.1 through 211.208 provides cogent minimum current good manufacturing practice for preparation of drug products for administration to humans or animals.

SUBPART B—ORGANIZATION AND PERSONNEL

§ 211.22 Responsibilities of Quality Control Unit

(a) There shall be a quality control unit that shall have the responsibility and authority to approve or reject all components, drug product containers, closures, in-process materials, packaging material, labeling, and drug products, and the authority to review production records to assure that no errors have occurred or, if errors have occurred, that they have been fully investigated. The quality control unit shall be responsible for approving or rejecting drug products manufactured, processed, packed, or held under contract by another company.

(b) Adequate laboratory facilities for the testing and approval (or rejection) of components, drug product containers, closures, packaging materials, in-process materials, and drug products shall be available to the quality control unit.

(c) The quality control unit shall have the responsibility for approving or rejecting all procedures or specifications impacting on the identity, strength, quality, and purity of the drug product.

(d) The responsibilities and procedures applicable to the quality control unit shall be in writing; such written procedures shall be followed.

§ 211.25 Personnel Qualifications

(a) Each person engaged in the manufacture, processing, packing, or holding of a drug product shall have education, training, and experience, or any combination thereof, to enable that person to perform the assigned functions. Training shall be in the particular operations that the employee performs and in current good manufacturing practice (including the current good manufacturing practice regulations in this chapter and written procedures required by these regulations) as they relate to the employee's functions. Training in current good manufacturing practice shall be conducted by qualified individuals on a continuing basis and with sufficient frequency to assure that employees remain familiar with CGMP requirements applicable to them.

(b) Each person responsible for supervising the manufacture, processing, packing, or holding of a drug product shall have the education, training, and experience, or any combination thereof, to perform assigned fuctions in such a manner as to provide assurance that the drug product has the safety, identity, strength, quality, and purity that it purports or is represented to possess.

(c) There shall be an adequate number of qualified personnel to perform and supervise the manufacture, processing, packing, or holding of each drug product.

§ 211.28 Personnel Responsibilities

(a) Personnel engaged in the manufacture, processing, packing, or holding of a drug product shall wear clean clothing appropriate for the duties they perform. Protective apparel, such as head, face, hand, and arm coverings, shall be worn as necessary to protect drug products from contamination.

(b) Personnel shall practice good sanitation and health habits.

(c) Only personnel authorized by supervisory personnel shall enter those areas of the buildings and facilities designated as limited-access areas.

(d) Any person shown at any time (either by medical examination or supervisory observation) to have an apparent illness or open lesions that may adversely affect the safety or quality of drug products shall be excluded from direct contact with components, drug product containers, closures, in-process materials, and drug products until the condition is corrected or determined by competent medical personnel not to jeopardize the safety or quality of drug products. All personnel shall be instructed to report to supervisory personnel any health conditions that may have an adverse effect on drug products.

§ 211.34 Consultants

Consultants advising on the manufacture, processing, packing, or holding of drug products shall have sufficient education, training, and experience, or any combination thereof, to advise on the subject for which they are retained. Records shall be maintained stating the name, address, and qualifications of any consultants and the type of service they provide.

SUBPART C—BUILDINGS AND FACILITIES

§ 211.42 Design and Construction Features

(a) Any building or buildings used in the manufacture, processing, packing, or holding of a drug product shall be of suitable size, construction and location to facilitate cleaning, maintenance, and proper operations.

(b) Any such building shall have adequate space for the orderly placement of equipment and materials to prevent mixups between different components, drug product containers, closures, labeling, in-process materials, or drug products, and to prevent contamination. The flow of components, drug product containers, closures, labeling, in-process materials, and drug products through the building or buildings shall be designed to prevent contamination.

(c) Operations shall be performed within specifically defined areas of adequate size. There shall be separate or defined areas for the firm's operations to prevent contamination or mixups as follows:

(1) Receipt, identification, storage, and withholding from use of components, drug product containers, closures, and labeling, pending the appropriate sampling, testing, or examination by the quality control unit before release for manufacturing or packaging;

(2) Holding rejected components, drug product containers, closures and labeling before disposition;

(3) Storage of released components, drug product containers, closures, and labeling;

(4) Storage of in-process materials;

(5) Manufacturing and processing operations;

(6) Packaging and labeling operations;

(7) Quarantine storage before release of drug products;

(8) Storage of drug products after release;

(9) Control and laboratory operations;

(10) Aseptic processing, which includes as appropriate:

(i) Floors, walls, and ceilings of smooth, hard surfaces that are easily cleanable;

(ii) Temperature and humidity controls;

(iii) An air supply filtered through high-efficiency particulate air filters under positive pressure, regardless of whether flow is laminar or non-laminar;

(iv) A system for monitoring environmental conditions;

(v) A system for cleaning and disinfecting the room and equipment to produce aseptic conditions;

(vi) A system for maintaining any equipment used to control the aseptic conditions.

(d) Operations relating to the manufacture, processing, and packing of penicillin shall be performed in the facilities separate from those used for other drug products for human use.

§ 211.44 Lighting

Adequate lighting shall be provided in all areas.

§ 211.46 Ventilation, Air Filtration, Air Heating and Cooling

(a) Adequate ventilation shall be provided.

(b) Equipment for adequate control over air pressure, microorganisms, dust, humidity, and temperature shall be provided when appropriate for the manufacture, processing, packing, or holding of a drug product.

(c) Air filtration systems, including prefilters and particulate matter air filters, shall be used when appropriate on air supplies to production areas. If air is recirculated to production areas, measures shall be taken to control recirculation of dust from production. In areas where air contamination occurs during production, there shall be adequate exhaust systems or other systems adequate to control contaminants.

(d) Air-handling systems for the manufacture, processing, and packing of penicillin shall be completely separate from those for other drug products for human use.

§ 211.48 Plumbing

(a) Potable water shall be supplied under continuous positive pressure in a plumbing system free of defects that could contribute contamination to any drug product. Potable water shall meet the standards prescribed in the Public Health Service Drinking Water Standards set forth in Subpart J of 42 CFR Part 72. Water not meeting such standards shall not be permitted in the potable water system.

(b) Drains shall be of adequate size and, where connected directly to a sewer, shall be provided with an air break or other mechanical device to prevent back-siphonage.

§ 211.50 Sewage and Refuse

Sewage, trash, and other refuse in and from the building and immediate premises shall be disposed of in a safe and sanitary manner.

§ 211.52 Washing and Toilet Facilities

Adequate washing facilities shall be provided, including hot and cold water, soap or detergent, air driers or single-service towels, and clean toilet facilities easily accessible to working areas.

§ 211.56 Sanitation

(a) Any building used in the manufacture, processing, packing, or holding of a drug product shall be maintained in a clean and sanitary condition. Any such building shall be free of infestation by rodents, birds, insects, and other vermin (other than laboratory animals). Trash and organic waste matter shall be held and disposed of in a timely and sanitary manner.

(b) There shall be written procedures assigning responsibility for sanitation and describing in sufficient detail the cleaning schedules, methods, equipment, and materials to be used in cleaning the buildings and facilities; such written procedures shall be followed.

(c) There shall be written procedures for use of suitable rodenticides, insecticides, fungicides, fumigating agents, and cleaning and sanitizing agents. Such written procedures shall be designed to prevent the contamination of equipment, components, drug product containers, closures, packaging, labeling materials, or drug products and shall be followed. Rodenticides, insecticides, and fungicides shall not be used unless registered and used in accordance with the Federal Insecticide, Fungicide, and Rodenticide Act (7 U.S.C. 135).

(d) Sanitation procedures shall apply to work performed by contractors or temporary employees as well as work performed by full-time employees during the ordinary course of operations.

§ 211.58 Maintenance

Any building used in the manufacture, processing, packing, or holding of a drug product shall be maintained in a good state of repair.

SUBPART D—EQUIPMENT

§ 211.63 Equipment Design, Size, and Location

Equipment used in the manufacture, processing, packing, or holding of a drug product shall be of appropriate design, adequate size, and suitably located to facilitate operations for its intended use and for its cleaning and maintenance.

§ 211.65 Equipment Construction

(a) Equipment shall be constructed so that surfaces that contact components, in-process materials, or drug products shall not be reactive, additive, or absorptive so as to alter the safety, identity, strength, quality, or purity of the drug product beyond the official or other established requirements.

(b) Any substances required for operation, such as lubricants or coolants, shall not come into contact with components, drug product containers, closures, in-process materials, or drug products so as to alter the safety, identity, strength, quality, or purity or the drug product beyond the official or other established requirements.

§ 211.67 Equipment Cleaning and Maintenance

(a) Equipment and utensils shall be cleaned, maintained, and sanitized at appropriate intervals to prevent malfunctions or contamination that would alter the safety, identity, strength, quality, or purity of the drug product beyond the official or other established requirements.

(b) Written procedures shall be established and followed for cleaning and maintenance of equipment, including utensils, used in the manufacture, processing, packing, or holding of a drug product. These procedures shall include, but are not necessarily limited to, the following:

(1) Assignment of responsibility for cleaning and maintaining equipment;

(2) Maintenance and cleaning schedules, including, where appropriate, sanitizing schedules;

(3) A description in sufficient detail of the methods, equipment, and materials used in cleaning and maintenance operations, and the methods of disassembling and reasembling equipment as necessary to assure proper cleaning and maintenance;

(4) Removal or obliteration of previous batch identification;

(5) Protection of clean equipment from contamination prior to use;

(6) Inspection of equipment for cleanliness immediately before use.

(c) Records shall be kept of maintenance, cleaning, sanitizing, and inspection as specified in § § 211.180 and 211.182.

§ 211.68 Automatic, Mechanical, and Electronic Equipment

(a) Automatic, mechanical, or electronic equipment or other types of equipment, including computers, or related systems that will perform a function satisfactorily, may be used in the manufacture, processing, packing, and holding of a drug product. If such equipment is so used, it shall be routinely calibrated, inspected, or checked according to a written program designed to assure proper performance. Written records of those calibration checks and inspections shall be maintained.

(b) Appropriate controls shall be exercised over computer or related systems to assure that changes in master production and control records or other records are instituted only by authorized personnel. Input to and output from the computer or related system of formulas or other records or data shall be checked for accuracy. A backup of data entered into the computer or related system shall be maintained except where certain data, such as calculations performed in connection with laboratory analysis, are eliminated by computerization or other automated processes. In such instances a written record of the program shall be maintained along with appropriate validation data. Hard copy or alternative systems, such as duplicates, tapes, or microfilm, designed to assure that backup data are exact and complete and that it is secure from alteration, inadvertent erasures, or loss shall be maintained.

§ 211.72 Filters

Filters for liquid filtration used in the manufacture, processing, or packing of injectable drug products intended for human use shall not release fibers into such products. Fiber-releasing filters may not be used in the manufacture, processing, or packing of these injectable drug products unless it is not possible to manufacture such drug products without the use of such filters. If use of a fiber-releasing filter is necessary, an additional non-fiber-releasing filter of 0.22 micron maximum mean porosity (0.45 micron if the manufacturing conditions so dictate) shall subseqently be used to reduce the content of particles in the injectable drug product. Use of an asbestos-containing filter, with or without subsequent use of a specific non-fiber-releasing filter, is permissible only upon submission of proof to the appropriate bureau of the Food and Drug Administration that use of a non-fiber-releasing filter will, or is likely to, compromise the safety or effectiveness of the injectable drug product.

SUBPART E—CONTROL OF COMPONENTS AND DRUG PRODUCT CONTAINERS AND CLOSURES

§ 211.80 General Requirements

(a) There shall be written procedures describing in sufficient detail the receipt, identification, storage, handling, sampling, testing, and approval or rejection of components and drug product containers and closures; such written procedures shall be followed.

(b) Components and drug product containers and closures shall at all times be handled and stored in a manner to prevent contamination.

(c) Bagged or boxed components or drug product containers, or closures shall be stored off the floor and suitably spaced to permit cleaning and inspection.

(d) Each container of grouping of containers for components or drug product containers, or closures shall be identified with a distinctive code for each lot in each shipment received. This code shall be used in recording the disposition of each lot. Each lot shall be appropriately identified as to its status (i.e., quarantined, approved, or rejected).

§ 211.82. Receipt and Storage of Untested Components, Drug Product Containers, and Closures

(a) Upon receipt and before acceptance, each container or grouping of containers of components, drug product containers, and closures shall be examined visually for appropriate labeling as to contents, container damage or broken seals, and contamination.

(b) Components, drug product containers, and closures shall be stored under quarantine until they have been tested or examined, as appropriate, and released. Storage within the area shall conform to the requirements of § 211.80.

§ 211.84 Testing and Approval or Rejection of Components, Drug Product Containers, and Closures

(a) Each lot of components, drug product containers, and closures shall be withheld from use until the lot has been sampled, tested, or examined, as appropriate, and released for use by the quality control unit.

(b) Representative samples of each shipment lot shall be collected for testing or examination. The number of containers to be sampled, and the amount of material to be taken from each container, shall be based upon appropriate criteria such as statistical criteria for component variability, confidence levels, and degree of precision desired, the past quality history of the supplier, and the quantity needed for analysis and reserve where required by § 211.170.

(c) Samples shall be collected in accordance with the following procedures:

(1) The containers of components selected shall be cleaned where necessary by appropriate means.

(2) The containers shall be opened, sampled, and resealed in a manner designed to prevent contamination of their contents and contamination of other components, the drug product containers, or closures.

(3) Sterile equipment and aseptic sampling techniques shall be used when necessary.

(4) If it is necessary to sample a component from the top, middle, and bottom of its container, such sample subdivisions shall not be composited for testing.

(5) Sample containers shall be identified so that the following informaiton can be determined: name of the material sampled, the lot number, the container from which the sample was taken, the data on which the sample was taken, and the name of the person who collected the sample.

(6) Containers from which samples have been taken shall be marked to show that samples have been removed from them.

(d) Samples shall be examined and tested as follows:

(1) At least one test shall be conducted to verify the identity of each component of a drug product. Specific identity tests, if they exist, shall be used.

(2) Each component shall be tested for conformity with all appropriate written specifications for purity, strength, and quality. In lieu of such testing by the manufacturer, a report of analysis may be accepted from the supplier of a component, provided that at least one specific identity test is conducted on each component by the manufacturer, and provided that the manufacturer establishes the reliability of the supplier's analyses through appropriate validation of the supplier's test results at appropriate intervals.

(3) Containers and closures shall be tested for conformance with all appropirate written procedures. In lieu of such testing by the manufacturer, a certificate of testing may be accepted from the supplier, provided that at least a visual identification is conducted on such container/closures by the manufacturer and provided that the manufacturer establishes the reliability of the supplier's test results through the appropriate validation of the supplier's test results at appropriate intervals.

(4) When appropriate, components shall be microscopically examined.

(5) Each lot of a component, drug product container, or closure that is liable to contamination with filth, insect infestation, or other extraneous adulterant shall be examined against established specifications for such contamination.

(6) Each lot of a component, drug product container, or closure that is liable

to microbiological contamination that is objectionable in view of its intended use shall be subjected to microbiological tests before use.

(e) Any lot of components, drug product containers, or closures that meets the appropriate written specifications of identity, strength, quality, and purity and related tests under paragraph (d) of this section may be approved and released for use. Any lot of such material that does not meet such specifications shall be rejected.

§ 211.86 Use of Approved Components, Drug Product Containers, and Closures

Components, drug product containers, and closures approved for use shall be rotated so that the oldest approved stock is used first. Deviation from this requirement is permitted if such deviation is temporary and appropriate.

§ 211.87 Retesting of Approved Components, Drug Product Containers, and Closures

Components, drug product containers, and closures shall be retested or reexamined, as appropriate, for identity, strength, quality, and purity and approved or rejected by the quality control unit in accordance with § 211.84 as necessary, e.g., after storage for long periods or after exposure to air, heat, or other conditions that might adversely affect the component, drug product container, or closure.

§ 211.89 Rejected Components, Drug Product Containers, and Closures

Rejected components, drug product containers, and closures shall be identified and controlled under a quarantine system designed to prevent their use in manufacturing or processing operations for which they are unsuitable.

§ 211.94. Drug Product Containers and Closures

(a) Drug product containers and closures shall not be reactive, additive, or absorptive so as to alter the safety, identity, strength, quality, or purity of the drug beyond the official or established requirements.

(b) Container closure systems shall provide adequate protection against foreseeable external factors in storage and use that can cause deterioration or contamination of the drug product.

(c) Drug product containers and closures shall be clean and, where indicated by the nature of the drug, sterilized and processed to remove pyrogenic properties to assure that they are suitable for their intended use.

(d) Standards or specifications, methods of testing, and, where indicated, methods of cleaning, sterilizing, and processing to remove pyrogenic properties shall be written and followed for drug product containers and closures.

SUBPART F—PRODUCTION AND PROCESS CONTROLS

§ 211.100 Written Procedures; Deviations

(a) There shall be written procedures for production and process control designed to assure that the drug products have the identity, strength, quality, and purity they purport or are represented to possess. Such procedures shall include all requirements in this subpart. These written procedures, including any changes, shall be drafted, reviewed, and approved by the appropriate organizational units and reviewed and approved by the quality control unit.

(b) Written production and process control procedures shall be followed in the execution of the various production and process control functions and shall be documented at the time of performance. Any deviation from the written procedures shall be recorded and justified.

§ 211.101 Charge-in of Components

Written production and control procedures shall include the following, which are designed to assure that the drug products produced have the identity, strength, quality, and purity they purport or are represented to possess:

(a) The batch shall be formulated with the intent to provide not less than 100 percent of the labeled or established amount of active ingredient.

(b) Components for drug product manufacturing shall be weighed, measured, or subdivided as appropriate. If a component is removed from the original container to another, the new container shall be identified with the following information:

(1) Component name or item code;

(2) Receiving or control number;

(3) Weight or measure in new container;

(4) Batch for which component was dispensed, including its product name, strength, and lot number.

(c) Weighing, measuring, or subdividing operations for components shall be adequately supervised. Each container of component dispensed to manufacturing shall be examined by a second person to assure that:

(1) The component was released by the quality control unit;

(2) The weight or measure is correct as stated in the batch production records;

(3) The containers are properly identified.

(d) Each component shall be added to the batch by one person and verified by a second person.

§ 211.103 Calculation of Yield

Actual yields and percentages of theoretical yield shall be determined at the conclusion of each appropriate phase of manufacturing, processing, packaging, or holding of the drug product. Such calculations shall be performed by one person and independently verified by a second person.

§ 211.105 Equipment Identification

(a) All compounding and storage containers, processing lines, and major equipment used during the production of a batch of a drug product shall be properly identified at all times to include their contents and, when necessary, the phase of processing of the batch.

(b) Major equipment shall be identified by a distinctive identification number or code that shall be recorded in the batch production record to show the specific equipment used in the manufacture of each batch of a drug product. In cases where only one of a particular type of equipment exists in a manufacturing facility, the name of the the equipment may be used in lieu of a distinctive identification number or code.

§ 211.10 Sampling and Testing of In-Process Materials and Drug Products

(a) To assure batch uniformity and integrity of drug products, written procedures shall be established and followed that describe the in-process controls, and tests, or examinations to be conducted on appropriate samples of in-process materials of each batch. Such control procedures shall be established to monitor the output and to validate the performance of those manufacturing processes that may be responsible for causing variability in the characteristics of in-process material and the drug product. Such control procedures shall include, but are not limited to, the following, where appropriate:

(1) Tablet or capsule weight variation;

(2) Disintegration time;

(3) Adequacy of mixing to assure uniformity and homogeneity;

(4) Dissolution time and rate;

(5) Clarity, completeness, or pH of solutions.

(b) Valid in-process specifications for such characteristics shall be consistent with drug product final specifications and shall be derived from previous acceptable process averages and process variability estimates where possible and determined by the application of suitable statistical procedures where appropriate. Examination and testing of samples shall assure that the drug product and in-process material conform to specifications.

(c) In-process materials shall be tested for identity, strength, quality, and purity as appropriate, and approved or rejected by the quality control unit, during the production process, e.g., at commencement or completion of significant phases or after storage for long periods.

(d) Rejected in-process materials shall be identified and controlled under a quarantine system designed to prevent their use in manufacturing or processing operations for which they are unsuitable.

§ 211.111 Time Limitations on Production

When appropriate, time limits for the completion of each phase of production shall be established to assure the quality of the drug product. Deviation from established time limits may be acceptable if such deviation does not compromise the quality of the drug product. Such deviation shall be justified and documented.

§ 211.113 Control of Microbiological Contamination

(a) Appropriate written procedures, designed to prevent objectionable microorganisms in drug products not required to be sterile, shall be established and followed.

(b) Appropriate written procedures, designed to prevent microbiological contamination of drug products purporting to be sterile, shall be established and followed. Such procedures shall include validation of any sterilization process.

§ 211.115 Reprocessing

(a) Written procedures shall be established and followed prescribing a system for reprocessing batches that do not conform to standards or specifications and the steps to be taken to insure that the reprocessed batches will conform with all established standards, specifications, and characteristics.

(b) Reprocessing shall not be performed without the review and approval of the quality control unit.

SUBPART G—PACKAGING AND LABELING CONTROL

§ 211.122 Materials Examination and Usage Criteria

(a) There shall be written procedures describing in sufficient detail the receipt, identification, storage, handling, sampling, examination, and/or testing of labeling and packaging materials; such written procedures shall be followed. Labeling and packaging materials shall be representatively sampled and examined or tested upon receipt and before use in packaging or labeling of a drug product.

(b) Any labeling or packaging materials meeting appropriate written specifications may be approved and released for use. Any labeling or packaging materials that do not meet such specifications shall be rejected to prevent their use in operations for which they are unsuitable.

(c) Records shall be maintained for each shipment received of each different labeling and packaging material indicating receipt, examination or testing, and whether accepted or rejected.

(d) Labels and other labeling materials for each different drug product, strength, dosage form, or quantity of contents shall be stored separately with suitable identification. Access to the storage area shall be limited to authorized personnel.

(e) Obsolete and outdated labels, labeling, and other packaging materials shall be destroyed.

(f) Gang printing of labeling to be used for different drug products or different strengths of the same drug product (or labeling of the same size and identical or similar format and/or color schemes) shall be minimized. If gang printing is employed, packaging and labeling operations shall provide for special control procedures, taking into consideration sheet layout, stacking, cutting, and handling during and after printing.

(g) Printing devices on, or associated with, manufacturing lines used to imprint labeling upon the drug product unit label or case shall be monitored to assure that all imprinting conforms to the print specified in the batch production record.

§ 211.125 Labeling Issuance

(a) Strict control shall be exercised over labeling issued for use in drug product labeling operations.

(b) Labeling materials issued for a batch shall be carefully examined for identity and conformity to the labeling specified in the master or batch production records.

(c) Procedures shall be utilized to reconcile the quantities of labeling issued, used, and returned, and shall require evaluation of discrepancies found between the quantity of drug product finished and the quantity of labeling issued when such discrepancies are outside narrow preset limits based on historical operating data. Such discrepancies shall be investigated in accordance with § 211.192.

(d) All excess labeling bearing lot or control numbers shall be destroyed.

(e) Returned labeling shall be maintained and stored in a manner to prevent mixups and provide proper identification.

(f) Procedures shall be written describing in sufficient detail the control procedures employed for the issuance of labeling; such written procedures shall be followed.

§ 211.130 Packaging and Labeling Operations

There shall be written procedures designed to assure that correct labels, labeling, and packaging materials are used for drug products; such written procedures shall be followed. These procedures shall incorporate the following features:

(a) Prevention of mixups and cross-contamination by physical or spatial separation from operations on other drug products.

(b) Identification of the drug product with a lot or control number that permits determination of the history of the manufacture and control of the batch.

(c) Examination of packaging and labeling materials for suitability and correctness before packaging operations, and documentation of such examination in the batch production record.

(d) Inspection of the packaging and labeling facilities immediately before use to assure that all drug products have been removed from previous operations. Inspection shall also be made to assure that packaging and labeling materials not suitable for subsequent operations have been removed. Results of inspection shall be documented in the batch production records.

§ 211.134 Drug Product Inspection

(a) Packaged and labeled products shall be examined during finishing operations to provide assurance that containers and packages in the lot have the correct label.

(b) A representative sample of units shall be collected at the completion of finishing operations and shall be visually examined for correct labeling.

(c) Results of these examinations shall be recorded in the batch production of control records.

§ 211.137 Expiration Dating[a]

(a) To assure that a drug product meets applicable standard of identity, strength, quality, and purity at the time of use, it shall bear an expiration date determined by appropriate stability testing described in § 211.166.

(b) Expiration dates shall be related to any storage conditions stated on the labeling, as determined by stability studies described in § 211.166.

(c) If the drug product is to be reconstituted at the time of dispensing, its labeling shall bear expiration information for both the reconstituted and unreconstituted drug products.

(d) Expiration dates shall appear on labeling in accordance with the requirements of § 201.17 of this chapter.

(e) Homeopathic drug products shall be exempt from the requirements of this section.

(f) Pending consideration of a proposed exemption, published in the FEDERAL REGISTER of September 29, 1978, the requirements in this section shall not be enforced for human OTC drug products if their labeling does not bear dosage

[a]EFFECTIVE DATE NOTE: The expiration dating requirements under these amendments that have not been previously in effect shall apply to drug products packaged after September 28, 1979. See 44 FR 11064, Feb. 27, 1979.

limitations and they are stable for at least 3 years as supported by appropriate stability data.

SUBPART H—HOLDING AND DISTRIBUTION

§ 211.142 Warehousing Procedures

Written procedures describing the warehousing of drug products shall be established and followed. They shall include:

(a) Quarantine of drug products before release by the quality control unit.

(b) Storage of drug products under appropriate conditions of temperature, humidity, and light so that the identity, strength, quality, and purity of the drug products are not affected.

§ 211.150 Distribution Procedures

Written procedures shall be established, and followed, describing the distribution of drug products. They shall include:

(a) A procedure whereby the oldest approved stock of a drug product is distributed first. Deviation from this requirement is permitted if such deviation is temporary and appropriate.

(b) A system by which the distribution of each lot of drug product can be readily determined to facilitate its recall if necessary.

SUBPART I—LABORATORY CONTROLS

§ 211.160 General Requirements

(a) The establishment of any specifications, standards, sampling plans, test procedures, or other laboratory control mechanisms required by this subpart, including any change in such specifications, standards, sampling plans, test procedures, or other laboratory control mechanisms, shall be drafted by the appropriate organizational unit and reviewed and approved by the quality control unit. The requirements in this subpart shall be followed and shall be documented at the time of performance. Any deviation from the written specifications, standards, sampling plans, test procedures, or other laboratory mechanisms shall be recorded and justified.

(b) Laboratory controls shall include the establishment of scientifically sound and appropriate specifications, standards, sampling plans, and test procedures designed to assure that components, drug product containers, closures, in-process materials, labeling, and drug products conform to appropriate standards of identity, strength, quality, and purity. Laboratory controls shall include:

(1) Determination of conformance to appropriate written specifications for the acceptance of each lot within each shipment of components, drug product containers, closures, and labeling used in the manufacture, processing, packing, or holding of drug products. The specifications shall include a description of the sampling and testing procedures used. Samples shall be representative and adequately identified. Such procedures shall also require appropriate retesting of any component, drug product container, or closure that is subject to deterioration.

(2) Determination of conformance to written specifications and a description of sampling and testing procedures for in-process materials. Such samples shall be representative and properly identified.

(3) Determination of conformance to written descriptions of sampling pro-

cedures and appropriate specifications for drug products. Such samples shall be representative and properly identified.

(4) The calibration of instruments, apparatus, gauges, and recording devices at suitable intervals in accordance with an established written program containing specific directions, schedules, limits for accuracy and precision, and provisions for remedial action in the event accuracy and/or precision limits are not met. Instruments, apparatus, gauges, and recording devices not meeting established specifications shall not be used.

§ 211.165 Testing and Release for Distribution

(a) For each batch of drug product, there shall be appropriate laboratory determination of satisfactory conformance to final specifications for the drug product, including the identity and strength of each active ingredient, prior to release. Where sterility and/or pyrogen testing are conducted on specific batches of shortlived radiopharmaceuticals, such batches may be released prior to completion of sterility and/or pyrogen testing, provided such testing is completed as soon as possible.

(b) There shall be appropriate laboratory testing, as necessary, of each batch of drug product required to be free of objectionable microorganisms.

(c) Any sampling and testing plans shall be described in written procedures that shall include the method of sampling and the number of units per batch to be tested; such written procedure shall be followed.

(d) Acceptance criteria for the sampling and testing conducted by the quality control unit shall be adequate to assure that batches of drug products meet each appropriate specification and appropriate statistical quality control criteria as a condition for their approval and release. The statistical quality control criteria shall include appropriate acceptance levels and/or appropriate rejection levels.

(e) The accuracy, sensitivity, specificity, and reproducibility of test methods employed by the firm shall be established and documented. Such validation and documentation may be accomplished in accordance with § 211.194(a)(2).

(f) Drug products failing to meet established standards or specifications and any other relevant quality control criteria shall be rejected. Reprocessing may be performed. Prior to acceptance and use, reprocessed material must meet appropriate standards, specifications, and other relevant criteria.

§ 211.166 Stability Testing

(a) There shall be a written testing program designed to assess the stability characteristics of drug products. The results of such stability testing shall be used in determining approximate storage conditions and expiration dates. The written program shall be followed and shall include:

(1) Sample size and test intervals based on statistical criteria for each attribute examined to assure valid estimates of stability;

(2) Storage conditions for samples retained for testing;

(3) Reliable, meaningful, and specific test methods;

(4) Testing of the drug product in the same container-closure system as that in which the drug product is marketed;

(5) Testing of drug products for reconstitution at the time of dispensing (as directed in the labeling) as well as after they are reconstituted.

(b) An adequate number of batches of each drug product shall be tested to determine an appropriate expiration date and a record of such data shall be maintained. Accelerated studies, combined with basic stability information on the components, drug products, and container-closure system, may be used to support tentative expiration dates provided full shelf life studies are not available and are being conducted. Where data from accelerated studies are used to project a tentative expiration date that is beyond a date supported by actual shelf life studies, there must be stability studies conducted, including drug product testing at appropriate intervals, until the tentative expiration date is verified or the appropriate expiration date determined.

(c) For homeopathic drug products, the requirements of this section are as follows:

(1) There shall be a written assessment of stability based at least on testing or examination of the drug product for compatibility of the ingredients, and based on marketing experience with the drug product to indicate that there is no degradation of the product for the normal or expected period of use.

(2) Evaluation of stability shall be based on the same container-closure system in which the drug product is being marketed.

§ 211.167 Special Testing Requirements

(a) For each batch of drug product purporting to be sterile and/or pyrogen-free, there shall be appropriate laboratory testing to determine conformance to such requirements. The test procedures shall be in writing and shall be followed.

(b) For each batch of ophthalmic ointment there shall be appropriate testing to determine conformance to specifications regarding the presence of foreign particles and harsh or abrasive substances. The test procedures shall be in writing and shall be followed.

(c) For each batch of controlled-release dosage form, there shall be appropriate laboratory testing to determine conformance to the specifications for the rate of release of each active ingredient. The test procedures shall be in writing and shall be followed.

§ 211.170 Reserve Samples

(a) An appropriately identified reserve sample representative of each lot in each shipment of each active ingredient shall be retained for at least 1 year after the expiration date of the last lot of the drug product containing the active ingredient or, in the case of certain OTC drug products lacking expiration dating because they meet the criteria for exemption under § 211.137, 3 years after distribution of the last drug product lot containing the active ingredient. It shall consist of at least twice the quantity necessary for all tests required to determine whether the active ingredient meets its established specifications, except the quantity requirement shall not apply for sterility and pyrogen samples.

(b) A properly identified reserve sample representative of each lot or batch of drug product shall be stored under conditions consistent with product labeling and shall be retained for at least 1 year after the expiration date of the drug product or in the case of certain OTC drug products lacking expiration dating because they meet the criteria for exemption under §211.137, 3 years after distribution of the lot or batch of drug product. The sample shall be stored in the same immediate container-closure system in which the drug product is marketed or an immediate container-closure system having essentially the same characteristics. The sample shall consist of at least twice the quantity necessary to perform all the required tests, except those for sterility and pyrogens. Such samples shall be at least visually examined annually for evidence of deterioration unless such examination would affect the integrity of the samples. The results of such examination shall be recorded and maintained with other stability data on the drug product. Samples of compressed medical gases need not be retained.

§ 211.173 Laboratory Animals

Animals used in testing components, in-process materials, or drug products for compliance with established specifications shall be maintained and controlled in a manner that assures their suitability for their intended use. They shall be identified, and adequate records shall be maintained showing the history of their use.

§ 211.176 Penicillin Contamination

If a reasonable possibility exists that a non-penicillin drug product has been exposed to cross-contamination with penicillin, the non-penicillin drug product shall be tested for the presence of penicillin. Such drug product shall not be marketed if detectable levels are found when tested according to procedures specified in "Procedures for Detecting and Measuring Penicillin Contamination in Drugs."[a]

SUBPART J—RECORDS AND REPORTS

§ 211.180 General Requirements

(a) Any production, control, or distribution record that is required to be maintained in compliance with this part and is specifically associated with a batch of the drug product shall be retained for at least 1 year after the expiration date of the batch or, in the case of certain OTC drug products lacking expiration dating because they meet the criteria for exemption under § 211.137, 3 years after distribution of the batch.

(b) Records shall be maintained for all components, drug product containers, closures, and labeling for at least 1 year after the expiration date or, in the case of certain OTC drug products lacking expiration dating because they meet the criteria for exemption under § 211.137, 3 years after distribution of the last lot of drug product incorporating the component or using the container, closure, or labeling.

(c) All records required under this part, or copies of such records, shall be readily available for authorized inspection during the retention period at the establishment where the activities described in such records occurred. These records or copies thereof shall be subject to photocopying or other means of reproduction as part of such inspection. Records that can be immediately retrieved from another location by computer or other electronic means shall be considered as meeting the requirements of this paragraph.

(d) Records required under this part may be retained either as original records or as true copies such as photocopies, microfilm, microfiche, or other accurate reproductions of the original records. Where reduction techniques, such as microfilming, are used, suitable reader and photocopying equipment shall be readily available.

(e) Written records required by this part shall be maintained so that data therein can be used for evaluating, at least annually, the quality standards of

---

[a]Copies may be obtained from: Director, NCAA (HFD-430), Food and Drug Administration, 200 C St. SW., Washington, D.C. 20204.

each drug product to determine the need for changes in drug product specifications or manufacturing or control procedures. Written procedures shall be established and followed for such evaluations and shall include provisions for:

(1) A review of every batch, whether approved or rejected, and, where applicable, records associated with the batch.

(2) A review of complaints, recalls, returned or salvaged drug products, and investigations conducted under § 211.192 for each drug product.

(f) Procedures shall be established to assure that the responsible officials of the firm, if they are not personally involved in or immediately aware of such actions, are notified in writing of any investigations conducted under § § 221.198, 211.204, or 211.208 of these regulations, any recalls, reports of inspectional observations issued by the Food and Drug Administration, or any regulatory actions relating to good manufacturing practices brought by the Food and Drug Administration.

§211.182 Equipment Cleaning and Use Log

A written record of major equipment cleaning, maintenance (except routine maintenance, such as lubrication and adjustments), and use shall be included in the individual equipment logs that show the date, time, product, and lot number of each batch processed. If equipment is dedicated to manufacture of one product, then individual equipment logs are not required, provided that lots of batches of such product follow in numerical order and are manufactured in numerical sequence. In cases where dedicated equipment is employed, the records of cleaning, maintenance, and use shall be part of the batch record. The persons performing and double-checking the cleaning and maintenance shall date and sign or initial the log indicating that the work was performed. Entries in the log shall be in chronological order.

§ 211.184 Component, Drug Container, Closure, and Labeling Records

These records shall include the following:

(a) The identity and quantity of each shipment of each lot of components, drug product containers, closures, and labeling; the name of the supplier; the supplier's lot number(s) if known; the receiving code as specified in § 211.80; and the date of receipt. The name and location of the prime manufacturer, if different from the supplier shall be listed if known.

(b) The results of any test or examination performed (including those performed as required by § 211.82(a), § 211.84(d), or § 211.122(a), and the conclusions derived therefrom.

(c) An individual inventory record of each component, drug product container, and closure and, for each component, a reconciliation of the use of each lot of such component. The inventory record shall contain sufficient information to allow determination of any batch or lot of drug product associated with the use of each component, drug product container, and closure.

(d) Documentation of the examination and review of labels and labeling for conformity with established specifications in accord with § 211.122(c) and § 211.130(c).

(e) The disposition of rejected components, drug product containers, closure, and labeling.

§ 211.186 Master Production and Control Records

(a) To assure uniformity from batch to batch, master production and control records for each drug product, including each batch size thereof, shall be prepared, dated, and signed (full signature, handwritten) by one person and independently checked, dated, and signed by a second person. The preparation of master production and control records shall be described in a written procedure and such written procedure shall be followed.

(b) Master production and control records shall include:

(1) The name and strength of the product and a description of the dosage form;

(2) The name and weight or measure of each active ingredient per dosage unit or per unit of weight or measure of the drug product, and a statement of the total weight or measure of any dosage unit;

(3) A complete list of components designated by names or codes sufficiently specific to indicate any special quality characteristic;

(4) An accurate statement of the weight or measure of each component, using the same weight system (metric, avoirdupois, or apothecary) for each component. Reasonable variations may be permitted, however, in the amount of components necessary for the preparation in the dosage form, provided thay are justified in the master production and control records;

(5) A statement concerning any calculated excess of component;

(6) A statement of theoretical weight or measure at appropriate phases of processing;

(7) A statement of theoretical yield, including the maximum and minimum percentages of theoretical yield beyond which investigation according to § 211.192 is required;

(8) A description of the drug product containers, closures, and packaging materials, including a specimen or copy of each label and all other labeling signed and dated by the person or persons responsible for approval of such labeling;

(9) Complete manufacturing and control instructions, sampling and testing procedures, specifications, special notations, and precautions to be followed.

§ 211.188 Batch Production and Control Records

Batch production and control records shall be prepared for each batch of drug product produced and shall include complete information relating to the production and control of each batch. These records shall include:

(a) An accurate reproduction of the appropriate master production or control record, checked for accuracy, dated, and signed;

(b) Documentation that each significant step in the manufacture, processing, packing, or holding of the batch was accomplished, including:

(1) Dates;

(2) Identity of individual major equipment and lines used;

(3) Specific identification of each batch of component or in-process material used;

(4) Weights and measures of components used in the course of processing;

(5) In-process and laboratory control results;

(6) Inspection of the packaging and labeling area before and after use;

(7) A statement of the actual yield and a statement of the percentage of theoretical yield at appropriate phases of processing;

(8) Complete labeling control records, including specimens or copies of all labeling used;

(9) Description of drug product containers and closures;

(10) Any sampling performed;

(11) Identification of the persons performing and directly supervising or checking each significant step in the operation;

(12) Any investigation made according to § 211.192.

(13) Results of examinations made in accordance with § 211.134.

§ 211.192 Productions Record Review

All drug product production and control records, including those for packaging and labeling, shall be reviewed and approved by the quality control unit to determine compliance with all established, approved written procedures before a batch is released or distributed. Any unexplained discrepancy (including a percentage of theoretical yield exceeding the maximum or minimum percentages established in master production and control records) or the failure of a batch or any of its components to meet any of its specifications shall be thoroughly investigated, whether or not the batch has already been distributed. The investigation shall extend to other batches of the same drug product and other drug products that may have been associated with the specific failure or discrepancy. A written record of the investigation shall be made and shall include the conclusions and followup.

§ 211.194 Laboratory Records

(a) Laboratory records shall include complete data derived from all tests necessary to assure compliance with established specifications and standards, including examinations and assays, as follows;

(1) A description of the sample received for testing with identification of source (that is, location from where sample was obtained), quantity, lot number or other distinctive code, date sample was taken, and date sample was received for testing.

(2) A statement of each method used in the testing of the sample. The statement shall indicate the location of data that establish that the methods used in the testing of the sample meet proper standards of accuracy and reliability as applied to the product tested. (If the method employed is in the current revision of the United States Pharmacopeia, National Formulary, Association of Official Analytical Chemists, Book of Methods,[a] or in other recognized standard references, or is detailed in an approved new drug application and the referenced method is not modified, a statement indicating the method and reference will suffice.) The suitability of all testing methods used shall be verified under actual conditions of use.

(3) A statement of the weight or measure of sample used for each test, where appropriate.

(4) A complete record of all data secured in the course of each test, including all graphs, charts, and spectra from laboratory instrumentation, properly identified to show the specific component, drug product container, closure, in-process material, or drug product, and lot tested.

(5) A record of all calculations performed in connection with the test, including units of measure, conversion factors, and equivalency factors.

(6) A statement of the results of tests and how the results compare with

---

[a]Copies may be obtained from: Association of Official Analytical Chemists, P.O. Box 540, Benjamin Franklin Station, Washington, D.C. 20204.

established standards of identity, strength, quality, and purity for the component, drug product container, or drug product tested.

(7) The initials, or signature of the person who performs each test and the date(s) the tests were performed.

(8) The initials or signature of a second person showing that the original records have been reviewed for accuracy, completeness, and compliance with established standards.

(a) Complete records shall be maintained of any modification of an established method employed in testing. Such records shall include the reason for the modification and data to verify that the modification produced results that are at least as accurate and reliable for the material being tested as the established method.

(b) Complete records shall be maintained of any testing and standardization of laboratory reference standards, reagents, and standard solutions.

(c) Complete records shall be maintained of the periodic calibration of laboratory instruments, apparatus, gauges, and recording devices required by § 211.160(b)(4).

(d) Complete records shall be maintained of all stability testing performed in accordance with § 211.166.

§ 211.196 Distribution Records

Distribution records shall contain the name and strength of the product and a description of the dosage form, name and address of the consignee, date and quantity shipped, and lot or control number of the drug product.

§ 211.198 Complaint Files

(a) Written procedures describing the handling of all written and oral complaints regarding a drug product shall be established and followed. Such procedures shall include provisions for review by the quality control unit, or any complaint involving the possible failure of a drug product to meet any of its specifications and, for such drug products, a determination as to the need for an investigation in accordance with § 211.192.

(b) A written record of each complaint shall be maintained in a file designated for drug product complaints. The file regarding such drug product complaints shall be maintained at the establishment where the drug product involved was manufactured, processed, or packed, or such file may be maintained at another facility if the written records in such files are readily available for inspection at that other facility. Written records involving a drug product shall be maintained until at least 1 year after the expiration date of the drug product, or 1 year after the date that the complaint was received, whichever is longer. In the case of certain OTC drug products lacking expiration dating because they meet the criteria for exemption under § 211.137, such written records shall be maintained for 3 years after distribution of the drug product.

(1) The written record shall include the following information, where known: The name and strength of the drug product, lot number, name of complainant, nature of complaint, and reply to complainant.

(2) Where an investigation under § 211.192 is conducted, the written record shall include the findings of the investigation and followup. The record or copy of the record of the investigation shall be maintained at the establishment where the investigation occurred in accordance with § 211.180(c).

(3) Where an investigation under § 211.192 is not conducted, the written

record shall include the reason that an investigation was found not to be necessary and the name of the responsible person making such a determination.

SUBPART K—RETURNED AND SALVAGED DRUG PRODUCTS

§ 211.204 Returned Drug Products

Returned drug products shall be identified as such and held. If the conditions under which returned drug products have been held, stored, or shipped before or during their return, or if the condition of the drug product, its container, carton, or labeling, as a result of storage or shipping, casts doubt on the safety, identity, strength, quality or purity of the drug product, the returned drug product shall be destroyed unless examination, testing, or other investigations prove the drug product meets appropriate standards of safety, identity, strength, quality, or purity. A drug product may be reprocessed provided the subsequent drug product meets appropriate standards, specification, and characteristics. Records of returned drug products shall be maintained and shall include the name and label potency of the drug product dosage form, lot number (or control number or batch number), reason for the return, quantity returned, date of disposition, and ultimate disposition of the returned drug product. If the reason for a drug product being returned implicates associated batches, an appropriate investigation shall be conducted in accordance with the requirements of § 211.192. Procedures for the holding, testing, and reprocessing of returned drug products shall be in writing and shall be followed.

§ 211.208 Drug Product Salvaging

Drug products that have been subjected to improper storage conditions including extremes in temperature, humidity, smoke, fumes, pressure, age, or radiation due to natural disasters, fires, accidents, or equipment failures shall not be salvaged and returned to the marketplace. Whenever there is a question whether drug products have been subjected to such conditions, salvaging operations may be conducted only if there is (a) evidence from laboratory tests and assays (including animal feeding studies where applicable) that the drug products meet all applicable standards of identity, strength, quality, and purity and (b) evidence from inspection of the premises that the drug products and their associated packaging were not subjected to improper storage conditions as a result of the disaster or accident. Organoleptic examinations shall be acceptable only as supplemental evidence that the drug products meet appropriate standards of identity, strength, quality, and purity. Records including name, lot number, and disposition shall be maintained for drug products to this section.

WORK SHEET

The master formula card and work sheet must never be removed from the control of the pharmacy office. Therefore, a means must be devised whereby the manufacturing pharmacist will have available all of the necessary data for the production and packaging of the finished product, as well as having a form to record the necessary information obtained from the control laboratories.

This can be easily accomplished by the use of any of the modern day duplicating devices. A stencil can be cut, showing all the essential data on the master formula and work sheet, and readily duplicated within the hospital. These sheets when completed must be filed since they represent the detailed history of the manufactured product.

A good control system record will provide the hospital pharmacist with the following informaiton on each product manufactured:

1. Name
2. Strength
3. Date of manufacture
4. Formula
5. Ingredients
   a. Manufacturer
   b. Lot number
6. Method of compounding
7. Person who prepared finished product
8. Person who checked the materials and process
9. The hospital lot number assigned to the product
10. Its disposition
11. Its packaging
12. Laboratory control data
13. Percentage yield
14. Time consumed in its preparation
15. Raw material cost
16. Packaging cost

In addition to the above, some authors recommend the use of a receiving number for all raw materials as a means of completely identifying each raw material container. In those hospitals where serially numbered receiving slips ar utilized, the number on the receiving slip constitutes a suitable receiving number. (For information on the use of a receiving memo the reader is referred to Chapter 9 dealing with purchasing and inventory control.)

Also suggested as an additional means of control is a so-called "Identification Number" which is issued to each raw material, whether it be a chemical, bottle, cap, tube or drug.

If all these numbers are used, they should be attached to the raw material container and shown on the pharmacy inventory card. Although some hospital pharmacists write the numbers on the fiber drum containing the chemicals or on the label, if the material is in a glass bottle, the use of an ancillary colored adhesive label is suggested, one color to indicate the receiving number and a second color to identify the raw materials identification number.

Prior to the release of a manufactured product, it should be subjected to chemical or bacteriological analysis. In some hospitals, this control work is performed within the department of pharmacy by a group of pharmacists specifically assigned to the control laboratory. This, of course, is the ideal situation and those institutions with sufficient volume to support such a unit are strongly advised to do so.

On the other hand, small or medium sized hospitals that cannot afford this luxury are nonetheless not excused from the obligation of checking formulas for purity and accuracy produced in the pharmacy or central sterile supply room. This can be done through the close cooperation of the department of pathology (pyrogen testing), the chemistry laboratory (chemical analyses utilizing the spectrophotometer) and the bacteriology laboratory (for sterility determinations).

After all is said and done, none of the above described procedures will guarantee the purity and integrity of every product every time it is produced, unless the individuals concerned with the manufacturing program can be adequately supervised and trained.

With this in mind, it is of interest to present at this point the philosophy of Sr. Francis[9] on how to avoid troubles in the manufacture of parenteral solutions in the hospital pharmacy.

"1. *Pharmaceutical Supervision:*
    a. of the formulae prepared
    b. of the procedures
    c. of the cleaning process
    d. of controls
2. *Exacting cleanliness:*
    a. of the manufacturing room
    b. of flasks and other glassware
    c. of rubber tubings
    d. of flask closures
    e. of stored chemicals
3. Routine cleaning of water still
4. Careful selection of chemicals
5. Production of a pure, pyrogen-free distillate which is checked electrically before and after each operation of the still, and which is sterilized within 8 hours
6. *Accurate measurements:*
    a. of original chemicals
    b. of the finished solution
7. Controlled sterilization process guided by exhaust line thermometer readings
8. Hermetically sealed flasks
9. Prompt and proper filling
10. Inspection and checking of finished products."

MAINTENANCE OF MANUFACTURING EQUIPMENT

Because of the hospital's high investment in pharmaceutical manufacturing equipment and the expense associated with frequent repairs, it behooves the pharmacist to develop an equipment maintenance program which will ensure maximum performance with the lowest possible repair cost.

This can be accomplished by establishing an Equipment Maintenance Record (Fig. 77) which may be kept by the pharmacist or the plant engineer. In addition to identifying clearly the equipment as to name, vendor, serial number and cost, the Equipment Maintenance Record provides the interested parties with a quick history of the repairs required on the apparatus. Furthermore, the routine or preventive

HOSPITAL PHARMACY

EQUIPMENT MAINTENANCE RECORD

EQUIPMENT: _____   INITIAL COST $ _____

DATE OF PURCHASE	VENDOR	SERIAL NUMBER	EXPIRATION OF WARRANTY	SERVICE CONTRACT YES | NO	DATE OF REPAIR	TYPE OF REPAIR	COST OF REPAIR

MISCELLANEOUS DATA OR COMMENTS

1979   1980

	1	2	3	4	5	6	7	8	9	10	11	12	13	14	15	16	17	18	19	20	21	22	23	24	25
Grease																									
Oil																									

Fig. 77

monthly maintenance required by the equipment can be recorded and checked off when performed. Omission of the monthly service can be easily detected by reference to this record and corrected prior to the onset of mechanical difficulties.

Parenteral Hyperalimentation

Parenteral hyperalimentation is the intravenous administration of sufficient nutrients above the usual basal requirements to achieve tissue synthesis, positive nitrogen balance and anabolism.[10]

The preparation of parenteral hyperalimentation solutions must be considered as an integral part of the pharmacy department's manufacturing program irrespective of its size. The procedures employed are not unduly complicated and do not require extensive capital outlay for equipment.

Most hospital pharmacists prepare these solutions by using a technique described as the "wet method" through the extemporaneous compounding techniques of an intravenous admixture program.[10] This consists of mixing the dextrose solution from one flask with the fibrin hydrolysate solution in another flask utilizing a solution transfer set. In the "dry method" the pharmacist adds the appropriate amount of anhydrous glucose to the fibrin hydrolysate solution. Both methods must be carried out under a laminar flow hood.

Because of the nature of these products, the pharmacy must have available appropriate refrigeration equipment and the pharmacist must become familiar with membrane filtration processes in view of the fact that the heat associated with the normal sterilization process will cause caramelization of the dextrose contained in each formula.

INTRAVENOUS ADDITIVE PROGRAM

One writer has stated that an *intravenous additive program* and an *intravenous additive service* may not be the same.[11] The differentiation cited is that an IV additive program consists of policies and procedures for both the preparation and administration of intravenous fluids to which drugs are to be added under aseptic conditions, on an around-the-clock basis, and controlled as to location and person preparing the product. On the other hand, the IV additive service usually refers only to the preparation of the product by individuals who may not necessarily be the same as those who will administer them and assume the responsibility for the monitoring of its clinical effects. The conclusion

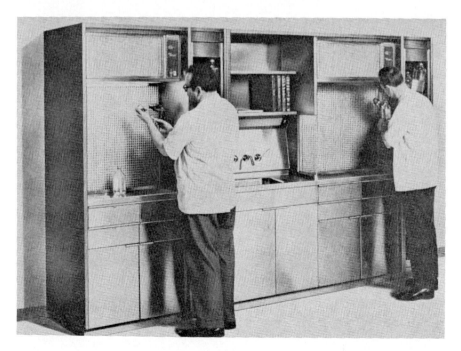

Fig. 78. The Market Forge IV Prep Station. Units such as this offer the pharmacist and the nurse an area for the preparation of intravenous additives in a controlled environment. (Courtesy of Market Forge Co., Everett, Massachusetts.)

arrived at is that an IV additive service is a part of an IV additive program.

Through the implementation of an IV additive service, the hospital pharmacist might be expected to achieve the following objectives:[11] *(a)* that the preparation of the final product be accomplished under aseptic conditons; *(b)* that drug interactions be avoided through the judicious choice of additive and mixing techniques; and *(c)* that the final product is appropriately labeled, dispensed and stored.

In the not too distant past, the preparation of intravenous solutions with their additives was a task performed on the nursing floor by nurses

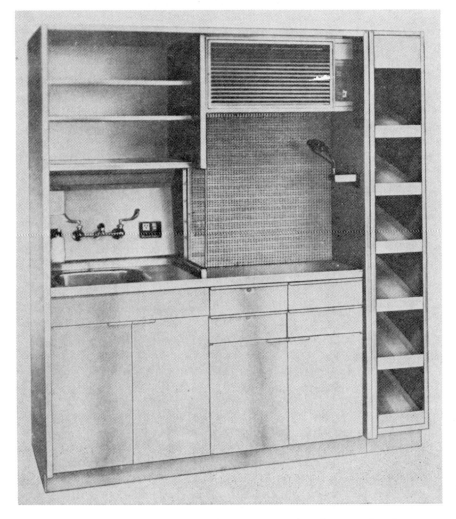

Fig. 79. The Market Forge IV Prep Station. (Courtesy of Market Forge Co., Everett, Massachusetts.)

or interns and residents. The concept that the preparation of these products requires the skills of a pharmacist has raised many other questions not the least of which is availability of the product at odd hours particularly if the site of preparation is moved to the main pharmacy. Thus, has evolved the satellite pharmacy, staffed by a clinical pharmacist and pharmacy technicians. (See Figs. 78, 79, and 80 for medication station for IV preparation.) On final analysis, it is irrelevant where the additives are added so long as definite policies are formulated which spell out responsibilities. In addition, it is imperative that the pharmacist become involved in the preparation of these products in an environment conducive to the efficient and safe preparation of them.[12]

PREPARATION OF IV ADDITIVE SOLUTIONS

In the preparation of these solutions, the pharmacist should work from the physician's original order sheet or from a direct copy. Upon receipt of the order, a pressure-sensitive label must be prepared which provides the following information: *(a)* patient identification; *(b)* patient location; *(c)* physician's name; *(d)* name of drugs with quantities added; *(e)* date of compounding; *(f)* expiration date; and *(g)* identification of the pharmacist preparing the product. If necessary, any ancillary labeling should also be prepared at this time. When applying

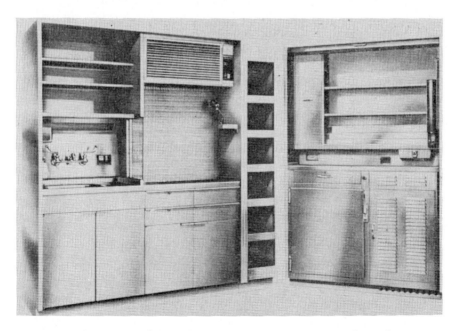

Fig. 80. Combination installation of a Market Forge IV Prep Station and a Medi-Prep Unit. (Courtesy of Market Forge Co., Everett, Massachusetts.)

the label to the container, it must be positioned in an upside down order to facilitate reading when the container is hung from an intravenous solution pole on the patient's bed.

Preparation of the solution should always take place under a laminar flow hood using sterile needles and syringes or double ended transfer needles. In some instances, a Cornwall syringe is useful in reconstitution procedures.

Once the transfer is made, the metal disc must be replaced and a new seal crimped on to the container. As a safety device, a different colored seal should be used in view of the fact that it warns individuals that drugs have been added.[13]

Before permitting the admixture to leave his control, the pharmacist must carry out a final inspection of the product. The inspection should include a review of the label, clarity of the solution, and the mathematics involved in the preparation.[14]

ASHP GUIDELINES FOR PHARMACIST PARTICIPATION IN HOME PARENTERAL NUTRITION PROGRAMS[18]*

Home parenteral nutrition (HPN) programs have been developed to meet the needs of patients who require prolonged or lifelong intravenous feeding. In many hospitals, pharmacists have assisted in solution preparation and supply; in patient training in solution preparation, infusion technique, and catheter care; and in monitoring side effects of HPN. Hospital pharmacists may question under what circumstances they should become involved in the care of patients requiring HPN. Certain institutional, personnel, and patient-resource needs are necessary to provide services to these patients safely. The following guidelines will assist pharmacists in deciding whether they should develop an HPN program.

Institutional Qualifications

The hospital should have an i.v. admixture program. Because HPN is an around-the-clock, long-term form of therapy, the institution must be able to provide for 24-hour service. While a nutrition support service is not a prerequisite for provision of HPN, a team approach is helpful. A formalized nutritional support service is desirable. The institution should be able to respond to HPN-related concerns, such as catheter and pump repair, fluid and electrolyte imbalance, sepsis, and support

---

*Approved by the ASHP Board of Directors, June 6, 1983. Developed by the ASHP Council on Clinical Affairs.

of the patient's underlying disease. Reimbursement arrangements for supplies and services should be established.

The institution must have criteria by which patients can be selected for HPN. Criteria should embrace a patient's learning ability, physical capability, family support, medical condition, and prognosis. A written protocol for training patients should be prepared.

Personnel Qualifications

The pharmacist should have an understanding of parenteral feeding therapy, including a knowledge of acid-base balance, nitrogen balance, fluid and electrolyte therapy, metabolic and mechanical complications, total parenteral nutrition delivery systems, catheter care and management, and drug-nutrient and drug-laboratory interactions. Good aseptic technique and experience in preparing intravenous admixtures is essential. A sufficient understanding of infectious disease is needed to differentiate HPN-related sepsis from underlying disease or drug reaction. The pharmacist should also be aware of current standards and recommendations on sterile admixtures and quality assurance. Assessment skills sufficient to allow monitoring of a patient's progress on a specific nutritional regimen and to recognize emergent problems, such as fever, emesis, and hematemesis, are important.

The pharmacist should be knowledgeable in the unique aspects of HPN, such as chronic infections, nutrient requirements, and effects of parenteral nutrition. A caring, patient-oriented attitude and good teaching skills are important in teaching HPN techniques to patients.

Other personnel such as physicians, nurses, dieticians, and medical social workers are important in assuring success with a patient on HPN. Working together, these health-care professionals must have interests and abilities to meet the needs of HPN patients in their particular areas of expertise.

Resource Requirements

Substantial personnel and equipment are needed for HPN programs. Though the time will vary, available information indicates that 7–44 hours are required to train a patient. Staff must be available on a 24-hour basis to answer questions for inpatients and outpatients. Teaching procedures may extend from early morning to late evening so as to involve both patients and families. Therefore, involvement of more than one pharmacist may be required. The institution must plan for and support the long-term obligation its staff will have to HPN patients.

The following types of equipment are required as a minimum for HPN programs.

- Infusion devices;
- HPN base solutions;
- Drug additives;
- Needles, syringes, and alcohol wipes;
- Dressing-change kits;
- I.V. sets, cassettes, and filters;
- I.V. pole; and
- Catheter accessories

Knowledge of alternate sources of HPN drugs and supplies is important. Procedures for dealing with emergency shortages must be established.

Most patients can be taught at least some aspects of nutritional self-care. This is worthwhile because it enhances feelings of self-esteem and increases quality of life. Given this philosophy, some special patients will require more than the expected amount of teaching time and personnel resources.

Summary

Pharmacists must make their own decisions as to whether they elect to participate in HPN programs. They need to determine the financial, social, and professional impact of an HPN program upon their institution. They need to consider the availability of these services from other hospitals or through private providers of home-health care. These guidelines are intended to help pharmacists make these decisions.

REFERENCES

1. Schneider P.J., Cipponeri, G.J.: Cost savings resulting from home hyperalimentation and third party reimbursement for training program. Infusion, 1979; *3*:179–82.
2. Wateska, L.P., Sattler, L.L., Steiger E.: Cost of a home parenteral nutrition program. JAMA., 1980; *244*:2303–4.

SAMPLE HOSPITAL INTRAVENOUS ADMIXTURE PROGRAM

Hospital intravenous admixture programs vary by institution due to the lack of space, personnel or equipment. This suggests a word of caution—an intravenous admixture program must have sufficient controls to assure the safety of the product for patient use.

The following is an intravenous admixture program utilized by one hospital.[15] Note the double component; one section outlines the responsibilities of physicians and nurses whereas the second features the pharmacy duties.

Action	*Responsibility*	*Notes*
1. Intravenous solutions with or without additives are ordered on the Doctor's Order Form.	Physician	A legible and complete copy of the Doctor's Order is sent to the Pharmacy. The rate of administration must be indicated by the physician. When no infusion rate is indicated, the solutions will be administered at the rate of 75 to 100 ml per hour. "Keep Open" I.V. solutions will be administered at the rate of 30 to 50 ml per hour, unless otherwise indicated by the physician. Children under the age of 12 must have the rate of infusion indicated without exception.
2. Forward a carbonless copy of the original Doctor's Order Form to the Pharmacy Department.	Nursing Personnel	Intravenous solution orders not requiring additives will be administered from the patient unit floor stock and charged accordingly. Orders containing intravenous solution admixture requests will be forwarded to the Pharmacy for compounding.
3. Add medications to running I.V. solutions.	Nurse	The system in no way prevents or prohibits a nurse or physician from adding medications to an I.V. bottle which is already hanging (when appropriate), or from adding drugs into the tubing or a running I.V., or from preparing I.V. admixtures when emergency situations arise.
4. Telephone the Pharmacy for I.V. solution admixtures needed "STAT."	Nurse or Physician	When an intravenous admixture is needed immediately, the nurse or physician telephones the Pharmacy and dictates the admixture order to the pharmacist.

Action	Responsibility	Notes
5. Reduce to writing the nurse's or physician's verbal request for "STAT" I.V. solution admixtures.	Pharmacist	The pharmacist immediately reduces the verbal order to writing, using the I.V. Admixture Worksheet, and proceeds to prepare the admixture. Before dispensing the admixture, the pharmacist must check it against the copy of the physician's original order to verify its accuracy.
6. Reduce to writing on Doctor's Order Form all physician's verbal orders pertaining to I.V. solution therapy.	Nurse	A carbonless copy of the I.V. solution order must be forwarded to the Pharmacy
7. Interpretation of the physician's I.V. admixture order.	Pharmacist	Upon receipt, the pharmacist interprets the order, checks the dosage, and checks for incompatibilities. Problems in incompatibilities or stability arising from an order should be immediately directed to the prescribing physician by the pharmacist.
8. Preparation of I.V. solution label.	Pharmacy Personnel	All intravenous admixtures prepared are labeled according to the I.V. admixture label format. Infusion rate conversion from ml/hr to gtts/min is determined by the use of the conversion table located in the admixture room.

Action	*Responsibility*	*Notes*
9. Assembly and preparation of the I.V. admixture.	Pharmacy Personnel	Routine orders with at least 24-hour stability are filled in two peak work periods during working hours. Orders needed for administration from 12 noon until 12 midnight are filled during mid-morning. Orders needed from 12 midnight until 12 noon the following day are filled during the mid-afternoon. The Admixture Schedule Worksheet, labels, additives, I.V. solution bottle, needles and syringes are assembled together on a small tray prior to preparation. The assembled tray is placed in the hood and the I.V. admixture is aseptically prepared. Only one admixture should be prepared at any one time. Work flow in the hood is from the right side to the left side. Particular attention is given to the order in which drugs (a) must be protected from light, (b) must be reconstituted with non-preserved water, (c) must be buffered and (d) have limited stabilty.

Action	Responsibility	Notes
10. Delivery of I.V. admixtures to the patient units.	Pharmacy Transport Nursing	Intravenous admixtures prepared by the Pharmacy are usually delivered by Pharmacy personnel. When the I.V. admixtures are brought to the nursing unit, they are placed in the nursing unit refrigerator. The Pharmacy technician places them on the designated shelf in a neat and orderly manner by patient name according to bottle number. He also checks all admixtures on the unit noting all expiration dates on the admixtures. All outdated or discontinued admixtures are removed from the refrigerator and returned to the Pharmacy for credit and/or disposition.
11. Preparing emergency intravenous solution admixtures on the patient units.	Nursing Personnel	Nursing personnel will retain the responsibility for preparing I.V. solution admixtures in emergency situations when time is critical.
12. Preparing intravenous admixtures on the patient units for orders received after the Pharmacy closes for the day.	Nursing Personnel	Indicate on the carbonless copy forwarded to the Pharmacy that the admixture was prepared on the patient unit.
13. Prepare own I.V. solution admixtures.	Operating Room Recovery Room	
14. Discontinue administration of any admixture exhibiting a color change, turbidity or precipitate.	Nurse	Return admixture to Pharmacy for replacement.
15. Check intravenous solution admixtures prepared by the Pharmacy for accuracy against the physician's order.	Nurse	

Action	Responsibility	Notes
16. Forward to the patient units sufficient I.V. solution admixtures to maintain the patient during those hours that the Pharmacy is closed.	Pharmacy Personnel	All I.V. solution admixture orders received before the Pharmacy closes for the day will be processed, compounded and delivered to the patient unit.

Pharmacy Procedure

Action	Responsibility	Notes
1. Prepare a separate Admixture Worksheet for each different admixture.	Pharmacy Technician	The Admixture Worksheet and a copy of the original Doctor's Orders are then brought to a pharmacist for checking. The expiration date placed on the label must be 24 hours after actual admixture compounding time unless the solution is stable for less than 24 hours when an appropriate time adjustment must be made. One admixture worksheet may be used for more than one I.V. in a series provided that the solutions are identical.
2. Initial Admixture Worksheet in designated area to indicate technician's accuracy of transcription from the copy of the original Doctor's Order to the Admixture Worksheet.	Pharmacist	The copy of the original Doctor's Order is to be filed once the Admixture Worksheet has been initialed by the pharmacist. The Admixture Worksheet now becomes the reference document.
3. Assemble supplies and medications.	Pharmacy Technician	The special I.V. admixture compounding trays are to be used to hold all supplies, medications, labels and Admixture Worksheets.

Action	Responsibility	Notes
4. Compound admixture.	Pharmacy Technician	Hands are to be washed with antiseptic detergent. The entire compounding tray is brought into the hood. Attention should be given to the method of assembly so that no additional items are needed once preparation begins. Only one admixture should be compounded at any one time.
5. Perform visual check on completed admixture.	Pharmacy Technician	The admixture should be checked for particulate matter, cores, precipitates, unusual color changes. If any of the above is seen, it should be brought to the attention of a pharmacist. The pharmacist will determine if it is necessary to prepare a replacement.
6. Place label on finished infusion.	Pharmacy Technician	The label is to be stamped with the expiration date before being placed on the admixture bottle.
7. Check the admixture.	Pharmacist	The check list includes: (a) Check the label against the Admixture Worksheet (no strikeovers are permitted on the label). (b) Check expiration date. (c) Check amount of additive used against empty or partially empty vials or ampuls. (d) Check used syringes, noting distance plunger is pulled out. (e) Check basic solution and quantity used. (f) Check for particulates, color change or physical incompatibilities.

Action	*Responsibility*	*Notes*
8. Approve admixture.	Pharmacist	The pharmacist will place his initials opposite the compounding technician's initials signifying the admixture is acceptable and is ready for dispensing or storage in the refrigerator. The pharmacist will reject suspicious admixtures and request the technician to again compound the admixture.
9. Forward to patient units all I.V. admixtures needed during those hours that the Pharmacy is closed.	Pharmacy Technician	All admixture orders received before the Pharmacy closes for the day will be processed and delivered before closing.

Technician Duties

Action	*Responsibility*	*Notes*
1. Transcribe all necessary information, prior to making morning rounds, to the "I.V. Check List" after reviewing each Admixture Worksheet.	Pharmacy Technician	Information to be transcribed includes: (a) Patient's last name and room number. (b) Basic solution. (c) Additives and amounts. (d) Solution volume and infusion rate. (e) I.V. solution series number (if any).
2. Check the patient unit medication refrigerators for unused intravenous solution admixtures.	Pharmacy Technician	Outdated, discontinued, changed, unusable, soiled or contaminated admixtures should be returned to the Pharmacy for disposition.
3. Check patient's room to determine status of admixture therapy.	Pharmacy Technician	Confirm that the information on the bottle or bag corresponds with the information on the I.V. Check List. In addition, the volume remaining and the expiration date of the admixture should be noted.

Action	Responsibility	Notes
4. Process the I.V. Admixture Worksheet when the admixture has been discontinued or changed.	Pharmacy Technician	A changed order constitutes modification of the: (a) Basic solution (b) Volume (c) Additive (d) Additive volume or strength.
5. Prepare new I.V. Admixture Worksheet to accommodate new or changed orders.	Pharmacy Technician	A registered pharmacist must initial the Admixture Worksheet to verify the accuracy of the technician's transcription.
6. Prepare admixture labels.	Pharmacy Technician	The number of labels prepared will correspond with the number of admixtures to be compounded.
7. Prepare sufficient admixtures to cover the time increment through the next scheduled rounds.	Pharmacy Technician	Usually sufficient for a period of 24 to 26 hours.
8. Deliver completed I.V. admixtures to the patient units.	Pharmacy Technician	Those solutions that are not needed immediately are placed in the patient unit medication refrigerator.
9. Dispose of or salvage returned admixtures.	Pharmacy Technician	Returned preparations must be kept in the Pharmacy refrigerator until utilized or expired. Issue credit to patients whose preparations have been utilized.

SELECTED READINGS

Fink, III, J.L.: Application of the FDA's Current Good Manufacturing Practices Regulations to Pharmacy Practice: A Legal View. Contemp. Pharm. Pract., 2:4:202, (Fall) 1979.

Stolar, M.H.: National Survey of Hospital Pharmacy Services—1978. Am. J. Hosp. Pharm., 36:315–325, (Mar.) 1979.

Brown, T., Clark, D., Cloyd, M.M., Cloyd, N.T., and Pennington, G.: Unit Dose I.V. Antibiotic Additive Program. Infusion, 3:35–37, 40–42, (Mar.–Apr.) 1979.

Leach, R.: Presentation of Medicines: Label Design. Pharm. J., 222:79–82, (Feb.) 1979.

REFERENCES

1. Francke, Don, Latiolais, Clifton, J., Francke, Gloria, N., and Ho, Norman H.: *Mirror to Hospital Pharmacy,* Washington, D.C., American Society of Hospital Pharmacists, p. 122.
2. Ibid., p. 123.

3. *Webster's New Collegiate Dictionary,* Springfield, Mass., G. & C. Merriam Co., 1973.
4. Klemme, Carl J.: Manufacturing Control Systems in Hospital Pharmacy. The Bulletin, A.S.H.P., *6*:278, 1949.
5. Osol, Arthur and Hoover, J.E.: *Remington's Practice of Pharmacy,* 12th Ed. Easton, Pa., The Mack Publishing Co., 1975.
6. Egool, E., and Bogash, R.C.: Hospital Mouthwash: An Examination of Direct and Indirect Costs. Hosp. Topics, *41*:119, 1963.
7. Skolaut, Milton W.: Quality Control Procedures for the Hospital Pharmacy, Hospitals. J.A.H.A., *38*:83, 1964.
8. Bogash, Robert C.: Why are Administrators and Physicians Reluctant and Sometimes Hostile to a Proposal for Making Sterile Solutions in the Pharmacy? Hosp. Topics, *41*:75, 1963.
9. Francis, Sr. M. Clara: Parenteral Fluids Prepared in the Hospital Pharmacy. The Bulletin, A.S.H.P., *5*:114, 1948.
10. Flack, Herbert L., Gans, John A., Serlick, Stanley E., and Dudrick, Stanley J.: The Current Status of Parenteral Hyperalimentation. Am. J. Hosp. Pharm., *28*:5:326, (May) 1971.
11. Ravin, R.L.: An IV Additive Program—Suggested Procedures. Hosp. Formulary Management, *3*:35, 1968.
12. Durgin, J.M.: Developing Policies and Procedures for an IV Additive Service. Hosp. Topics, *48*:47, 1970.
13. Brown, R.G.: IV Additive Program Belongs in the Pharmacy, Hospitals. J.A.H.A., *43*:92, 1969.
14. Pulliam, S.C. and Upton, J.H.: A Pharmacy Coordinated Intravenous Admixture and Administration Service. Am. J. Hosp. Pharm., *28*:92, 1971.
15. Pharmacy Procedural Manual Affiliated Hospitals Center, Inc. (Robert B. Brigham div.) Boston, Mass. 02115, 1979.
16. Title 21 Sect. 211 Code of Federal Regulations, West Publishing Co., Mineola, N.Y. 11501.
17. ASHP Technical Assistance Bulletin on Hospital Drug Distribution and Control. Am. J. Hosp. Pharm., *37*:1097–1103, (Aug.) 1980.
18. ASHP Guidelines for Pharmacist Participation in Home Parenteral Nutrition Programs. Am. J. Hosp. Pharm., *40*:1386–1387, (Aug.) 1983.

22|

The Pharmacy—
Central Sterile Supply Room

The Central Supply Department of a hospital has been defined as—

"... a centralized unit ... which provides professional supplies and equipment (sterile and non-sterile), to all specialized departments. ..."

A review of the literature will reveal that this specialized area of hospital operation is also known by other names, such as Central Sterile Supply Room, C.S.R., C.S.S.R., and Sterile Supply Room.

The "special departments" which are served include all nursing pavilions, clinics, certain specialized laboratories, such as the Cardiac Catheterization Laboratory, and the operating rooms.

In the early days of development, the majority of the items dispensed by the central supply room consisted of re-usable material. Today, with the advent of the age of plastics and disposables the reverse is true. Disposable drapes, syringes, tubing, urine collection sets, intravenous administration sets, needles, gloves and blood bags are an example of the inroads made by the plastic industry into the field of supplying hospitals with single use items.

In addition to the dispensing of the above mentioned items, the modern central sterile supply room may be involved in the cleaning, storage and dispensing of specialized equipment such as suction pumps, cardiac catheters, monitoring equipment, surgical dressing carts, resuscitation carts, and a myriad of special kits and trays.[2]

In 1960, the central sterile supply room was a relatively modern innovation in the hospital.[3,4] From its beginning as an equipment washroom with autoclaving facilities, it has adapted itself to modern production line technics with automatic control recording devices to insure sterility, modern washing, drying and powdering equipment for surgical gloves as well as taking an active role in developing the various gas and cold sterilization technics.

As to the management function of the central supply room, there are three schools of thought. One group[5,6] is of the opinion that the procurement, storage and distribution of supplies as well as the preparation

470

of the various sterile solutions, when necessary, lend themselves to the training of a pharmacist. In fact, the pharmacist is performing these very same functions within the department of pharmacy; therefore, if only from an economic point of view, it is feasible to incorporate into the pharmacist's duties the responsibility for the management of the central sterile supply room.

A second group contends that the majority of the items dispensed are ultimately used by nurses in the care of their patients and therefore since a nurse fully comprehends the intended use of the products, she logically should be responsible for the operation of the central sterile supply room.

The third group accepts the fact that the central sterile supply room has a dual function, namely, the cleaning, packaging and distribution of medical equipment and supplies as well as the manufacture of sterile fluids. Accordingly, it is the consensus that a nurse should be responsible for the former and a pharmacist should be responsible for the latter.

In actual practice, all three of these views are accepted and each can claim a representative number of hospitals which have adopted the respective ideology of each group.

CSSR—PHILOSOPHY AND OBJECTIVES

The Central Sterile Supply Room (Central Processing Department) is a centralized system practicing total decontamination and gives professional support and service for improved patient care by maintaining high processing standards.

The objectives of the department generally encompass the following:

1. Assume total responsibility for direct Operating Room supply.
2. Assume total responsibility for processing hospital items, thereby assuring that all of them receive the same degree of cleaning and sterilization.
3. Strive for uniformity and simplicity in preparation of procedural trays and sets used in the care and treatment of patients.
4. Maintain accurate and current inventory of supplies and equipment in the department.
5. Maintain an accurate record of the effectiveness of the various processes of cleaning, disinfecting and sterilization.
6. Contribute educational programs within the hospital relating to infection control.
7. Develop a cost effective program by cost analysis of personnel, supplies and equipment.

CSSR IN THE HOSPITAL ORGANIZATION

Unlike the pharmacy which has been accorded full departmental status, the central sterile supply room is, in many hospitals, considered as a sub-department. In these institutions, the department may fall under the aegis of the Operating Room Supervisor or the Nursing Service. Under this type of organization, the director, supervisor or manager of the unit does not report to the administrator or his assistant but to some major department head.

In some hospitals, a division of surgical care is established as a section of the general nursing service. Within this division are the central sterile supply room, operating rooms, recovery rooms and intensive surgical care unit. Here again, the head of the central sterile supply room is operating at a sub-departmental level.

In still other hospitals, the manufacture of sterile injectable or irrigating solutions is separated from the central sterile supply room and this "solution room" is placed within the administrative scope of the pharmacist. Under this arrangement, the pharmacist reports directly to the administrator or to one of his assistants. The same rung in the organizational structure of the hospital is retained if the pharmacy and central sterile supply room are considered as one unit.

It is of interest to note at this point that pharmacy and central sterile supply may have a joint responsibility. The situation is brought about when the pharmacy (1) prepares the solutions in bulk and transports the tanks to the central sterile supply room for bottling and sterilization, (2) prepares and packages the solutions for sterilization by the central sterile supply room, (3) prepares a concentrated solution which is then diluted, packaged and sterilized in the central sterile supply room, or (4) prepares a mixture of the chemicals in the dry state which when dissolved in a specified volume of distilled water results in the desired product which is then packaged and sterilized by the central sterile supply room personnel.

Although it may seem strange to the reader to have the pharmacy prepare and bottle the various solutions and the central sterile supply room assume the responsibility for their sterilization, it is, in effect, a very practical solution to the dilemma of whether or not identical sterilization equipment may be installed in both the pharmacy and the central sterile supply room.

QUALIFICATIONS OF THE HOSPITAL PHARMACIST TO MANAGE THE CSSR

Because the modern pharmacy curriculum provides the student with an exposure to bacteriology, the principles of sterilization, accounting and management, the hospital pharmacist is educationally better qualified to manage the central sterile supply room than is the nurse. Admittedly, the nurse has a better knowledge of the ultimate use of the products dispensed, and, in some instances, the experience required for an efficient operation. This is not a reflection upon the nurse who may be presently in charge of a central sterile supply room nor upon the nursing profession as a whole. It is merely a comparison of two different callings—one is devoted to the direct care of the ill patient and therefore does not require training in the principles of procurement, packaging, storage and dispensing, whereas the other is a profession devoted to providing the various services associated with the needs of doctors, nurses and ill patients and therefore requires a thorough grounding in the above principles in addition to certain areas of scientific knowledge.

The pharmacist, as a part of his daily practice in the operation of the hospital pharmacy, performs many functions which are either identical to or closely resemble those which are performed by his counterpart in the central sterile supply room. These duties consist of:

  a. Interviewing sales personnel
  b. Purchasing of supplies
  c. Meeting with and discussing procedures or specific problems with the medical staff
  d. Dispensing of supplies in small lots
  e. Distributing of supplies to pavilions
  f. Receiving and storing of supplies
  g. Charging, inventory and accounting procedures
  h. Teaching or lecturing to various groups
  i. Practicing the principles of standardization
  j. Manufacturing in bulk
  k. Manufacturing in small lots, both sterile and non-sterile products.

Clearly then, it would appear that the pharmacist is qualified both by education and experience to supervise the activities of the central sterile supply room. It is also reasonable to state that such a consolidation of responsibility will result in more economical management as well as savings which result from a reduction in certain strata of personnel, fuller utilization of space and equipment and consolidation of inventories.

PERSONNEL

Staffing this department is difficult in view of the fact that most applicants have not had any prior experience and must receive on-the-job training. Individuals must be trained in the principles of sterilization, monitoring autoclaves, operating gas sterilizers and aerators, identification of surgical instruments, assembly of treatment trays, disassembly, cleaning and assembling equipment, decontamination, basic bacteriology and biological testing. Clearly an on-the-job training program is time consuming, varies from hospital to hospital and is costly to the institution. Therefore, the pharmacist-director of the CSSR should undertake a technician training program in order to develop personnel who are qualified in theory and technology.[8,9]

The materials handling aspect of the CSSR operation should be coordinated with those of the departments of pharmacy, purchasing and distribution. By so doing a duplication of services or function will be eliminated or, at least, minimized.

LOCATION

Ideally, the central sterile supply room should be centrally located in relation to the areas requiring the greatest utilization of its services. Consideration must also be given to the fact that the central sterile supply room must be able to receive large quantities of linen from the laundry, surgical dressings from the storeroom and large shipments of sterile intravenous and irrigating fluids if these are not manufactured by the hospital. If an ideal central location is not readily available, then resort must be made to utilize types of conveyor and pneumatic tube systems.

If the pharmacy and central sterile supply room management are to be combined, then, where possible, the two units should be physically combined or at least adjacent to one another. By so doing, there can be closer supervision of the personnel as well as a consolidation of duties and coverage of both services on a twenty-four-hour basis.

PLANNING THE CSSR

A close look at a modern central sterile room quickly reveals that it consists of a series of special work stations in a "dirty area" which is separated from the "clean area" by autoclaving and sterilizing equipment.

In effect then, we have all contaminated or non-sterile material and supplies entering one end of the room, passing through the various work stations and sterilizers and finally reposing in a sterile storage area ready to be dispensed from the clear side of the room. This concept is best illustrated by Figure 81.

The purpose of such a layout is to minimize the cross-flow of contaminated or non-sterile goods with those that are clean or sterile thereby eliminating the possibility of cross contamination or even the dispensing of a "dirty" kit for a clean one.

The number, type and size of work stations required will, of course,

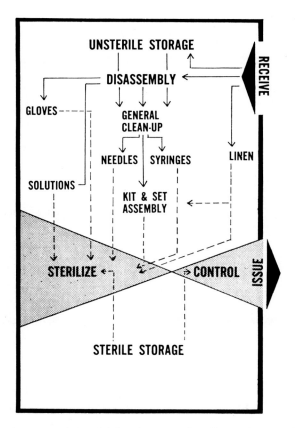

Fig. 81. General concept of material flow in a central sterile supply room. (From *Macbick/CSR Equipment* brochure published by the Macbick Co., Wilmington, Massachusetts.)

depend upon the size and nature of the hospital, the quantity of disposable materials used, the number of work shifts per day, the type of sterilization required, and whether or not the hospital purchases or manufactures sterile intravenous and irrigating fluids.

Because the planning of a central sterile supply room's space requirements cannot be reduced to a square foot per bed formula, any hospital pharmacist who undertakes to assist in the development, planning and construction of a central sterile supply room should avail himself of the technical know-how and experience that can be provided by the design staff of a reputable producer of such equipment.

In order that the student and the pharmacist have an idea as to typical plans for central sterile supply rooms for various size hospitals, Figures 82A, 82B, 83, and 84, are provided.

TYPICAL PLAN –
CENTRAL SUPPLY FOR THE SMALLER HOSPITAL

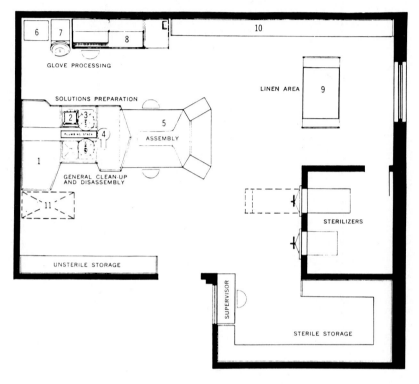

1   Clean-Up and Disassembly Station
2. Flask Washer (set in sink)
3. Flask Rinser (set in sink)
4. Still
5. Kit Assembly Station

6. Glove Washer-Drier
7. Glove Powderer
8. Glove Packaging Station
9. Linen Inspection and Folding Station
10. Linen Storage
11. CSR Truck

Fig. 82.   *A.* Typical plan of a central sterile supply room for a small hospital. (From *Macbick/ CSR Equipment* brochure published by the Macbick Co., Wilmington, Massachusetts.) *(Figure continues on next page.)*

LAMINAR FLOW HOODS

Although many hospitals have abandoned the preparation of large volume, sterile intravenous fluids, a large number have commenced other programs, such as the intravenous solutions additive procedure, which require sterile technics to be performed in an atmosphere of microfiltered air.

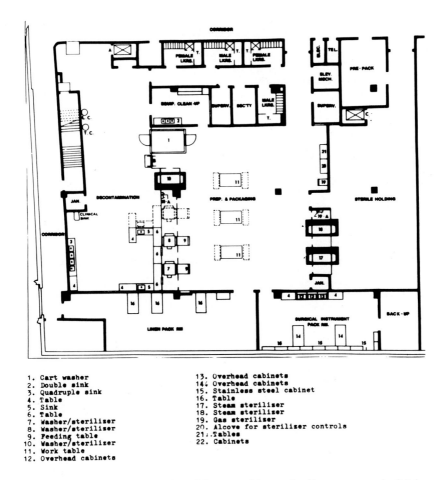

1. Cart washer
2. Double sink
3. Quadruple sink
4. Table
5. Sink
6. Table
7. Washer/sterilizer
8. Washer/sterilizer
9. Feeding table
10. Washer/sterilizer
11. Work table
12. Overhead cabinets

13. Overhead cabinets
14. Overhead cabinets
15. Stainless steel cabinet
16. Table
17. Steam sterilizer
18. Steam sterilizer
19. Gas sterilizer
20. Alcove for sterilizer controls
21. Tables
22. Cabinets

Fig. 82 (Continued). *B.* Floor plan of the Central Processing Department at the Brigham and Women's Hospital in Boston, Massachusetts.

In order to create such an atmosphere, various manufacturers of hoods have incorporated into them the laminar flow principle.

Laminar air flow is defined by Federal Standard 209[7] as:

". . . air flow in which the entire body of air within a confined area moves with uniform velocity along parallel flow lines, with a minimum of eddies."

By providing a constant outward flow of microfiltered air over the entire face of the hood's work area opening, dust particles may be kept from entering the work area from the ambient atmosphere.

Hospital pharmacists who plan to commence intravenous solutions

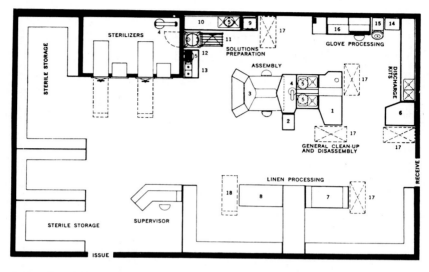

1. Clean-Up and Disassembly Station	10. Solutions Clean-Up
2. Utility Washer	11. Flask Drain Truck
3. Kit Assembly Station	12. Batch Tank
4. Still	13. Flask Filling and Capping Station
5. Storage Tank	14. Glove Washer-Drier
6. Clean-Up and Disassembly	15. Glove Powderer
7. Linen Inspection and Folding	16. Glove Packaging Station
8. Linen Packaging	17. CSR Truck
9. Flask Washer	18. Autoclave Truck

Fig. 83. Typical plan of a central sterile supply room for a medium size hospital. (From *Macbick/CSR Equipment* brochure published by the Macbick Co., Wilmington, Massachusetts.)

additive programs or those who are called upon to produce special sterile research products should investigate the possibilities which such an installation offers.

Pharmacy-Central Sterile Supply Rooms that still produce parenteral fluids should install laminar flow hoods in order to ensure safe, sterile products.

STANDARDIZATION COMMITTEE

The Standardization Committee may be defined as that group within the hospital which is commissioned with the responsibility to investigate, to develop and to standardize procedures and equipment. In some institutions, this group is also known as the Current Practices Committee.

If such a committee is not in existence, it behooves the Director of Pharmacy and Central Sterile Supply Services to take the initial steps to have such a committee formed. By so doing, he will be assured of

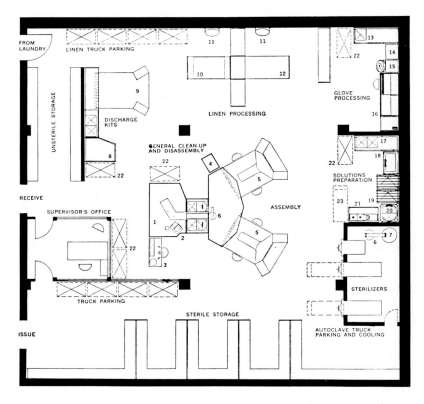

1. Clean-Up and Disassembly Station
2. Needle Washer
3. Needle Packaging Station
4. Utility Washer
5. Kit Assembly
6. Still
7. Storage Tank
8. Clean-Up and Disassembly Station (CD-0)
9. Kit Assembly Station
10. Linen Inspection
11. Linen Hamper
12. Linen Packaging
13. Accumulation Counter
14. Glove Washer-Drier
15. Glove Powderer
16. Glove Packaging Station
17. Solutions Clean-Up
18. Flask Washer-Rinser
19. Flask Drain Truck
20. Batch Tank (50 gal.)
21. Flask Filling and Capping Station
22. CSR Truck
23. Autoclave Truck

Fig. 84. Typical plan of a central sterile supply room for a large hospital. (From *Macbick/CSR Equipment* brochure published by the Macbick Co., Wilmington, Massachusetts.)

the creative thinking of a group of individuals who are intimately associated with the use of the supplies and products to be dispensed from the central sterile supply room. In addition, the Director of Pharmacy and Central Sterile Supply Services can then assure the hospital administration that a concerted effort is being made to reduce duplication of inventory and produce standardization of procedures.

Membership on this committee should be by appointment of interested staff members, the appointment being made jointly by the chief of staff and the administrator of the hospital. Each major discipline in the hospital should be represented on the committee. Ideally, the following represents a good working group.

Administration (1)	Nursing Service (2)
Director of Laboratories	Nursing School (1)
Surgery (2)	Director of Pharmacy
Medicine (2)	and Central Sterile
Radiology (1)	Supply
Pathology (1)	

Other areas such as Dietary, Engineering and Maintenance should be invited to attend the meetings during which subjects pertaining to their services are discussed.

A chairman and a secretary should be appointed from the committee membership. Meetings should be held according to a set schedule throughout the year. The secretary of the committee should be assigned the responsibility of gathering all samples and prices of material as well as other pertinent data dealing with a particular procedure or type of equipment.

The chairman of the committee may then assign the responsibility for the investigation and development phases of the problem under discussion to a sub-group of the master committee. Once this smaller group has reached a decision as to equipment or developed a new procedure, the secretary should write up the material in accordance with a predetermined format and submit it to the master committee for approval. Once approved, the report should be distributed to the staff and pavilions.

To encourage proper filing of these documents, some hospitals provide each recipient with a binder and appropriate separators to demarcate the various divisions of the hospital—*i.e.,* surgery, medicine, nursing, pharmacy, etc.

An index should be published periodically and distributed to all those on the mailing list. The bound volume of "bulletins" may then be referred to as the Standardization Manual or the Current Practices Manual and should serve as an authoritative procedural manual.

SELECTED READINGS

Avis, K.E. and Levchuk, J.W.: Special Considerations in the Use of Vertical Laminar-flow Workbenches. Am. J. Hosp. Pharm., *41*:81–87, 1984.

Bryan, D. and Marback, R.C.: Laminar-airflow Equipment Certification: What the Pharmacist Needs to Know. Am. J. Hosp. Pharm., *41*:1343–1349, 1984.

REFERENCES

1. Teresa, Sr. M.: Hospital Pharmacy and Central Supply Combination Service. Am. Prof. Pharm., *23*:4:358, 1957.
2. Skolaut, M.W.: Pharmacy-Central Sterile Supply Services. Am. J. Hosp. Pharm., *17*:710, 1960.
3. ———: Pharmacy-Central Sterile Supply Services—History. Am. J. Hosp. Pharm., *17*:11:244, 1960.
4. ———: Pharmacy-Central Sterile Supply Services—Historical Background. Am. J. Hosp. Pharm., *17*:6:364, 1960.
5. Pierpaoli, Paul J.: Some Administrative Considerations in Assigning Responsibility for Central Sterile Supply Service. Am. J. Hosp. Pharm., *20*:8:370, 1963.
6. Hassan, Wm. E., Jr.: Who Should Manage Central Sterile Supply? Hosp. Management, *75*:5:76, 1963.
7. Clean Room and Work Station Requirements, Environment, Controlled Federal Standard 209 General Services Administration, December 16, 1963.
8. Baker, B.M.: A Central Supply Technician Training Program. Hospital Topics, *55*::3, (Jan.–Feb.) 1977.
9. Schwertner, T.A.: An Improved Approach; Programmed Instruction for Central Service Technicians. Hospital Topics, *55*:5:27, (Sept.–Oct.) 1977.

23|

The Nuclear Pharmacy

With the increased use of radioactive isotopes in the hospital, many administrators and isotope users have felt the need to develop a means whereby there is a centralized responsibility for the dissemination of information, purchase, use, storage, disposal and monitoring of these potentially hazardous materials.

Hospital pharmacists have been quick to recognize this situation as one whereby they may fill the void and expand the professional services rendered by the pharmacy department. In addition, the American Society of Hospital Pharmacists in order to guide this movement established a Committee on Isotopes which was staffed by a group of hospital pharmacists who had already gained considerable experience in this new phase of hospital pharmacy.

In 1955 the committee submitted a comprehensive report[1] with a proposed outline for a course in isotope pharmacy. This report was followed by the report of the 1958 committee in which the following objectives were proposed.[2]

1. To develop suggestions for special courses for hospital pharmacists in the handling of isotopes in hospitals.
2. To determine the feasibility of an isotope section operated by the hospital pharmacy.
3. To determine layout and design for a radioactive branch of a pharmacy department.
4. To compile a bibliography on isotopes.

In the meantime, hospital pharmacists were publishing articles dealing with the fundamentals of radioactivity,[3] the various aspects of radiologic health,[4] and descriptions of programs within hospitals having an established radioisotope pharmacy.[5,12]

Simultaneously the hospital literature began to publish articles concerning facilities and equipment for isotope programs[6] and data on the types of facilities required for the use of isotopes in the general hospital.[7]

Simultaneously, the American Hospital Association developed and distributed a *Manual on the Use of Radioisotopes in Hospitals*[8] with the following stated purpose.[9]

482

"... for use by hospitals when setting up a radioisotopes program or when reviewing their current procedures for handling radioisotopes. It is intended to guide the administrator of the general hospital in the procurement procedures for radioactive materials, in the radiation protection measures necessary for their handling, in the allocation of space and equipment for isotopes laboratories, and in the organization and training of the hospital staff for the utilization of radioactive materials."

Thus, it becomes necessary to expose the student in hospital pharmacy to the licensing requirements of the Atomic Energy Commission, the radioisotope committee and its function and the role which the alert hospital pharmacist can assume in this rapidly developing phase of therapeutics and diagnosis.

Because of the limited scope of this text, and the highly technical nature of the equipment, no data concerning the various types of monitoring, handling or measuring devices in current use will be presented or the physical facilities needed to establish a radioisotope pharmacy.

A large number of hospitals and clinics in the United States are currently using radioisotopes for diagnostic, therapeutic and research purposes. The use of those potentially dangerous materials is subject to the control and supervision of the Atomic Energy Commission, a governmental agency established by the United States Congress under the **Atomic Energy Act of 1954.**

Jurisdiction of the AEC

The Act provides that the Atomic Energy Commission has jurisdiction over all "by-product material" which is further defined by the Act as—

"... any radioactive material (except special nuclear material) yielded in or made radioactive by exposure to the radiation incident to the process of producing or utilizing special nuclear material."

Perusal of the Federal regulations reveals that jurisdiction of the AEC applies not only to radioisotopes produced in the United States, but also to those imported into this country.

Radioactive isotopes may be used only by duly licensed individuals who have complied with the statutory provisions of the Atomic Energy Act and the latest AEC regulations appearing in the *Federal Register.*

LICENSURE INFORMATION

In order that the hospital pharmacist render a high quality, knowledgeable service with regard to isotope materials, it is necessary for him to have a general understanding of the basic requirements which must be met, by both individuals and institutions, before they may become licensed for the medical use of radioisotopes.

Accordingly, the following discussion relates to the types of licenses that can be issued, the types of applications which should be submitted to obtain the licenses, and the information which should be included in the application.

Licenses may be issued to institutions or to private practitioners. The type of licenses available and their characteristics are as follows:

Institutional License

This type of license is specific in that it limits the use of the isotopes to those listed on the license. It also restricts the clinical use and the physicians who may use the material to those named on the license document.

In addition, the regulations require that an institutional licensee have a medical isotope committee to evaluate all proposals for research, diagnostic, and therapeutic uses of isotopes within the hospital.

One advantage of such a license is that it provides a means whereby physicians desiring licensure for the use of radioisotopes may obtain basic and clinical isotope training to meet the criteria required to qualify as an individual user.

Broad Medical Licenses Issued to Institutions

This type of license is issued to those institutions that meet the following criteria:

   a. previous experience operating under a specific institutional license and,
   b. are engaged in medical research, as well as routine diagnosis and therapy.

Although a medical isotope committee is required, no physicians are listed as individual users on the license, nor are the radioisotopes limited to specified users.

This type of license also permits physicians to obtain basic and clinical radioisotope training and experience.

Specific Licenses Issued to Physicians for Their Private Practice

This license is usually issued to the private practitioner of medicine irrespective of whether or not his office is or is not located on the hospital premises. The license usually specifies the isotope and its clinical use. These licenses do not permit or provide for other physicians to obtain basic and clinical radioisotope training and experience. In addition, the licenses are limited to well-established uses of by-product materials and require that the physician, so licensed, personally conduct the program.

TYPES OF APPLICATION FORMS

Form AEC 313 and Form AEC 313a are two application forms upon which information concerning a proposed medical radioisotope program may be submitted.

Form AEC 313MC may be appropriate for a specific institutional or for a specific private practice license. In addition, this form should be used only by physicians who are qualified to handle one entire category of uses. If the physician does not so qualify, application should be made upon Form AEC 313.

Form AEC 313a must be submitted for each physician who is to be listed on an institutional license or for each physician applying for a private practitioner's license.

RADIOISOTOPE COMMITTEE

The regulations of the Atomic Energy Commission require that a radioisotope committee be established for the supervision and control of the hospital isotope program. The committee should include a radiation physicist, a clinical radiologist, an internist, a hematologist and a surgeon. Other members or specialties to be represented on the committee should be determined by the type and scope of program being undertaken by the hospital.

In addition to the above, it is also suggested that a representative from nursing service, administration and pharmacy be included on the committee roster.

The reasons for the participation of nursing and administrative representatives are that the nurses will become familiar with the type of work carried out on the pavilions, the associated dangers and the means whereby the patient, doctor and nurse may protect themselves. The administrator can contribute to the development of the entire program through his efforts with the board of trustees and the pharmacist may be of assistance in the purchasing, receiving and storage of isotopes until such time as the theory of a centralized isotope pharmacy within the hospital materializes.

Generally the radioisotope committee should have the following responsibilities:[9]

1. Review, grant permission for, or disapprove the use of isotopes within the institution.
2. Prescribe special conditions as may be necessary, such as training of

personnel, designation of limited areas of use, disposal methods and the like.

3. Receive reports from the radiation protection officer and review his records.
4. Recommend remedial action when an individual fails to observe protection recommendations, rules, regulations.
5. Keep a record of actions taken in approving the use of isotopes.

In order to acquaint the hospital pharmacist with the type of instructional and precautionary literature prepared by the committee, the following bulletin entitled *Protective Procedures for Personnel Caring for Patients Receiving Therapeutic Isotopes* is presented.[10]

"Radioactive isotopes are administered to patients for treatment of various conditions, *e.g.,* radioactive iodine for hyperthyroidism, radioactive gold for malignant effusions, radioactive phosphorus for malignant hematological conditions. These emit beta and gamma rays and exposure should be reduced to the minimum by:

a. avoiding contamination of clothing and skin from body secretions of the patient.
b. keeping the time close to the patient as short as possible.
c. keeping as great a distance from the patient as possible when in the unit.

General Precautions

1. A radioisotope administration sheet (Fig. 85) is placed in the medical record by the isotope administrator at the time of treatment and is to remain there permanently. Particular precautions required by the specific isotope used will be listed on this sheet by the isotope administrator and called to the attention of the medical and nursing staff caring for the patient. These will be written in the Doctor's Order Book by the physician in charge of the patient.
2. An isotope sign is placed at the entrance of the room or unit by the isotope administrator.
3. The isotope administrator will provide the name of a substitute who may be contacted in case the administrator is not readily available.

Care of the Patient: for most patients, these precautions should be taken:

1. No nurse should care for more than one radioactive patient at a time.
2. The patient should be encouraged to do as much as possible for himself so that close bedside nursing can be reduced to the minimum.
3. Gloves are to be worn when the nurse handles the patient's linen, skin or excreta utensils.
4. A plastic apron or sheet of expendable plastic is to be worn for bedside nursing (to protect from spoilage). If an apron is worn, it should be used for one patient only and marked clearly which is the inside of the apron.
5. Excreta utensils should be marked with a "radioactive" sign and reserved for one patient's use. These utensils should be flushed clean with a superfluous amount of water; dilution is the best protection. If the radioactive element is difficult to flush, carrier solution (the ordinary substance such as iodine, not radioactive) will help and can be supplied by the isotope administrator.

PETER BENT BRIGHAM HOSPITAL

RADIOACTIVE ISOTOPE ADMINISTRATION

TRACER ☐
THERAPY ☐

RADIOACTIVE ISOTOPE FORM

Addressograph Plate

Isotope:_____ Effective Half-Life:_____

Dose _____

Route of Administration_____

The patient received_____ mc. of radioactive

isotope_____ at_____M on_____19_____

The following special precautions are to be meticulously observed.

All personnel responsible for the medical or nursing care of this patient must review and be familiar with the special procedures and requirements outlined in the Current Practice Manual, Peter Bent Brigham Hospital, Bulletin_____

In the event of spillage or isotopic contamination notify at once the undersigned and the Radiologic House Officer on duty. Make no attempt to clean the area or to remove any item touched by the isotope.

RADIOACTIVE
ISOTOPE FORM   Form 71

Signed_____ M. D.
:   Responsible Isotope Administrator

RADIOACTIVE
ISOTOPE FORM

Fig. 85. Radioactive Isotope Administration form which is placed in the medical record of each patient receiving radioactive isotopes. The sheet is a canary yellow in color and the Atomic Energy Commission insignia is printed in red ink.

6. The House Officer will notify the isotope administrator of any draining wound.
7. Anything soiled with body discharge is to be retained in a plastic bag until monitored and appropriate disposal directed by the isotope administrator. Linen is to be kept in large plastic bags. Dressings, tissues and small disposable articles in small plastic envelops are to be placed in a yellow dump-lid waste container with radioactive marker provided by the isotope administrator and will be removed by him to the decay area properly labeled.

Visitors

No visitors are permitted for the first two weeks except by special dispensation by the isotope administrator. Children and pregnant women are not permitted at any time.

Therapeutic Procedures

Thoracentesis or paracentesis within fifteen days of isotope administration should be carried out only after specific approval of the isotope administrator and with his explicit direction for disposal of material and utensils.

Urine should be collected or sent to the laboratory only under the specific conditions imposed by the administrator.

Routine Post-Operative Orders

1. Usual diet and medication may be resumed on return to the ward unless otherwise specified.
2. Patients receiving therapeutic isotopes are to be cared for in a specified radiation area and to be confined to this area unless bathroom privileges are definitely assigned by the isotope administrator.
3. Soiled or wet dressings are to be brought to the attention of the House Officer immediately.
4. The Radiation Safety Officer should be contacted if the patient has a long distance to travel on discharge.
5. If any doubt arises about the procedure for these patients, contact the isotope administrator whose name is signed on the yellow Form #71 or his deputy as indicated.

INCREASED DISTANCE AND REDUCTION IN THE TIME OF EXPOSURE ARE ALWAYS THE BEST PROTECTION. THE NEED FOR HANDWASHING CANNOT BE OVER-EMPHASIZED.

RESPONSIBILITY OF PERMIT HOLDERS

Those persons who are granted a permit to use radioisotopes have an obligation and a responsibility for the safe use of radiation sources by individuals under their control. Permit holders are therefore generally responsible for the following:[11]

1. Compliance with all rules and regulations for the safe use and handling of radioactive materials.
2. Insuring that employees under their control are instructed in the use of safety devices and procedures.
3. Adequate planning of an experiment, or procedure, to assure that the necessary safety precautions are taken.
4. Informing the Radiation Safety Officer of the hospital, of the names of all personnel involved in operational procedures, and of changes in such personnel; radioactive materials being used; procedures of handling; changes in the laboratory arrangement which could lead to changes in personnel exposure or contamination levels.
5. Direction of personnel under their control to comply with all recommendations by the Radiation Safety Officer relative to dosimeters, and other recommendations to control or to reduce exposure to radiation hazards.
6. Limitation of use of radioisotopes under their permit to those over whom they have direct supervision.
7. Maintenance of required current records of receipt, use, storage and disposal of radioisotopes.

RESPONSIBILITY OF INDIVIDUAL USERS

From the point of view of self-preservation and moral obligation for the safety of others, each person who uses sources of ionizing radiation has the following responsibilities:[11]

1. To receive instruction in radiation safety as determined appropriate by the Radiation Safety Officer.
2. To keep his exposure to radiation at the lowest possible level and specifically below the maximum permissible exposure.
3. To wear recommended radiation dosimeters for personnel, such as film badges, pocket ionization chambers, and finger dosimeters.
4. To survey his hands, shoes, body, and clothing for radioactivity and remove all loose contamination before leaving the laboratory when appropriate.
5. To use all appropriate protective measures such as protective clothing, respiratory protection, remote pipetting devices, ventilated and shielded glove box and hoods.
6. To prohibit smoking and eating in radioisotope laboratories.
7. To check working areas daily, or after each radioisotope procedure.
8. To maintain good laboratory practices, such as keeping work areas and equipment clean and orderly.
9. To use proper labels on equipment being used with radioactive materials.
10. To place all active waste in proper containers, equipped with proper labels.
11. To report immediately the details of a "spill" or other accident involving radioactive substances to the Radiation Safety Officer.
12. To conduct decontamination procedures as directed by the Radiation Safety Officer.

The National Association of Boards of Pharmacy (NABP) has issued a set of Model Regulations for Nuclear Pharmacy.© The following material[13] is excerpted from this document which is available from the publications desk of the NABP.

NABP MODEL REGULATIONS FOR NUCLEAR PHARMACY

Section 3. General Requirements for Pharmacies Providing Radiopharmaceutical Services

(a) The application for a permit to operate a pharmacy providing radiopharmaceutical services shall only be issued to a qualified nuclear pharmacist. All personnel performing tasks in the preparation and distribution of radioactive drugs shall be under the direct supervision of a qualified nuclear pharmacist. A qualified nuclear pharmacist shall be responsible for all operations of the pharmacy and shall be in personal attendance at all times that the pharmacy is open for business. In emergncy situations, in the pharmacist's absence, designated qualified licensed professionals may have access to the licensed area. These individuals may prepare single doses of radiopharmaceuticals for the immediate emergency and must document such withdrawls in the quality control records.

(b) Nuclear pharmacies shall have adequate space, commensurate with the scope of services required and provided, meeting minimal space requirements established for all pharmacies in the state. The nuclear pharmacy area shall be separate from the pharmacy areas for non-radioactive drugs and shall be secured from unauthorized personnel. All pharmacies handling radiopharmaceuticals shall provide a radioactive storage and product decay area, occupying at least 25 square feet of space, separate from and exclusive of the hot laboratory, compounding, dispensing, quality assurance and office area. A nuclear pharmacy handling radioactive drugs exclusively may be exempted from the general space requirements for pharmacies by obtaining a waiver from the State Board of Pharmacy. Detailed floor plans shall be submitted to the State Board of Pharmacy and the Radiation Control Agency or NRC before approval of the license.

(c) Nuclear pharmacies shall only dispense radiopharmaceuticals which comply with acceptable professional standards of radiopharmaceutical quality assurance and nuclear pharmacy practice.

(d) Nuclear pharmacies shall maintain records of acquisition, inventory and disposition of all radioactive drugs in accordance with the appropriate pharmacy and radiological control agency or NRC.

(e) Nuclear pharmacies shall comply with all applicable laws and regulations of federal and state agencies, including those laws and regulations governing non-radioactive drugs.

(f) Radiopharmaceuticals are to be dispensed only upon a prescription or medication order, from a licensed medical practitioner authorized to possess, use and administer radiopharmaceuticals.

(g) A nuclear pharmacist may transfer to authorized persons radioactive materials not intended for drug use, in accordance with the appropriate regulations of the radiological control agency. A nuclear pharmacy may also furnish radiopharmaceuticals for office use to these practitioners for individual patient use.

(h) In addition to any labeling requirements of the State Board of Pharmacy for non-radioactive drugs, the immediate outer container of a radioactive drug to be dispensed shall also be labeled with:

(1) The standard radiation symbol;
(2) The words "Caution-Radioactive Material";
(3) The radionuclide;
(4) The chemical forms;
(5) The amount of radioactive material contained, in millicuries or microcuries;
(6) If a liquid, the volume in cubic centimeters;

(7) The requested calibration time for the amount of radioactivity contained.

(i) The immediate container shall be labeled with:

(1) Standard radiation symbol;

(2) The words "Caution-Radioactive Material";

(3) The name, address and telephone number of the nuclear pharmacy;

(4) The prescription number.

(j) The amount of radioactivity shall be determined by radiometric methods for each product immediately prior to dispensing.

(k) Nuclear pharmacies may re-distribute NDA Approved radioactive drugs if the pharmacy does not process the radioactive drugs in any manner nor violate the product packaging.

(l) The permit to operate a nuclear pharmacy is conditioned upon an approved Radiation Central Agency or Nuclear Regulatory Commission license. Copies of RCA or NCR inspection reports shall be made available for Board inspection.

Section 4. General Requirements for Nuclear Pharmacists to Obtain a Nuclear Pharmacy Permit

A qualified nuclear pharmacist shall:

(a) Be a currently licensed pharmacist in the state; and

(b) Be certified as a nuclear pharmacist by the Board of Pharmaceutical Specialties; or

(c) Meet the following standards:

(1) Meet minimal standards of training for medical uses of radioactive material (cite radiological control agency or NRC licensure guide);

(2) Have received a minimum of 200 contact hours of didactic instruction in nuclear pharmacy from an accredited college of pharmacy;

(3) Attain a minimum of 500 hours of clinical nuclear pharmacy training under the supervision of a certified nuclear pharmacist in a nuclear pharmacy providing nuclear pharmacy services in a certified nuclear pharmacy residence program or in a structured nuclear pharmacy training program in an accredited college of pharmacy;

(4) Submit an affidavit of experience and training to the State Board of Pharmacy.

Section 5. Library

Each nuclear pharmacy shall have the following reference books. All books must be current editions or revisions:

(a) United States Pharmacopeia/National Formulary with supplements.

(b) State laws and regulations relating to pharmacy.

(c) State and/or Federal Regulations governing the use of applicable radioactive materials.

(d) United States Public Health Service, Radiological Health Handbook.

Section 6. Minimum Equipment Requirements

(a) Laminar flow hood.
(b) Dose calibrator.
(c) Refrigerator.
(d) Class A prescription balance or balance of greater sensitivity.
(e) Single or multiple channel scintillation counter.
(f) Microscope.
(g) A radiochemical hood and filter system.
(h) Other equipment necessary for radiopharmaceutical services provided as required by the Board of Pharmacy.

ROLE OF THE PHARMACIST IN THE HOSPITAL WITH AN ISOTOPE PHARMACY

In hospitals which have established a radioisotope pharmacy, the pharmacist purchases, stores and dispenses the various isotopes required by the medical staff licensed to use these materials.

In these institutions, the physician, upon deciding to prescribe radioactive material, calls the pharmacist and provides him with all of the necessary information.

The pharmacist then makes the necessary calculations in order to arrive at the required dosage, transfers same from the stock container, using a remote control pipette, places it in a paper cup within a lead container and transports it to the patient for administration.

From this point on, the responsibility for radiation protection, contamination, and disposal of waste products will fall under the aegis of the radiation safety officer.

ROLE OF THE PHARMACIST IN THE HOSPITAL WITHOUT AN ISOTOPE PHARMACY

The mere fact that the majority of the hospitals using radioisotopes have not established, as yet, an isotope pharmacy is no criterion for the hospital pharmacist not to make some contribution toward the administrative aspects of the hospital's isotope program. In this regard, the hospital pharmacist may assume the responsibility for the ordering, receiving and storage of all isotopes in current use throughout the hospital. The purchasing phase of such a program is relatively simple and does not differ from the purchase of other pharmaceutical products. In fact, a number of the commonly used radioisotopes are usually purchased in pre-determined quantities for automatic shipment on a standing order basis.

The receiving aspect of radioisotopes differs from the receiving phase of purchased pharmaceuticals in that all packages coming to the pharmacy must be stored in a lead vault and a record maintained which indicates the date of receipt, the purchase order number, the ordering physician, the name of the isotope and the quantity of isotope received. Upon receipt, the appropriate physician or technician is notified to remove the material from the pharmacy vault.

The radiation safety officer monitors the pharmacy vault and the surrounding area as part of his safety program; therefore, there is little possibility of harmful radiation within the environs of the pharmacy. All records of isotope materials received are to be maintained in the pharmacy office and are made available to the radiation safety officer and the Atomic Energy Commission inspector when necessary.

TRAINING STUDENTS IN NUCLEAR PHARMACY

Because more pharmacists are exhibiting an interest in this branch of pharmaceutical practice, the ASHP developed an Accreditation Standard for Residency Training in Nuclear Pharmacy (With Guide to Interpretation).[14] This document establishes the following standards:

STANDARD I. QUALIFICATIONS OF THE TRAINING HOSPITAL

A. Nuclear pharmacy residency training programs shall be oriented to institutional practice and shall be based, in large part, in a hospital. The hospital shall be accredited by the Joint Commission on Accreditation of Hospitals or the American Osteopathic Association. Further, the hospital shall operate an organized nuclear medicine department and shall be licensed by the Environmental Protection Agency or the Nuclear Regulatory Commission and other appropriate agencies, for all categories of radioactive byproduct materials used in humans.

B. Two or more institutions may join together to provide nuclear pharmacy residency training, provided that each meets the intent of this Standard.

C. Nuclear pharmacy residencies shall be conducted only in those institutions in which the educational benefits to the resident are considered of paramount importance in relation to the service benefits which the institution may obtain from the resident.

D. The institutions must provide a wide range of nuclear medicine studies.

E. The institution shall be staffed with at least one board-certified nuclear medicine physician and one nuclear medicine technologist.

Where two or more institutions are used as training sites, at least half of the participating institutions shall be staffed by at least one board-certified nuclear medicine physician and one board-certified nuclear medicine technologist.

STANDARD II. QUALIFICATIONS OF THE NUCLEAR PHARMACY SERVICE

A. The nuclear pharmacy service shall be organized in accordance with the principles of good management under the immediate supervision of a legally qualified pharmacist. It shall have sufficient staff, both professsional and supportive, to carry out a broad scope of radiopharmaceutical services, and shall comply (where applicable) with all federal, state and local laws, codes, statutes, and regulations.

B. The nuclear pharmacy shall have physical facilities that are adequate to permit activities over a broad range of services including, but not limited to, the following professional and administrative areas:

1. Nuclear pharmacy administration,
2. Radiopharmaceutical distribution and inventory control,
3. Technology and quality control,
4. Radiotracer development and evaluation,
5. Radiopharmaceutical chemistry and tracer methodology,
6. Radiological health activities, and
7. Clinical services.

It is necessary that a regular and continuing experience be provided in these activities, and it is not sufficient to create artificial situations for residents to obtain this experience. If any of the designated activities or divisions of pharmaceutical practice are not available in the parent training site, arrangements shall be made with another nuclear pharmacy unit (or other facility acceptable to the American Society of Hospital Pharmacists) to provide the necessary experience.

C. The director of the nuclear pharmacy unit shall have the responsibility and the authority to carry out a broad scope of radiopharmaceutical services.

STANDARD III. QUALIFICATIONS OF THE RESIDENCY DIRECTOR AND PRECEPTORS

A. The director of the nuclear pharmacy service shall be the overall director of the residency training program and shall be subject to general administrative control and guidance by the director of pharmacy services, college dean, institutional director, or appropriate executive officer.

B. The residency director shall be a pharmacist, shall have completed a nuclear pharmacy residency accredited by the ASHP, and shall have had two years of administrative and clinical experience; or, if lacking a residency, shall have five years of experience in a nuclear pharmacy, a substantial part of which should have been of an administrative nature.

C. The residency director shall have demonstrated superior capabilities in the operation of a nuclear pharmacy service and shall have made significant contributions to the development or improvement of nuclear pharmacy practice.

D. The residency director shall have considerable latitude in delegating preceptorial responsibilities to the staff. Each individual designated as a preceptor must have demonstrated outstanding strengths in one or more areas of nuclear pharmacy practice. The residency director, however, is ultimately accountable for the overall quality of the residency training program.

E. There shall be at least one preceptor employed for each resident in the program.

F. The residency director shall be an active member of the American Society of Hospital Pharmacists. Other designated preceptors should also be members of the Society.

STANDARD IV. QUALIFICATIONS AND SELECTION OF THE APPLICANT

A. The applicant should be a graduate of a school of pharmacy accredited by the American Council on Pharmaceutical Education.

B. The applicant should have a thorough grounding in patient-oriented (clinical) pharmacy services; further, the applicant should demonstrate some degree of knowledge and skills in nuclear pharmacy practice.

C. The applicant should be recommended by his college faculty, previous employers, or professional colleagues.

D. The applicant should be a member of the American Society of Hospital Pharmacists; or, if not, he should become a member of the Society if accepted as a resident.

E. Final approval of the qualifications of the applicant and his acceptance shall be the responsibility of the nuclear pharmacy service director.

STANDARD V. RESIDENCY TRAINING PROGRAM

A. Objectives for the residency program shall be set out in writing and shall be provided to each resident at the beginning of his program. The objectives shall relate both to the administrative and professional practice skills required in contemporary good nuclear pharmacy practice and shall describe the terminal competencies to be striven for in the residency program. Objectives for training in each of the following areas shall be included:

1. Nuclear pharmacy administration,
2. Radiopharmaceutical distribution and inventory control,
3. Technology and quality control,
4. Radiotracer development and evaluation,
5. Radiopharmaceutical chemistry and tracer methodology,
6. Radiological health activities,
7. Clinical services,
8. Educational experience and activities, and
9. Research methodology.

B. Each resident's activities shall be scheduled in advance and shall be planned to make possible the attainment of the predetermined objectives. The overall schedule shall consist of a minimum of 2000 hours of training (residency-related) time, extending over a period of no less than 12 months.

C. Each resident shall maintain a record of his training activities which clearly delineates the scope and period of training. The residency director shall keep such records on file for review by the ASHP accreditation survey team.

D. Provision shall be made for formalized and regularly scheduled evaluation of the resident's achievement in terms of the objectives previously established.

STANDARD VI. CERTIFICATION

A. An appropriate certificate indicative of successful completion of the residency shall be awarded to the resident by the training institution on the recommendation of the nuclear pharmacy residency program director.

SOURCES OF INFORMATION

Current copies of Atomic Energy Commission regulations may be obtained from the Division of Licensing and Regulation, U.S. Nuclear Regulatory Commission, Washington, D.C. 20555

SELECTED READINGS

Ulackas, E.: Nuclear Pharmacy: A Red Hot Specialty. Apothecary 93:4:32, (April) 1981.
Levine, G. and Goodman, C.: Radiopharmacist Profile—Baseline 1974–1975. Contemp. Pharm. Practice, 2:3:123, (Summer) 1979.
Kawada, T., Wolf, W., and Seibert, S.: Unit-dose Dispensing of Radiopharmaceuticals. Hospitals, 48:145–160, (Jul.) 1974.

Kavula, M.M.: Centralized Radiopharmaceutical Services of the Indiana University Medical Center. Am. J. Hosp. Pharm., *31*:158–164, (Feb.) 1974.

Pollock, M.L., Strane, T.R., Brown, G.J., and McNeil, K.F.: Nuclear Pharmacy: A Student's Perspective. Contemp. Pharm. Pract., *2*:4:190, (Fall) 1979.

REFERENCES

1. Latiolias, Clifton J., Parker, Paul F., Hutchinson, George, and Statler, Robert A.: Radioisotopes in Hospital Pharmacy. The Bulletin, A.S.H.P., *12*:4:72, 1955.
2. Solyom, Peter: Report of the Committee on Isotopes. Am. J. Hosp. Pharm., *15*:8:712, 1958.
3. Latiolais, Clifton J.: Fundamentals of Radioactivity. The Bulletin, A.S.H.P., *13*:3:220. 1956.
4. Briner, William H.: Certain Aspects of Radiological Health. Am. J. Hosp. Pharm., *15*:1:44, 1958.
5. Solyom, Peter: Pharmacy Service University of Chicago Clinics. Am. J. Hosp. Pharm., *15*:1:52, 1958.
6. Morgan, G.W.: Facilities and Equipment for Isotopes Program. Hospitals, *29*:3:103, 1955.
7. Ingraham, S.C. and Taylor, W.R.: Radioisotope Facilities in the General Hospital. Hospitals, *26*:12:74, 1952.
8. Manual on Use of Radioisotopes in Hospitals. American Hospital Association, Chicago, Ill.
9. Ibid. p. 12.
10. Greene, Allan: Protective Procedures for Personnel Caring for Patients Receiving Therapeutic Isotopes. Current Practice Bulletin 6-1-3 of the Peter Bent Brigham Hospital, Boston, Mass.
11. Radioisotope Manual of the Peter Bent Brigham Hospital, Boston, Mass., January, 1969.
12. Barker, L.F. and Evans, W.E.: Unit-dose Radiopharmaceutical Service as a Component of Total Pharmacy Practice. Am. J. Hosp. Pharm., *33*:61–63, (Jan.) 1976.
13. Model Regulations for Nuclear Pharmacy 1984. National Association of Boards of Pharmacy, 1 East Wacker Drive, Chicago, Ill. 60601.
14. ASHP Accreditation Standard for Residency Training in Nuclear Pharmacy (With Guide to Interpretation). Am. J. Hosp. Pharm., *38*:1964–1971, (Dec.) 1981.

24

The Physical Plant and Its Equipment

The Minimum Standard for Pharmacies in Hospitals provides as follows:[1]

"Adequate pharmaceutical and administrative facilities shall be provided for the pharmacy department, including especially: (A) the necessary equipment for the compounding, dispensing and manufacturing of pharmaceuticals and parenteral preparations, (B) bookkeeping supplies and related materials and equipment necessary for the proper administration of the department, (C) an adequate library and filing equipment to make information concerning drugs readily available to both pharmacists and physicians, (D) special locked storage space to meet the legal requirements for storage of narcotics, alcohol and other prescribed drugs, (E) a refrigerator for the storage of thermolabile products, (F) adequate floor space for all pharmacy operations and the storage of pharmaceuticals at a satisfactory location provided with proper lighting and ventilation."

Accordingly, this chapter is presented for consideration of the student as well as those seeking information which may be useful in developing plans either for the renovation of an existing department or the construction of a new facility, data concerning location, floor space, general equipment, refrigeration and storage facilities and general construction information relating to lighting, ventilation, plumbing and surface finishes.

FUNCTIONAL PLANNING

Many competent authorities have stated that before the architect's pencil touches paper, he must become thoroughly familiar with the hospital's objectives, plan of operation and operational policies relating to the area to be designed.

The architect may gather this information by attending various meetings with the hospital administrator, the department head and the Building Committee. During these sessions, many questions will be asked and at their conclusion it is possible that a special study or survey will be conducted to confirm or establish the need.

498

Because hospital pharmacists new to the field have seldom become involved in this aspect of the hospital planning, they are often frightened and confused at the prospect of having to meet with the architect and the trustees with regard to pharmacy construction or remodeling. This is especially so because they do not know what to expect during such sessions.

Prior to exposure to the architect and trustees, the hospital pharmacist should become acquainted with the overall planning process. Basically, it consists of three parts: (1) a master program, (2) functional programming, and (3) equipment planning and architectural design. The master program sets forth goals and objectives. The functional program specifies the operational demands upon the facilities. The architectural design and equipment programming translates these into physical space, equipment and furnishings.[2]

Steps for developing a functional program and supporting materials for the architect are:[3]

1. Identify hospital purposes and goals.
2. Determine pharmacy objectives and plan of operation.
3. Determine functions to be performed.
4. Determine workflow and procedures.
5. Estimate workload.
6. Determine work areas needed.
7. Determine personnel to be accommodated in each work area.
8. Determine space, shape, furniture, equipment and service needs of each work area.
9. Determine interrelationships between work areas and between the pharmacy and other departments. Consider shared services.
10. Arrange work areas to maximize the performance functions.
11. Design one or more schematic floor plans to meet requirements; then reconcile these with "real life" limitations.
12. Evaluate effectiveness of each design for meeting requirements.
13. Review the above steps until an optimal design emerges.

The three broad general functions have been identified as **utility, amenity** and **expression.** Utility is the service the pharmacy provides to the hospital; amenity is the satisfaction of the personal satisfaction of the pharmacy staff and expression is the symbolized significance of the pharmacy to the hospital and its community.[3]

In order to acquaint these pharmacists with the type of information which they will be asked to present, the following questions, although not exhaustive on the subject, are abstracted from a U.S. Public Health Service publication[5] and are herewith presented.

On the right side of the questionnaire are check lines in columns headed A, B, and C. These are intended to help the functional programming team in evaluating and rating the relative significance of all questions and subfactors to be considered in accordance with the following:[4]

1. Checkmark in Column "A"—indicates the question deserves essential consideration and/or certain of its subparts call for definitive answers.
2. Checkmark in Column "B"—calls for further study before being included or excluded as a program consideration. Following appropriate review, if the factor is to be included in the program, it would be marked "A." If it is to be excluded, it would become a "C."
3. Checkmark in Column "C"—indicates the question will be excluded as a program consideration because it is either impractical or unnecessary.

WORKLOADS AND WORKFLOWS

	A	B	C
(1) Will the inpatient pharmacy be operative 24-hours a day? If not, what will be its hours of operation? What provisions will be made for issuance of medications when the pharmacy is closed	—	—	—
(2) How will physicians order medications so the pharmacy will receive copies of original orders?			
☐ Use of carbonized paper?	—	—	—
☐ Use of automated devices?	—	—	—
Input/output device?	—	—	—
Photocopier?	—	—	—
Telewriter?	—	—	—
Voice recorder?	—	—	—
Other?	—	—	—
(3) How will patient medication profiles be maintained in the pharmacy and on the nursing unit?			
☐ Duplicate orders stored together in individual patient file?	—	—	—
☐ Transcribed onto cards or suitable form?	—	—	—
☐ Use of automated devices?	—	—	—
(4) Will there be a bulk compounding program?			
☐ Where and how will distilled water be obtained?	—	—	—
☐ What type of sterile area will be required?	—	—	—
☐ What equipment will be needed?	—	—	—
☐ What type of quality control programs will be instituted?	—	—	—
(5) Will there be a packaging program?			
☐ Will an outside contractor be used?	—	—	—
☐ What equipment and supplies will be needed?	—	—	—
☐ What type of quality control program will be instituted?	—	—	—
(6) What types of pharmacy educational programs will be developed?			
☐ In-service?	—	—	—
☐ Nursing education?	—	—	—
☐ Interns?	—	—	—

	A	B	C
☐ Residents?	—	—	—
☐ Students?	—	—	—
☐ Technicians?	—	—	—
☐ Patients and families?	—	—	—
☐ Cooperative clinical pharmacy program with school of pharmacy?	—	—	—

(7) What type of pharmacy research program will be developed?

	A	B	C
☐ Administrative or behavioral?	—	—	—
☐ Bench type?	—	—	—
☐ Clinical?	—	—	—

(8) Will the pharmacy be concerned with radio-pharmaceuticals? If so, where located?

	A	B	C
Pharmacy?	—	—	—
Radiology?	—	—	—
Other/	—	—	—

(9) Will there be a drug information center? If so, what will be its hours of operation? Which of the following functions will it have?

	A	B	C
☐ Drug information?	—	—	—
To Pharmacy and Therapeutics Committee?	—	—	—
Within pharmacy department?	—	—	—
On patient care areas?	—	—	—
Regulate activities of drug company representatives?	—	—	—
Answer specific requests, verbal and written?	—	—	—
Prepare periodical bulletins and newsletters?	—	—	—
☐ Poison control?	—	—	—
Respond to calls?	—	—	—
Coordinate poison control with drug information?	—	—	—
Coordinate communications with medical personnel?	—	—	—
Maintain consultant panel?	—	—	—
Coordinate information with treatment center?	—	—	—
☐ Investigational drugs?	—	—	—
Search literature?	—	—	—
Review protocols?	—	—	—
Establish control measures for the hospital?	—	—	—
☐ Drug surveillance?	—	—	—
Conduct current and retrospective reviews of all drug practices (drug selection and utilization, adverse reactions, drug usage studies)?	—	—	—
☐ Education?	—	—	—
Present lectures, consultations, surveys, reports?	—	—	—
☐ Research?	—	—	—

Where would the drug information center be located?

	A	B	C
☐ Pharmacy?	—	—	—
☐ Medical library?	—	—	—
☐ Other?	—	—	—

What staff would be required?

                   A   B   C

☐ Drug information pharmacists?   — — —
☐ Pharmacy residents, interns, students?   — — —
☐ Technicians?   — — —
☐ Secretarial personnel?   — — —

(10) What type of drug distribution system will be employed?
    ☐ Individual prescription?   — — —
    ☐ Individual prescription-floor stock combination?   — — —
    ☐ Centralized unit-dose?   — — —
    ☐ Decentralized unit-dose?   — — —
    ☐ Combination centralized-decentralized unit-dose?   — — —
    ☐ Automated?   — — —
    ☐ Other?   — — —

(11) If individual prescription or combination system is employed:
    ☐ How will orders be transmitted to the pharmacy?
      Pharmacy messenger?   — — —
      Other messenger?   — — —
      Pneumatic tube or drop chute?   — — —
      Automated device?   — — —
      Telephone (under what circumstances acceptable)?   — — —
    ☐ How will drugs be packaged?
      Single unit packages?   — — —
      Number of doses per package?   — — —
    ☐ How will orders be filled?   — — —
      Plastic bags or envelopes?   — — —
      Individual patient drawer?   — — —
    ☐ How will orders be delivered to nursing unit?
      Pharmacy messenger?   — — —
      Other messenger?   — — —
      Pneumatic tube?   — — —
      Conveyor or dumbwaiter?   — — —
    ☐ How will *stat* orders be handled?
      Sent to pharmacy by automatic device?   — — —
      Telephone?   — — —
      Intercom?   — — —
      Picked up by pharmacy messenger?   — — —
      Delivered to pharmacy by nursing unit personnel?   — — —
    ☐ How will individual prescription orders be stored on the nursing unit?
      Cart with individual patient drawers?   — — —
      Cabinets with individual patient compartments?   — — —
      Pass-through closet with doors or other storage area in patient rooms?   — — —
    ☐ What will be the administrative procedures on nursing unit for:
      Administering medications?   — — —
      Charting?   — — —
      Maintaining patient medication profile?   — — —
      Recording charges?   — — —
    ☐ How will *prn* orders be refilled?

	A	B	C
Regular exchange interval?	—	—	—
Special requisition by nursing unit?	—	—	—
Suspense file in pharmacy?	—	—	—

☐ How will routine orders be refilled?

	A	B	C
Regular exchange interval?	—	—	—
Requisition by nursing unit?	—	—	—
Suspense file in pharmacy?	—	—	—

☐ How will written or recorded orders be changed after conference between pharmacist and physician?

	A	B	C
Change noted on all copies of order form?	—	—	—
Computer correction made by physician or pharmacist?	—	—	—
Change card prepared and signed by parties involved?	—	—	—

☐ How will narcotics and controlled drugs be handled?

	A	B	C
Individual prescription with prescription or portion thereof stored in patient's compartment or drawer?	—	—	—
Regular floor stock?	—	—	—
Other?	—	—	—

☐ How will IV additives be handled?

	A	B	C
Solution with additive prepared in pharmacy?	—	—	—
Additives sent to nursing unit ready to add to solution?	—	—	—
Complete procedure handled on nursing unit?	—	—	—

☐ How will cancelled orders and out-of-date prescriptions be handled?

	A	B	C
Returned to pharmacy when cancellation order is written?	—	—	—
Returned to pharmacy when located on nursing unit?	—	—	—

☐ How will absence of medication in usual storage area be noted?

	A	B	C
Reminder card of location (e.g., refrigerator, floor stock, narcotic cabinet)?	—	—	—

☐ How will limited floor stock be replenished?

	A	B	C
Use of preprinted requisition form by nursing unit?	—	—	—
Routine inventory check by pharmacy?	—	—	—

☐ How will charges be handled?

	A	B	C
At nursing unit (doses administered)?	—	—	—
At pharmacy (doses dispensed)?	—	—	—

(12) If centralized unit-dose system is employed:

☐ How will orders be transmitted to main pharmacy?

	A	B	C
Pharmacy messenger?	—	—	—
Other messenger?	—	—	—
Pneumatic tube?	—	—	—
Drop chute?	—	—	—
Automated device?	—	—	—

☐ How will patient medication profiles be maintained?

	A	B	C
Visible card file?	—	—	—
Envelope?	—	—	—
Card?	—	—	—
Automated device?	—	—	—

A   B   C

☐ How many unit-doses are expected to be dispensed per day, assuming that a unit-dose may consist of one or more single unit packages?   — — —
☐ How will unit-doses be packaged? (Procurement of all possible commercially packaged items?)
    Large packaging program?   — — —
    Small packaging program?   — — —
    Outside contractor?   — — —
    Extemporaneous packaging, including sterile?   — — —
☐ How will unit-doses be dispensed?
    Supervised pickers?   — — —
    Automated devices?   — — —
☐ How will unit-doses be prepared for delivery?
    Individual patient containers (envelopes and bags)?   — — —
    Individual patient drawers?   — — —
☐ After routine dosage times have been established (for example, q.i.d. 9,1,5,9-h.s.—10 p.m.) how many dosage intervals will be covered by each delivery, or how many deliveries per day will be scheduled?
    Morning?   — — —
    Noon?   — — —
    Afternoon?   — — —
    Evening?   — — —
☐ What is the expected number of orders to be processed by time of day? (Consider *regularly scheduled meds, prns, IVs, stats,* and *pre-ops* separately.)   — — —
☐ What is the expected number of prescriptions or unit-doses to be dispensed by time of day? (Consider required scheduled drugs, IVs, IV additives added later, those requiring reconstitution and those requiring varying amounts of compounding.)   — — —
☐ How will unit-doses be delivered?
    Pharmacy messenger?   — — —
    Other messenger?   — — —
    Pneumatic tube?   — — —
    Conveyor, dumbwaiter, other automated devices?   — — —
☐ How will unit-doses be stored on the nursing units?
    Patient drawers in carts?   — — —
    Nurserver or other storage area in patient room?   — — —
    Patient compartment in cabinet?   — — —
    Other storage area?   — — —
☐ What administrative procedures will be established on nursing units for drug administration?
    Nurse, licensed, practical nurse, pharmacy employee?   — — —
    Chart with schedule, visible card file?   — — —
    Patient profile?   — — —
☐ How will charges be handled?
    Nursing unit, doses administered?   — — —
    Pharmacy, doses dispensed?   — — —
☐ How will *stat* orders be handled?

	A	B	C
Sent to pharmacy by automated device (e.g., pneumatic tube, conveyor, computer, electrowriter)?	—	—	—
Telephone?	—	—	—
Intercom?	—	—	—
Picked up by pharmacy messenger?	—	—	—
Sent to pharmacy by nursing unit personnel?	—	—	—

☐ How will nonroutine doses be handled?

☐ How will narcotics be handled?

	A	B	C
Unit-dose?	—	—	—
Floor-stock?	—	—	—

☐ How will IV additives be handled?

	A	B	C
Prepared in advance or on order by pharmacy?	—	—	—
Ready-to-use additives sent to nursing unit by pharmacy?	—	—	—
Prepared on nursing unit?	—	—	—

(13) If decentralized unit-dose system is employed: Because pharmacy substations on nursing units are used in this system, answer all questions for centralized unit-dose system wherever applicable after first answering the following questions.

☐ Where will the pharmacy substations be installed and how many patients will each cover?   — — —

☐ What will be the operating hours of the various substations?   — — —

☐ How will the substations be staffed?   — — —

☐ What will be the activities of the substation pharmacist?

	A	B	C
Review charts?	—	—	—
Consult with physicians on orders?	—	—	—
Consult with nurses?	—	—	—
Conduct patient interviews?	—	—	—
Make round with physicians?	—	—	—
Maintain and review patients' medication profile?	—	—	—
Supervise dispensing and dose preparation on floor?	—	—	—

(14) Will a centralized-decentralized unit-dose system be employed?   — — —

(After first establishing the parameters of the extent of use of both systems, proper answers to the applicable questions for centralized and decentralized unit-dose systems should supply all of the information required for establishment of a centralized-decentralized unit-dose system.)

(15) If automated systems are employed

☐ What type of system will be used:

	A	B	C
Automated dispensing, pharmacist activated?	—	—	—
Automated dispensing, computer activated?	—	—	—

☐ How will the system be inspected?   — — —

☐ Where will automated devices be located?

	A	B	C
Main pharmacy?	—	—	—
Pharmacy substation?	—	—	—
Each nursing unit?	—	—	—
Combination of nursing units?	—	—	—

	A	B	C

☐ How will the pharmacist receive a direct copy of the physician's order?
☐ What type of packages will be used?   — — —
☐ How will devices be filled?   — — —
☐ How will the automated system be backed up during failures?   — — —

(16) Will the pharmacy department include out-patient prescriptions?   — — —

(17) Who will be entitled to use outpatient services?
☐ Hospital outpatients?   — — —
☐ Patients treated by physicians whose offices are located in the hospital?   — — —
☐ Hospital employees?   — — —

(18) Where will the cashier be located?   — — —

(19) Will there be a separate outpatient pharmacy?   — — —

(20) Will there be partitioned spaces and/or offices for pharmacist interviews with outpatients?   — — —

(21) What administrative procedures will be established for:
☐ Maintenance for outpatient medication profiles?   — — —
☐ Prescription files, including records of refills for outpatients?   — — —

Work Areas

(1) What are the office space requirements for the following personnel:
☐ Chief pharmacist?   — — —
☐ Assistant chief pharmacist?   — — —
☐ Other section chiefs?   — — —
☐ Clerical?   — — —
☐ Clinical pharmacist (inpatient care areas)?   — — —

(2) What are the other work space requirements?
☐ Extemporaneous compounding?   — — —
☐ Inpatient dispensing, centralized?   — — —
☐ Bulk compounding?   — — —
☐ Packaging?   — — —
☐ Drug information center?   — — —
☐ Sterile compounding, including IV additive services?   — — —
☐ Editing or order review center?   — — —
☐ Storage of drugs and supplies (e.g., refrigeration, alcohol and other flammables, narcotics and regular active and inactive)?   — — —
☐ Quality control and research?   — — —
☐ Educational activities?   — — —
☐ Radiopharmacy?   — — —
☐ Outpatient dispensing?   — — —
☐ Cart storage?   — — —

	A	B	C
☐ Staff lockers and lounge area?	—	—	—
☐ Waiting areas (inpatient, outpatient, and offices)?	—	—	—

(3) What are the space requirements for the pharmacy sub-stations in the following areas?

	A	B	C
☐ Administration			
Office?	—	—	—
Education?	—	—	—
Drug information?	—	—	—
☐ Dispensing?	—	—	—
☐ Compounding (extemporaneous and sterile)?	—	—	—
☐ Editing or order review?	—	—	—
☐ Storage			
Active?	—	—	—
Bulk?	—	—	—
Refrigeration?	—	—	—
Medication cart?	—	—	—
Narcotics?	—	—	—

Staffing Requirements

Decisions arising from considering questions posed in previous sections will bear importantly on factors presented in this section.

(1) Based on the drug distribution system chosen, to what extent will nonprofessionals be used in the pharmacy for the following activities?

	A	B	C
☐ Label typing?	—	—	—
☐ Other clerical duties?	—	—	—
☐ Bulk compounding?	—	—	—
☐ Packaging?	—	—	—
☐ Pickup and delivery?	—	—	—
☐ Inventory control?	—	—	—
☐ Equipment maintenance?	—	—	—
☐ Housekeeping?	—	—	—
☐ Dispensing?	—	—	—
☐ Purchasing?	—	—	—

(2) What supervision will nonprofessionals require?   — — —

(3) What will be the education and training requirements for nonprofessionals and how will they be trained?

	A	B	C
☐ Inhouse training program?	—	—	—
☐ On-the-job training?	—	—	—
☐ Formal outside training?	—	—	—

(4) How will coverage be provided during meal hours, days off, vacations, and sick leave?   — — —

(5) With the increasing use of nonprofessionals, what additional professional duties will be given to pharmacists?

☐ Conduct patient interviews (admission and discharge)?   — — —

	A	B	C
☐ Maintain patient medication profiles?	—	—	—
☐ Edit all medication orders?	—	—	—
☐ Discuss drug regimen with physicians?	—	—	—
☐ Provide information to physicians, nurses, and aides?	—	—	—
☐ Supervise preparation of all medication doses?	—	—	—
☐ Supervise medication administration?	—	—	—
☐ Maintain IV additive program?	—	—	—

(6) Will there be a clinical pharmacy training program in conjunction with a school of pharmacy? If so, what will be the student/preceptor ratio?   — — —

(7) If 24-hour service is to be given, how will the workload be distributed?   — — —

(8) Will volunteers be used? If so, what tasks will they perform? At what hours and on what days?   — — —

(9) What are the estimated staffing patterns and hours for:

	A	B	C
☐ Full-time pharmacist?	—	—	—
☐ Part-time pharmacist?	—	—	—
☐ Technician?	—	—	—
☐ Helpers?	—	—	—
☐ Clerical?	—	—	—
☐ Other?	—	—	—
Shifts			
8:00 a.m.–4:00 p.m.	—	—	—
4:00 p.m.–12:00 a.m.	—	—	—
12:00 a.m.–8:00 a.m.	—	—	—

Mechanical and Other Requirements for Built-In Equipment

(1) What mechanical systems will be required for carrying supplies and requisitions between the inpatient pharmacy and the following activities:

Activity	*Pneumatic Tube (and size)*	*Vertical Conveyor*	*Horizontal Conveyor*	*Other*
Nursing Unit	_____	_____	_____	_____
Outpatient Pharmacy	_____	_____	_____	_____
Central Service	_____	_____	_____	_____
Operating Room	_____	_____	_____	_____
Emergency	_____	_____	_____	_____
General Stores	_____	_____	_____	_____
Clinical Laboratories	_____	_____	_____	_____
X-Ray	_____	_____	_____	_____
Mailroom	_____	_____	_____	_____
Accounting	_____	_____	_____	_____
Data Processing	_____	_____	_____	_____

	A	B	C

(2) If there is to be a separate outpatient pharmacy, what will be its needs in regard to the above activities? — — —

(3) What will be the preferred pharmacy locations for the pneumatic tube and/or conveyor stations? — — —

(4) Will the pharmacy require gas, vacuum, and compressed air; if so, where will the outlets be placed? — — —

(5) Where will 110–120v electrical outlets be placed? — — —
Will there be any special lighting requirements? — — —
Will high voltage voltage lines be required? — — —

(6) Will the pharmacy require its own still? — — —

(7) Will the pharmacy require its own autoclave? — — —

(8) Where will sinks be required and placed? (State type and size.) — — —

(9) Will special flooring be required? — — —
What type? — — —
Where? — — —

(10) What functional elements and service outlets within the pharmacy must be provided with standby power? — — —

(11) What special requirements will be needed in the sterile area?
A/C vents near laminar flow hoods? — — —
UV light? — — —
Other? — — —

(12) Will any special plumbing fixtures, such as floor drains be required?

(13) What will be the storage and fixed equipment requirements for each of the following:
☐ Refrigerated drugs? — — —
☐ Alcohol? — — —
☐ Narcotics and other controlled drugs? — — —
☐ Bulk supplies? — — —
☐ Active supplies? — — —
☐ Documents? — — —

(14) What will be the cabinet, shelving, and work counter requirements for:
☐ Extemporaneous compounding area? — — —
☐ Inpatient dispensing area? — — —
☐ Sterile production area? — — —
☐ Bulk compounding area, including quality control? — — —
☐ Packaging area? — — —
☐ Administrative areas:
  Office? — — —
  Education? — — —
  Drug information? — — —
  Conference room/library? — — —

	A	B	C
Staff lockers?			
☐ Radiopharmaceutical?	—	—	—
☐ Outpatient dispensing area?	—	—	—
☐ Storerooms?	—	—	—
☐ Pharmacy substations:			
Administrative areas?	—	—	—
Dispensing areas?	—	—	—
Compounding areas?	—	—	—
Editing areas?	—	—	—
Storage areas?	—	—	—

(15) Will drinking fountains be required? — — —
Where? — — —

(16) If bulletin boards are needed, what size and where will they be placed? — — —

(17) Where will central vacuum cleaning outlets be located? — — —

(18) What clocks will be needed? — — —
Where? — — —

(19) What signs will be needed? — — —
Type and size? — — —
Illuminated? — — —
Where located? — — —

(20) What equipment listed below will be required? (Indicate floor area needed for item and operator and where item will be placed.)
☐ Duplicating? — — —
☐ Dictating? — — —
☐ Transcribing? — — —
☐ Imprinting? — — —
☐ Computer terminals? — — —
☐ Direct writing intercom? — — —
☐ Teletype? — — —
☐ Calculators? — — —
☐ Closed circuit TV? — — —
☐ Files? — — —

Interrelationships

What will be the interrelationship between the pharmacy department and the following major departments and/or services relative to the factors listed?

(1) Nursing Units
☐ Ordering medications (routine prescriptions, refills, *stats, prns,* investigational drugs, back orders, telephone orders, and non-formulary drugs)? — — —
☐ Delivery of written medication orders? — — —
☐ Delivery of medications? — — —
☐ Ordering, delivering, and record keeping of controlled drugs? — — —
☐ Credits for unused medications? — — —

	A	B	C

☐ Control of medications brought in by patient? ___ ___ ___
☐ Information on patient census status? ___ ___ ___
☐ Patient medication charges? ___ ___ ___
☐ Replacement of emergency drug boxes? ___ ___ ___
☐ Procedures for discharge medications? ___ ___ ___
☐ Procedures for obtaining medications when pharmacy is closed? ___ ___ ___

(2) Administration
☐ Pharmacy's place in hospital organizational structure? ___ ___ ___
☐ Authority of chief pharmacist? ___ ___ ___
☐ Hours of service for pharmacy? ___ ___ ___
☐ Committees on which chief pharmacist and other pharmacists will serve? ___ ___ ___

(3) Medical Staff
☐ Pharmacy and Therapeutics Committee? ___ ___ ___
☐ Formulary? ___ ___ ___
☐ Automatic stop orders? ___ ___ ___
☐ Narcotics control? ___ ___ ___
☐ Drug informaiton service? ___ ___ ___
☐ Handling of physician's samples? ___ ___ ___

(4) Procurement
☐ Ordering and receiving supplies and equipment for pharmacy? ___ ___ ___
☐ Setting standards for drugs and supplies? ___ ___ ___

(5) Central Service
☐ Common use of delivery equipment and services? ___ ___ ___
☐ Supply of freshly distilled water? ___ ___ ___
☐ Common use of sterilizing equipment? ___ ___ ___

(6) Inpatients
☐ Medication history? ___ ___ ___
☐ Patient medication profile? ___ ___ ___
☐ Discharge interview? ___ ___ ___

(7) Business Office
☐ Budget status reports? ___ ___ ___
☐ Charges to patients? ___ ___ ___
☐ Credits for unused medications? ___ ___ ___
☐ Procedure for paying for pharmacy materials? ___ ___ ___

(8) Personnel Department
☐ Job descriptions policy? ___ ___ ___
☐ Awards policy? ___ ___ ___
☐ Pharmacy staffing patterns? ___ ___ ___
☐ Staff promotions? ___ ___ ___

(9) Clinical Support Activities
☐ How will supplies be requisitioned, issued, delivered, and charged routinely and irregularly to such areas as the laboratory, surgery, and X-ray? ___ ___ ___

	A	B	C

(10) General Stores
☐ Requisitioning pharmacy supplies and equipment?   — — —
☐ Delivering pharmacy supplies and equipment?   — — —
☐ Will a special storage area in general stores be required for pharmacy items?   — — —

(11) Data Management
☐ How will the pharmacy used EDP?
Patient information for drug distribution system?   — — —
Patient medication profiles?   — — —
Ward medication schedules?   — — —
Patient information for drug utilization reviews?   — — —
Patient information for adverse action reporting?   — — —
Charges and credits?   — — —
Inventory?   — — —
Ordering supplies?   — — —
Drug formulary?   — — —
Drug utilization review?   — — —

(12) Housekeeping
☐ How will cleaning supplies be handled?   — — —
☐ How will housekeeping for pharmacy department be handled?   — — —

(13) Outpatient Department
☐ Supervision of outpatient pharmacy?   — — —
☐ Required office space for outpatient pharmacy?   — — —
☐ Processing of outpatient prescriptions?   — — —
☐ Payment method for outpatient prescriptions (Cashier in pharmacy?)   — — —
☐ Extent of outpatient department use of different stock (e.g., nonunit dose), thus requiring duplicate inventory contract systems, purchasing, and charging?   — — —
☐ Processing of employee prescriptions?   — — —

(14) Medical Records Department
☐ Review of charts for adverse actions and drug utilization review?   — — —
☐ Prescriptions filled directly from charts?   — — —

Communication and Transport

(1) How many telephones will be required?   — — —
What type?   — — —
Location?   — — —

(2) Will there be direct audio-intercom between pharmacy department and the following:
☐ Nursing units?   — — —
☐ Emergency department?   — — —
☐ Central service?   — — —
☐ Drug storage area?   — — —
☐ Outpatient pharmacy?   — — —

          A   B   C

(3) Will the pharmacy be tied into general paging and piped music system?

Location of terminals?   — — —

(4) Will pharmacy be tied into emergency alert?
- ☐ Cart?   — — —
- ☐ Other equipment?   — — —
- ☐ Signal apparatus?   — — —

(5) What are the materials handling needs of the pharmacy?

Vertical?   — — —

Horizontal?   — — —

Demand by time of day?   — — —

(6) What type of transportation system will be used for drug distribution?
- ☐ Large carts?   — — —
- ☐ Individual patient drawer carts?   — — —
- ☐ Automated?

  (automated cart conveyor—pneumatic tube—dumb-waiter)   — — —
- ☐ Other?   — — —

(7) Will there be computer input-output devices in the inpatient and/or outpatient pharmacies and, if so, where will they be located?   — — —

Location

(1) Where will pharmacy department be located in relation to:
- ☐ Main entrance and lobby?   — — —
- ☐ Outpatient area?   — — —
- ☐ Elevators?   — — —
- ☐ Information desk?   — — —
- ☐ General stores?   — — —
- ☐ Central service?   — — —
- ☐ Business office?   — — —
- ☐ Physician's lounge?   — — —
- ☐ Loading dock?   — — —
- ☐ Other?   — — —

(2) Will there be more than one inpatient pharmacy substation?

Locations?   — — —

(3) Will there be a separate outpatient pharmacy?   — — —

Location?   — — —

(4) Will the pharmacy receive supplies directly into its area?

Loading platform?   — — —

Other?   — — —

A   B   C

(5) In the traffic flow, what will be the nature and number of commerce units between the pharmacy department and

☐ Nursing units?   — — —
☐ Outpatient area?   — — —
☐ General stores?   involving   — — —
☐ Central service?   people,   — — —
☐ Elevators?   materials, and   — — —
☐ Clinical support services?   information.   — — —
☐ Extended care facility?   — — —

When will peak traffic occur relative to above?

Environmental Requirements

(1) Will carpeting be required in any or all areas?   — — —

(2) Where and to what extent should acoustical treatment be given?   — — —

(3) What type of temperature and humidity controls will be required?   — — —

(4) What is the preferred color scheme by functional areas?   — — —

(5) What door-keying system and controls will be used?   — — —

(6) What will be the air filtration requirements?   — — —

Although the foregoing list provides the hospital pharmacist with a reasonable check on the subjects and areas to be planned for, it is important for the planner to give consideration to the changes that have taken place within the practice of hospital pharmacy since the list was prepared. As a result of the changes made in the health care delivery system during the past 10 years, consideration must now be given to the following subjects and areas in order that the end product be a modern hospital pharmacy.

1. Will the pharmacy have need for a quality control laboratory?
2. Will the hospital pharmacy become involved in the handling and dispensing of radioisotopes?
3. Will the hospital's Allergy Department require the hospital pharmacy to become involved in the preparation of allergenic extracts and subsequent dilutions?
4. Is there a need for a research laboratory?
5. Has consideration been given to providing space for certain specialized functions, *i.e.* unit dose dispensing; I.V. solution additive program; drug information service; patient drug control system (patient profile); unit-dose packaging area and required equipment?

6. Will the pharmacy become involved with educational programs for the benefit of medical, nursing and pharmacy students; interns and residents; graduate physicians, nurses and pharmacists; co-operative clinical pharmacy programs with schools or colleges of pharmacy?

7. Will the pharmacy and its staff be an integral part of the local poison control center? If so, facilities planning should include space for information gathering, storage and a suitable communications system. Consideration must also be given to its location and staffing requirements.

8. With the improvements that have been made in electronic data processing systems, consideration should be given to the use of a computer by the pharmacy. If this is determined to be feasible, planning must include specialists from administration, pharmacy, nursing, medical staff and data processing in order to ascertain the extent of the program required as well as the selection and placement of appropriate equipment. In developing the system, all parties concerned should give consideration to building into it a system of inspections and checks as well as to provide for adequate back-up service in case of mechanical failure.

9. Consideration must be given to the means by which pharmacy supplies and requisitions will be carried between the pharmacy and nursing stations. These mechanical systems may be any one or combination of pneumatic tube, vertical conveyor or horizontal conveyor.

10. Because of the nature of the modern practice of pharmacy, large medical center type operations may require that the planners provide space for direct writing intercoms, teletype, closed circuit television, printing and/or duplicating equipment.

In addition to the above cited questions, the hospital pharmacist should be prepared to furnish answers which pertain to such areas as pre-packaging, methods and statistics involving the volume of dispensing, the number of people who will be in any one sector of the pharmacy at any single time, the peak dispensing hours, the measurements of the various carts or trucks used in the pharmacy, the department's provisions for night emergency service, the number of nursing stations and other departments to be serviced and finally a plan which will allow for a continuation of service to the hospital and yet permit forward progress for the construction crew.

LOCATION

The hospital pharmacy should be located in an area which is convenient for providing service to the many departments and personnel who make daily use of such service. Therefore, since this is a primary consideration, it is irrelevant where the pharmacy is located in the hospital so long as it meets the test of convenience.

Milne and Taylor[10] in their article dealing with suggested plans for hospital pharmacies have stated:

"In hospitals of less than 200 beds the pharmacy should be located on the first floor, in the center of the activities it is called upon to service frequently, easily accessible to the elevator, and near or adjoining the out-patient department, if such is maintained by the hospital. This will provide the most efficient service and conserve man-hours of work.

Though it is recommended that the pharmacy be all located on one floor, it may be varied in larger hospitals when first floor space is at a premium.

The basement is not desirable for a pharmacy."

Because most hospital pharmacies were designed and constructed during an era before out-patient facilities had developed to their present status, many clinic administrators feel that they are poorly located insofar as the out-patient department is concerned. Since the majority of the hospital pharmacies serving clinic patients combine out-patient and in-patient facilities, the pharmacists concur with the observation made by the clinic administrative personnel.

The *Mirror to Hospital Pharmacy,*[11] in discussing this subject, states:

"If a hospital provides out-patient pharmacy service then, if possible, pharmacy facilities should be located either in or immediately adjacent to the out-patient department. It is not suitable for a cashier, nurse or other hospital personnel to accept the prescription from the patient and send it by pneumatic tube or by other means to the pharmacy located in some other section of the hospital and return the medication to this person for delivery to the patient. Although man-hours may be conserved by combining in-patient dispensing units, this advantage should not take precedence over locating the out-patient pharmacy facility in the immediate area serving out-patients. If a low volume of work does not justify such a location, then it would seem best either to not offer out-patient pharmacy service or to have the patient carry his prescription to the in-patient pharmacy."

In general, the in-patient pharmacy appears to be reasonably well situated to render the services required of it. Where possible, all sections of the in-patient pharmacy—storage, dispensing, manufacturing, parenteral solutions, etc. should be contiguous. When these functions are separated from the main pharmacy, it is recommended that they be in a direct vertical relationship if possible. In addition, this concept of direct vertical relationship should be extended between the pharmacy and the various divisions of the hospital utilizing pharmaceutical services.

With the advent of clinical pharmacy programs, many hospitals have found it advisable to develop *satellite pharmacies* on the patient pavilions. In effect, these are sub-pharmacies that receive their supplies from the main pharmacy but have the advantage of being able to respond to the clinical needs of the patient on a current basis. In addition, such a system makes available to the patient, physician, and nurse the services of a pharmacist in a clinical capacity rather than as just a dispenser of medications. By being on the nursing floor, the pharmacist is available for the taking of patient drug histories, maintaining patient drug policies, observing the patient for drug reactions and toxicity and dispensing unit-doses and intravenous products with additives.

FLOOR SPACE

Milne, Taylor and their Public Health Service Associates recommend the following floor space and its distribution within the pharmacy area:

AREA DISTRIBUTION FOR GENERAL HOSPITAL PHARMACIES

Areas in Square Feet	50 Bed	100 Bed	200 Bed
Compounding and Dispensing Laboratory	205	320	495
Parenteral Solutions Laboratory		185	200
Active Store Room		125	200
Manufacturing Laboratory			120
Office and Library			105
Circulation			60
TOTAL	205	630	1180

The areas shown in the above chart are net areas and do not include walls and partitions. Additional storage space of approximately 170 square feet per 100 beds is provided for bulk storage in an area directly beneath the pharmacy and separate from the main hospital store room.

Translating the above figures into a square foot per bed ratio, the following is noted:

AREA DISTRIBUTION—SQUARE FEET PER BED

Areas in Square Feet	50 Bed	100 Bed	200 Bed
Compounding and Dispensing Laboratory	4.1	3.20	2.48
Parenteral Solutions Laboratory		1.85	1.00
Active Store Room		1.25	1.00
Manufacturing Laboratory			0.60
Office and Library			0.53
Circulation			0.30
TOTAL	4.1	6.30	5.91

In contrast, Francke *et al.*[12] in their survey requested the survey participants to indicate the number of additional square feet of space

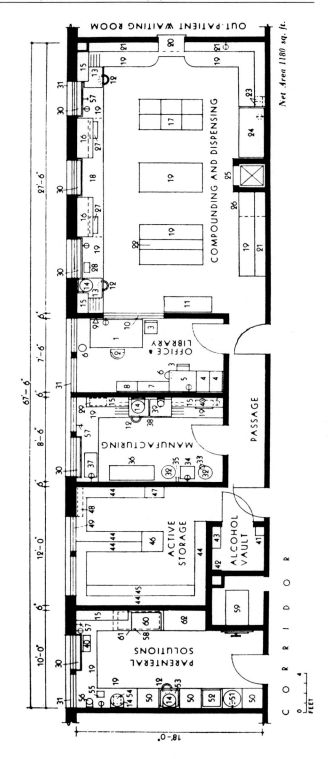

1. Desk, executive
2. Chair, executive
3. Chair, straight
4. File, 4 drawer
5. Table, writing
6. Receptacle, waste paper
7. Case, book
8. Rack, magazine
9. Outlet, telephone
10. Glass panel
11. Rack, carboy
12. Can, sanitary waste
13. Sink, with goose neck spout and drainboard, graduate rack above, cabinets below
14. Tank, glass, distilled water, 12 gallon
15. Cabinets, adjustable shelves
16. Cabinet, drug, sectional type, with shelf above counter
17. Cabinets, drug, sectional type

18. Counter, prescription, cabinets and drawers below
19. Counter, cabinets and drawers below
20. Window, dispensing
21. Shelves, adjustable, open, starting 18 inches above counter
22. Shelf, above counter
23. File, prescription
24. Refrigerator, with biological drawers, 32 cubic feet
25. Dumbwaiter
26. Safe, narcotic, under counter
27. Scale, prescription, class A
28. Scale, prescription, heavy duty
29. Scale, counter
30. Heat outlet grill, inlet grill in base of cabinet
31. Guards, at all windows
32. Tank, mixing or storing, 20 gallons, mounted on stand with casters

33. Mixer, portable, electric
34. Filter press, suction-pressure type, mounted on casters
35. Outlets, hot and cold water
36. Rack, filter
37. Mill, colloidal
38. Sink, two compartment, with drainboard, goose neck spout, cabinets below
39. Still, 2 gallon per hour
40. Hot Plate, double element
41. Vent, outlet, 8 inches above floor to atmosphere
42. Vent, inlet, near floor to atmosphere
43. Shelves, starting 42 inches above, floor
44. Shelves, 12 inches wide, adjustable, open
45. Shelves, 24 inches wide, 36 inches high, adjustable

46. Rack, barrel
47. Locker, clothes
48. Radiator, above shelving
49. High windows
50. Rack, bottle
51. Cleaner, bottle, pressure type
52. Sink with goose neck spout
53. Sink, with distilled water rinser, omit hot & cold water supply
54. Drip pan with waste connection in counter top
55. Pump, suction and pressure
56. Still, 10 gallon per hour
57. Outlet, gas
58. Carriage, sterilizer, under counter
59. Sterilizer, 21 x 36 x 48 inches
60. Oven, hot air, 21 x 14 x 14 inches, on counter
61. Counter, open below
62. Cabinet, storage, open adjustable shelves

Pharmacy for a 200 bed general hospital

Fig. 86. The above plan for a pharmacy for a 200-bed general hospital may still be found in a large number of hospitals. With slight modification it is adaptable to modern day dispensing practices. (From Public Health Service Publication No. 891.)

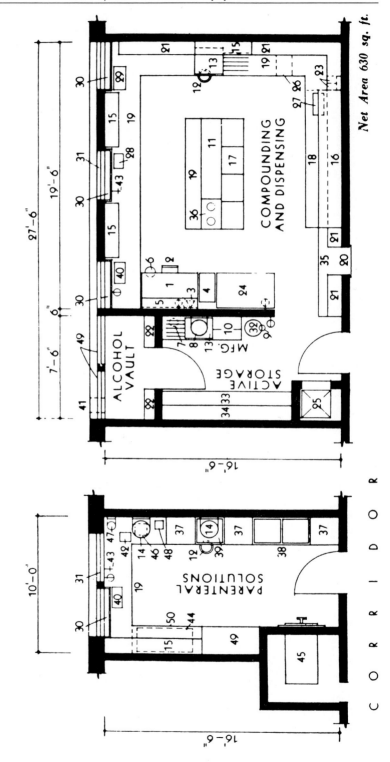

Pharmacy for a 100 bed general hospital

1. Desk
2. Chair
3. Outlet, telephone
4. File, 4 drawer
5. Shelves, book, over desk
6. Receptacle, waste paper
7. Still, 2 gallon per hour. Required if parenteral solution room is omitted
8. Tank, glass, distilled water, 5 gallon
9. Mixer, portable, electric
10. Counter, cabinets below, shelves above
11. Rack, carboy, above counter
12. Can, sanitary waste
13. Sink, with goose neck spout and drainboard. graduate rack above, cabinets below
14. Tank, glass, distilled water, 12 gallon
15. Cabinet, adjustable shelves
16. Cabinet, drug, sectional type, with shelf above counter
17. Cabinets, drugs, sectional type
18. Counter, prescription, cabinets. sectional type drawers below

19. Counter, cabinets and drawers below
20. Window, dispensing
21. Shelves, adjustable, open, starting 18 inches above counter
22. Shelves, starting 42 inches above floor
23. File, prescription
24. Refrigerator, 16 cubic feet, with biological drawers
25. Dumbwaiter
26. Safe, narcotic. under counter
27. Scale, prescription, class A
28. Scale, prescription, heavy duty
29. Scale, counter
30. Heat outlet grill, inlet grill in base of cabinet
31. Guards, at all windows
32. Tank, mixing, 20 gallons, mounted on stand with casters
33. Shelves, 24 inches wide. 36 inches high. adjustable, open
34. Shelves, 12 inches wide, adjustable. open

35. Counter, 18 inches wide, adjustable shelves below
36. Rack, filter, above counter
37. Rack, bottle
38. Sink, two compartment, goose neck spout. cabinets below
39. Sink, with distilled water rinser, omit hot and cold water supply, cabinets below
40. Hot plate. double element
41. Vent, at ceiling and floor
42. Scale, metric, solution
43. Outlet, gas
44. Carriage. sterilizer, under counter
45. Sterilizer, 24 x 36 x 48 inches
46. Drip pan with waste connection in counter top
47. Still, 5 gallon per hour
48. Pump, suction and pressure
49. Cabinet, storage. open. adjustable shelves
50. Counter. open below

Fig. 87. The above design for a pharmacy for a 100-bed hospital was recommended by the Division of Hospital and Medical Facilities in the early 1950s. (From Public Health Service Publication No. 891.)

they felt would be necessary for them to give the type of service the pharmacy should provide and obtained the following results which are compared with the Public Health Service recommendations for short-term hospitals.

# Beds	Public Health Service Recommendations	Survey Findings
100	6.3 sq. ft./bed	8.12 sq. ft./bed
200	5.9 sq. ft./bed	6.62 sq. ft./bed
300		5.39 sq. ft./bed
400		5.00 sq. ft./bed

Before utilizing the above figures, it should be remembered that the Public Health Service plans provide an additional 170 square feet per 100 beds for reserve storage of bulk pharmaceuticals outside the pharmacy and that the survey findings make no provisions for this additional storage facility.

Exclusive of the survey conducted by Francke *et al.,* little has been published relative to area distribution for general hospital pharmacies since the work of Milne and Taylor in 1950. Therefore, it is important to recognize the fact that in the intervening years pharmaceutical services in the hospital have expanded considerably thereby suggesting that, until more up-to-date information is developed, the recommendations of the Public Health Service for floor space in hospital pharmacies should be considered minimal for the construction of today's hospital pharmacy.

Furthermore, it is important to note that today's practice of pharmacy provides its practitioners the opportunity to perform variable functions ranging from standard type dispensing methods to unit dose dispensing methodologies. Involvement with intravenous additive programs, drug information centers and clinical pharmacy endeavors simply means that pharmacy floor space requirements must be determined by factors other than bed capacity and ambulatory clinic patient load. Also, no two hospitals should be compared for the purpose of determining the square footage requirements of the other in spite of the fact that both appear to have similar pharmaceutical involvement. It is not the similarity of involvement that determines space requirements but the degree or scope of involvement coupled with the type of equipment used in the programs.

EQUIPMENT PLANNER'S RESPONSIBILITY

The pharmacist, administrator, purchasing agent and architect, as a group, assume the responsibility for the planning and the subsequent purchase of the major equipment items to be located in the pharmacy.

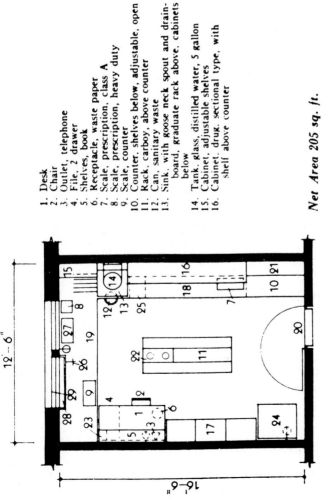

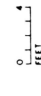

CORRIDOR

1. Desk
2. Chair
3. Outlet, telephone
4. File, 2 drawer
5. Shelves, book
6. Receptacle, waste paper
7. Scale, prescription, class A
8. Scale, prescription, heavy duty
9. Scale, counter
10. Counter, shelves below, adjustable, open
11. Rack, carboy, above counter
12. Can, sanitary waste
13. Sink, with goose neck spout and drainboard, graduate rack above. cabinets below
14. Tank, glass, distilled water, 5 gallon
15. Cabinet, adjustable shelves
16. Cabinet, drug, sectional type, with shelf above counter
17. Cabinets, drug, sectional type
18. Counter, prescription, cabinets and drawers below
19. Counter, cabinets and drawers below
20. Dutch door
21. Shelves, adjustable, open, starting 18 inches above counter
22. Rack, filter, above counter
23. File, prescription, on desk
24. Refrigerator, 8 cubic feet, with biological drawers
25. Safe, narcotic
26. Outlet, gas
27. Hot plate, double element
28. Heat outlet grill, inlet grill in base of cabinet
29. Guards, at both windows

Net Area 205 sq. ft.

Pharmacy for a 50 bed general hospital

Fig. 88. The above design for a pharmacy for a 50-bed hospital was adequate for the type of pharmacy practiced in the period 1950–60. Many hospitals today still have similarly designed units. (From Public Health Service Publication No. 891.)

The less expensive items, commonly used in the daily practice of the profession, are usually purchased by the purchasing agent after he has consulted with the pharmacist.

In selecting the equipment, all parties must exercise extreme care in choosing those items which will provide good service, with minimal maintenance, at a price within the hospital's equipment budget. All too often, many pharmacists succumb to the temptation of equipping a particular section of the pharmacy with elaborate and expensive equipment and then purchase equipment of a lower quality for another division of the pharmacy in order to remain within the budgetary allowance.

The cost of equipment should not be estimated nor should a percentage of the building construction cost be used. Whenever such short cuts are taken, experience has demonstrated that insufficient funds are available for the purchase of the desired equipment. Clearly then, once the equipment list is prepared, it behooves the pharmacist to consult freely with the purchasing agent, manufacturer's representatives and vendors as well as to peruse through the latest editions of the catalogues.

Equipment is segregated into two groups: fixed and movable.

FIXED EQUIPMENT

Fixed equipment is defined as that which requires installation and becomes attached to the building. The single connection of electric power lines into the building's electric system or temporary attachment to a utility system does not qualify the item as fixed equipment. Fixed equipment is usually included in construction contracts and must be purchased and installed in accord with the requirements of the contract. Examples of fixed equipment are cabinets, counters, sinks, dumbwaiters and elevators.[6]

MOVABLE EQUIPMENT

Movable equipment is defined as that equipment which is capable of being moved and is not intended to be permanently affixed to the building. This group includes large items of furniture and equipment having a reasonable fixed position in the building but which can be moved. Examples of movable equipment are carts, desks, balances, mixers etc.[6]

SUGGESTED EQUIPMENT LISTS

Because the scope of service rendered by each hospital pharmacy will vary from one section of the country to the other or, for that matter, from hospital to hospital, it is an impossible task to attempt to prepare a standard list of equipment which will meet every need.

The Equipment Planning Branch of the United States Public Health Service has prepared a suggested equipment list[13] which may be used as a guide. For the convenience of the student and the hospital pharmacist who may wish to use the said equipment list as a check list for the inventory of basic pharmaceutical equipment within the department, the suggested list is hereinafter published.

The symbols used in these lists have definite meaning as follows.[7]

1. " indicates that the item is required but the quantity is not determined. Quantity is dependent upon correlation of the schematic plans."
2. "— indicates the item is not applicable to the particle size group."
3. "Supplies are not included in the term 'equipment' as they are not participated in for hospital projects constructed under the "Hospital and Medical Facilities (Hill-Burton) Program'."

DRUG DISTRIBUTION

| | *Suggested Quantity* *Number of Beds* | | |
| | 100 | 300 | 500 |

Order Review

	100	300	500
Fixed			
Bookshelves, adjustable.	—	—	1
Pneumatic tube station.	1	1	2
Utility pole, phone, electric.	2	2	4
Movable			
Cabinet, filing			
Letter size, 3-drawer	2	2	4
Card size, two-level, revolving.	1	1	2
Visible index type.	1	1	2
Cart, for photocopier, storage shelf.	—	1	1
Chair, swivel, with arms.	2	5	10
Desk			
Office, double pedestal.	2	3	6
Editing, special.	—	2	4
File, swinging panel, strip, insert.	2	2	3
Photocopier, bound volumes, desk type.	—	1	1
Table, writing 2' × 2'	2	—	—
Time/date stamp, electric.	1	1	2
Typewriter, electric, nonmovable carriage.	2	3	6
Waste receptacle.	2	2	4

Inpatient Dispensing

	100	300	500
Fixed			
Cabinets, wall-mounted.			
Counter, prescription, cabinets, bins and drawers below.	1	3	6

	Suggested Quantity Number of Beds		
	100	300	500
Dumbwaiter.	1	1	1
Pneumatic tube station.	0	1	1
Shelving, adjustable, 12", starting 18" above counter	1	2	3
Ledge, fixed.	0	1	1
Movable			
Cabinet, filing, 5-drawer, letter size.	1	1	0
Cart, delivery, large.	0	1	2
Refrigerator			
Biological type, with freezer.	1	0	0
Pass-through, cafeteria type, for IV solutions.	0	1	1
Open front, refrigerated case type.	0	1	1
Typewriters, electric, nonmovable carriage.	1	2	4
Stool, operator's, adjustable.	1	2	4

Receiving and Storage

Fixed			
Counter, with adjustable shelving beneath.	1	1	1
Safe.	1	0	0
Shelving, adjustable, wall-mounted, 9"	1	1	1
Rail-mounted			
in narcotic vault. Back 24", sides 12".	—	1	1
in flammables room, 12".	—	1	1
Vent, inlet and outlet, in flammables room.	1	1	1
Movable			
Cradle, drum.	1	1	1
Waste receptacle.	1	1	1

Purchasing and Inventory Control

Fixed			
Bookshelves, wall-mounted above desk.	1	1	—
Movable			
Cabinet, filing, visible index type			
One section.	1	—	—
Three section.	—	1	—
Letter size, 5-drawer.	1	1	—
Chair, swivel, with arms.	—	1	—
Desk, office, double pedestal.	1	1	—
File, swinging, strip insert.	—	1	—
Waste receptacle.	—	1	—

Extemporaneous Preparations

Fixed			
Cabinet, wall-mounted.			
Counter with sink, drainboard, adjustable shelves beneath.	2	2	2
Counter, with open adjustable shelving beneath.	1	2	5
Shelving, fixed ledge.	0	1	1

	Suggested Quantity Number of Beds		
	100	300	500
Movable			
Bins, autoclavable.	10	10	20
Cart, flask transport.	1	1	2
Cart, utility, flat top, locking wheels.	2	2	2
Chair, swivel.	1	1	1
Desk, office, single pedestal, file drawer.	1	1	1
Hood, laminar airflow, horizontal or vertical.	1	1	2
Waste receptacle.	2	2	4

Outpatient Dispensing

	100	300	500
Fixed			
Cabinet, wall-mounted.	—	1	—
Counter, with sink, drainboard, file drawer.	—	1	—
Counter, with file drawer, bins, and shelf beneath.	1	1	—
Door, flexible, pulldown type for outpatient dispensing counter window.	1	1	—
Panels, acoustical.	—	1	—
Shelving, adjustable, wall-mounted, 12".	1	—	—
Movable			
Cabinet, filing, rotary, mechanical.	—	1	—
Chairs, guest, for waiting area.	—	4	—
File, swinging panel, strip insert.	1	1	—
Refrigerator, biological, with freezer.	—	1	—
Waste receptacle.	1	—	—

OUTPATIENT PHARMACY (Separate)

Dispensing

	100	300	500
Fixed			
Counter, with drawers and adjustable shelving beneath.	—	—	—
Counter, with drawer and knee space.	—	—	1
Panel, acoustical.	—	—	6
Pneumatic tube stations.	—	—	1
Shelving, adjustable, wall-mounted, 12".	—	—	—
Movable			
Cabinet, steel, double locks plus alarm buzzer.	—	—	1
Cabinet, filing, letter size, 5-drawer.	—	—	1
Cabinet, filing, rotary, mechanical.	—	—	1
File, swinging panel, strip insert.	—	—	2
Refrigerator, biological, with freezer.	—	—	1
Stool, operator's, adjustable.	—	—	1
Typewriter, electric, nonmovable carriage.	—	—	2
Waste receptacle.	—	—	3

Extemporaneous Preparations (Outpatient)

	100	300	500
Fixed			
Cabinet, wall-mounted.	—	—	4

	Suggested Quantity Number of Beds		
	100	300	500
Counter, with drawers and open adjustable shelving beneath.	—	—	—
Sink unit, with drainboard.	—	—	1
Movable			
Hood, laminar airflow, vertical or horizontal.	—	—	1
Waste receptacle.	—	—	1

PHARMACY SUBSTATION

Order Review

	100	300	500
Fixed			
Counter, desk height, with drawers and adjustable shelves beneath.	—	—	1
Shelving, adjustable, wall-mounted, 12".	—	—	—
Movable			
Chair, swivel, with arms.	—	—	1
Waste receptacle.	—	—	1

Distribution

	100	300	500
Fixed			
Counter, with open adjustable shelving beneath.	—	—	—
Counter, hinged.	—	—	1
Shelving, adjustable, wall-mounted, 12"	—	—	—
Sink unit, with drainboard.	—	—	1
Movable			
Cart, with cassette storage.	—	—	1
Hood, laminar airflow, vertical or horizontal.	—	—	1
Refrigerator, with freezer, beneath counter.	—	—	1
Waste receptacle.	—	—	1

MANUFACTURING AND PACKAGING

Cleanup Room

	100	300	500
Fixed			
Counter, stainless steel, with adjustable shelves and doors beneath, double sink.	—	—	1
Shelving, adjustable, 12".	—	—	—
Wash area, 6" high curb with 1" sill.	—	—	1
Window, pass-through into Injections Filling room.	—	—	1
Movable			
Cart, utility, stainless steel, 23" × 46", with locking wheels, for solution flasks.	—	—	1

	Suggested Quantity Number of Beds		
	100	300	500
Table, utility, stainless steel, 23" × 46", with locking wheels.	—	—	1
Washer, automatic, laboratory type, pass-through on rails into Injections Filling room, to accommodate 25 l flasks per batch, plus two headers for l flasks and one for small glassware, test tubes, and pipettes.	—	—	1

Injections Filling Room and Still Room

Fixed

Autoclave, steam, fast exhaust, pass-through into Central Service autoclave area, size suited to solution workload.	—	—	1
Counter, stainless steel, with open adjustable shelving beneath.	—	—	—
Still, capacity 25 gal per hour (mounted in still room).	—	—	2
Storage tank, glass lined or similar, heated, 150-gal capacity, ceiling suspended (mounted in still room).	—	—	1

Movable

Carriage, autoclave.	—	—	1
Cart, autoclave.	—	—	1
Cart, solution flask drain type.	—	—	2
Conductivity meter, recording.	—	—	2
Filling machine, automatic, dual nozzle type, type, foot operated, for amps and vials.	—	—	1
Hood, laminar airflow, horizontal or vertical.	—	—	1
Stool, operator's, adjustable.	—	—	1
Table, utility, stainless steel, 35" × 70", with locking wheels.	—	—	1
Tank, premix, 50-gal capacity, with pump agitator unit and hand-operated filler mechanism with filter, fitting under table.	—	—	1
Filter, membrane type.	—	—	2

Sterile Preparation

Fixed

Counter, with storage cabinets beneath.	—	—	—
Kettle, steam,jacketed, 5-gal capacity.	—	—	1
Shelving, wall-mounted, 12".	—	—	—
Sink unit, laboratory type, corner.	—	—	1
Window, pass-through, to Injections Filling room and Aseptic Filling room.	—	—	2

Movable

Balance, prescription, type A, with weights.	—	—	1
Balance, single beam, capacity 4.5 kg.	—	—	1
Chair, swivel.	—	—	1

	Suggested Quantity Number of Beds		
	100	300	500
Cabinet, filing, letter size, 5-drawer.	—	—	1
Cart, utility, laboratory type with railed top.	—	—	1
Desk, office, single pedestal.	—	—	1
Filter, membrane type.	—	—	1
Hot plate, electric, double element, heavy duty, variable heat.	—	—	1
Lockers (in air lock).	—	—	3
pH meter.	—	—	1
Pump, suction and pressure, with gauges.	—	—	1
Stirrer, small volume, counter top.	—	—	1
Stool, operator's, adjustable.	—	—	1
Waste receptacle.	—	—	2

Sterile Area Storage

Fixed
Counter, 1' × 2', for writing.	—	—	1
Shelving, adjustable, 18", for storage of materials, containers, and supplies.	—	—	—

Movable
Stool, 2 steps.	—	—	1

Aseptic Filling

Fixed
Counter, stainless steel, open beneath.	—	—	3
Shelving, wall-mounted, 12".	—	—	3
Window, pass through to Labeling and Inspection room.	—	—	1

Movable
Hood, laminar airflow, horizontal or vertical.	—	—	2
Pipetting machine, automatic, foot operated.	—	—	1
Stool, operator's, adjustable.	—	—	2
Syringe, e.g., Cornwall type with Swinney adapter.	—	—	4

Labeling and Inspection

Fixed
Cabinet, floor	—	—	1
Counter drawer units.	—	—	3
Counter top units.	—	—	1
Cupboard drawer units	—	—	3
Corner unit.	—	—	1
Desk height.	—	—	1
Small drawer.	—	—	1
Sink unit, corner.	—	—	1
Shelving, wall-mounted, 12".	—	—	—

Movable
Labeling machine, automatic, with foot operated clutch, plain worktable and offset pad, plus attachments for pressure sensitive labels.	—	—	1

	Suggested Quantity Number of Beds		
	100	300	500
Labeling machine, hand operated.	—	—	1
Light-dark inspection box.	—	—	1
Stool, operator's, adjustable.	—	—	1
Plate imprinting machine, low capacity, for making imprinting plates for use with labeling machines.	—	—	1
Typewriter, manual, ½ line advance, 16 characters per inch.	—	—	1
Waste receptacle.	—	—	1

Quarantine Storage

Fixed
Shelving, adjustable, 18".	—	—	—

Prepackaging

Fixed
Cabinet, e.g., Schwartz type.	—	—	3
Counter, wall-mounted, open beneath.	—	—	—
Counter, with drawer and storage cabinet beneath.	—	—	1

Movable
Filling machine, automatic, dual type, capacity 0.025 to 100 ml, with suck back device, foot operated.	—	—	1
Heat sealer, electric, stick-resistant covered shoe.	—	—	2
Packager, pouch-type, with imprinter and heat sealer.	—	—	1
Stool, operator's, adjustable.	—	—	1
Strip packaging machine, low volume, quick changeover, imprinting.	—	—	1
Table, utility, stainless steel, flat surface 25" × 70", with locking wheels.	—	—	1

Nonsterile Mixing and Filling

Fixed
Cabinets, e.g., Schwartz type.	—	—	3
Counter, with drawers and storage cabinets beneath.	—	—	—
Kettle, steam-jacketed, capacity 20 gal	—	—	1
Rack, filter.	—	—	2
Range, electric, variable heat, heavy duty, installed flush with counter.	—	—	1
Shelving, adjustable, 18".	—	—	1
Shelving, adjustable, wall-mounted, 12".	—	—	1
Sink unit, laboratory type.	—	—	2
Wash area, 6" curb with 1" sill.	—	—	1

Movable
Balance, prescription, type A, plus weights.	—	—	1
Balance, single beam, capacity 4.5 kg, weights.	—	—	1
Blender, electric, multispeed.	—	—	1
Chair, swivel, with arms.	—	—	1

	Suggested Quantity Number of Beds		
	100	300	500
Desk, office, single pedestal, with file drawer.	—	—	1
Filter press, suction pressure type, 10 gal per minimum capacity on casters.	—	—	1
Homogenizer.	—	—	1
Mixer, large, tank-mounted.	—	—	2
Mixer-blender, e.g., Hobart type, for semisolids.	—	—	1
Ointment mill, three roller.	—	—	1
Rheostat, variable, for 110-volt line.	—	—	1
Tank, mixing and storage, 50-gal capacity, with spigot, filter attachment, on wheels	—	—	2
Timer, electric	—	—	1
Washer, laboratory type, automatic, for small glassware and control laboratory items, distilled water rinse.	—	—	1
Waste receptacle, large.	—	—	1

ADMINISTRATION

Chief Administrative Officer

	100	300–500
Movable		
Bookcase.	—	1
Chair, guest.	2	3
Chair, swivel, arms.	1	1
Credenza.	—	1
Desk, double pedestal.	1	1
Dictating machine, recorder.	1	1

Secretary/Receptionist

Movable		
Cabinet, filing, 5-drawer.	1	4
Cabinet, storage.	1	1
Chair, guest.	3	3
Chair, swivel, typist's.	1	2
Desk, single pedestal, secretarial.	1	2
Dictating machine, transcriber.	1	1
Table, corner.	1	—
Typewriter, electric.	1	2
Waste receptacle.	1	2

Conference Room

Fixed		
Blackboard, wall-mounted.	—	1
Movable		
Cabinet, storage.	—	1
Chairs, conference, folding.	—	8

	Suggested Quantity Number of Beds	
	100	300–500
Projection screen.	—	1
Table, conference.	—	2
Table, corner.	—	1
Waste receptacle.	—	1

Assistant for Business Affairs

Movable

Adding machine, electric, printing	—	1
Bookcase.	—	1
Chair, guest.	—	1
Chair, swivel, arms.	—	2
Table, desk type.	—	1
Waste receptacle.	—	1

CONTROL

Control Laboratory

	300–500
Fixed	
Counter, with drawers and storage cabinet beneath.	
Fume hood, with sink, distilled water, and electric gas outlets.	1
Shelving, wall-mounted, 12".	
Sink unit, corner.	1
Sink unit.	1
Movable.	
Balance, analytical, one-pan, substitution weighing, reading to 0.1 mg.	1
Battery jar, cylindrical, e.g., Pyrex, 16" diameter by 12" high, for use with constant temperature unit.	1
Burets, micro, class A, 3-way stopcock, e.g., Teflon and stopcock plug, 10 ml.	2
Burets, automatic, class A, e.g., Kimax or e.g., Pyrex with stopcock and plug, 10 ml.	2
Burner, e.g., Fisher, high temperature.	5
Burner, e.g., Terrill, natural gas.	2
Cabinet, e.g., Schwartz type.	1
Centrifuge, clinical, 15- and 40-ml tubes.	1
Chromatography apparatus, thin layer type, for 8" × 8" plates	1
Chromatography cabinet, bench type.	1
Constant temperature unit, e.g., Tecam Tempunit.	1
Electrode, silver billet, combination type, for pH meter.	1
Extraction apparatus with, e.g., Friedrichs condenser.	1
Freezer, upright, to include capacity for storing frozen unit-dose injectables.	1
Heating mantle, hemispherical, for 125-ml flask.	1

	Suggested Quantity Number of Beds 300–500
Hotplate, electric, square, thermostatic.	1
pH meter, line operated, direct reading.	1
Incubator, gravity convection, large size.	1
Melting point apparatus, e.g., Fisher-Johns or equivalent, for determining melting point of paraffix wax.	1
Microscope, polarizing, e.g., Uniton type.	1
Nitrogen distillation apparatus, micro.	1
Oven, gravity convection, 200° range.	1
Power supply for hydrogen lamp.	1
Refrigerator, home type.	1
Shaker, wrist action, e.g., Burrell type.	1
Silica cells for spectrophotometer, set of two.	1
Spectrophotometer, for use in visible and ultraviolet ranges, with deuterium lamp.	1
Stirring apparatus, magnetic, variable speed.	1
Stool, laboratory type, with back.	1
Support stands, various sizes.	
Table, for balances, adjusting level.	1
Table, utility.	1
Transformer, variable, e.g., Powerstat type.	1
Waste receptacle.	1

Control Office

Movable

Bookcase.	1
Cabinet, filing, 5-drawer.	4
Chair, guest.	2
Chair, swivel, with arms.	1
Costumer.	1
Dictating machine, transcriber.	1
Table, desk type.	1
Waste receptacle.	2

DRUG INFORMATION

Drug Information/Conference Area

	100
Fixed	
Bookshelves, wall-mounted, 12".	1
Blackboard, wall-mounted.	1
Movable	
Cabinet, filing, side opening, 5-drawer	4
Calculator, electronic, statistical, printing.	1
Chair, library.	4
Shelving, adjustable, 12".	4
Table, reading/conference.	1
Table, desk type.	1

	Suggested Quantity *Number of Beds* 300–500
Typewriter, electric, wide carriage, ½ line advance, *changeable type.*	1
Waste receptacle.	1

Reception

	300–500
Movable	
Chair, guest.	2
Chair, swivel.	1
Costumer.	1
Desk, secretarial, single pedestal, typing return.	1
Table, corner.	1
Typewriter, electric, wide carriage, ½ line advance.	1
Waste receptacle.	1

Drug Information Officer

Fixed	
Blackboard, wall-mounted.	1
Bookshelves, wall-mounted, 12".	
Counter, desk-height, open beneath.	2
Movable	
Cabinet, filing, under counter, 2-drawer.	1
Calculator, electronic, statistical, printing.	1
Chair, library.	2
Chair, swivel, with arms.	1
Waste receptacle.	1

Library

Movable	
Cabinet, filing, side opening, 5-drawer.	4
Chairs, library.	3
Microfilm reader.	1
Shelving, adjustable, 12".	1
Table, reading.	1

Processing and Records

Fixed	
Counter, with storage cabinets beneath.	1
Pneumatic tube station.	1
Movable	
Cabinet, filing, tab card, 8-drawer.	2
Chair, swivel, operator.	1
Collator, punchcard.	1
Keypunch, printing.	1
Photocopier, capable of copying from bound vol- *umes.*	1
Photographic equipment, slidemaking.	1

	Suggested Quantity *Number of Beds* *300–500*
Sorter, electronic, punchcards.	1
Waste receptacle.	1

TEACHING

Student Work Area

Fixed

Desk-height counter, built-in, open beneath, with *book shelves above, one desk drawer below.*	2
Bulletin board, wall-mounted.	1
Blackboard, wall-mounted.	1

Movable

Cabinet, filing, 5 drawer.	2
Chair, swivel, with arms.	2
Locker.	2
Lamp, desk type, fluorescent, 2-bulb.	2
Typewriter, electric, wide carriage, ½ line advance.	1
Waste receptacle.	1

Instructor Work Area

Fixed

Bulletin board, wall-mounted.	1
Blackboard, wall-mounted.	1

Movable

Cabinet, filing, 5-drawer.	2
Chair, swivel, with arms.	1
Chair, guest.	2
Costumer.	1
Desk, double pedestal, office.	1
Dictating machine, transcriber.	1
Table, desk type.	1
Waste receptacle.	1

EQUIPMENT ELECTRICAL SAFETY

Electrical safety within the hospital has become a topic of major interest amongst physicians, planners, engineers and safety experts. This has arisen because of the inherent danger involved in the use of some of the commonly used equipment in the hospital. At one time or another, articles have been written commenting on electrical hazards in electric beds, monitoring equipment, x-ray machines and cleaning equipment.

Thus it behooves the hospital pharmacist to select all equipment used in the pharmacy with care. In general compliance with the N.F.P.A.

standards (National Fire Protective Association) is a start in the right direction.

Electrical safety in the hospital pharmacy could be improved if consideration is given to the following guiding principles:[15]

1. Keep electrical power cords as short as possible in order to eliminate electrical leakage.
2. Use equipment with proper ground lines. (Three-prong plugs)
3. Purchase equipment with power on-off switches which have clearly visible indication of power status (on or off).
4. Eliminate slow blow fusing whenever possible since this type of fusing increases the exposure time of the operator to the electrical hazards.
5. Before permitting personnel to operate new equipment, be sure that they are properly trained in its use. In addition, it is important that they read the instructional manual—particularly the section dealing with safe use and possible hazards.
6. Train operators to disconnect the power receptacle from the power source by pulling on the connector, not on the cable.
7. Avoid the use of extension cords.
8. Do not attempt to make repairs to the equipment.
9. Cooperate with in-house maintenance programs.

CLEANUP AREA

A pharmacy that is involved in a reasonable volume of extemporaneous compounding or manufacturing should have a cleanup room. A cleanup room designed for joint use by CSSR and pharmacy is the most efficient and economical. Appropriately located pass-through windows and a curbed floor area with floor drain are desirable features.

NONSTERILE MIXING AND FILLING ROOM

The area for mixing and filling ointments should be separate from that for liquids, although both may be in the same room. Provision shold be made for weighing and measuring, mixing and stirring (sometimes over heat), blending, homogenization, filtration and filling. Adequate storage space must be provided.[8]

PREPACKAGING AREA

The prepackaging room is for the packaging of oral solid dosage forms into containers. In hospitals of 300 beds or less without a manufacturing program and without unit dose dispensing it may be possible to prepackage oral solids in the extemporaneous preparations area.[9]

INJECTION RECONSTITUTION AREA

The area for the reconstitution of injections should be equipped with two or more Class 100 laminar airflow hoods. Such units are available with horizontal, vertical, converging 90-degree and converging 180-degree flow patterns.[9]

LABELING AND INSPECTION ROOM

The labeling and inspection room should be adjacent to the filling areas so that the unlabeled drug products can be transferred directly through a pass-through window to eliminate the chance of their being used prematurely. Adequate storage space for labels, printing machine accessories, forms etc., must be provided.[9]

QUARANTINE STORAGE

Products manufactured and filled in the pharmacy are subject to quarantine until appropriate chemical and bacterial testing is complete. Finished products should be transferred directly to the quarantine storage area.[9]

REFRIGERATION FACILITIES

Most hospital pharmacists and architects when developing plans for a new pharmacy are quite cognizant of the desirability and the need for air conditioning and large biological refrigerators in the hospital pharmacy. More often than not, little thought is given to the need of a freezer and a cold room.

A review of the storage requirements for drugs in the National Formulary XIII shows that the thermal storage requirements vary from "cold place" to "store in refrigerator" or "avoid excessive heat or excessive temperature."

The complete list of storage temperature terms and the definitions are as follows:

Cold Place—A cold place is one having a temperature not exceeding 8° (46° F).

Refrigerator—A refrigerator is a cold place in which the temperature is held between 2° and 8° (36° and 46° F).

Cool Place—A cool place is one having a temperature between 8° and 15° (46° and 59° F).

Room Temperature—Room temperature is between 15° and 30° (59° and 86° F).

Excessive Heat—The expression "excessive heat" designates temperatures above 40° (104° F).

Since many of the drugs, so described, are in common use in the hospital, the pharmacist should make every effort to see that proper storage facilities are made available. This is easily done in most hospitals by the purchase of a large biological refrigerator and a freezer. In the small hospital, these two units or, as is usually the case, the refrigerator with a built-in freezer compartment, provide adequate facilities. The problem which usually arises in the larger hospital is that the refrigerator is too small to accommodate the inventory requiring refrigeration. Some pharmacists have tried to solve this problem by purchasing additional refrigerators or by borrowing space in the large dietary walk-in "iceboxes."

Although both of these arrangements are workable, it would seem that a less expensive and a less inconvenient method of cold storage within the pharmacy could be had by the construction of a cold room.

For the purpose of this section, a cold room is defined as an artificially cooled room with a regulated temperature range of 12° to 15° C (53.6° to 59° F).

CONSTRUCTING A COLD ROOM[a]

In existing facilities, a cold room may be inexpensively constructed if the parties involved will use a little imagination. A little-used corner of the basement storage area should be selected and the necessary area marked off. If windows are present, they should be bricked-up or at least double-paned and sealed against the outside atmosphere with caulking compound.

An electric light fixture and the required number of electrical outlets should be installed with the switch controlling the light fixture being on the outside wall nearest the entrance to the room.

The necessary additional walls of the room may be constructed of concrete, cinder block, concrete blocks, or brick. Where the use of the above building materials is not feasible, a similar result may be had by the use of wood studs with aluminum foil insulation. The inner side of this type of wall should be cement plastered and the outer side "finished-off" by covering with masonite or other inexpensive material. The door should fit tightly, be no larger than necessary, and be provided with a good automatic door closer.

An electric motor-driven air cooled Freon compressor unit with a remote blower-type cooling coil will provide the necessary refrigeration. This unit should be installed with the necessary thermostat and expansion valve required to maintain the desired temperature range.

The blower is mounted in the cold room. To it, a small waste line is installed to drain away the condensate which collects on the refrigerator coil. The compressor may be installed outside of the cold room in order to conserve space within.

---

[a]Adapted from an article entitled "A Cold Room for the Hospital Pharmacy" by William E. Hassan, Jr., and George Stilgoe. Am. J. Hosp. Pharm., *16*:3:120, 1959.

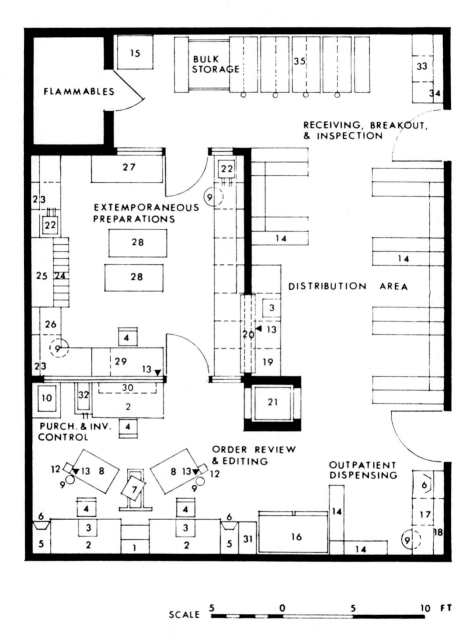

Fig. 89. Pharmacy Department in a 100-Bed Hospital. This plan is to be considered as one example of a modern pharmacy design. (From Planning for Hospital Pharmacies, U.S. Dept. HEW, Health Services & Mental Health Administration, Health Care Facilities Services, Washington, D.C.) (*Legend continues on following page.*)

Legend for Figure 89 (Continued)

1. Pneumatic tube station
2. Desk
3. Typewriter, electric, nonmovable carriage
4. Chair
5. Files, intermediate height
6. Files, swinging panel, strip insert type
7. File, revolving on two levels
8. Table, movable, 2 feet by 3 feet
9. Waste receptacle
10. Photocopier
11. File, 2-drawer
12. Utility pole
13. Telephones
14. Shelving, adjustable, 12 inches
15. Safe
16. Refrigerator, with freezer
17. Counter, with file drawer, bins
18. Shelving, adjustable, 7 inches
19. Counter, dispensing
20. Two-shelf unit above counter
21. Dumbwaiter, open both sides
22. Cabinet, with sink, drain board
23. Cabinet, wall-mounted
24. Bins
25. Hood, laminar airflow, vertical or horizontal
26. Counter, with open adjustable shelving beneath
27. Cart, storage
28. Carts, utility
29. Desks, small
30. Bookcase, wall-mounted
31. File cabinet, 5-drawer
32. File, visible index type
33. Counter, with adjustable shelves beneath
34. Shelving, wall-mounted, 9 inches
35. Shelving, adjustable, rail-mounted

Obviously the size of the cold room to be constructed will determine the capacity of the refrigeration unit to be installed. In general, a room approximately $10' \times 10' \times 10'$ would require one ton of refrigeration to maintain a temperature range of 50° to 60° F.

Once constructed, the room may be equipped with the necessary shelving, storage binds, cabinets, and work bench.

BUILT-IN EQUIPMENT

One of the most important aspects of a pharmacy modernization or construction program is that which involves the planning and selection of the built-in cabinets, counters and other types of casework. Due consideration must be given to such details as the height of the bench or cabinet, the size of the shelving or drawers, the types of handles on drawer and cabinet doors, whether or not the shelving is to be fixed or adjustable as well as the type of material which will be installed on the counter top.

The materials used in the construction of built-in equipment must be reviewed by the hospital pharmacist in the light of the activity to which the equipment will be subjected. Thus it is not sufficient to specify that the equipment will be constructed of stainless steel. One should specify whether it is expected to be constructed of mild, cold rolled, annealed furniture steel; the gauges of the metal to be used; the gauge of the metal to be used in the shelving and whether or not the face of the shelf should be turned back up under the shelf and brought into contact with it in order to provide additional support; and details relative to the doors, adjustability of the shelving, etc. Much of this

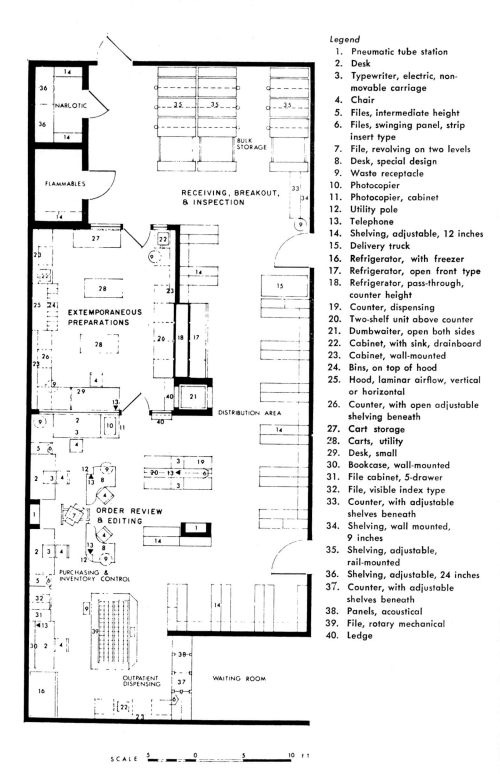

SCALE 5 ___ 0 _____ 5 ____ 10 FT

Fig. 90. Pharmacy Department in a 300-Bed Hospital. This plan is to be considered as one example of a modern pharmacy design. (From Planning for Hospital Pharmacies, U.S. Dept. HEW, Health Services & Mental Health Administration, Health Care Facilities Services, Washington, D.C.)

542

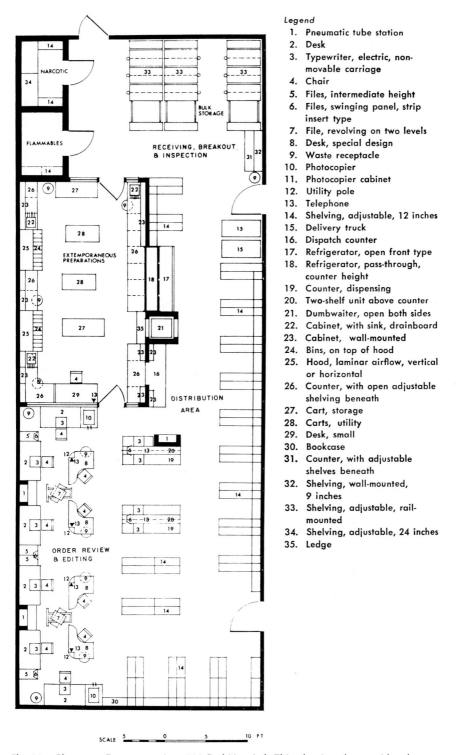

Legend
1. Pneumatic tube station
2. Desk
3. Typewriter, electric, non-movable carriage
4. Chair
5. Files, intermediate height
6. Files, swinging panel, strip insert type
7. File, revolving on two levels
8. Desk, special design
9. Waste receptacle
10. Photocopier
11. Photocopier cabinet
12. Utility pole
13. Telephone
14. Shelving, adjustable, 12 inches
15. Delivery truck
16. Dispatch counter
17. Refrigerator, open front type
18. Refrigerator, pass-through, counter height
19. Counter, dispensing
20. Two-shelf unit above counter
21. Dumbwaiter, open both sides
22. Cabinet, with sink, drainboard
23. Cabinet, wall-mounted
24. Bins, on top of hood
25. Hood, laminar airflow, vertical or horizontal
26. Counter, with open adjustable shelving beneath
27. Cart, storage
28. Carts, utility
29. Desk, small
30. Bookcase
31. Counter, with adjustable shelves beneath
32. Shelving, wall-mounted, 9 inches
33. Shelving, adjustable, rail-mounted
34. Shelving, adjustable, 24 inches
35. Ledge

SCALE 5 0 5 10 FT

Fig. 91. Pharmacy Department in a 500-Bed Hospital. This plan is to be considered as one example of a modern pharmacy design. (From Planning for Hospital Pharmacies, U.S. Dept. HEW, Health Services & Mental Health Administration, Health Care Facilities Services, Washington, D.C.)

type of detail is available from the manufacturer's catalogue and specification sheets.

Special attention should be given to the counter tops. All too often, excellent base cabinets are provided but the counter tops do not offer resistance to corrosion and abrasion. Accordingly, it is of importance for the pharmacist to inquire about the physical properties of the counter finishes. Some guidelines are the following:

1. To what degree can it be bent without cracking or breaking down?
2. How much of an impact will it withstand without flaking or peeling?
3. What effect will a high relative humidity have upon it?
4. Is it sufficiently hard to resist erosion?
5. If the material is colored, is the color retention quality sufficient to resist appreciable discoloration?
6. Is the finish coat abrasion resistant to the degree that prevents premature wearing through?
7. Is the finish coat reagent resistant? Bear in mind that it must resist acids, alkalies, oils and solvents.

Many of these units are available from the several manufacturers who specialize in the development and construction of such components.

ELECTRIC LIGHTING AND SERVICE

The availability of good electrical lighting and a sufficient number of grounded electrical outlets is mandatory for a smoothly functioning pharmacy.

Accordingly, sufficient lighting must be provided for the various work areas as well as the library and the offices. Although the present literature indicates that 30 foot candles are adequate for general illumination, and 50 foot candles for special areas, such as the prescription dispensing area, it is recommended that in any new construction the services of a lighting engineer be utilized. This is important because each hospital, or unit within the hospital, has particular needs based upon many factors some of which are characteristic of the operation, whereas others may be due to location and environment.

In selecting the type of lighting and light fixture, care should be given to the selection of a unit which will not become a housekeeping problem. That is to say that, when possible, a fixture which can be mounted in the ceiling is highly desirable since it will not gather dust and dirt. Fluorescent light is recommended; however, recent studies by the various manufacturers of lighting equipment seem to indicate that a combination of fluorescent tube and standard bulb in the same fixture provides a better light.

Grounded electrical outlets should be provided in all areas in which the use of electrical equipment may be indicated. In addition, thought must be given to the requirements of voltage in the range of 220 volts for some of the ovens or mixers in the manufacturing area.

If volatile solvents are used in the manufacturing areas or are stored in the pharmacy, consideration must be given to the installation of explosion proof fixtures and outlets.

VENTILATION

Air conditioning of the pharmacy is desirable for a number of reasons. First, it obviates the need for the opening of windows and doors through which dirt, dust and other environmental contaminants may enter the pharmacy. Second, the use of the various autoclaves, ovens and steam jacketed kettles may render the working environment too hot. Third, air conditioning permits the maintenance of a temperature which is compatible with the official storage requirements for drugs on a year round basis irrespective of the climatic conditions. Fourth, adequate ventilation is essential for the removal of the strong odors which are characteristic of the chemicals used in the manufacture of the various galenicals, preservative fluids and reagents. Fifth, because doors and windows can be kept closed, there can be effected a saving in the cost of housekeeping service in the pharmacy.

CONVEYOR AND PNEUMATIC TUBE SYSTEMS

Modern engineering technology has made available a means of transporting nearly every item from the pharmacy to its hospital destination. Accordingly, in order to conserve pharmaceutical manpower, thought should be given to the installation of dumbwaiters, pneumatic tube systems and other like devices for the movement of supplies from the pharmacy to their desired hospital destination. The type of combination of equipment necessary will vary with each hospital; therefore, it is recommended that the advice be sought from the hospital's architect and/or the various manufacturers and distributors of such devices.

PLUMBING

It is not expected that the pharmacist should be knowledgeable in the technicalities of the plumbing installation; however, he should be in a position to advise the architect and his plumbing consultant of the particular details and requirements of the pharmacy and the nature of the materials which will be disposed of through the various waste lines.

By so doing, the plans will properly specify acid resistant piping, adequate hot and cold water mixing valves, stainless steel or soapstone sinks, distilled water lines and faucets which will allow gallon jugs or carboys to be filled without the use of a connecting hose.

Type	Ease of Maintenance	Resistance			Advantages	Disadvantages
		To Moisture	To Alkali	To Oil & Solvents		
Asphalt	Fair*	Excellent	Excellent	Poor*	Lowest cost resilient tile Most resistant to cigarette burns Excellent choice for basement floors May be applied and used immediately	Least resilient and least comfortable tile Does not take as high polish as others Very poor indentation resistance Limited color range (dark)
Linoleum	Very Good	Poor	Fair to Poor	Excellent	More comfortable than asphalt Good warmth Low noise level	Can be used only as above-grade floors
Vinyl-Asbestos	Good	Excellent	Excellent	Good	Good wearing qualities at reasonable cost Inexpensive to maintain May be applied above, on or below grade Wider range of colors than asphalt	Only fair resilience and comfort
Cork	Fair	Fair	Fair	Fair	Excellent comfort, warmth, quietness	Can be used only on above-grade floors Soft, easily marred High cost
Rubber	Good	Good	Good	Poor	Almost as comfortable as cork Lustrous sheen Excellent indentation resistance Wide range of colors	High cost Usually unsuitable for below-grade locations Must be polished frequently to maintain high gloss
Vinyl	Very Good	Good	Excellent	Excellent	May be applied above, on or below grade Smooth and polished-looking Widest range of colors and styles	Most expensive of tiles

*New, grease-resistant variety shows good ease of maintenance and excellent solvent resistance.

FINISHES

a. Work Counters

Although many of the work counters will be constructed of stainless steel, others will not require such construction. For those units, Formica or a similar material is suggested as an efficient and durable surface.

b. Floors

The floors of the pharmacy proper should be resilient, smooth but not slippery, stain resistant and yet complimentary to the existing or proposed decor of the department. Many flooring materials are currently available which are highly satisfactory and economical. Some of the floor coverings currently in use are asphalt tile, vinyl tile, rubber tile and heavy duty linoleum. The Hospital Bureau, Inc.[14] has made available information on page 546.

In recent years, many architects and designers have introduced carpeting into the hospital pharmacy with aesthetic results. On the other hand, some of the installations have not been complementary to the operation of a hospital pharmacy. Carpeting has proven to be acceptable in the office, library, waiting room areas but has not been acceptable in the various work areas. Much of the complaint centers around the excessive generation of static electricity and the flammability of the carpet material.

Low relative humidity has always been the major problem in controlling static generation in carpets. The lower the relative humidity, the greater the problem. Thus, it is important to ascertain the kilovolts of static electricity that a carpet will generate at the normal building temperature and with a relative humidity of 10 to 20%. Clearly, the lower the kilovolts generated, the more acceptable the carpet will be for pharmacy installation. The student is cautioned to the fact that a high humidity will also produce low kilovolt readings of static electricity. Obviously, a high humidity does not lend itself to the pharmacy area for a number of reasons associated with drug storage and personal comfort. Also, carpets that are advertised as being "static free" or "static proof" must be viewed with a jaundiced eye in view of the fact that such material does not exist. Static electricity is present, to some degree, in all materials.

With respect to flammability, the United States Public Health Service has promulgated carpet standards for hospitals and nursing homes using Hill-Burton funds. Carpets in these facilities must have a rating of not less than 75 using the Tunnel Test (ASTM Standard #E-84-61).

The floors of the manufacturing and parenteral solutions room should be supplied with a floor drain covered with a durable paint or enamel. Recent literature describes the application of a vinyl epoxy latex coating to concrete floors which permits the routine use of soap and water for cleaning and yet does not crack and lift as do ordinary paints and enamels.

c. Walls

The walls of the pharmacy should be painted with a material which permits periodic washing without the danger of losing its original color. The selection of the appropriate color scheme is here left to the taste and discretion of the parties involved.

In the manufacturing and parenteral products rooms, painted wall surfaces do not usually withstand the constant washing necessary for the maintenance of the desired degree of asepsis. Accordingly, it is suggested that a ceramic tile, or other comparable material, be utilized in these areas.

SELECTED READINGS

Barker, Kenneth N.: Planning a Hospital Pharmacy Facility. Am. J. Hosp. Pharm., *28*:6:423, 1971.

Brown, Thomas R., Barker, Kenneth N., Rowland, F. Herron, Smith, Mickey C., and Mikeal, Robert L.: A National Survey of Planning for Hospital Pharmacy Facilities. Am. J. Hosp. Pharm., *28*:6:532, 1971.

Osterberger, David J.: Layout and Design for Mechanized Centralized Unit Dose Dispensing. Am. J. Hosp. Pharm., *28*:6:447, 1971.

Miller, R.F. and Herrick, J.D.: Modernizing an Ambulatory Care Pharmacy in a Large Multiclinic Institution. Am. J. Hosp. Pharm., *36*:371–375, Mar., 1979.

Swensson, Earl S.: An Innovative Design in Hospital Pharmacy Facilities. Am. J. Hosp. Pharm., *28*:6:440, 1971.

REFERENCES

1. Minimum Standard for Pharmacies in Hospitals with Guide to Application. Am. J. Hosp. Pharm., *15*:11:992, 1958.
2. Planning For Hospital Pharmacies, Dept. HEW Publication No. (HRA)-77-4003, August, 1977, Superintendent of Documents, U.S. Government Printing Office, Washington, D.C. 20402, p. 1.
3. Ibid: page 2
4. Ibid: page 3
5. Ibid: pages 5–26
6. Ibid: page 85
7. Ibid: pages 86–98
8. Ibid: page 64
9. Ibid: page 67
10. Milne, A.M. and Taylor, W.R.: Suggested Plans for Hospital Pharmacies, 50, 100 and 200-Bed General Hospitals, Bull. Am. Soc. Hosp. Pharm., *7*:3:122, 1950.
11. Francke, D.E., Latiolais, C.J., Francke, G.N., and Ho, N.F.H.: *Mirror to Hospital Pharmacy*, p. 62. American Society of Hospital Pharmacists, Washington, D.C.
12. Ibid: page 65
13. Milne, A.M., Burgoon, D.F., Sim, M. and Donovan, A.C.: Hospital Equipment and Planning Guide, pages 23–26, Public Health Service Publication No. 930-D-4 (Revised 1964), U.S. Government Printing Office, Washington, D.C.
14. Selecting Floor Tile, Bureau Research News, Hospital Bureau Inc., New York 19, N.Y., Vol. VII No. 5, May, 1960.
15. Von Der Mosel, Hans A.: Electrical Safety and Our Hospitals. Medical Instrumentation, *4*:1:2, (Jan.–Feb.) 1970.

25|

The Pharmacy Library—
Drug Information Center

In planning the hospital pharmacy of tomorrow, some thought should be given to the library. Too often, this segment is totally neglected and winds up as a file cabinet and a shelf of 6 to 12 books either in the pharmacy office or in some out of the way corner of the department.

Some hospital administrators refuse to allow the pharmacist a budget for the pharmaceutical library, arguing that the hospital already maintains a central professional library or that the hospital is associated with a university and therefore facilities of the university are readily available. To a certain extent this is a valid argument until examined in the light of modern thinking.

Many prominent medical librarians are of the opinion that hospital libraries possess a great potential for continuing medical education. If this is true for the hospital library *per se*, then it should also be true for the pharmaceutical library.

In a study commonly referred to as the Dryer report[1] there are two major observations:

1. Continuing education of physicians is a major problem which confronts medical education.
2. The results of basic research are not brought to bear clinically quite as fast as they should because of the problem of disseminating research results to the person who is to apply them.

The American Hospital Association has conducted surveys amongst member hospitals in an attempt to learn more about their libraries and has devoted a special section on health communications in the June 16, 1964 issues of *Hospitals,* the Journal of the American Hospital Association.

Therefore, it would seem that a well-planned pharmaceutical library can play a major role in the continuation of medical education, the rapid dissemination of basic pharmacologic research and as a source of research reference material.

This chapter will be concerned with the location, organization and contents of a pharmaceutical library.

LOCATION

Ideally, the pharmaceutical library should be located within and as an integral division of the department of pharmacy. Although, if it becomes necessary for one reason or another to consolidate it with the regular hospital library then, rather than risk the chance of having no worthwhile facility, this alternative should be accepted.

The reasons for placing the pharmaceutical library in the pharmacy are many, but probably the most worthy is that an individual using the facility would have available to him on-the-spot consultation with individuals whose forte is information concerning drugs. Also, whenever a clinician's work requires data concerning drugs or drug therapy, he is, more likely than not, inclined to go to the pharmacy for the desired information. Clearly then, it is advantageous to both doctor and pharmacist to have the reference material at hand rather than consume more valuable time in going to the hospital library.

In addition, the pharmacy is the logical repose of all worthwhile drug related literature: the various journals, product reference and price catalogues, and special releases concerning withdrawal, toxicity or contraindications to the use of existing products.

PHYSICAL FACILITIES

Because the pharmaceutical library is usually restricted to the medical and nursing staffs, its dimension will be determined by the size of the utilizing staff, the type of hospital, the number of textbooks, monographs and journals subscribed to as well as accessibility to the hospital library (if any) or to other medical libraries in the area.

Garland[2] quoting the *Handbook of Medical Library Practice*[3] provides the following measurements as being useful in determining space requirements.

1. The reading area should allow 25 to 30 square feet per reader.
2. If rectangular tables are selected, they should measure 36 × 60 feet. These would then require 100 square feet of floor space for each. (Accommodates 4 readers.)
3. Circular tables measuring 48 inches in diameter and accommodating 4 readers also require 100 square feet of floor space.
4. Aisles:
   a. between tables—not less than 5 feet.
   b. between tables and walls—3 to 4 feet.
5. Shelf space:
   a. bound volumes—4 to 5 volumes per foot of shelf.
   b. reference tools—3 to 4 volumes per foot of shelf. An allowance of 7 inches per 3 foot shelf should be made for additions.

SELECTION OF CONTENTS

The pharmaceutical library should contain in it those volumes, monographs and journals dealing with pharmacy and its allied sciences. Volumes and other published materials dealing with the various clinical and pre-clinical subject areas should be reserved for the hospital medical library.

As a nucleus around which to add volumes, the library should contain the *United States Pharmacopeia* and the *National Formulary* and their supplements.

Pharmaceutical subjects which should be represented in the library include pharmacology, toxicology, pharmaceutical organic chemistry, pharmacognosy, physiology, anatomy and bacteriology. In addition, there should be included a dictionary, medical dictionary, abstract journals, and selected journals dealing with the above subjects. The various types of drug reference books should not be overlooked.

Most drug manufacturers provide in addition to their catalogues comprehensive literature concerning each of their products. It is strongly recommended that these be filled for ready reference. Those hospitals using the *American Hospital Formulary System* often file this type of literature according to the system of classification of drugs employed in the *Formulary.*

In January 1964, the American Society of Hospital Pharmacists commenced a new abstract publication entitled *International Pharmaceutical Abstracts.* In keeping with the recommendations of the Commission on Pharmaceutical Abstracts of the International Pharmaceutical Federation, the Society publishes the journal in English, issues it 24 times per year and provides a cumulative index twice annually.

International Pharmaceutical Abstracts includes abstracts of articles on product formulation and formulas; drug stability and storage; drug synthesis; pharmaceutical technology; pharmacognosy; pharmacology; biopharmaceutics; physical pharmacy; investigational drugs; drug evaluations; and history, ethics and sociology.

Some drug companies also produce films and projection slides covering a number of points of clinical interest. Certainly, a listing of these should be available in the pharmacy library and the pharmacist should be acquainted with the procedure for obtaining them for various clinical and nursing groups.

Of late, producers of pharmaceuticals have made available excellent plastic reproductions of various body organs which possess excellent teaching qualities. A collection of these should certainly be available from the pharmacy library to the school of nursing.

Federal publications, particularly those of the U.S. Department of Health and Human Services (HHS), should always be obtained. One of the most recent issues for which every hospital pharmacist should have his hospital's name placed on the mailing list is *Investigational Drug Circular* issued by the Bureau of Medicine, Food and Drug Administration.

The Federal Food and Drug Administration publishes a journal containing its decisions and views. The name of the journal is *FDA Papers* and is available on a subscription basis from the Government Printing Office in Washington, D.C.

Many house organs contain excellent review articles of clinical interest to both nurse and physician. Accordingly, these should also be part of the pharmacy library.

The American Society of Hospital Pharmacists' *Drug Products Information File* (DPIF) is also a valuable addition to the library. The DPIF is a data bank composed of terms and code numbers for commercially available drug products. The drug data bank is organized to facilitate automatic processing of drug data. This multi-functional drug coding system is based on a 5-digit generic drug product number that identifies the generic product, a 6-digit brand drug product number which identifies a specific manufacturer's brand of drug, and a 5-digit brand drug product package number which extends the information to a specific package of a manufacturer's brand of drug product. In addition, each aspect of a drug product description such as route of administration, dosage form, strength, etc. is systematically coded.

Because of the versatility of the data bank, DPIF has been incorporated into applications such as inventory control; purchasing of drugs; formulary preparation; patient billing; drug therapy auditing; experimental drug information program; adverse drug reaction programs; patient medication records, orders, summaries, charges and labeling.

With the trend towards the utilization of audio-cassettes for continuing education, the American Society of Hospital Pharmacists introduced VOICES 12/60. This is a monthly cassette tape communications program designed specifically for pharmacists, with particular emphasis on clinical and institutional pharmacy practice. Since this is a monthly continuing service, it constitutes the basis for an audio reference library.

The hospital pharmacist desirous of a single source to serve as a check list of possible publications is referred to the *Basic List of Books and Journals for Veterans Administration Medical Libraries,*[4] *The Guide To Information Sources for the Hospital Pharmacist*[5] and to the *World List of Pharmacy Periodicals.*[6]

The decision as to which textbook or journal is necessary for rendering good drug information service is a difficult one to make. Each hospital offering such a service may well have a different source library. The following is a listing used by one hospital and is offered as a guide to the practitioner seeking to create a drug information library. (Use latest available editions.)

American Drug Index
(Billups, N.F.) (J.B. Lippincott Co., Philadelphia)
An alphabetical listing of drugs with cross-indexing by generic, brand and chemical names. Also included are the product composition, dosage forms and use.

American Hospital Formulary Service
(American Society of Hospital Pharmacists, Washington)
Comprehensive presentation of drug monographs on selected commercially available drugs.

Dangerous Properties of Industrial Materials
(Reinhold Publishing Co., New York)
The synonyms, descriptions, physical characteristics, hazards and counter-measures for approximately 12,000 common industrial and laboratory materials are listed.

deHaen Drugs In Use
(Paul deHaen, New York)
Abstracts of clinical studies providing basic clinical data along with product information which is added by the abstract service.

The United States Dispensatory
(Osol, A., Pratt, R. and Gennaro, A.R.) (J.B. Lippincott Co., Philadelpha)
A collection of alphabetically arranged presentations on drugs and classes of drugs. Included in the descriptive matter is data on pharmacology, uses, contraindications, adverse effects and dosage.

Documenta Geigy Scientific Tables
(Konrad Diem, Editor)
(Geigy Pharmaceuticals, Ardsley, New York)
Contains tables of mathematical, physical and chemical data.

Extra Pharmacopoeia—Martindale Edition
(The Pharmaceutical Press, 17 Bloomsbury Sq., London, W.C. 1)
Drug monographs containing the usual information pertaining to physical and chemical properties, pharmacological activity and posology. A source of information for British and foreign drugs.

Facts and Comparisons
(P.O. Box 8, Baden Station, St. Louis)
Comparative listing of drugs to show composition, dosage forms and relative cost. Products are listed by therapeutic use.

FDA Clinical Experience Abstracts
(Dept. HHS, Food and Drug Administration, Washington)
Abstracts of clinical studies on drugs, devices, cosmetics, food additives, pesticides and nutrients with emphasis on adverse effects, hazards and efficacy.

FDA Suspected Adverse Reactions
(Dept. HHS, Food and Drug Administration, Washington)
Abstracts of unusual adverse reactions in single patients.

Handbook of Non-Prescription Drugs
(American Pharmaceutical Association, Washington)
Compilation in tabular form of composition of over-the-counter products with accompanying descriptive monograph on each group of drugs.

Merck Index
(Merck & Co., Rahway, New Jersey
Monographs of physical and chemical data about chemicals and drugs.

Organisch-Chemische Arzneimittel und ihre Synonyma
(Negwe, M., Editor)
(Akademia-Verlag, Berlin, Germany)
Tables of chemical structures, names and synonyms, and uses of organic chemicals. The book provides for a source of information on German drug products.

The Pharmacological Basis of Therapeutics
(Goodman, L.S. and Gilman, A.)
(The Macmillan Co., New York)
Provides information relative to the activity, use and doses of drugs with particular emphasis upon the relationship of pharmacology to clinical practice.

PharmIndex
(Skyline Publishers, P.O. Box 1029, Portland, Oregon)
A compilation of product information including composition, dosage forms, use and cost. Also included are review articles and investigational drug information.

Symptomatology and Therapy of Toxicological Emergencies
(Academic Press Inc., New York)
Provides an alphabetical listing of toxic substances giving expected reactions and suggested treatment.

Unlisted Drugs
(Unlisted Drugs, Box 401, Chatham, New Jersey)
Contains a numeric and/or alphabetical listing of old and new drug items and for each is presented data pertaining to composition, action, dosage, manufacturer and pertinent reference source.

Drug Interactions
(Hansten, Philip D.)
(Lea & Febiger, Philadelphia)
A clinically useful guide to drug-drug interactions and the effects of drugs on clinical laboratory results.

Clinical Toxicology
(Thienes, C.H. and Haley, T.J.)
(Lea & Febiger, Philadelphia)
A grouping of poisons according to their major toxic actions with accompanying method of treatment.

Hazards of Medication
(Martin, E.W., Editor)
(J.B. Lippincott Co., Philadelphia)
A manual on drug interactions, incompatibilities, contraindications and adverse effects of drugs and drug products.

Drug Interactions—
(American Society of Hospital Pharmacists, Washington)
A compilation of abstracts pertaining to drug interactions.

Handbook of Drug Interactions
  (Hartshorn, E.A.)
  (Hamilton Press Inc., Hamilton, Illinois)
  A compilation of articles on drug interactions which have been published
in Drug Intelligence.

USP, NF and USP-DI (Latest editions)
  (USPC Inc., P.O. Box 2248
  Rockville, MD, 20852)

Drug Intelligence & Clinical Pharmacy
  (Drug Intelligence & Clinical Pharmacy
  P.O. Box 42435, Cincinnati, Ohio 45242)
  A journal on drug therapy.

Clinical Pharmacy
  (American Society of Hospital Pharmacists
4630 Montgomery Avenue, Bethesda, MD 20814)
  A journal containing review articles on drug therapy and experiences.

DRUG INFORMATION CENTER

Of late, editors,[7] physicians,[8] pharmacists,[9,11] and administrators[12] have published much data concerning the use and need for adequate drug information in the treatment and care of patients. Many elaborate systems have been developed and put into use by pharmacists in the large teaching centers. In the small community hospital, it is not possible to install or staff such a drug information center. However, it is not impossible to provide the clinical staff with much vital information concerning the use and abuse of drugs, as well as information concerning the drug's chemical nature, mode of action, side effects, dosage forms, cost, and literature pertinent to its clinical use.

In addition, the hospital pharmacist is in a position to alert the physician of any untoward reactions encountered within the hospital from the use of the particular drug. All of this information can be provided the physician by the hospital pharmacist through the pharmacy library. This is possible because, in addition to the latest texts and journals, the hospital pharmacist is in daily touch with the medical service representatives of the major drug producers. Much vital literature and information can be gathered from this source if the hospital pharmacist will only avail himself of it. Once gathered, it should be properly catalogued and filed in such a manner as to make it readily available to all those desirous of making use of it.

Large university affiliated hospitals have developed and staffed a new division of the department of pharmacy which is commonly referred to as the **Drug Information Center.** This new concept in hospital pharmacy operations is usually located in a separate section of the pharmacy, contains a large number of reference texts, journals, reprints and brochures, may be equipped with electronic data processing equipment, and has a full-time director and adequate secretarial assistance.

In order to file the vast number of sources of information that are received by the unit, many hospital pharmacists have adopted the classification of drugs employed in the *American Hospital Formulary Service* and thus have a cross-reference between the files and the *Formulary.*

The Drug Information Center may also assume the responsibility of gathering information on all investigation use drugs in current use in the hospital; record all data on drug reactions in the institution; and may participate in the program of the local Poison Information Center. In some hospitals, the Drug Information Center publishes an Investigational Drug Bulletin and an Adverse Drug Reaction Report for the clinical staff.

The need for a reliable local source of drug information within a medical community is of inestimable importance in rendering effective clinical care to the patient. Thus, it behooves every hospital pharmacist to develop a local source of drug information irrespective of whether it be a modest pharmaceutical library or a comprehensive Drug Information Center. The main theme of either type unit should be—providing drug information when it is needed.

Recognizing the need for this type of service to be rendered by the hospital pharmacist, the American Society of Hospital Pharmacists, in 1968, issued a statement entitled *The Hospital Pharmacist and Drug Information Services.* In justification of the involvement of the hospital pharmacists in this endeavor, the statement cites the following:[13]

"1. Traditionally the service orientation of the pharmacist has been related to drugs—their efficacy, safety and control. Therefore, pharmacy encumbers by reason of tradition a special obligation to accept these challenges.

2. Pharmacy is unique among the health professions in that it possesses an established, but unchallenged, capability to adapt its services for specific contributions to drug therapy. Full utilization of the hospital pharmacist's professional potential represents a more efficient and economical application of health manpower resources.

3. There exists today a nucleus of hospital pharmacy practitioners who are engaged in the functional establishment of a service foundation for drug information activities and responsibilities. Increasing clinical involvement of the heretofore cloistered hospital pharmacist has precipitated a growing demand for this drug information support to those in immediate contact with drug care needs of the patient.

4. Increasingly sophisticated concepts of pharmacodynamic and biochemical complexities of drug actions, a burgeoning drug literature, and the scientific and medicolegal difficulties attending clinical surveillance of drug experiences constitute adequate grounds for advocacy of interprofessional teamwork in the clinical use of drugs. Pharmacy's acceptance of its share of responsibility will lessen the formidable burden placed on other components of the health care community."

Clearly, if the profession of pharmacy is to accept the challenge and accompanying responsibility, its practitioners must be capable of performing in their new role. Within the ASHP's statement, the following performance guidelines are presented:[13]

"1. He demonstrates professional and technical competence in the evaluation, critical selection, and utilization of the drug literature. He presents to those whom he serves the maximum relevant information with a minimum volume of pertinent supporting documentation so as to permit independent, informed conclusions and decisions.
2. His knowledge of institutional and extramural library facilities, literature utilization, and librarian services will permit his taking full advantage of all such resourses available to him.
3. He possesses written and verbal communication skills which enable him to contribute effectively to intra- and inter-institutional dialogue relative to pharmacotherapeutic information.
4. He has the capacity for substantial contributions to the continuing education of all health professions.
5. He is involved directly and indirectly in patient care with drugs as a contributor to its continuing quality and as a monitor of its characteristics.
6. He is familiar with electronic data processing methodology to the extent necessary for him to utilize its services for information storage, processing and retrieval.
7. He is qualified to provide professional services in support of the pharmacy and therapeutics committee.
8. He supports, complements and supplements the efforts of colleagues in pharmacy who are now attempting to marshal the knowledge, skills, scientific acumen and professional judgment necessary to bring appropriately effective pharmaceutical services of all types into the mainstream of patient care with drugs. Thus he contributes to and is an integral part of clinical pharmacy practice and the education of clinical pharmacy practitioners.
9. He contributes to the drug literature through appropriate participation in research activities which include, but are not restricted to, (a) clinical and pre-clinical drug studies, (b) surveillance of clinical drug experiences in his institution, and (c) experimentation in professional services."

A review of the literature reveals that drug information services within a hospital are beginning to be created on a more widespread basis. Some of these units are not as well developed as others, however they represent a trend. A good model of a comprehensive in-hospital drug information service is the unit operated within the University of Alabama Hospitals and Clinics.[14]

Regional drug information service or networks are, as yet, not very common. One that is in operation is the Michigan Regional Drug Information Network.[14] Some of the goals of the regional network include the development of a reproducible, standardized reporting system for auditing drug therapy, supplying of information to all hospitals, institutions and health professionals in the region and serving as a prototype for other medical centers and community hospitals wishing to develop similar services.

Specific objectives related to the latter goals were designed to provide:[14]

(1) An analysis of drug information and drug therapy relating to heart disease, cancer, stroke and related diseases and provision of this information to the physician;

(2) A drug information abstract service to physicians in the region regarding new developments in drug therapy and heart disease, cancer, stroke and related diseases;

(3) An analysis and evaluation of the regional utilization of drugs in the institutions served by the network and dissemination of this information to the respective medical staffs for audit; and

(4) A reduction in the lag time existing between the development of new information and the practical application of this information to patient care—.

Of interest to the student are the criteria set forth for participation by other units in the progam.[14] They are as follows:

(1) That the director of the pharmacy department be interested in establishing a drug information center, be interested in the possibilities of affiliation with a larger center and be willing to continue the drug information center after the period of grant funding.

(2) That the hospital, in particular the pharmacy department, be willing to accept calls from physicians in the surrounding community and other health professionals and to answer these questions to the best of their ability.

(3) That the affiliated drug information center service an area of sizeable population and not impinge on other affilitate's area of coverage. It was also important that the surrounding community physicians related to this particular hospital for the health care of the community.

(4) That the administrative head of the hospital support a drug information center affiliated with the main center and be willing to continue support to the drug information center at the conclusion of the grant.

(5) That the members of the medical staff, preferably those affiliated with the Pharmacy and Therapeutics Committee, show an interest in support of the network.

(6) That the affiliate be willing to provide twenty-four hours a day, seven days a week coverage.

In summary, the drug information function is primarily concerned with pharmaceutical advice and consultation regarding drug therapy, and is involved in the following activities:[15]

1. Establishing and maintaining:
   a. A system for retrieving information from drug literature.
   b. A system for surveillance of the use of drugs in the hospital, including patient drug histories and profiles and reporting adverse drug reactions.
   c. A panel of drug consultants.

2. Answering requests for specific items of drug information for the drug therapy of individual patients.
3. Offering unsolicited drug information for the drug therapy of individual patients.
4. Answering requests for comprehensive drug information complications or bibliographies for:
   a. In-service education programs.
   b. Poison control information centers.
   c. Pharmacy research projects.
   d. Pharmacy and therapeutics committee deliberations—literature searches and background papers on drugs and drug problems.
   e. Pharmacy research projects.
   f. Other pharmacy functions such as manufacturing, control, research and clinical pharmacy.
5. Producing and distributing periodic compilations of drug information directed toward special audiences such as drug information bulletins for physicians, nurses and pharmacists.
6. Maintaining the formulary and/or drug list.
7. Evaluating the detailing activities by drug vendors including promotional exhibits in the hospital.

ASHP SUPPLEMENTAL STANDARD AND LEARNING OBJECTIVES FOR RESIDENCY TRAINING IN DRUG INFORMATION PRACTICE[16]*

Preamble

Definition. A specialized residency in drug information practice is defined as a postgraduate program of organized education and training that meets the requirements set forth and approved by the American Society of Hospital Pharmacists. The ASHP Accreditation Standard for Specialized Residency Training,[1] together with this supplement, are the basic criteria used to evaluate drug information residency training programs in institutions applying for accreditation by the American Society of Hospital Pharmacists.

A specialized residency in drug information practice must be organized and conducted to develop a mastery of knowledge and an expert level of competency in this area of pharmacy, differentiated in scope, depth, and proficiency from the drug information activities of institutional pharmacy residents. Objectives of such training shall include extensive experiences in providing comprehensive drug information services in an institution or with several institutions, integrated with the institution's clinical pharmacy services, drug-distribution systems, and the appropriate committees dealing with drug use.

Qualifications of the Training Site. The parent facility for an ac-

---

*Approved by the ASHP Board of Directors, September 24, 1982. The initial draft was developed by a working group of the SIG on Drug and Poison Information Pharmacy Practice. The final document was approved by the Commission on Credentialing before submission to the Board of Directors.

credited residency in drug information pharmacy practice shall be a general hospital or a health science center that is formally affiliated with one or more general hospitals.

Two or more hospitals may collaborate in conducting a drug information residency program, provided that one hospital is identified as the primary site and one individual is designated as the residency program director.

Qualifications of the Pharmacy Service. The pharmacy department in which an accredited drug information practice residency is based must meet the requirements set forth in Standard II of the ASHP Accreditation Standard for Specialized Pharmacy Residency Training.[1] In addition, the pharmacy department must provide a comprehensive program of drug information services far beyond that required in the ASHP Minimum Standard for Pharmacies in Institutions.[2] The following specific requirements are established for the drug information service program.

Physical Facilities. There shall be a defined area for the drug information center. Space shall be adequate to house the furniture, equipment, literature resources, and personnel of the drug information center.

Resources. There shall be a comprehensive drug information library with appropriate holdings of primary, secondary, and tertiary literature. Scientific and professional practice journals in pharmacy and medicine shall be available in the drug information center or quickly accessible in another location. At least two secondary information services (indexing or abstracting services) shall be available in the drug information center. Reference texts shall be current and provide detailed information in at least the following areas of drug information: administration, adverse effects, availability, bioavailability, chemistry, cost, dose, drugs of choice, efficacy, excretion, formulations, incompatibilities, identifications (foreign and American), indications, interactions, laws, mechanisms of action, nonprescription drugs, pathophysiology, pharmacokinetics, statistics, teratogenicity, tissue distribution, and toxicology.

The drug information center should be located near a medical library that, in turn, has access to a regional medical library.

Computer-search capabilities shall be available in the drug information center or through the medical library.

Staffing. At least one full-time drug information specialist shall be employed in the drug information center. Secretarial and clerical support shall be readily available to the drug information center staff, including typing of communications, filing, and related duties.

Availability of Service. The drug information center shall be open for service at least eight hours per day, Monday through Friday, with off-hours service capability through a paging system, answering service, or other mechanism.

Scope of Service. The drug information service program shall be oriented toward patient-specific requests, and it shall respond to at least five (minimum average) such requests per day. Documentation of all responses shall be maintained. The drug information center shall also provide the following services on a regular basis: development of drug monographs for use by the pharmacy and therapeutics committee, participation in ongoing drug-use review and medical audits, publication of therapeutics newsletters, and formal instruction of students or residents. The following additional services should be provided where feasible: investigational drug information clearinghouse, adverse drug reaction reporting, drug information support service to other institutions, and formulary revision.

Location. Drug information centers located outside the pharmacy department (e.g., a medical library or college of pharmacy) may be used as training sites, provided that they meet the requirements set forth in this section (Qualifications of the Pharmacy Service) and are routinely used in the hospital pharmacy's drug information service program.

Qualifications of the Preceptor. The area of specialization of the preceptor shall be drug information pharmacy practice. He shall have had a minimum of three years of experience operating a drug information center. In addition, he shall maintain an active patient-care involvement, either through clinical consultations and other patient-oriented services provided through the drug information center or through other routinely provided clinical pharmacy services.

Qualifications of the Applicant. In addition to meeting the requirements set forth in Standard IV, the applicant should have completed formal academic instruction in the following subject areas or their equivalents: drug-literature evaluation, pathophysiology, statistics, and toxicology.

The following learning objectives shall be approved by the Commission on Credentialing following review annually by a committee appointed from the Special Interest Group on Drug and Poison Information Practice of the American Society of Hospital Pharmacists.

Learning Objectives and Areas of Emphasis

I. **Learning Objectives.** A resident who completes an accredited program in drug information practice shall be able to:

    A. Develop a plan for the organization and operation of a drug information service, including physical accommodations, reference sources, professional and supportive personnel, budgeting, relationships with other health-care departments, work flow, assumed or designated responsibilities, and documentation of services.

    B. Make effective use of institutional and extramural library facilities and librarian services.

C. Select the most appropriate drug information literature sources for any given question.
D. Use the primary literature, including the pharmacy practice literature, in providing drug information services.
E. Demonstrate a mastery of drug information filing systems.
F. Evaluate written and verbal promotional material about drugs provided by pharmaceutical representatives.
G. Apply a knowledge of biopharmaceutics in selecting drug products and in solving patient-specific drug-therapy problems.
H. Evaluate the study design of research articles in the drug literature, and state an opinion on the validity of the published results.
I. Communicate effectively, in person and by telephone, with pharmacists, nurses, physicians, patients, and pharmaceutical representatives in solving drug information problems.
J. Obtain appropriate patient, drug, and disease information from an inquirer initiating a patient-oriented drug information request.
K. Write concise, authoritative, grammatically correct, and clinically applicable consultations, drug monographs, and other drug-related manuscripts.
L. Respond to patient-specific inquiries in time for maximum clinical usefulness.
M. Provide rapid and accurate information relating to poison treatment.
N. Respond with authority to questions relating to drug induced disorders.
O. Provide a pharmacy and therapeutics committee with drug information support, including comparative drug-monograph reviews.
P. Take charge of the organization, preparation, and dissemination of an in-house periodic bulletin or newsletter (e.g., drug information bulletin/newsletter, or P&T committee newsletter).
Q. Contribute to the practice of pharmacy-based drug information services through publication of a therapeutic review, drug monograph, case report, or the results of original research.
R. Make a clear statement about the organization and role of a hospital's institutional review board, the relationship of the pharmacist to its activities, and the role of the pharmacist in distribution and control of investigational drugs.
S. Initiate a drug-use review or medical audit.
T. Participate in the formal inservice training or continuing education of physicians, pharmacists, nurses, or other health-care professionals in therapeutic areas, and conduct classes and training sessions dealing with drug information skills and knowledge for appropriate groups of learners.
U. Develop and defend a proposal for implementing a research project or a new drug information service or other clinical service.
V. Participate in research activities that include, but are not restricted to, clinical and preclinical drug studies, surveillance of clinical drug experiences in the institution, evaluation of new and innovative services, and drug-use review.

II. *Areas of Emphasis.* The resident's training program shall be structured around practical applications of drug-literature retrieval and analysis in solving clinical problems, and associated communications skills. It must be organized in a way that makes possible the attainment of the learning objectives. Experiences must be provided in each of the following areas:

A. *Use of drug information literature.*
    1. Primary literature (journals). The resident must receive extensive experience in the use of journals in pharmacy, medicine, and the pharmaceutical and biomedical sciences.
    2. Secondary sources. The resident must have an expert knowledge in the use of at least two of the following sources and be capable of using the others when necessary: *Current Contents, de Haen Drugs in Research, de Haen Drugs in Use, Index Medicus, Inpharma, Iowa Drug Information Service, International Pharmaceutical Abstracts, Reactions,* and *Service Citation Index.* Skill in using the following special information systems is also expected: *Drugdex, Poisindex,* and *Unlisted Drugs.*
    3. Tertiary literature (reference books). The resident must have experience in using current, standard textbooks or reference volumes in solving drug information problems. The resident's experience should include use of books in each of the following subject areas: adverse effects, administration, availability, bioavailability, chemistry, drug cost, dose, drugs of choice, efficacy, excretion, formulations, incompatibilities, identifications (foreign and American), indications, interactions, laws, mechanism of action, nonprescription drugs, pathophysiology, pharmacokinetics, statistics, teratogenicity, tissue distribution, and toxicology.
B. *Drug-induced (iatrogenic) disease.* The resident shall receive instruction and training in evaluating the pathophysiology, mechanism of action, and treatment of drug-induced disorders.
C. *Toxic drug ingestion.* The resident shall receive instruction and training in evaluating potentially toxic drug ingestions and providing information to patients and to other health professionals concerning signs and symptoms, general supportive care, and specific treatment.
D. *Information storage.* The resident shall receive training in proper storage (filing) of special drug information, such as formulation contents of pharmaceuticals and drug distribution to specialized body compartments.
E. *Communications skills.* The resident shall have numerous assignments throughout the year aimed at developing written and verbal communications skills. The residency preceptor shall be specifically responsible for setting goals for the resident's growth and development in these areas, monitoring the resident's progress, and counseling the resident on a regular basis concerning communication abilities.
F. *Clinical practice skills.* The resident shall have adequate experiences throughout the year to maintain a good level of expertise in clinical practice.

Extramural Experiences

When appropriate, rotations or visitations to other institutions should be scheduled to augment the resident's training (e.g., a poison control center, a pharmacokinetics consultation service, a federal drug information agency, a pharmaceutical company information center, and a medical library or pharmacy school information center). If the drug information service does not answer poison information inquiries, a rotation in a poison control center shall be required. Special rotations may also be arranged to strengthen the resident's clinical, communications, and research skills.

Extramural rotations may be conducted either as full-time training activities (e.g., a one-month block), or on a regularly scheduled part-time basis. If extramural rotations are scheduled for the purpose of pursuing one or more of the fundamental learning objectives, there must be a pharmacist preceptor who has defined responsibilities for monitoring the progress and evaluating the accomplishments of the resident. A detailed set of of objectives for extramural rotations must be prepared in advance. The qualifications of the extramural training site are subject to review and approval by the American Society of Hospital Pharmacists.

Research Projects

The residency training schedule shall make provision for the resident's participation in a self-directed or collaborative research project. The final report of the project should be of such quality to merit presentation at a national professional meeting or publication in an appropriate journal.

REFERENCES

1. American Society of Hospital Pharmacists. ASHP accreditation standard for specialized pharmacy residency training (with guide to interpretation). Am. J. Hosp. Pharm., 1980; *37*:1229–32.
2. American Society of Hospital Pharmacists. ASHP minimum standard for pharmacies in institutions. Am. J. Hosp. Pharm., 1977; *34*:1356–8.

SELECTED READINGS

Ensom, R.J. and McCollom, R.A.: Regional Hospital Pharmacy Information Index. Am. J. Hosp. Pharm., *42*:119–121, 1985.
Thompson, D.F. and Kaczmarek, E.R.: Literature Filing System for Hospital Pharmacy Practice. Am. J. Hosp. Pharm., *41*:2392–2395, 1984.
Robins, R.V. and King, C.M.: Revised Classification and Filing System for Hospital Pharmacy. Am. J. Hosp. Pharm., *18*:31–41, 1983.

REFERENCES

1. Dryer, B.V.: Lifetime Learning for Physicians. J. Med. Ed., *37*: pt. 2, 1962.
2. Gartland, Henry J.: Blue Print for a Professional Hospital Library, Hospitals. J.A.H.A., *38*:12:58, 1964.

3. Doe, J. and Marshall, M.L.: *Handbook of Medical Library Practice.* Chicago, American Library Association, 1956.
4. U.S. Veterans Administration, Basic List of Books and Journals for Veterans Administration Medical Libraries. Program Guide G-14 (Revised), Washington, D.C.: U.S. Government Printing Office.
5. Guide to Information Sources for the Hospital Pharmacist, 1960 Revision. Am. J. Hosp. Pharm., *18*:1:15, 1961.
6. Andrews, Theodora: World List of Pharmacy Periodicals (From a Preliminary Listing by Sinifred Sewell). Am. J. Hosp. Pharm., *20*:2:43, 1963.
7. Francke, Don E.: The Expanding Role of the Hospital Pharmacist in Drug Information Services. Am. J. Hosp. Pharm., *22*:1:32, 1965.
8. Pellegrino, E.D.: Drug Information Services and the Clinician. Am. J. Hosp. Pharm., *22*:1:38, 1965.
9. Parker, Paul F.: The University of Kentucky Drug Information Center. Am. J. Hosp. Pharm., *22*:1:142, 1965.
10. Burkholder, David F.: Operation of the Drug Information Center at the University of Kentucky. Am. J. Hosp. Pharm., *22*:1:48, 1965.
11. Anderson, R. David and Latiolais, Clifton J.: The Drug Informaiton Center at the Ohio State University Hospitals. Am. J. Hosp. Pharm., *22*:1:52, 1965.
12. Wittrup, Richard D.: The Responsibility of the Hospital for Drug Information Services. Am. J. Hosp. Pharm., *22*:1:58, 1965.
13. The Hospital Pharmacist and Drug Information Services. Am. J. Hosp. Pharm., *26*:7:381, 1968.
14. Drug Information Services: Two Operational Models, DHEW Publication No. (HSM) 72-3030 Stock No. 1721-0004 Superintendent of Documents, U.S. Printing Office, Washington, D.C. 20402.
15. Planning for Hospital Pharmacies DHEW Publication No. (HRA) 77-4003 Superintendent of Documents, U.S. Government Printing Office, Washington, D.C. 20402 Aug., 1977, pp. 70–71.
16. ASHP Supplemental Standard and Learning Objectives for Residency Training in Drug Information Practice. Am. J. Hosp. Pharm. *39*:1970–1972, 1982.

26|

The Role of the Hospital Pharmacist in Educational and Training Programs

Because of the pharmacist's scope of activity, his usually high professional standards, his academic accomplishments, and his willingness to assume a teaching role, hospitals have been catapulted into a wide variety of teaching programs. These include undergraduate and graduate programs in medicine, teaching student nurses, licensed practical nurse programs, and the training of technologists, physiotherapists, dietitians, administrative residents, social service workers and pharmacists.

Being an integral part of this academic setting, the hospital pharmacist is usually involved in one or more of these programs, It has been reported[1] that the major contribution made by the pharmacist to the hospital's teaching program is his role in the education of student nurses. The same publication further states that hospital pharmacists also take active roles in the training of graduate nurses, undergraduate pharmacy students as well as graduate students in hospital pharmacy programs.

As a matter of fact, the hospital pharmacist, because of his education, training and experience, does partake in both "internal" and "external" teaching ventures. This novel classification of the hospital pharmacist's teaching activity requires further elaboration.

Internal teaching programs are considered to be those which involve the training of student nurses; the conducting of seminars in therapeutics for graduate nurses, house staff members and senior medical staff; and assisting in the education of undergraduate pharmacy students, graduate pharmacy students and residents in hospital administration.

External teaching programs are considered to be those in which the hospital pharmacist is the guest lecturer or speaker, or possibly the sole instructor in charge of a specific course in a school or college. Examples of external type programs are courses in colleges of pharmacy, refresher courses under the auspices of a college of pharmacy, seminars, institutes or conventions which are sponsored by professional associations.

PROFESSIONAL EDUCATION OF THE HOSPITAL PHARMACIST

In order that the hospital pharmacist effectively become engaged in the teaching and training of other personnel, he must himself be qualified by virtue of degrees as well as by experience.

Francke *et al.*[2] have shown that the majority of the chief pharmacists practicing today hold either a Graduate in Pharmacy (Ph.G.), Pharmaceutical Chemist (Ph.C.), or Bachelor of Science degree. A small number of practitioners also hold Master of Science, Doctor of Pharmacy, Doctor of Science, or Doctor of Philosophy degrees.

Because of the efforts of the colleges of pharmacy to graduate competent practitioners, it should not be too long before the trend will be toward the opposite end of the spectrum, namely, that the majority of the chief pharmacists will hold graduate degrees.

In the meantime, there does exist a shortage of hospital pharmacy practitioners and an attempt must be made to satisfy the need with what is available. In fact, the present graduate of the 5-year curriculum, although holding only a Bachelor of Science degree, is reasonably well qualified to assume a certain amount of teaching responsibility particularly in those non-metropolitan, non-university affiliated community institutions. It is safe to say that, in these hospitals, relatively few members of the staff, with the exception of the medical and dental staff, hold graduate degrees.

The modern 5-year program provides the pharmacist with a broad training in the biological, chemical, and pharmaceutical sciences. In addition an opportunity is provided for the acquisition of knowledge in the areas of statistics, management, marketing, and higher mathematics.

Those practitioners who presently hold the Master of Science degree (the present graduate degree in hospital pharmacy) have completed, in addition to the courses referred to in a sample 5-year summary,[3] at least 30 credit hours of graduate work in courses in hospital pharmacy, physical chemistry and advance pharmacology. In addition, the curriculum requires a minimum of 2,000 clock hours of practice in hospitals to meet the *Accreditation Standard for Pharmacy Residency in a Hospital* of the American Society of Hospital Pharmacists.[14]

ASHP ACCREDITATION STANDARD FOR PHARMACY RESIDENCY IN A HOSPITAL[a]
(With Guide to Interpretation)

Preamble

Definitions. A pharmacy residency in a hospital is defined as a postgraduate program of organized training that meets the requirements set forth and approved by the American Society of Hospital Pharmacists in this Standard.

The Accreditation Standard for Pharmacy Residency in a Hospital is the basic criterion used in evaluation of pharmacy residency training programs in hospitals applying for accreditation by the American Society of Hospital Pharmacists. The interpretative narrative following each element of the Standard is intended to illustrate how the Standard will be interpreted by the accreditation site surveyors and the Society's Commission on Credentialing in evaluation of residency programs. The companion document to the Standard, the Statement on Accreditation of Pharmacy Residencies in Hospitals,[1] sets forth the policies governing the accreditation program and describes the procedures to be followed in applying for accreditation of pharmacy residency programs.

Objectives of Pharmacy Residency Training in Hospitals. Pharmacy residency programs in hospitals should be organized and conducted in such a manner as to develop special skills and competency in hospital pharmacy far beyond the legal requirements for licensure. A *residency* in pharmacy is distinguished from an *internship* in pharmacy in that the latter term describes the type of training program meeting the requirements of boards of pharmacy for licensure. Residency programs also meet requirements for licensure, but internship programs do not meet requirements for residency programs as defined by this Standard. An internship is essentially an on-the-job training program given a recent graduate to develop him into a legally competent practitioner. A residency program on the other hand, should seek to provide an already legally competent practitioner with expert skills in institutional pharmacy practice.

The objectives of internships are to provide experience in basic practice situations and to develop the ability to coordinate the various functions and divisions within the hospital pharmacy so that a meaningful service can be provided. The objectives of residency training programs, however, are to provide experience in learning how to coordinate the total pharmacy service with the needs of the total insti-

---

[a]Approved by the ASHP Board of Directors November 8, 1962; revised December 6, 1965, April 11, 1970, November 8, 1972, November 21, 1974, and November 16, 1978.

tution and to provide a broad scope of in-depth experiences leading to an advanced level of knowledge and fostering the ability to conceptualize new and improved pharmacy services.

Application of the Standard. A fundamental principle of this Standard is that the residency program is structured to insure the achievement of certain predetermined competencies. While the Standard requires a minimum of 2000 hours training time for the residency, there is no set way in which this time is to be allotted. Standard V, below, specifies eight areas in which the resident's competence must be developed. Obviously, the amount of time required to accomplish a minimum level of competence in each of these areas will vary from one resident to another. The time remaining in the program *after* the achievement of these basic competencies may be distributed evenly over administrative and professional practice areas *or* may be applied to developing special competence in either administration or professional practice (e.g., clinical practice). Experience has shown that the minimum requirement of 2000 hours must generally be exceeded in order to accomplish the basic intent of the Standard plus provide for special training in an area of emphasis.

The Accreditation Standard for Pharmacy Residency in a Hospital applies only to the nonacademic aspects of residency training programs, that is, those aspects for which no academic credit is ordinarily given. The American Society of Hospital Pharmacists assumes no authority for evaluation of the academic components of residency training programs.

Standard I—Qualification of the Training Hospital

A. The hospital shall be accredited by the Joint Commission on Accreditation of Hospitals or the American Osteopathic Association.

B. Pharmacy residencies shall be conducted only in those hospitals in which the educational benefits to the resident are considered of paramount importance in relation to the service benefits which the hospital may obtain from the resident.

Interpretation

I-A. Only those hospitals whose governing bodies, personnel, and professional staffs have collaborated to seek excellence, which have accepted outside appraisal, and which have demonstrated substantial conformance with professionally developed and nationally applied criteria, should serve as training facilities for pharmacy residents. The Joint Commission on Accreditation of Hospital's Standards for Pharmaceutical Services,[2] or the Accreditation Requirements of the American Osteopathic Association,[3] will serve as the basic guides in evaluating the qualifications of the training hospital.

I-B. A residency training program should provide experience in the technological aspects of institutional pharmacy practice, in all aspects of total drug-use control in the hospital, and in the clinical application of drugs in the treatment of patients. Participation by the resident in the activities of the department lends understanding, confidence, and purpose to his academically attained professional background. A significant portion of this participation must, of necessity, involve on-the-job training since only through actual performance of some activities can the resident be expected to gain an appreciation and an understanding of the knowledge and skills required to carry out these activities. Through actual experience the resident learns how these activities interrelate and are best coordinated with other activities and functions throughout the department and the institution. The greater emphasis in residency training, however, should be concentrated upon developing in the resident the ability to coordinate activities and conceptualize, integrate and transform accumulated experiences and knowledge into improved pharmacy services.

Standard II—Qualifications of the Pharmacy Service

A. The pharmacy department shall be organized in accordance with the principles of good management under the direction of a legally qualified pharmacist and with sufficient appropriate personnel to carry out a broad scope of pharmacy services within the hospital and for the patient, and shall comply (where applicable) with all federal, state and local laws, codes, statutes and regulations.

B. There shall be at least one full-time, legally qualified pharmacist for each resident.

C. The pharmacy department shall have adequate facilities to carry out a broad scope of services including but not limited to the following areas of professional and administrative activity:

1. Departmental administration;
2. Ambulatory patient services;
3. Inpatient drug distribution and control;
4. Technology and quality control activities;
5. Clinical services; and
6. Drug information services.

It is necessary that a regular and continuing experience be provided in these activities and it is not sufficient to create "artificial situations" for residents to obtain this experience.

If any of the designated activities or divisions of pharmaceutical practice are not available in the training hospital, arrangements shall be made with a hospital or facility acceptable to the American Society of Hospital Pharmacists to provide the necessary experience.

D. The pharmacy director shall have the responsibility and the authority to carry out a broad scope of professional service.

E. The pharmacy director, or his designee, shall be a member of and actively participate in the pharmacy and therapeutics committee of the medical staff.

Interpretation

II-A. The pharmacy service should comply with the requirements of the Minimum Standard for Pharmacies in Institutions approved by the American Society of Hospital Pharmacists.

Although the organizational plans of hospitals may vary, depending upon the type, size and ownership of the institution, the pharmacy service should have departmental status and the pharmacy director should be classified as a department head. He should be responsible to administrative authority of the hospital for developing, supervising and coordinating all activities of the department and should regularly participate in the appropriate administrative meetings in the hospital.

There should be an organizational chart for the pharmacy illustrating the chain of authority and responsibility for departmental personnel and depicting what functions the pharmacy presumes to carry out. Departmental objectives should be clearly defined in a written statement and all pharmacy staff members should be familiar with the intent and substance of the objectives. As a department head in the hospital, the pharmacy director is responsible for determining departmental objectives and these should be in accord with the established objectives of the hospital. They will become criteria for evaluating progress on departmental projects.

Written policies to govern the procedures and conduct of the pharmacy should exist and these should be kept current. Adequate measures to implement promulgated policies should be established and all departmental staff should have a clear understanding of them and comply with them as applicable. There should be written procedures for all routine transactions, functions and operations in the department, and these should be kept current. Orientation of all new pharmacy personnel should include a review of the policy and procedure manual, its scope and use.

All personnel in the department should be thoroughly familiar with the procedures applicable to their respective areas of responsibility and should comply with them.

The professional personnel complement should be adequate to carry out the stated objectives for the department and to provide legally competent pharmacy service at all times. The pharmacy director, his assistant(s) and staff pharmacists should be graduates of colleges of pharmacy accredited by the American Council on Pharmaceutical Education and currently licensed to practice in one of the jurisdictions of the United States. Professional staff members should have had experience in hospital pharmacy and supervisory pharmacists should, preferably, have completed a pharmacy residency in a hospital accredited by the American Society of Hospital Pharmacists. Professional staff members should demonstrate their interest in maintaining professional competency by attendance at continuing education programs, reading the professional literature, and participation in their local, state and national professional organizations

The supportive staff complement should be adequate to support the professional staff. The number of supportive staff members should ordinarily equal or exceed the number of qualified professional staff. The basic criterion for determining the required number of supportive staff members is whether or not the supportive staff complement is adequate to relieve pharmacist staff members from performing a significant number of responsibilities and functions which can be appropriately assigned to paraprofessional personnel.

Job responsibilities for all professional and supportive personnel should be clearly delineated in current job descriptions. Each staff member should be thoroughly familiar with the job description for his respective position and, preferably, will have actively participated in writing it.

II-B. The ratio of one full-time legally qualified pharmacist for each resident is prescribed to assure that the number of professional staff members is adequate to provide the requisite amount of supervisory and tutorial time for effective training of the resident(s) and to obviate the exploitation of trainees.

II-C. A broad scope of service is essential to a well-rounded residency program. The ability of the institution to provide an appropriate scope of experiences for the resident is determined in large part by the organizational adequacy of the hospital and the pharmacy department to provide well-operated, patient-oriented service programs in each of the specified areas of professional practice. It is not acceptable to synthesize training experience to substitute for nonexistent service programs. Neither is it acceptable to substitute academic college courses for experience in service programs in the hospital. Required experience may be obtained in another hospital, but a written protocol for this training experience and a survey of the facility must be approved by the American Society of Hospital Pharmacists.

The following service functions are some of the more important recommended minimal requirements for any hospital offering a pharmacy residency training program meeting the requirements of the Accreditation Standard:

Departmental Administration. The functions performed in administration of the pharmacy department are basically the same as those of any other major hospital department and include directing, organizing, staffing, planning, budgeting, controlling, coordinating, supervising and reporting. There are administrative aspects associated with all departmental functions, thus it is difficult to consider departmental administration as an isolated group of functions. Of primary importance is the existence of and compliance with formalized policies and procedures for administrative activities such as purchasing and inventory control, cost accounting, budgeting, personnel selection and management, policy and procedures development, handling correspondence, committee participation, indexing and filing, control of regulated drugs and supplies, interdepartmental relationships, periodic reporting to administration and related activities.

The official ASHP documents, Minimum Standard for Pharmacies in Institutions,[4] and Statement on Hospital Drug Control Systems,[5] will serve as guides in evaluation of administrative service activities.

Ambulatory Patient Services. The functions of the outpatient pharmacy including dispensing medications to outpatients and employees and counseling patients on the safe and appropriate use of the medication. An adequate data base should be maintained on all outpatients. Adequate controls should exist to permit supportive personnel to handle the mechanics of filling prescription orders, including selecting the drugs, typing labels, retrieving and filing patient records, and other appropriate activities. Only pharmacists, however, should issue medications to patients and provide consultation. A counseling station, which provides privacy and protects the patient's dignity, should be available.

The pharmacist should be guided by the ASHP Statement on Pharmacist-conducted Patient Counseling[6] in providing service to outpatients.

Inpatient Drug Distribution and Control. An adequate level of drug-use control is the prime consideration in inpatient drug distribution. For this reason, a unit dose drug distribution system must be operational in any hospital desiring to maintain an accredited pharmacy residency program. The floor stock system or any other system which does not provide for product identity up to the point of administration, must be considered unacceptable.

Associated with the drug distribution system employed must be appropriate provision for pharmacists' review of physicians' medication orders before administration of the drugs. This implies also that the pharmacy should maintain a drug profile on each patient and establish policy and procedures for screening for potential drug related problems.

The drug distribution system must provide for pharmacy for pharmacy preparation of all parental admixtures on an around-the-clock basis.

Twenty-four hour staffing for the pharmacy department is rapidly becoming standard operating procedure and is especially needed in hospitals where the unit dose drug distribution system is in operation.

In evaluation of the inpatient drug distribution service function, the ASHP Statement on Hospital Drug Control Systems[5] will be used.

Technology and Quality Control. The primary purposes of these service activities are:

1. To provide a product, special dosage form, or package size or type not commercially available (this includes parenteral admixtures, total parenteral nutrition fluids, and other sterile dosage forms);
2. To control the quality of all drugs manufactured, extemporaneously compounded, packaged, repackaged or labeled within the pharmacy department;
3. To monitor the precision and accuracy of all staff members involved in product manipulation (e.g., aseptic techniques);
4. To control the storage and distribution of investigational use drugs;
5. To implement suitable systems for the storage, handling and distribution of controlled substances, ethyl alcohol, and other dangerous substances; and
6. To comparatively evaluate the pharmaceutical quality of drug products under consideration for purchase by the hospital.

The pharmacy must have adequate personnel, space and facilities to carry out these activities. When facilities are not immediately available, arrangements may be made with other departments in the hospital in which suitable facilities are found (examples: use of autoclaves in central supply for terminal sterilization of irrigating fluids; use of culture media and incubators in microbiology for sterility tests).

Clinical Services. Being a health care profession, pharmacy is inherently clinical. The use of the term *clinical pharmacy,* however, has served a useful purpose in recent years—it has reminded us that the focal point of the practice of pharmacy is the control of the interaction of patients and drugs, not just the delivery of a drug product. Although most, if not all, of the service functions of the hospital pharmacy department have clinical components associated with them, clinical services are taken to be, for the purpose of this Standard, those functions identified in the ASHP Statement on Clinical Functions in Institutional Pharmacy Practice.[7] These are:

1. Preparation of patient medication histories entered in patients' permanent medical records and/or data bases.
2. Monitoring drug therapy including routine analysis of patients' drug therapy, medical problems, laboratory data, and special procedures, as well as correlating these analyses with direct patient observation and communicating these analyses with other clinicians responsible for the patients' care.
3. Patient education and counseling.
4. Participation in management of medical emergencies, e.g., cardiopulmonary resuscitation and drug overdosage.
5. Provision of written consultations in such areas as total parenteral nutrition, intravenous therapy, clinical pharmacokinetics, selection of drug therapy, and determination of therapeutic endpoints.
6. Management of patients with chronic diseases such as hypertension, diabetes mellitus, chronic obstructive pulmonary disease, arthritis and cancer, in cooperation with the medical staff.

7. Initiation of and participation in clinical drug investigations in collaboration with appropriate members of the institution's medical staff.
8. Detection and reporting of adverse drug reactions.
9. Control of medication administration and drug distribution in the patient care area.
10. Conducting drug utilization reviews and participation in patient care audits.
11. Participation in the education of medical, pharmacy and nursing personnel in the patient care areas.

Although it is not expected that every pharmacy department in which a residency program is conducted will necessarily be involved in each of these activities, there must be a comprehensive program of clinical services, sufficient to meet the hospital's specific needs. In evaluating clinical service activities the Society considers only those services performed by hospital pharmacy department staff members or clinical facility members who are accountable to the director of pharmacy, and only those services which are continuously performed even in the absence of students and residents.

The provision of clinical services should be a stated objective of the pharmacy department and should be addressed in the departmental policies and procedures, in position descriptions for the professional staff, and in the pharmacy director's management reports to hospital administration. Further, the director should have some system for evaluating the quality of clinical services provided by his staff.

Drug Information Services. The term drug information service encompasses those activities involved with accumulating, organizing, retrieving and evaluating drug information. By broader definition, the ability to provide close and continuing support to the information user, thereby increasing his potential for efficiency and effectiveness, is also implied. Such a service must offer critical analyses of information of drugs so that clinicians have available essential information necessary to reach informed and intelligent conclusions concerning a particular problem in drug therapy. Further, a responsibility for active participation in drug utilization review and control is implied.

The functions involved in a drug information service are (1) establishing and maintaining a system for retrieving information from drug literature; (2) answering requests for comprehensive drug information compilations or bibliographies for inservice education programs, poison control in information centers, clinical drug investigations, pharmacy research projects and other pharmacy functions; (3) producing and distributing periodic compilations such as bulletins for physicians, nurses and pharmacists; (4) providing informational support to the hospital's Pharmacy and Therapeutics Committee; and (5) evaluating the detailing activities by drug vendors.

The drug information function interrelates with the teaching function by providing the content for teaching programs and with the other pharmacy functions by providing bibliographies, literature searches and background papers.

Where shared drug information services on a regional or city-wide basis are available, the required facilities and resources within a given hospital may be modified considerably, as long as the ability of the pharmacy to respond to drug information requests is not seriously impaired.

The philosophy and basic concepts put forth in the ASHP document, The Hospital Pharmacist and Drug Information Services,[8] will serve as guides in evaluating the drug information service.

II-D. As director of the residency program, the pharmacy director must have a wide latitude of freedom to coordinate and integrate the service and training functions, both intradepartmentally and interdepartmentally. This is only possible if he has total responsibility and authority as a department head to manage the department and coordinate its services and functions with the other departments in the hospital.

II-E. The ASHP Statement on the Pharmacy and Therapeutics Committee[9] states that the pharmacist (pharmacy director) is generally designated secretary of this committee. As the one individual ultimately responsible for total drug-use control in the hospital, as manager of all drug-related resources in the institution, and as the administrative head of the department best qualified to provide drug information and consultation as required, the pharmacy director logically earns his roles as a member of, and secretary to, the pharmacy and therapeutics committee.

The pharmacy director has the option of designating another pharmacist on his staff to represent him as a member of, and secretary to, the pharmacy and therapeutics committee. This designee is usually a pharmacist with special training or qualifications in the area of drug information and clinical practice.

Standard III—Qualifications of the Residency Director

A. The director of the hospital pharmacy shall be the overall director of the residency training program and shall be subject to similar general administrative control and guidance employed by the hospital for medical, dental, dietetic and other similar training programs.

B. The residency director shall have completed a pharmacy residency in a hospital accredited by the American Society of Hospital Pharmacists and have had two years of administrative experience in a hospital pharmacy, or have had at least five years experience in a pharmacy meeting the requirements of the Minimum Standard for Pharmacies in Institutions, a significant part of which experience should have been of an administrative nature.

C. The residency director shall have demonstrated superior capabilities in the operation of a pharmacy service and made significant contributions to the development or improvement of hospital pharmacy practice.

D. The residency director shall be an active member of the American Society of Hospital Pharmacists and the state affiliated chapter of the Society. All other pharmacists on the staff should also hold active membership in these organizations.

E. The residency director shall have considerable latitude in delegating preceptorial responsibilities for the residency program to others on his staff. Each individual designated as a preceptor must have demonstrated outstanding strengths in one or more areas of pharmacy practice. The residency director, however, is ultimately accountable for the overall quality of the residency training program.

Interpretation

III-A. Pharmacy residency training programs conforming to the Accreditation Standard for Pharmacy Residency in a Hospital are designed to train institutional pharmacy practitioners who are competent to provide a wide range of professional services and to provide administrative support and direction to others. The only appropriate director of such a program, therefore, is the director of the pharmacy department in which the residency is based. It is he who sets the tone of the program, and he does so by the personal philosophy he professes, by what he stands for, by the contributions he makes to his profession, and by his sense of values.

Since pharmacy residency programs conforming to the Accreditation Standard are hospital-based programs (as opposed to programs academically based in a college of pharmacy), they are subject to administrative control by the hospital.

III-B. Administrative experience is interpreted to mean experience as a department head (pharmacy director), or as an assistant department head with responsibilities largely commensurate with those of the pharmacy director. Experience as supervisor of a professional service section or division (e.g., parenteral admixture service, inpatient drug distribution service) is not acceptable as administrative experience for purposes of meeting this requirement.

In place of having completed an accredited an accredited pharmacy residency, five years of hospital pharmacy experience is required, three years of which must meet the definition of acceptable administrative experience given above.

III-C. Besides possessing the attributes of a residency director stated in the interpretation for section III-A, and in addition to having demonstrated his administrative capabilities as interpreted in section III-B, the residency director must also have demonstrated professional competence through publications, attendance at and participation in continuing education programs, and involvement in interprofessional programs in the hospital.

III-D. As a professional person, the residency director has an obligation to his profession, as well as to himself, to support his professional organizations. As director of the residency program he has a special opportunity to set an example for the resident through membership in, and active leadership participation in, professional organizations at all levels.

Standard IV—Qualifications and Selection of the Applicant

A. The applicant should be a graduate of a school of pharmacy accredited by the American Council on Pharmaceutical Education.

B. The applicant should be recommended by his college faculty and/or previous employers.

C. The resident should be a member of the American Society of Hospital Pharmacists.

D. Final approval of the qualifications of the applicant and his acceptance shall be the responsibility of the residency director.

Interpretation

IV-A. It is permissible to admit foreign graduates of schools not accredited by the American Council on Pharmaceutical Education to accredited residency programs, if other qualified residents are concurrently in training.

IV-B. It is advisable also to conduct a personal interview with each qualified applicant before making final decisions.

IV-C. As a professional person, the resident has an obligation to his profession and himself to support his professional organizations. Membership and active participation in professional organizations not only demonstrate a favorable attitude toward his profession, but are most effective in broadening his professional horizons by fostering a better understanding of the role of the profession in society and the profession's obligations to the public it serves.

IV-D. Since residents become, in effect, members of the pharmacy department's staff, the director of the pharmacy department must have authority to accept or reject any applicant. To do otherwise is to usurp his authority as a department head.

Standard V—Residency Training Program

A. Objectives for the residency program shall be in writing and shall be provided to each resident at the beginning of his program. The objectives shall relate both to the administrative and professional practice skills required in contemporary good practice and shall describe the terminal competencies to be striven for in the residency program. Objectives for training in each of the following areas shall be included:

1. Departmental administration;
2. Ambulatory patient services;
3. Inpatient drug distribution and control;
4. Technology and quality control activities;
5. Clinical services;
6. Drug information services;
7. Collateral and interdepartmental activities; and
8. Continuing education.

B. Each resident's activities shall be scheduled in advance and shall be planned to make possible the attainment of the predetermined objectives. The training schedule shall consist of a minimum of 2000 hours of training (contact) time, extending over a period of 50 weeks or longer.

C. Each resident shall maintain a record of his training activities which clearly delineates the scope and period of training. The residency director shall keep such records on file for review by the Society's accreditation survey team.

D. Provision shall be made for formalized and regularly scheduled evaluation of the resident's achievement in terms of the objectives previously established.

Interpretation

V-A. The specific training activities and experiences in which the resident will participate under each of the eight training areas listed are subject to considerable variation because of the difference existing between hospitals, between training programs, between residency directors and between residents. Furthermore, there are no clear lines of distinction between the eight major training areas in regard to the discrete activities which each encompasses. For the purpose of this Accreditation Standard, however, each of these areas is taken to include the specific training activities outlined below. The residency director should use these lists of activities as guidelines in developing training objectives for his program. The objectives should specify the attitudes, skills and knowledge the resident should be expected to gain from each activity. These objectives then serve as guides for the residency director and other persons responsible for the resident's training in developing and supervising training experiences and in evaluating achievement.

Since the Accreditation Standard stresses outcomes more than the process by which those outcomes are achieved, the residency director should make every effort to assess the entering resident's baseline knowledge and skills in each of the eight major areas of training, thereby identifying the resident's proper entry level in each area and avoiding unnecessary repetition of training which he has previously received.

Once the residency director has satisfied himself that a resident has achieved a predetermined minimum level of competence in each of these areas, he may arrange for that resident to concentrate, during the time remaining in his program, on either administrative affairs or professional practice. This does not provide, however, for a major emphasis in one narrow or specialized practice area. If an area of emphasis is to be pursued, an understanding on this point should be agreed upon in advance by the residency director and the resident, and the predetermined objectives for training should identify the additional competencies to be achieved in the area of emphasis, above and beyond that expected of another resident whose program does not concentrate on that area.

Departmental Administration. The objectives for the resident's training in departmental administration are to orient him, not only to the functions and concepts of depaprtmental management, but also to the department head's philosophy of total pharmacy service and to increase his knowledge, refine his skills, mold his attitudes, and develop his problem-solving abilities relating to personnel management, organizational management, communications and management of all drug-related resources. He must learn to make judgments, set priorities, and assume responsibilities. The director of pharmacy department must serve as the principal preceptor in this area of training.

The resident should receive orientation, instruction and experience leading to competence in, but not restricted to, the following specific areas and activities.

1. Organization of hospital and pharmacy department;
2. Administrative policies;
3. Professional policies;
4. Development and maintenance of policy and procedure manual;
5. Interdepartmental administrative activities;
6. Hospital staff meetings and administrative conferences;
7. Hospital committee (pharmacy and therapeutics committee, infections committee, etc.);
8. Departmental staff meeting;
9. Intra- and interdepartmental communications;
10. Local, state, and federal laws and regulations;
11. Personnel management;
12. Drug procurement and inventory control;
13. Accounting and bookkeeping procedures;
14. Departmental budgeting;
15. Contract services to subscribers;
16. Department records and reports;
17. Office procedures (filing, handling correspondence, etc.);
18. Professional organization participation;
19. Interdepartmental orientations;
20. Safety practices.
21. Space and facilities planning; and
22. Departmental quality assurance programs.

Ambulatory Patient Services. The objectives for training in this service area are to develop the resident's clinical skills in primary health care and maintenance care of patients. The objectives also include in-depth orientation of the resident in the functions of education, service and research associated with ambulatory patient services. Of least importance to the resident's needs are the mechanics of outpatient dispensing, and caution should be taken to assure that the resident's time spent in this activity is meaningful.

The resident should receive orientation, instruction and experience leading to competence in, but not restricted to, the following activities and areas.

1. Providing drug counseling and education to patients;
2. Providing drug information to the professional staffs;
3. Maintaining drug profile systems;
4. Taking medication histories;
5. Providing drug and toxicology information;
6. Providing emergency services;
7. Outpatient dispensing procedures;
8. Outpatient prescription pricing;
9. Extemporaneous compounding;
10. Outpatient pharmacy policies;
11. Local, state and federal laws and regulations;
12. Processing public assistance, Medicaid and other prepaid services; and
13. Records, reports, and budgets.

Inpatient Drug Distribution and Control. The objectives for the resident's training in inpatient drug distribution and control are to develop his abilities in all aspects of drug-use control in the hospital and to develop his philosophy about the responsibilities of the hospital pharmacists in providing optimum pharmaceutical care for patients.

The resident should receive orientation, instruction and experience leading to competence in, but not restricted to, the following areas and activities:

1. Inpatient pharmacy service policies and procedures;
2. Standards, laws and regulations;
3. Drug product selection and the formulary system;
4. Physicians' orders and their transmission;
5. Containers and labeling;
6. Drug profiles and patient records;
7. PRN, Stat, and emergency stocks;
8. Logistics of drug distribution;
9. Medication administration;
10. Drug samples;
11. "Bring-in" medications;
12. Investigational drugs;
13. "After-hours" service;
14. Adverse drug reaction reporting;
15. Medication error reporting;
16. Hospital committees concerned with drug control;
17. Electronic data processing applications;
18. Drug recalls;
19. Patient charges and drug pricing;
20. Parenteral admixture and total parenteral nutrition services;
21. Space and facilities planning;
22. Discharge medications handling; and
23. Patient self-medication programs.

Technology and Quality Control Activities. The major objectives for the resident's training in this area are to enable him to procure or produce good quality pharmaceutical products for use in the hospital to protect the quality of these products until they are consumed, and to protect against the patient's receiving a mislabeled, misbranded or adulterated drug. This area of training, then, will develop or reinforce the resident's understanding of the physical, chemical and compounding principles which influence dosage forms and govern their selection; factors affecting drug product stability; and systems used to minimize compounding, packaging and labeling errors.

Note: The pharmacist's undergraduate training in such areas as physical pharmacy, technology, and biopharmaceutics may go a long way toward achieving those objectives stated above, and it may not be necessary to dwell on these activities to achieve the desired competencies. The residency director should not overlook the need, however, to assess the resident's latent knowledge and skills in these areas and to schedule training activities as appropriate to complement the resident's baseline abilities. The director should give special attention to the resident's ability to compound prescriptions for intravenous administration and other dosage forms requiring aseptic technique.

The resident should receive orientation, instruction and experience leading to competence in, but not limited to, the following activities and areas;

1. Product formulation principles and theory;
2. Product procurement specifications;
3. Good manufacturing practices;
4. Use and operation of compounding, packaging and labeling equipment;
5. Packaging and labeling;
6. Storage and stability considerations;
7. Quality control procedures;
8. Records and reports;

and in the following activities and areas relating specifically to sterile products:

9. Principles and methods of sterilization;
10. Aseptic techniques and procedures;
11. Use and limitations of the laminar air flow hood;
12. Formulation, production and control of intravenous and irrigating fluids;
13. Preparation and control of parenteral admixture and total parenteral nutrition fluids;
14. Preparation of sterile ophthalmic products;
15. Distilled water production and pyrogen testing and control;
16. Storage problems for sterile products;
17. Tonicity and *p*H adjustments and control;
18. Commercial i.v. administration systems;
19. Sterile syringe packaging;
20. Reconstitution of injectables;
21. Sterility testing;
22. Records and reports;
23. Standards, laws and regulations; and
24. Space, equipment and facilities planning.

Clinical Services. The objectives for training in clinical services are to strengthen and reinforce the resident's clinical and therapeutic knowledge and to develop his abilities in the clinical application of drugs in patient care. Central to this area of the resident's training is the evaluation of drug therapy problems in relation to the special needs of individual patients.

The resident should receive orientation, instruction and experience leading to competence in, but not limited to, the following areas and activities:

1. Patient medication histories;
2. Monitoring drug therapy;
3. Patient counseling and education;
4. Participation in management of medical emergencies;
5. Drug therapy consultations;
6. Participation in management of the chronically ill;
7. Clinical research;

8. Adverse drug reaction reporting;
9. Routine consultation with nursing service personnel on drug use and administration;
10. Drug utilization review (DUR) and patient care audit activities; and
11. Interdisciplinary educational activities.

Drug Information Services. The objectives of training in this activity are to improve the resident's skills in assimilating and disseminating drug information, and to prepare him to manage a drug information service program.

The resident should receive orientation, instruction and experience leading to competence in, but not limited to, the following areas and activities:

1. Organization, philosophy and procedures;
2. Capabilities and limitations of the service;
3. Economic considerations in initiating and maintaining the service;
4. Operational problems encountered in operating the service;
5. Criteria for selection of reference material;
6. Operation of communication and retrieval systems;
7. Utilization of specific professional consultants;
8. Taking the request for specific information;
9. Procedures for answering a request efficiently (how to collect and analyze data);
10. Utilization of the medical library and other informational sources (e.g., manufacturers, faculty personnel, public agencies, governmental agencies);
11. Preparation of oral and written reports regarding requests for information;
12. Poison control procedures;
13. Preparation of clinical follow-up reports;
14. Methods of analyzing the effectiveness of the service;
15. Foreign drug information services;
16. Preparation of drug evaluations for the P & T committee;
17. Instruction of interns and other students in procedures of the service;
18. Preparation of newsletter;
19. Preparation and/or revision of hospital formulary;
20. Investigational drug programs;
21. Adverse reaction reporting programs; and
22. Conducting inservice and/or continuing education programs.

Collateral and Interdepartmental Activities. The objectives for training in these activities are to involve the resident in in-depth professional experience intended to familiarize him with the external professional environment; to motivate him to participate independently in activities which will broaden his professional horizons; and to stimulate him to develop a personal philosophy of, and commitment to, his professional role and responsibilities.

The resident should receive orientation, instruction and experience leading to competence in, but not limited to, the following areas and activities:

1. Observation of the procedures and operation of departments of pharmacy in other hospitals;
2. Observation of other departments within the hospital through a planned program of rotation;
3. Observation of the functions of the pharmacy and therapeutics committee and participation in its activities through service as its acting secretary for a meeting if possible;
4. Participation in the teaching of pharmaceutical and therapeutic subjects

to interdisciplinary groups such as pharmacy technicians, nurses, nursing
students, dieticians, inhalation therapists and members of the house staff;

5. Investigation of some particular pharmacy problem should be completed
   as one of the requirements for the residency.

Continuing Education. The objectives of training in this area are to instill in
the resident the attitude that it is his responsibility as a professional person to
maintain his competnce through a planned program of self-education and continuing education. An important corollary objective is to develop the resident's
communications skills and his skill as a teacher.

The resident's training in this area should include, but not be limited to, the
following:

1. Lecture and conference or case study topics presented to and with the
   residents by the residency director and other preceptors whom he designates;
2. Review on a continual basis of current and past literature related to
   hospital pharmacy practice;
3. Review of principles of education (learning objectives, lesson plans, evaluation instruments, etc.);
4. Formal presentation of information to various groups of learners (e.g., at
   staff development programs, medical grand rounds, or to various groups
   of undergraduate students—pharmacy, nursing, medical, respiratory therapy);
5. Conferences with residency director on a weekly basis for discussion and
   counsel (if more than one resident in program, a weekly group conference
   between the residency director and residents);
6. Attendence at and participation in seminars and continuing education
   programs on a local, state, regional and national basis as much as possible;
   and
7. Development of a personal philosophy and strategy for life-long continuing education.

V-B. The minimum total training hours and training period may be exceeded
without limit, but they may not be reduced.

It is important that a schedule of activities for the residency training program
be planned in advance of the resident's arrival. The schedule should be written
in sufficient detail to give the resident a clear understanding of each assignment
and activity. The schedule must reflect the predetermined learning objectives
and make possible their achievement. In fact, it may be desirable to integrate
the learning objectives and the training schedule into one syllabus.

It is recognized that detail planning of time schedules in advance is at best
difficult, and frequently almost impossible. The important aspect of this element of the Standard is not the existence of a detailed time (clock or calendar)
schedule but, rather, that careful and conscientious planning has gone into the
development of the residency training program in advance of its initiation. The
schedule may be thought of as the planning tool by which the objectives are
achieved, and which aids in insuring that no objective is overlooked.

V-C. It is important that the resident maintain sufficient documentation of
his training activities so that the residency director and other preceptor(s) can
monitor his progress. Documentation for any given period of time (one month,
for example) should relate to the predetermined learning objectives for that
period. Such records can thus serve as a basis for evaluation of the resident by
his preceptors and for periodic self-evaluation by the resident himself.

V-D. The periodic evaluation must relate to the resident's progress in achieving the pre-set learning objectives, and *not* be based solely on personality traits and other similar subjective criteria. When deficiencies are noted, appropriate remedial action must be taken. A written record of the periodic evaluation must be maintained and must be reviewed with the resident.

Standard VI—Certification

A. An appropriate certificate indicative of successful completion of the prescribed residency shall be awarded to the resident by the hospital.

Interpretation

VI-A. Certification of completion of the pharmacy residency training program is the responsibility of the hospital. The American Society of Hospital Pharmacists certifies the hospital (residency program) only—not the resident.

REFERENCES

1. ASHP statement on accreditation of pharmacy residencies in hospitals with policies and procedures. Am. J. Hosp. Pharm., *36*:72–74, Jan. 1979.
2. Accreditation manual for hospitals 1978, Joint Commission on Accreditation of Hospitals, 645 North Michigan Avenue, Chicago, IL 60611.
3. Accreditation requirements of American Osteopathic Association, Feb. 1976, American Osteopathic Association, 212 East Ohio Street, Chicago, IL 60611.
4. ASHP minimum standard for pharmacies in institutions. Am. J. Hosp. Pharm., *34*:1356–1358, Dec. 1977.
5. ASHP statement on hospital drug control systems. Am. J. Hosp. Pharm., *31*:1198–1207, Dec. 1974.
6. ASHP statement on pharmacist-conducted patient counseling. Am. J. Hosp. Pharm., *33*:644–645, Jul. 1976.
7. ASHP statement on clinical functions in institutional pharmacy practice. Am. J. Hosp. Pharm., *35*:813, Jul. 1978.
8. ASHP statement on the hospital pharmacist and drug information services. Am. J. Hosp. Pharm., *25*:381–382, Jul. 1968.
9. ASHP statement on the pharmacy and therapeutics committee. Am. J. Hosp. Pharm., *35*:813–814, Jul. 1978.

Having established a pharmacy residency program in the hospital, it is desirable to have the program accredited. The American Society of Hospital Pharmacists maintains an accreditation program for this purpose. In March, 1980, the ASHP issued a revised *Statement on Accreditation of Pharmacy Residencies in Hospitals.* Because of its value to the practitioner in determining the quality of his educational program, it is hereinafter reproduced.[13]

ASHP STATEMENT ON ACCREDITATION OF PHARMACY RESIDENCIES IN HOSPITALS[a] (WITH POLICIES AND PROCEDURES)

Preamble

Hospital pharmacists have from the beginning of their formal association recognized the need for perpetuating and improving their specialty through organized training programs. Early in its history the American Society of Hospital Pharmacists supported the development of training programs in hospital pharmacy and promulgated standards for residency in hospital pharmacy. To insure adherence to the principles and philosophy of these standards, an accreditation program is established by the Society.

Objectives

The accreditation program shall have as its objectives: (1) to improve the professional competence of hospital pharmacy practitioners through organized educational training programs; (2) to guide, assist and recognize those hospitals that wish to support the profession by operating such programs; (3) to provide criteria for the prospective resident in the selection of a program by identifying those hospitals conducting accredited residency programs; (4) to provide hospitals and related health agencies a basis for determining the level of competency of pharmacists in hospitals by identifying those pharmacists who have successfully completed accredited residency programs.

Definition

For the purpose of accreditation, a pharmacy residency in a hospital is defined as a postgraduate program of organized training that meets the requirements set forth and approved by the American Society of Hospital Pharmacists in the Accreditation Standard for Pharmacy Residency in a Hospital with Guide to Interpretation.

Authority

The program for accreditation of pharmacy residency programs in hospitals is established by authority of the Board of Directors of the American Society of Hospital Pharmacists under the direction of the Commission on Credentialing. All matters of policy relating to the accreditation program considered by the Commission on Credentialing will be submitted for approval to the Board of Directors of the Society. The Commission on Credentialing shall review and evaluate applications and survey reports submitted, and shall be specifically delegated by the Board of Directors to take final action on all applications for accreditation, in accordance with the policies and procedures set forth herein. The minutes of all transactions of the Commission on Credentialing shall be submitted to the Board of Directors for its review.

---

[a]Approved by the ASHP Board of Directors November 8, 1962; revised April 11, 1970, November 19, 1973, November 16, 1977, and March 20, 1980.

Policies

The following policies shall apply to the accreditation program:

1. *Initial Evaluation of Residency Programs*
   a. The accreditation program shall be conducted as a service of the American Society of Hospital Pharmacists to any hospital or other organized health care setting (hereafter referred to as the institution) voluntarily requesting evaluation of its program.
   b. To be eligible for accreditation, a program must have been in operation for one year and have at least one graduate. (If accreditation is granted, it shall be retroactive to the date on which a valid and complete application, including all requested supporting documents, is received by the Society's Director of Accreditation Services.)
   c. Program evaluation shall be by site survey for which an appropriate fee, established by the Board of Directors, shall be assessed to the institution.
   d. Programs shall be reviewed by an accreditation survey team consisting of at least two individuals, one of whom shall be the Society's Director of Accreditation Services or his designee. The other may be a member of the Commission on Credentialing or an individual designated by the Director of Accreditation Services, who is not from the same geographic area as the hospital being surveyed, and who has no conflict of interest with respect to the institution.
2. *Certificate of Accreditation*
   a. A certificate of accreditation will be issued for a period not to exceed six years; however, the certificate remains the property of the American Society of Hospital Pharmacists and shall be returned to the Society at any time accreditation is withdrawn.
   b. Any reference by an institution to accreditation by the Society in certificates, catalogues, bulletins, communications or other form of publicity shall state only the following: "(Name of Institution) is accredited for pharmacy residency in (a category) by the American Society of Hospital Pharmacists."
3. *Continuing Evaluation of Accredited Programs*
   a. The Society regards evaluation of accredited residency programs as a continuous process; accordingly, the Commission on Credentialing shall request directors of accredited programs to submit periodic written status reports to assist the Commission in evaluating the continued conformance of individual programs to the Accreditation Standard, Written reports shall be required from program directors at least every two years.
   b. Accredited programs shall be reexamined by site visit at least every six years.
   c. Any major change in the organization of a program will be considered justificaiton for reevaluation.
   d. A survey fee, as established by the ASHP Board of Directors, shall be assessed to the institution for reaccreditation site visits.
4. *Withdrawal of Accreditation*
   a. Accreditation of a pharmacy residency program may be withdrawn by the Society for any of the reasons stated below
      (1) Accredited programs which no longer meet the requirements of the Accreditation Standard under which they were approved shall have accreditation withdrawn.

(2) Accredited programs without a resident in training for a period of three consecutive years shall have accreditation withdrawn.

(3) Accreditation shall be withdrawn if the director of an accredited program is replaced by another individual whose qualifications do not meet the requirements of the Accreditation Standard.

b. The institution shall submit a new application and undergo reevaluation to regain accreditation.

c. Accreditation shall not be withdrawn without first notifying the institution of the specific reasons why its program does not meet the requirements of the Accreditation Standard. In such instances, the institution shall be granted an appropriate specific period of time to correct deficiencies.

d. The institution shall have the right to appeal the decision of the Commission on Credentialing.

Accreditation Procedures

1. *Application for Accreditation*
   a. Application forms may be requested from: American Society of Hospital Pharmacists, Director of Accreditation Services, 4630 Montgomery Avenue, Washington, DC 20014. These should be filled out in duplicate. One copy of the application should be signed by the administrator and the director of pharmacy of the insitution and submitted, along with the supporting documents specified in the application instructions, to the Society's Director of Accreditation Services. The duplicate copy should be retained for the applicant's files.
   b. The Director of Accreditation Services will acknowledge receipt of the application and review it to make a preliminary judgment about the applicant's conformance to the basic requirements of the Accreditation Standard. If the Director feels that the program fails to meet the criteria of the Accreditation Standard in some fundamental way, he will notify the signatories of the application accordingly and advise against scheduling a site visit until the problems have been corrected. The applicant is not bound, however, to accept the Director's advice to delay the accreditation site visit.

2. *The Site Visit*
   a. At a mutually convenient time, the Society will send a survey team to review the pharmacy service and the residency program. Instructions for preparation for the site visit (list of documents to be made available to the survey team, suggested itinerary for the surveyors, etc.) will be sent to the director of pharmacy service well in advance. Normally, the site visit is conducted in two working days.
   b. After concluding its on-site evaluation, the survey team will present a verbal report of its findings to the institution administrator and director of pharmacy.

3. *The Survey Report*
   a. Following the site visit, the survey team will prepare a written report which will be sent to the institution administrator and the director of pharmacy service for review of factual accuracy and comment. Any written comments which either wishes to make must be submitted to the Director of Accreditation Services within 30 days after receipt of the report. Any comment respecting the factual accuracy of the report must set forth specifically the facts contested, the reasons therefor, and the institution's contentions with respect to the facts.

   b. The institution's residency accreditation application file, including the surveyor's report, plus any written comments received from the institution will be reviewed by the Commission at its next meeting. The Commission will resolve any factual issues at that time.

   c. Notice of action taken by the Commission will be sent to the institution administrator and director of pharmacy, along with a list of any deficiencies which the Commission considered in arriving at its decision and recommendations for overcoming those deficiencies. The report will indicate that the Commission has acted either (1) to accredit or reaccredit the program for a period not to exceed six years, or (2) to withhold or withdraw accreditation.

4. *Appeal from Commission Decision*

   a. *Notification of Intent to Appeal.* In the event the Commission shall fail to fully accredit or reaccredit a program, the institution administrator may appeal the decision of the Commission to an Appeal Board on the grounds that the decision of the Commission was arbitrary, prejudiced, biased, capricious, or incorrect application of the standards to the institution. The institution administrator must notify the Director of Accreditation Services, in writing by registered or certified mail, within 10 days after receipt of the Commission's decision, of the institution's intent to appeal. The institution administrator must state clearly on what grounds the appeal is being made. The institution shall then have an additional 30 days in which to prepare for its presentation to an Appeal Board.

   b. *Appeal Board.* Upon receipt of an appeal notice, the Director of Accreditation Services shall proceed to constitute an ad hoc Appeal Board. The Appeal Board shall consist of one member of the Society's Board of Directors, to be appointed by the President of the American Society of Hospital Pharmacists, and who shall serve as Chairman; and two preceptors of accredited pharmacy residency programs, neither of whom are members of the Commission on Credentialing, one to be named by the appellant and one by the Chairman of the Commission. The Director of Accreditation Services shall serve as Secretary of the Appeal Board. As soon as appointments to the Appeal Board shall have been made, the Director of Accreditation Services shall forward immediately to all Appeal Board members copies of all written documentation considered by the Commission in rendering its decision.

   c. *The Hearing.* The Appeal Board shall have convened in not less than 30 days nor more than 60 days from the date of receipt by the Director of Accreditation Services of an appeal notice. The Director of Accreditation Services shall notify appellants and Appeal Board members, at least 30 days in advance, of the date, time and place of the hearing. The institution filing the appeal may be represented at the hearing by one or more appropriate officials and shall be given the opportunity at such hearing to present written or written and oral evidence and argument tending to refute or overcome the findings and decision of the Commission on Credentialing. The Director of Accreditation Services shall represent the Commission at the hearing.

   The Appeal Board shall advise the appellant institution of the Board's decision, in writing by registered or certified mail, within 10 days of the date of the hearing. The decision of the Appeal Board shall be final and binding on both the appellant and the American Society of Hospital Pharmacists.

    d. *Appeal Board Expenses.* The appellant shall be responsible for all expenses incurred by its own representatives at the Appeal Board hearing, and shall pay all reasonable travel, living and incidental expenses incurred by its appointee to the Appeal Board. Expenses incurred by the other Board members and the Director of Accreditation Services shall be borne by the American Society of Hospital Pharmacists.

Having established a sufficient background to permit the hospital pharmacist to assume a role in the teaching function of the hospital, it is necessary to dwell briefly upon the specific areas of internal and external teaching in which the hospital pharmacist may or should become involved.

INTERNAL TEACHING PROGRAMS

Training of Student Nurses

Much has been written concerning the role of the pharmacist in the teaching of student nurses. Some advocate that the hospital pharmacist should teach student nurses the entire course of pharmaceutical calculations and pharmacology; others propose that he undertake to teach certain aspects of these courses in conjunction with the nursing instructor.

How much or how little a hospital pharmacist teaches will depend upon the individual and the environment in which he operates. If the individual is capable and has so impressed the nurse educators by his daily actions and deeds, he will be invited, more likely than not, to assist in the teaching program. Once appointed to this responsibility, it behooves the hospital pharmacist to develop his phase of the program in strict compliance with the requirements set forth by the nursing accreditation authorities.

Furthermore, the prepared lectures should be updated each year—to include the latest developments in pharmacology and therapeutics; the nomenclature used and all references to weights and measures should be in accord with the hospital's drug formulary; and finally any reference to dosage, contraindications or cautions should also comply with the formulary unless the information to be presented supersedes the latest revision of the hospital formulary.

Many authors[4-6] have published special texts on the subject of pharmacology and therapeutics for nurses. These texts are in use in various schools of nursing and may serve as an excellent guide to the hospital pharmacist who undertakes the responsibility to teach these courses to student nurses.

In addition, hospital pharmacists should consult the various textbooks in pharmacology which are written for basic nursing students.

Failure to do this may result in the preparation of a course, so sophisticated in content, that it will defeat the purpose of its presentation.

Seminars for Graduate Nurses, House Staff and Medical Staff

Although most pharmacists disseminate information to the members of the medical and nursing staffs via a pharmacy publication, there is still need for the direct or personal presentation which is afforded by conducting a seminar on the latest available therapeutic agents to the medical staff.

With regard to such a program, Sperandio[7] has stated that:

"The key to its success would be proper organization and presentation of the material. Ideally, the talk should be short (not over twenty minutes), complete, and concise. The subject should be covered in such a way that the audience can integrate all the factors and thereby obtain an appreciation of the many facets of drug therapy. Time should be allowed for discussion."

Frazier *et al.*[8] functioning as the 1954 Committee on Minimum Standards of the American Society of Hospital Pharmacists developed an outline of four lectures which may be presented by the hospital pharmacist to the resident staff.

Lecture One of this series concerns itself with an orientation to pharmacy services and covers such subject matter as:

  a. Location of the pharmacy
  b. A description of the physical plant
  c. Personnel
  d. Hours of operation
  e. Services provided by the department
  f. Hospital policies governing:
     i. Formulary
     ii. Use of generic names
     iii. Use of the metric system
     iv. Use of abbreviations
     v. Use of research drugs
     vi. Automatic stop orders
     vii. Discharge medications
     viii. Ordering narcotics and liquors

Lecture Two of the series is devoted to the philosophy and goals of the formulary system. In the course of the lecture, the hospital pharmacist should emphasize the composition of and the scope of the Pharmacy and Therapeutics Committee.

Lecture Three is suggested to take the form of a prescription clinic. Basically, this is an excellent suggestion and is highly recommended in view of the fact that very little attention is devoted to prescription writing in medical school classes. In the course of the lecture, the pharmacist should stress any Federal, state and hospital regulations governing the prescribing of drugs and the refilling of prescriptions. Past experience has also demonstrated that a short period of time devoted to a group criticism of prescriptions (projected onto a screen) which contain illegible writing, non-standard abbreviations, misplaced decimal points, misspelling of drug names and a mixture of English and Latin directions is extremely helpful in emphasizing the importance of accuracy in writing a prescription.

Lecture Four is reserved for a discussion of any topic of current interest to the staff. Suggested topics for this discussion include the following:

    i. Cost of medication
   ii. Incompatabilities of intravenous fluids
       and other injectable drugs
  iii. The new drug regulations
   iv. Drug interactions

Graduate nurses are encouraged to attend all in-service training programs offered within the hospital. These sessions are devoted to a wide spectrum of professional subjects. The hospital pharmacist should avail himself of the opportunity to present a few of the programs. His subject matter may consist of a discussion of new classes of therapeutic agents, incompatibilities of various drugs when added to intravenous solutions, drug storage and control, a review of the mathematics of pharmacy, or drug interactions.

Whatever the subject matter, it behooves the pharmacist to prepare the lecture adequately and where possible supplement the talk with slides, a short film, the distribution of an outline of the lecture, or the distribution of reprints or selected brochures describing the drugs lectured upon.

In addition, whenever new drugs are discussed, one should bring into the lecture room sample containers of the various forms which are commercially available. It is assumed that by actually handling, observing, smelling and where possible tasting the product, the nurse will be in a better position to detect an error should a mix-up in medication occur.

Training Undergraduate Students in Hospital Pharmacy

Blauch and Webster,[9] in The Pharmaceutical Curriculum, published in 1952 by the American Council on Education as a report for the Committee on Curriculum of the American Association of Colleges of Pharmacy, state:

"It is a source of considerable surprise to note that only a few colleges of pharmacy have developed working arrangements with hospitals for teaching purposes. One finds colleges of pharmacy in universities which have also large teaching hospitals but in which the colleges have no connection whatever with the pharmaceutical service. No doubt this situation reflects the traditional educational emphasis on the retail pharmacy, which for a long time has been the principal means of pharmaceutical service. With the changes which are apparently impending in health service, the hospital pharmacy will almost certainly play an increasing role. Colleges of pharmacy may well note this fact and plan their instructions accordingly."

Since the publication of the above report, the American Association of Colleges of Pharmacy and the American Society of Hospital Pharmacists have approved a **Statement on the Abilities Required of Hospital Pharmacists.**[10] This statement lists six specialized areas of competence that should be considered in developing a curriculum for hospital pharmacy. These are as follows:

Specfically the well-qualified hospital pharmacist must have:

1. A thorough knowledge of drugs and their actions.
2. Ability to develop and conduct a pharmaceutical manufacturing program.
3. An intimate knowledge of control procedures.
4. Ability to conduct and participate in research.
5. Ability to conduct teaching and in-service training programs.
6. Ability to administer and manage a hospital pharmacy.

Therefore the Joint Committee of the American Association of Colleges of Pharmacy and the American Society of Hospital Pharmacists prepared, in January 1966, a **Syllabus for a Course in Hospital Pharmacy** and, in April 1966, these same organizations approved a **Suggested Guide to Curriculum Development for Hospital Pharmacy.**

With these tools in hand, the hospital pharmacist should take the initiative and meet with the college administration and faculty for the purpose of commencing a program in hospital pharmacy. At this meeting, the hospital pharmacist should point out the fact that his department offers the prospective student a wealth of experience in the professional practice of his profession.

Patient Teaching Program

In one study[15] patient's knowledge of their prescribed drug regimen was assessed in 78 patients randomly chosen and interviewed at home within 6 to 9 days after hospital discharge. The study included the following areas: (1) name and purpose of the medication; (2) precautions to consider while taking the medication; and (3) other medications, foods, and beverages to avoid. The study concluded that considerable lack of knowledge about prescription medication was apparent in view of the fact that 52% could not determine length of drug regimen, 23% were not aware of why medication had been prescribed for them,

56% did not know the name of the medication and 56% were not given instructions on how to administer the medication.

This is one area of in-hospital teaching where the pharmacist can make a valuable contribution to the long term posthospital care of the patient. More frequently than not, patients leave the hospital with a variety of discharge medications with a meager knowledge of how they are to be used or, more importantly, how to recognize signs of toxicity or adverse reaction. This brief exposure to the medications is generally provided by the busy practitioner or a nurse.

Of late, those hospitals who have recruited clinical pharmacists to their staffs have developed extensive programs for the orientation of the patient to the subject of drug use both in the hospital and in the patient's home. These programs have consisted of patient counseling, development of instructional brochures, group conferences and closed circuit television presentations. Where the instruction needs to be individualized—as in the use of an individual's specific medication—the direct counseling technique is employed. However, where instruction of a general nature is to be given—such as how to detect adverse drug effects—the group discussion or television methodology is employed.

Training Clinical Pharmacists

With the development of this specialty within the profession of pharmacy, hospital pharmacists should work closely with the college of pharmacy and the college of medicine faculties as well as the various medical staff specialists in the conduct of such programs. Insofar as the clinical pharmacy programs are concerned, many schools have created specialization within the broad area of clinical pharmacy—pediatrics, clinical pharmacology, toxicology, drug information analysis and interpretation, infectious disease and geriatrics.

The hospital pharmacist, if he himself is unable to provide the training, should arrange to have the student acquainted with the contents of the medical record, drug history procedures, patient drug profile program, drug information center, poison control center, adverse drug reaction program and the opportunity to interface with interdisciplinary health care personnel such as physicians, dentists, nurses, dietitians and therapists. Of paramount importance, is the pharmacist's exposure to the patient—both ambulatory and hospitalized. Thus, the training of clinical pharmacists need not be limited to the hospital proper but may include the satellite health care centers, nursing homes, extended care facilities, home care programs and clinics.

The importance of clinical pharmacy to the institution is supported by the following joint statement.[16]

ASHP AND AHA STATEMENT ON CLINICAL PHARMACY AND ITS RELATIONSHIP TO THE INSTITUTION[a]

In 1957, the American Hospital Association and the American Society of Hospital Pharmacists called for greater involvement by hospital pharmacists in the control of drugs in the institutional setting by voting:

To urge hospital pharmacists, through appropriate channels, to extend their responsibilities to include participation in programs dealing with the safe handling of drugs throughout the hospital.

Since then, traditional patterns for the delivery of pharmaceutical services have given way to new concepts. These new concepts have resulted in greater involvement by the pharmacist in the institution's patient-care areas and the recognition of a need for a clinical component to pharmaceutical services and drug control in the institution. *This clinical service component* recognizes the need for pharmacy students to be patient-oriented as well as product-oriented.

In 1975, the Study Commission on Pharmacy recognized that:

. . . among deficiencies in the health care system, one is the unavailability of adequate information for those who consume, prescribe, dispense and administer drugs. This deficiency has resulted in inappropriate drug use and an unacceptable frequency of drug-induced disease. Pharmacists are seen as health professionals who could make an important contribution to the health care system of the future by providing information about drugs to consumers and health professionals. Education and training of pharmacists now and in the future must be developed to meet these important responsibilities.

Schools of pharmacy recognize the need for a clinical component in the professional curriculum for future practitioners and are establishing viable working relationships with organized health care settings as clinical facilities for the training of students. Accrediting bodies, governmental agencies, and professional associations also are fostering role reconstruction in pharmacy which requires proper environments for the education and training of both degree-seeking and non-degree-seeking individuals.

In recognizing the concept of clinical pharmacy and its value in optimizing drug therapy in the institutional setting, and in keeping with the spirit of the AHA "Statement on Role and Responsibilities of

---

[a]This document was approved by the ASHP Board of Directors at its July 30–31, 1979, meeting, and by the ASHP House of Delegates on April 21, 1980. Approval by the American Hospital Association is required to make this an official document of the two organizations. An earlier version was approved by the ASHP Board of Directors at its March 13–14, 1970, meeting, and by the AHA General Council at its meeting of October 7–9, 1970.

the Hospital in Providing Clinical Facilities for a Collaborative Educational Program in the Health Field," the American Hospital Association and the American Society of Hospital Pharmacists encourage hospitals to (1) support the concept of clinical pharmacy as an integral component of comprehensive pharmaceutical services and drug control; and (2) make their facilities available to schools of pharmacy for clinical preparation of future pharmacy practitioners.

A program of clinical education and training requires close collaboration between a clinical institution and a college or school of pharmacy. In recognition of this, the American Association of Colleges of Pharmacy and the ASHP have developed the following agreement which can serve as the basis for negotiations:

NABP MODEL CLINICAL PHARMACY EDUCATION AND TRAINING AGREEMENT[a]

WHEREAS, the (Pharmacy school name), hereinafter referred to as (short school name), located at (address), (city), (state, zip) has established, as part of the requirements leading to a degree in pharmacy, a program of clinical education and training, which requires clinical facilities, equipment, services and personnel appropriate for students to obtain the necessary clinical experience; and

WHEREAS, (institution name), (description: hospital, nursing home, community pharmacy, etc.) hereinafter referred to as (short institution name), located at (address), (city), (state, zip) has the required facilities, equipment, personnel and services to provide this clinical experience.

NOW, THEREFORE, it is agreed by and between (short school name) and (short institution name) that:

I.   The (short school name) shall appoint representatives and (short institution name) shall appoint the Director of the (short institution name) Department of Pharmaceutical Services and/or a designee(s) (which may include member(s) of the health care team) to jointly plan for:
   (1) Student placement and orientation in the (short institution name).
   (2) Periodic review and preparation of objectives for the instructional program.
   (3) Evaluation of student performance.
   (4) Periodic review of program costs and payments. It is specifically agreed that neither party shall be responsible for costs or expenditures incurred by the other in the conduct of the clinical education and training program, other than those expenses defined in any sep-

---

[a]Approved by the ASHP Board of Directors (January 1979) and the AACP Board of Directors (March 1979). This agreement is *not* intended to be used in its present form. It is a model to be used as a guide by pharmacy schools and institutions and should be retyped to meet specific needs. The designation of the "Dean" and the "Director of Pharmaceutical Services" as the signing parties means that appropriately responsible persons are deemed necessary.

arate agreements that may be made between the (short school name) and (short institution name).

(5) Mutually acceptable criteria for faculty practitioners who have teaching responsibilities within the institution.

(6) (Additional clauses may be added to set forth further details of the agreement).

II. The (short school name) shall undertake the following:

(1) Appoint the Director of Pharmaceutical Services as a member of the clinical faculty of (short school name) and as the Director of the Clinical Pharmacy Education and Training Program at (short institution name), when deemed appropriate by the Dean and the Hospital Director.

(2) Provide information regarding dates for instruction, according to (short school name) calendar and forecasts of the number of students to be assigned to (short institution name).

(3) Arrange for the purchase of liability and malpractice insurance with coverage not less than ($) for each student and faculty member participating in the program or assure that such liability and malpractice coverage is provided by the University. Certificates indicating effective coverage will be furnished to the (short institution name) prior to commencement of instruction.

(4) Indemnify and hold harmless the (short institution name) for damages or injuries to patients or other persons not a party to this contract, caused by acts or omissions of students or faculty members participating in the clinical education and training program in pharmacy.

(5) Establish standards for selection and appointment of (short institution name) pharmacy staff members as faculty.

III. The (short institution name), consistent with its primary obligation to care for patients, and consistent with available space and facilities, assumes responsibility for implementation and conduct of the clinical pharmacy education and training program within the institution, under the authority of (short school name), by agreeing to:

(1) Provide educational experience opportunities for students in patient care areas, service departments and other selected areas.

(2) Accept for instruction up to (number) students at the same time.

(3) Maintain pharmacy services without reliance on assigned students.

(4) Cooperate with faculty members of (short school name) in the selection of student learning experiences.

(5) Provide equipment, facilities, supplies and services for students and faculty assigned to the (short institution name) necessary to meet the objectives of the program.

IV. When the Director of Pharmaceutical Services is appointed as Director of Clinical Pharmacy Education and Training at (short institution name) he/she shall be responsible to the Dean of (short school name) for the clinical pharmacy education and training program. (See II Section (1).) Clinical faculty assigned to (short institution name) by (short school name) will be responsible to the Director of Clinical Pharmacy Education and Training for their activities at (short institution name).

V. The (short school name) and (short institution name) will not discriminate against any employee or applicant for employment or enrollment in its source of study because of race, color, creed, sex or national origin.

VI. The students assigned to the (short institution name) shall in no sense be considered employees of the (short institution name) unless specifically agreed to. (E.G., for workmen's compensation purposes). Students and faculty shall adhere to the (short institution name) rules, regulations, procedures and policies during their period of clinical instruction.

The (short institution name) shall have the right to terminate the use of any of its facilities, equipment or supplies by any student or faculty member were flagrant or repeated violations of the (short institution name) rules, regulations, policies and procedures occur. Such action will not normally be taken until the grievance against any student or faculty member has been discussed with the appropriate representative of (short school name). The (short institution name) reserves the right to take immediate action to maintain its facilities free from disruption.

VII. All notices or official communications which may be required under this agreement shall be given as follows:
(1) Notice to the (short school name): (specify person, address)
(2) Notice to the (short institution name): (specify person, address)

VIII. This agreement may be amended by mutual agreement in writing, executed by officials executing this agreement or their successors.

IX. This agreement shall become effective (date) and shall continue indefinitely, except that either party may terminate the agreement by giving written notice to the other party at least (number) months in advance of the proposed termination date. Dates of termination should coincide with the end of semester or quarter instruction for students enrolled in the clinical experience program at (short institution name).

By: _____
Dean

_____
School Name

Date: _____
By: _____
Director of Pharmaceutical Services

_____
Institution Name

Date: _____
By: _____
Hospital Director

_____
Institution Name

Date: _____

Training Residents in Hospital Administration

Today, a relatively large number of universities maintain programs for the education of individuals desirous of a career in hospital administration. Candidates for the degree of *Master in Hospital Administration* must, in addition to the didactic requirements, serve a residency in an approved institution under the guidance of a preceptor.

While serving this residency, the neophyte administrator is exposed to the function and operation of every department in the hospital. Because it is at this time that the young administrator forms his opinion as to the organization and scope of the pharmacy department, as well as the responsibilities of the hospital pharmacist, the American Society of Hospital Pharmacists undertook, through its *Committee on Pharmacy in Hospital Administration Education,* to prepare a course outline to be used by the hospital pharmacist in presenting his image to the trainee in hospital administration.

In 1963, the then *Committee on Pharmacy in Hospital Administration Education* proposed an outline for the teaching of these students. The said outline is hereby presented in detail.[11]

I.   Development of Hospital Pharmacy
    1.   Influence of increased use of drugs
    2.   Influence of the newer pharmaceuticals on the pharmacist's skills
    3.   Influence of pharmaceutical associations
    4.   Influence of all levels of pharmaceutical educational programs
II.   Organization
    1.   Establish a hospital department or purchase an outside service
    2.   Personnel
        a. Education and qualifications
        b. Departmental organization
        c. Possibility of dual function in smaller hospitals: *e.g.* Pharmacist-Purchasing Agent; Pharmacist-Central Sterile Supply Coordinator
    3.   Interdepartmental Relationships
        a. Administration
        b. Nursing
        c. Laboratories
        d. Miscellaneous
    4.   Special relationship to the medical staff
        a. Pharmacy and Therapeutics Committee
        b. Control of research drugs
        c. Pharmacy bulletins
III. Physical Facilities and Design[a]
    1.   General considerations
        a. Location
        b. Size
    2.   Dispensing Areas
        a. In-patient
        b. Out-patient
        c. Ancillary supplies
    3.   Compounding Areas
        a. Extemporaneous compounding
        b. Bulk compounding
        c. Sterile preparations

---

[a]Minimum Standard for Pharmacies in Hospitals. Am. J. Hosp. Pharm., *15*:4:310, 1958.

      4.   Storage Areas
         a. General
         b. Narcotics
         c. Alcohol
         d. Special
      5.   Administrative Areas
         a. Offices
         b. Library

IV. Responsibilities of the Pharmacist
      1.   Administrative
         Budget, purchasing, inventory control, records, and reports
      2.   Professional
         Dispensing, compounding, drug consultant role, teaching and research
      3.   Legal
         Federal, state, local as they apply to alcohol, narcotics, dangerous drugs, poisons, pharmacy
      4.   Ethical
         a. The patient
         b. The physician
         c. The hospital
         d. The community pharmacists

V. The Hospital Formulary System
      1.   Guiding principles
      2.   Philosophy of the Pharmacy and Therapeutics Committee
      3.   The American Hospital Formulary Service
      4.   The private formulary, its advantages and disadvantages

VI. Sources of Information[a]
      1.   Pharmaceutical organizations
      2.   Pharmaceutical literature
         a. "Tentative Draft of An Outline for Teaching Students in Hospital Administration," Bull. Am. Soc. Hosp. Pharm., *8*:357, 1951.
         b. "Syllabus for a Course in Hospital Pharmacy," Bull. Am. Soc. Hosp. Pharm., *12*:261, 1955.

EXTERNAL TEACHING PROGRAMS

As has been previously stated, an external teaching program consists of any teaching activity performed by the pharmacist outside the hospital.

Most chief pharmacists in university-affiliated teaching hospitals hold appointments on the faculty of the associated college of pharmacy. In this capacity, the hospital pharmacist may and usually does teach courses other than hospital pharmacy. These include product development, preparation of parenteral products, sterilization technics and pharmacology.

---

[a]Special literature and reference material relative to the pharmacy department of a hospital are available to the administrative resident from the American Society of Hospital Pharmacists, 4630 Montgomery Avenue, Washington, D.C.

Participation in seminars, institutes and refresher courses is another way in which the hospital pharmacist may carry on a teaching program. The sponsors of these programs do not necessarily have to be pharmaceutical organizations. As a matter of fact, participation in the activities of nursing, dietary, oxygen therapist and medical technologist associations does much to improve the professional stature of the hospital pharmacist.

Teaching, in its broadest interpretation, need not be restricted to personal lectures but may include the preparation of manuscripts for publication in the professional press. The subject matter may consist of the results of original scientific research in product development, sterilization technics; or comprehensive literature surveys in a particular area of hospital pharmacy; or the results of a study which improves the managerial and service rendering aspects of the department.

Some hospital pharmacists have been sufficiently progressive to obtain various grants-in-aid to support research in drug distribution technics or in studying the prescribing habits of physicians associated with large hospital clinics. Certainly this kind of basic study, when completed and published, serves as teaching material, for it is in this way that other pharmacists learn to improve the service they render to their institutions.

SPECIALIZED PHARMACY RESIDENCY TRAINING

A specialized pharmacy practice residency is defined as a postgraduate program of organized training that meets the requirements set forth and approved by the ASHP for that specialty. Specialized pharmacy training programs are directed toward developing expert knowledge and skills in a given area of pharmacy practice, far beyond that which might be expected from clerkship experiences, internship training, or a general practice hospital pharmacy residency. On the other hand, a specialized residency will not, *per se*, develop the broad skills and competency in institutional pharmacy practice which general residency training affords.[17] Specialized pharmacy residency standards have been developed by the ASHP in oncology,[18] nutritional support,[19] gerontology[20] and psychiatry[21] amongst others.

DRUG ABUSE TEACHING PROGRAM

Hospital and clinical pharmacists can make a worthy contribution towards the education of the hospital's staff, employees, patients and students enrolled in the various teaching programs on the issues of drug abuse. In addition, the pharmacists should make themselves available to lecture on the subject to community agencies and other interested groups.

Generally, the drug information center of the department of pharmacy possesses the necessary drug abuse information as well as references to sources of additional teaching aids such as slides, films and film strips.

In addition to conducting lectures and conferences on the subject, displays can be prepared for showing in the hospital, local schools and in the library of the city or town. Also, training of out-of-hospital personnel who are interested in the drug abuse problem—school teachers, clergymen, law enforcement officials and members of the community at large—should be undertaken as part of the overall teaching program of the hospital pharmacy department.

TRAINING EMERGENCY MEDICAL TECHNICIANS

With the adoption of comprehensive statewide emergency medical services plans by many states, it became necessary to develop programs and centers charged with training emergency medicine personnel. As a service to assist in the training programs, hospital pharmacists have presented lectures covering (1) review of drug dosage forms, (2) brief review of drug action and basic pharmacokinetic principles, (3) review of the autonomic nervous system, (4) in-depth review of advanced cardiac life support drugs, and (5) a brief review of patient medications likely to be encountered in the field.[22]

SELECTED READINGS

Latiolais, Clifton J.: The Use of Management Tools in Hospital Pharmacy Internship Training. Am. J. Hosp. Pharm., *20*:4:194, 1963.

Flack, Herbert L.: A Planned and Scheduled Experience Program as One Characteristic of Strong Training Programs. Am. J. Hosp. Pharm., *20*:4:196, 1963.

Residency Accreditation Standards. Am. J. Hosp. Pharm., *37*:1220, (Sept.) 1980.

Kaul, A.F., Powell, S.H., and Wilson, J.A.: Postgraduate Fellowships (1982–1983). Drug Intel. and Clin. Pharm., *16*:949–951, (Dec.) 1982.

Edwards, R. and Adams, D.: Clinical Pharmacy Services in a Pediatric Ambulatory Care Clinic. Drug Intel. and Clin. Pharm., *16*:939–944, (Dec.) 1982.

Gorrell, John and Olszewski, Dell: The Role of the Hospital Pharmacist in the Education of Medical Interns and Residents. Am. J. Hosp. Pharm., *23*:3:151, 1966.

Stolar, M.H.: National Survey of Hospital Pharmacy Services. Am. J. Hosp. Pharm., *36*:316–325, (Mar.) 1979.

REFERENCES

1. Francke, D.E., Latiolais, C.J., Francke, G.N., and Ho, N.F.H.: *Mirror To Hospital Pharmacy*, Easton, Penna., Mack Printing Co., p. 132, 1964.
2. Ibid., page 158.
3. Massachusetts College of Pharmacy Bulletin, *56*:1:42, 1977–78.
4. Falconer, Mary W. and Patterson, R. Robert: *Current Drug Handbook*. Philadelphia, W.B. Saunders Co., 1960.
5. Wright, Harold N. and Montag, Mildred: *A Textbook of Pharmacology and Therapeutics*. Philadelphia, W.B. Saunders Co., 1959.

6. Mehta, H.R.: *Pharmacy for Nurses.* St. Louis, C.V. Mosby Co., 1961.
7. Sperandio, Glen J.: Pharmacy Seminars Within the Hospital, *Hospital Pharmacy Notes* No. 5, September/October, 1960, Eli Lilly & Co., Indianapolis, Ind.
8. Frazier, Walter *et al.*: 1954 Report of the A.S.H.P., Committee on Minimum Standards. The Bulletin, A.S.H.P., *12*:4:454, 1955.
9. Blauch, L.E. and Webster, G.L.: The Pharmaceutical Curriculum. A report prepared for the Committee on Curriculum of the American Association of Colleges of Pharmacy, American Council on Education, 1952.
10. Statement of Abilities Required of Hospital Pharmacists. Am. J. Hosp. Pharm., *19*:9:493, 1962.
11. Report of Committee on Pharmacy in Hospital Administration Education. Am. J. Hosp. Pharm., *20*:4:407, 1963.
12. Accreditation Standard for Pharmacy Residency in a Hospital. Am. J. Hosp. Pharm., *28*:3:189, 1971.
13. Statement on Accreditation of Pharmacy Residencies in Hospitals. Am. J. Hosp. Pharm., *37*:1221–1223, (Sept.) 1980.
14. ASHP Accreditation Standard for Pharmacy Residency in a Hospital (with guide to interpretation). Am. J. Hosp. Pharm., *36*:74–80, Jan., 1979.
15. Cyr, J.G. and McLean, W.M.: Patient Knowledge of Prescription Medication: Present Lack—Future Necessity. Can. Pharm. J., *111*:361–367, Oct., 1978.
16. ASHP and AHA Statement on Clinical Pharmacy and Its Relationship to the Institution. Am. J. Hosp. Pharm., *37*:1096–1097, (Aug.) 1980.
17. ASHP Accreditation Standard for Specialized Pharmacy Residency Training. Am. J. Hosp. Pharm., *37*:1229–1232, (Sept.) 1980.
18. ASHP Supplemental Standard and Learning Objectives for Residency Training in Oncology Practice. Am. J. Hosp. Pharm., *39*:1214–1215, (July) 1982.
19. ASHP Supplemental Standard and Learning Objectives for Residency Training in Nutritional Support Pharmacy Practice. Am. J. Hosp. Pharm., *38*:1971–1973, (Dec.) 1981.
20. ASHP Supplemental Standard and Learning Objectives in Geriatric Pharmacy Practice. Am. J. Hosp. Pharm., *39*:1972–1974, (Nov.) 1982.
21. ASHP Supplementary Standard and Learning Objectives for Residency Training in Psychiatric Pharmacy Practice. Am. J. Hosp. Pharm., *37*:1232–1234, (Sept.) 1980.
22. The White Sheet No. 9, (Oct.) 1984, P.O. Box 16532, Columbus, Ohio.

Preparation of the Annual Report

The preparation of an annual report to the Administrator of the hospital on the activities of the department of pharmacy is one of the most important responsibilities of the hospital pharmacist. In addition, it is the pharmacist's duty to prepare the report in such a manner as to make it an informative yet analytical document covering the activities of the past fiscal year.

Present day managerial practices dictate that there must be adequate communicaiton between all levels of management. It is said that without the free flow of proper information the particular enterprise cannot possibly progress to its maximum capacity. This basic principle of good management should obviously be applied in the hospital. Certainly, the hospital pharmacist can take the first step in the application of this basic principle by the preparation of a comprehensive annual report on the activities of his department.

Too many pharmacists, although they recognize this aspect of their work, refrain from the preparation of such a report because they feel that the administration is not interested in receiving one, or since no other department head submits a report, why should they be different?

The reader is hereby assured of the administration's desire for such a report and is also reminded that the pharmacist should be the leader in any movement, direct or indirect, which leads to improvement of the hospital and the care which it renders to its patients.

FORMAT

There is no specific format which can be recommended for general use. The format should reflect the creativeness and the ingenuity of the author; however, artwork and fancy design work should be avoided. Because the annual report properly belongs in the category of "business document," it should present such an appearance to the recipient.

In general, the report should be typewritten on white bond paper. The typewriter ribbon should be black and the use of red letters or underlining should be avoided.

It is also recommended that the report document be properly identified as to content and author, therefore a front page showing this information as well as a table of contents are in order. Once the body of the report document is completed, all tables and pages should be numbered for the convenience of the reader.

CONTENTS

Because each hospital and hospital pharmacy are different, so too are the contents of the reports submitted in each institution.

Accordingly, in the following discussion, a number of subjects will be covered which may be considered for incorporation into an annual report if they have application to the individual hospital or pharmacy department.

Some of the areas or subjects which may be incorporated into the pharmacist-in-chief's annual report are as follows:

I.   *Introduction*
The introductory remarks should be brief and be confined to a statement of introduction and transmittal.

II.   *The Pharmacy and Therapeutics Committee*
Because the pharmacist serves as the secretary of this committee he is in the best position to report on its activities The report should include a statement on the present membership, the number of meetings held, programs undertaken by the Committee and plans for the new fiscal year.

III.   *The Formulary*
A brief report on the hospital formulary is always in order. It should include a general review of the revisions made, that is, additions or deletions, and a statement concerning plans or the progress being made relative to a total revision and publication.

IV.   *The Pharmacy Bulletin*
Comments on the pharmacy publication are desirable as a means of keeping the administration informed of this extracurricular activity. The pharmacist should briefly relate the number of times the paper was published during the past year and any truly worthy comments concerning the publication or its contents made by the professional staff.

V.   *Teaching Activities*
If the pharmacist is engaged in the teaching programs of the hospital, the report should contain a resume of his activities in the teaching of student nurses, graduate nurses, interns and residents as well as the interns in the hospital pharmacy training program.

VI.   *Professional Activities*
Attendance at seminars, conferences or other professional meetings as well as a documentation of papers given or published are in order.

VII. *Personnel*
Additions or departures from the staff may well be reported, particularly if those who have left have been appointed to positions of prestige and merit and to stress the accomplishments and the quality of the newcomers to the hospital staff.

VIII. *Business Statistics*

This section of the report will probably comprise a large portion of the report if the pharmacist has had the foresight to accumulate the necessary data.

Although some of the financial data which will be included in this section may also be provided to the Administration by the Comptroller, it should nevertheless be repeated here in order to present a total picture rather than force the busy administrator to seek the informaiton in an ancillary document.

The following will serve to acquaint the student and the hospital pharmacist with the type of statistical data which can be accumulated and presented in an annual report:

GENERAL STATISTICS

Opening Inventory Value ....
Closing Inventory Value ....
Rate of Inventory Turn-over..
Income..
Expenses ....
Ratio of Income to Expenses ....
Pharmacist hours/week ....
Technician hours/week ....
Support hours/week ....
Average Income Generated/Pharmacist ....
Number of Hours of Service/Week ....
Gross Revenue/Hour of Service ....
Gross Revenue/Bed ....
Gross Review/Admission ....

IN-PATIENT PRESCRIPTION DATA

Number of Requisitions Dispensed ....
   a. Total Number of Items Ordered ....
   b. Average Number Items/Requisition ....
   c. Total Dollar Value of Items Dispensed ....
   d. Cost to Hospital of *(c)* ....

OUT-PATIENT PRESCRIPTION DATA

Number of Ambulatory Patient ....
Prescriptions Dispensed ....
   a. New Prescriptions ....
   b. Refill Prescriptions ....
   c. Total Gross Income ....
      i.   Cash ....
      ii. Charge..
      iii. Free..
   d. Average Price/Prescription ....

MANUFACTURING PROGRAM STATISTICS

Number of Products Manufacturered.....................................
Number of Gallons of Liquids ....

Number of Pounds of Powders ....

Number of Pounds of Ointments ....

Number of Capsules (Hand filled) ....

Number of Capsules (Machine filled) ....

Number of Vials of Sterile Injectables ....

Number of Units of Large Volume Parenterals ....

Number of Units of Irrigating Fluids ....

Difference between the potential purchase price and the cost of manufacturing within the Hospital Pharmacy resulted in a savings to the Hospital of .....

UNIT DOSE AND IV ADDITIVE SERVICE

Number of Solid Dose Units Packaged ....

Number of Liquid Single Dose Units Packaged ....

Number of Syringes Pre-filled ....

Number of IV Additive Solutions Prepared ....

Number of Hyperalimentations Prepared ....

GENERAL HOSPITAL
AND
LABORATORY REQUISITION DATA

Number of Requisitions Filled ....

Number of Items Dispensed ....

Average Number of Items per Requisition ....

Dollar Value (based on cost to hospital) ....

IX. *Drug Information Center*
A brief report concerning the addition of new subscriptions to journals or the purchase of new book or computer drug information services which may be of benefit to other segments of the hospital population should also be considered for inclusion.

X. *Drug Surveillance and Utilization Review*
Because of the importance of these two aspects of drug control, the pharmacist's annual report should inform the administration of its effectiveness. This can best be accomplished by abstracting the minutes of the Drug Utilization Review Committee, if one is in existence, or that portion of the minutes of the Pharmacy and Therapeutics Committee dealing with the subject.[1,2]

XI. *Training Programs*
In order to obviate the impression that the Department of Pharmacy is solely a service unit, it is important to highlight the various teaching roles and functions of the department.

XII. *DRG Impact*
With most hospitals being reimbursed under a prospective DRG-based system, the pharmacy manager must be alert as to the percent of the hospital's reimbursement is based on pharmacy expense. Thus, it is appropriate to include in the annual report a section showing the impact of the pharmacy operation and recommendations by the pharmacy manager to improve future performance. In the preparation of this segment of the report, the pharmacist should not only ascertain the institution's drug cost per DRG but should compare it as a percentage of total reimbursement on a national and regional level in order that the administrator may have a better understanding of it.[3]

XIII. *Proposed New Programs*

The report should be brought to a close with a brief discussion of proposed new programs or activities for the new fiscal year. These programs should not be discussed in detail in this report. The main purpose for including them here is to demonstrate that the pharmacist is always striving for better performance and higher goals and is not satisfied with a status quo policy no matter how satisfactory the past fiscal year may have been.

INCIDENTS INVOLVING MEDICATIONS AND PHARMACISTS

With the advent of the malpractice crisis, hospital management is increasingly aware of the need to develop loss control-risk management programs within the institution. The general theme of these is to co-ordinate the incident reports with the activities and reports of all of those committees involving patient care. Thus, it is advisable for the pharmacy department to keep an accurate record of incidents which involve medications and pharmacy staff as well as the corrective and preventive measures taken to occlude recurrence. Once accomplished, it is suggested that this matter be included in the annual report to the Administrator of the hospital.

From the preceding discussion, it should be apparent to all concerned that the preparation of an annual report requires a great deal of preparation and planning. Properly prepared, it will enchance the professional stature of the pharmacist in the hospital.

SELECTED READINGS

Rita, Sr. M.: Information Flow from Pharmacy to Administration. Hospitals, J.A.H.A., *38*:16:110, 1964.

Turnbull, R., Ashby, D.: Coping With DRGs: Harper-Grace Hospitals, Detroit, Michigan. Am. J. Hosp. Pharm., *40*:1499–1500, 1983.

Osborne, J.: Coping With DRGs: Baptist Medical Center of Oklahoma, Oklahoma City. Am. J. Hosp. Pharm., *40*:1506–1507, 1983.

Federal Register 48(171): September 1, 1983.

REFERENCES

1. Laventurier, Marc: Utilization and Peer Review by Pharmacists. J. A.PH.A., *NS12*:4:166, 1972.
2. Boisseree, Victor R.: A Case Study in Peer Review. J. A.PH.A., *NS12*:4:171, 1972.
3. Kolar, R., Stanaszek, W., Osborne, J. and Dougherty, K.: Identification of Drug Costs Within Diagnosis Related Groups. Hosp. Pharm., *19*:11:731, (Nov.) 1984.

28|

Safe Use of Medications in the Hospital

The legal literature is replete with cases of injury or death caused by errors in the administration of medications. These unfortunate incidents are not restricted to occurrences within hospitals, but also in doctor's offices, clinics, retail pharmacies and in the home. Furthermore, these mistakes do not always show doctors, nurses or pharmacists as the primary cause of the error. For example, a central sterile supply room aide dispensed a bottle of boric acid solution instead of dextrose solution to the baby formula room—result, several infants died; a pharmacy helper dispensed sodium nitrite solution for sodium phosphate solution—result, two adults died. In both of the above cases, non-professional employees of the hospital were involved.

It would appear that, in the above instances, clearly defined hospital policies governing the handling, dispensing or distribution of drugs or related products might have prevented both tragedies. Furthermore, the lack of these policies could place the trustees, administrator, nurse and pharmacist in a vulnerable position with regard to law suits, both criminal and civil.

Because the hospital pharmacist is the best judge of whether or not safe practices are being followed in the handling, storage, administration or dispensing of drugs and related products, he must assume the mantle of responsibility for the development of the required policies for adoption by the administration and the hospital's board of trustees.

On September 27, 1957, the Coordinating Committee and Board of Trustees of the American Hospital Association voted as follows:

"To urge through appropriate channels, that hospital pharmacists extend their responsibilities to include participation in programs dealing with the safe handling of drugs throughout the hospital."

MEDICATION ERROR—DEFINED

Seldom does a day pass in any large hospital but that some form of medication error is not reported. These errors, although not fatal or injurious to the patient, are nonetheless serious problems and must be coped with accordingly.

A review of the literature will reveal that there is a wide range given as to the definition of a medication error. Therefore, reports on the incidence of errors in one hospital or section of the country may not be comparable with those emanating from other hospitals in the same area or from another section of the country.

The ASHP Technical Assistance Bulletin on Hospital Drug Distribution and Control provides the following definitions and categories of medication errors:[1]

ASHP TECHNICAL ASSISTANCE BULLETIN ON HOSPITAL DRUG DISTRIBUTION AND CONTROL

Medication Errors. If a medication error is detected, the patient's physician must be informed immediately. A written report should be prepared describing any medication errors of clinical import observed in the prescribing, dispensing, or administration of a medication. This report, in accordance with hospital policy, should be prepared and sent to the appropriate hospital officials (including the pharmacy) within 24 hours. These reports should be analyzed, and any necessary action taken, to minimize the possibility of recurrence of such errors. Properly utilized, these incident reports will help to assure optimum drug use control. Medication error reports should be reviewed periodically by the pharmacy and therapeutics committee. (It should be kept in mind that, in the absence of an organized, independent error detection system, most medication errors will go unnoticed.)

The following definitions of medication errors are suggested.

A *medication error* is broadly defined as a dose of medication that deviates from the physician's order as written in the patient's chart or from standard hospital policy and procedures. Except for errors of omission, the medication dose must actually reach the patient; i.e., a wrong dose that is detected and corrected before administration to the patient is not a medication error. Prescribing errors (e.g., therapeutically inappropriate drugs or doses) are excluded from this definition.

Following are the nine categories of medication errors.

1. *Omission error:* the failure to administer an ordered dose. However, if the patient refuses to take the medication, no error has occurred. Likewise, if the dose is not administered because of recognized contraindications, no error has occurred.

2. *Unauthorized-drug error:* administration to the patient of a medication dose not authorized for the patient. This category includes a dose given to the wrong patient, duplicate doses, administration of an unordered drug, and a dose given outside a stated set of

clinical parameters (e.g., medication order to administer only if the patient's blood pressure falls below a predetermined level).

3. *Wrong-dose error:* any dose that is the wrong number of preformed units (e.g., tablets) or any dose above or below the ordered dose by a predetermined amount (e.g., 20%). In the case of ointments, topical solutions, and sprays, an error occurs only if the medication order expresses the dosage quantitatively, e.g., 1 inch of ointment or two 1-second sprays.

4. *Wrong-route error:* administration of a drug by a route other than that ordered by the physician. Also included are doses given via the correct route but at the wrong site (e.g., left eye instead of right).

5. *Wrong-rate error:* administration of a drug at the wrong rate, the correct rate being that given in the physician's order or as established by hospital policy.

6. *Wrong-dosage form error:* administration of a drug by the correct route but in a different dosage form than that specified or implied by the physician. Examples of this error type include use of an ophthalmic ointment when a solution was ordered. Purposeful alteration (e.g., crushing of a tablet) or substitution (e.g., substituting liquid for a tablet) of an oral dosage form to facilitate administration is generally not an error.

7. *Wrong-time error:* administration of a dose of drug greater than $\pm X$ hours from its scheduled administration time, X being as set by hospital policy.

8. *Wrong preparation of a dose:* incorrect preparation of the medication dose. Examples are incorrect dilution of reconstitution, not shaking a suspension, using an expired drug, not keeping a light-sensitive drug protected from light, and mixing drugs that are physically/chemically incompatible.

9. *Incorrect administration technique:* situations when the drug is given via the correct route, site, and so forth, but improper technique is used. Examples are not using Z-track injection technique when indicated for a drug, incorrect instillation of an ophthalmic ointment, and incorrect use of an administration device.

FACTORS CONTRIBUTING TO MEDICATION ERRORS

Many authors have published on this subject, and each has developed a check list by which the administrator or the pharmacist may evaluate the accident proneness of his pharmaceutical service.[2,3] Among the most commonly cited factors which are stated to contribute towards the making of medication errors by both pharmacists and nurses are the following:

   a. Lack of a hospital pharmacist.

 b. Use of non-professional personnel in areas which may require professional judgment.

 c. Inadequate labeling of drug and chemical packages for the nursing station.

 d. Inadequate drug stations on the pavilions.

 e. Inadequate policies governing the reporting of incidents.

CORRECTIVE MEASURES

Lack of a hospital pharmacist

It is a well known fact that approximately 50% of the hospitals in the United States do not employ a pharmacist on their staff.[4] This is a sad reflection upon the quality of care which most practitioners of medicine are forced to offer their patients. In addition, it is an open invitation for a serious medication error and subsequent litigation.

Recognition of the shortage of hospital pharmacists is hereby acknowledged, yet cannot be accepted as the excuse for not attempting to provide adequate pharmaceutical service.

Many solutions to this knotty problem have been described in the literature and include:

1. The sharing of a pharmacist by two or more small hospitals.
2. The combining of responsibilities which the pharmacist must carry such as pharmacist-purchasing agent, pharmacist-technician or pharmacist-administrator.
3. The purchase of pharmaceutical service from a community pharmacy or possibly from a nearby large hospital.
4. The use of consultant pharmacists.

Use of non-professional personnel in areas which may require professional judgment

Lay personnel should, under no circumstances, be placed in positions or areas which may require the exercise of professional judgment. On the other hand, lay personnel should be used in the hospital in areas where they will not be required to act in the capacity of a professional person or in those departments where their acts are under the direct supervision of a professional person.

It is strongly recommended that the director of the pharmacy service develop a strong policy governing the role of lay persons performing in the pharmacy department. Once prepared, the policy should be recorded in the form of job descriptions and sections within the procedural manual.

Inadequate labeling of drug and chemical packages for the nursing station

Unfortunately, too many individuals presume that the labeling of drugs and medications is a relatively simple matter and can, therefore, be assigned to lay employees. When this happens, medication containers become sloppy in appearance and lack the detail required by Federal and state laws, as well as the rules and regulations of the local boards of registration in pharmacy.

The basic concept of affixing a label to any container is to identify the contents and to relay to the user or consumer certain information which the manufacturer and the Government deem to be important. In fact, there should be little or no distinction between commercial medication containers and those dispensed by the hospital pharmacist to the nursing station. Both should bear information as to identity, strength, route of administration and cautions.

The medication label to be used in the hospital should be given considerable thought with respect to the information it is to convey, its size, color and adhesive quality. Many hospital pharmacists utilize only the generic name and metric system on the pharmacy label. Others use the generic name and immediately beneath place the trade name of the product. In addition, the apothecary weight equivalent to the metric system unit may also be displayed on the label. Some hospitals attempt to build into the label an additional safety factor through the use of a color coding system, namely labels printed with red ink on a white background indicate poisons; labels printed with blue ink on a white background indicate oral medications of a non-poisonous nature; green ink is reserved for topical products; black ink for nasal preparations; and purple ink for ophthalmic products.

The use of an auxiliary label is also encouraged in that it serves more readily to call attention to a specific point in relation to the medication. These auxiliary labels are readily available from a number of sources and may be affixed to the medication container in a variety of combinations.

Needless to point out, prescription container or other medication container labels must be neat, uniform, easy to read, unambiguous, comprehensive and factual. Labels should not be affixed one on top of the other for obvious reasons. Archambault[5] describes and pictures a "Label Position Indicator" which guarantees the uniform placement of labels upon containers. By use of this simple device, medication containers will be labeled in exactly the same position thereby creating a uniform appearance on the medication station.

Inadequate drug stations on the pavilions

Medication errors often occur when the nurse preparing the medication is distracted by the passing personnel, is unable to read adequately due to poor lighting, or is forced to go to several different cabinets to gather the materials necessary for the administration of the drug.

Many hospital architects and administrators have recognized this problem and in new construction provision is usually made for a medication room.

A medication room has been defined[6] as a room:

". . . used for the storage and preparation of medications."

Wagner[6] also provides that:

"This room should be enclosed for quiet, clear-glazed for observation both in and out, and sized to accommodate more than one person, because with team nursing, students, private-duty nurses, preoperative and postoperative care, several persons may often work here simultaneously."

The minimum requirements for a medication room are as follows:[6]

   i. Shallow or stepped shelves divided by some means for individual patient medication, with a system for readily changing patient identification.
  ii. A double-locked narcotics safe, with red warning light to indicate when the safe is unlocked, installed at eye level above the counter.
 iii. A counter having drawers underneath for storage of syringes and similar items, but open below without cabinets.
  iv. A bulletin board.
   v. A sink large enough for hand washing, equipped with gooseneck spout and blade handles, should be installed in the counter. This area should be equipped with paper towel dispenser, soap dispenser, and waste receptacle. A separate waste receptacle for broken glass and other non-burnable items should be provided.
  vi. A refrigerator mounted above the counter is more convenient, provides better visibility for drug storage, and allows greater ease in cleaning. An undercounter refrigerator with slide-out, removable tray shelves is acceptable.

In hospitals where a separate medication room is not possible, architects have seen fit to install commercial prefabricated drug stations off the main line of traffic or, where possible, to segregate the installation by a partition or sliding door arrangement.

These units are usually constructed of a non-magnetic stainless steel polished to a high finish. These are equipped with counter top space, sink, medicine shelves, medicine card rack, narcotic cabinet, biological refrigerator, medicine cup dispenser, illumination, syringe drawer and waste receptacles.

Although this type of unit is manufactured by a number of firms, probably the most widely known is the "Medi-Prep" unit (Fig. 92).

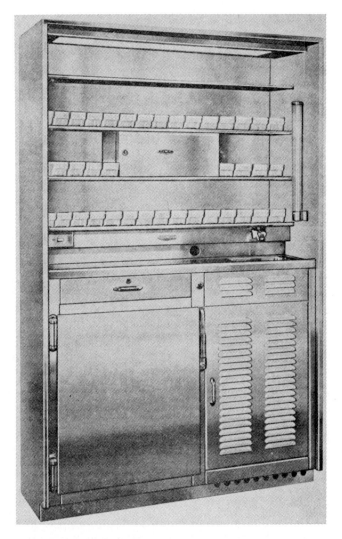

Fig. 92. An example of a type of nursing station medication cabinet. This unit is manufactured by the Market Forge Co., Everett, Massachusetts and is known as the Medi-Prep Unit. There are different models of this unit commercially available. (Courtesy of Market Forge Co., Everett, Massachusetts.)

Inadequate policies governing the reporting of incidents

Laxity in requiring a comprehensive report on each drug accident gives the employee the impression that nobody is interested, and therefore contributes toward the lowering of the standard of patient care. On the contrary, everybody from the nurse to the pharmacist, to the physician to the administrator is or should be interested in every single accident report in order to ascertain the extent of the injury to the patient as well as to initiate ways and means to prevent a recurrence.

This view is supported by the action taken by the Board of Trustees of the American Hospital Association on May 13, 1958[7] when it was voted—

"To urge hospitals to establish an incident reporting system; further to urge adoption of the Incident Report, for use in conjunction with the incident reporting system . . ."

When used in conjunction with the above vote, the word "incident" was defined as follows:

"An incident is any happening which is not consistent with the routine operation of the hospital or the routine care of the patient. It may be an accident or a situation which might result in an accident."

When possible, the medication error report form should be a separate form from that of the typical incident report form. This is necessary because of the very nature of the information which is required. A medication error report form should be able to elicit the following information concerning each drug error: patient's name, hospital number, and location; name of the drug, its strength and route of administration; the time and date of the error; the name and title of the person making the error; the type of error—(1) omission, (2) wrong dose, (3) extra dose given, (4) unordered drug given, (5) wrong dosage form, (6) wrong time of administration, (7) wrong route of administration; the name of the doctor to whom the incident was reported; the name of the nursing supervisor to whom the incident was reported; a brief description of the treatment or the orders given by the doctor as a result of the error; and a statement by the nursing supervisor as to the measures taken by the Nursing Service to prevent such error from recurring.

ASHP GUIDELINES RELATIVE TO THE SAFE USE OF MEDICATIONS IN HOSPITALS

The American Society of Hospital Pharmacists and its officers have always been concerned about safety practices and procedures in hospitals. Francke,[8] writing editorially, has summarized the history of the development of the Society's Committee on Safety Practices and Procedures and its subsequent publication of a series of guidelines for the safe use of drugs in the hospital.

This document represents one of the most important contributions made by the Society to improve and safeguard the care of hospitalized patients. Practitioners and students alike are urged to review its contents thoroughly and immediately proceed to implement its recommendations. Therefore, for the convenience of both, the *Guidelines Relative to the Safe Use of Medications in Hospitals,*[9] is hereby presented in full detail.

The following guidelines are presented for the use of professional personnel responsible for the safe handling of medications and diagnostic agents in hospitals. Recognizing that existing procedures may change, these guidelines are designed to provide a basis for formulating policies and procedures at the present time.

PREAMBLE

THE BOARD OF TRUSTEES OF THE AMERICAN HOSPITAL ASSOCIATION and the Executive Committee of the AMERICAN SOCIETY OF HOSPITAL PHARMACISTS in 1957 adopted the following significant position:

> To urge hospital pharmacists, through appropriate channels, to extend their responsibilities to include participation in programs dealing with the safe handling of drugs throughout the hospital.

Problems of medication safety are now the grave concern of the many persons involved with patient care. These include the hospital trustee, the physician, the administrator, the pharmacist, the nurse, and others. The multiplicity of drugs, the increased number and kinds of medications prescribed per patient, the increased number of both inpatients and outpatients who are being treated, and the ever-changing concepts of medical care make it mandatory that a system of safe medication practices be developed and maintained to insure that the patient receives the best possible care and protection.

In recent years, the rapid obsolescense of drugs, the availability of more specific drugs per disease entity, and the general increase in the prescribing of medications have placed a greater responsibility on pharmacy and nursing services in dispensing and administering medications.

The greatly increased use of medications has increased the hazard of possible error. The seriousness of the problem may be indicated by the fact that medication errors are among the leading causes of accidents in hospitals.

For the purpose of this statement, a medication error, though resulting from many possible causes, is defined as the administration of the wrong medicine or dose of medicine, diagnostic agent, or treatment requiring the use of such agent to a patient; or the administration of the medicine, agent, or treatment at the wrong time, or to the wrong patient; or the failure to administer such medication, agent, or treatment; or the failure to administer at the time specified or in the manner prescribed or normally considered as accepted practice.

SECTION I

LABELING AND MEDICATION CONTAINERS—GENERAL

1.1   Drug labeling should be performed by a pharmacist or under the supervision of a pharmacist. Prescription labels and pharmacy stock labels should be used only by the hospital pharmacy. (See 1.16 and 4.14.)

1.2   The pharmacist should be consulted and should make recommendations concerning labeling, containers and storage of housekeeping items, insecticides, cleaners, and such.

1.3 Medication labels should be typed or machine-printed. Labeling with pen or pencil, use of adhesive tape or china marking pencils should be prohibited. A label should not be superimposed on a label.

1.4 The label should be legible, easily read, and free from erasures and strike-overs. It should be firmly affixed to the container. The label for stock containers should be protected from chemical action or abrasion.

1.5 Labels should bear the name, address, and telephone number of the hospital.

1.6 One order or prescription should be filled and labeled at a time.

1.7 The following or similar accessory labels and caution statements should appear where indicated:

   a. Poison
   b. Not to be taken internally
   c. Shake well before using
   d. For external use only
   e. For the eye
   f. For the nose
   g. For the ear
   h. Refrigerate at 2°–10°C (35°–50°F)
   i. Refrigerate after reconstitution
   j. Warning: Not for injection
   k. Do not use after _____
   l. Not to be swallowed
   m. Keep out of reach of children
   n. Keep from freezing
   o. Keep below freezing
   p. Caution: Potent Drug
   q. Research Drug
   r. NONPROPRIETARY NAME[a]
   Note for information of staff:
   Prescription or order for *(Proprietary Name)* filled as per formulary policy; contents are same basic drug as prescribed, but may be of another brand.
   s. NONPROPRIETARY NAME[a]
   Note for informaiton of staff:
   Contents may be used per formulary policy, to fill prescriptions or orders for any of the following brands of the same basic drug:
   (Proprietary Name, Brand 1)
   (Proprietary Name, Brand 2)
   (Proprietary Name, Brand 3)
   t. Note change in color, size, and shape
   u. Other accessory labels providing special information such as dosage, side effects, or contraindications for investigational drugs may be used where necessary.

1.8 The metric system should be given prominence on all labels where both metric and apothecary systems are commonly used.

1.9 The name of the therapeutically-active ingredients should be indicated in compound mixtures.

---

[a]Applicable to those hospitals operating under the formulary system as outlined in AHA-ASHP *Statement of Guiding Principles on the Operation of the Hospital Formulary System. See* AM. J. HOSP. PHARM., *17*:609, Oct., 1960.

1.10 Labels for medications should indicate the amount of drug or drugs in each dosage form unless otherwise indicated.

1.11 Drugs and chemicals in forms intended for dilution or reconstitution should carry directions for so doing. Whenever possible, dilutions and labeling should be done in the pharmacy.

1.12 Perishable drugs, such as antibiotics and biologicals, should clearly indicate the expiration date on the label.

1.13 The routes of administration should be indicated for parenteral medications whenever possible.

1.14 Numbers, letters, coined names, and unofficial synonyms and abbreviations should not be used to identify medications with the exception of approved letter or number codes for investigational drugs.

1.15 Only light-resistant, tight containers meeting U.S.P. standards should be used.

1.16 Medications if brought into the hospital by the patient or physician should be positively identified before use. Such medications should be checked by the hospital pharmacist with the originating pharmacy by prescription serial number. A supplemental label should be attached in the hospital pharmacy providing information required in Section II. Where no pharmacist is on duty, the physician should check with the issuing pharmacy and attach the supplemental label described above.

1.17 Containers presenting difficulty in labeling, such as small tubes, should be labeled with no less than the prescription serial number, name of drug, strength, and name of the patient, and should then be placed in a larger carton or container bearing a label with the necessary information indicated in Sections II and III.

1.18 The label should conform with all applicable Federal, state, and local laws and regulations.

1.19 Floor stock medication labels should carry codes to identify source and lot number of medication.

SECTION II

LABELING AND DISPENSING IN-PATIENT PRESCRIPTIONS

2.1 In addition to the recommendations outlined in Section I, the in-patient prescription labels should bear, as a minimum, the following information:
   a. Patient's full name
   b. Nonproprietary and/or proprietary name of the drug actually dispensed
   c. Strength
   d. Date of issue
   e. Name or initials of dispensing pharmacist

2.2 The prescription or in-patient order should have noted thereon, at the time dispensed, the source and batch identifying number of the medication and the initials of the dispenser.

2.3 For in-patient self-care medications, label as in Section III.

SECTION III

LABELING AND DISPENSING OUT-PATIENT PRESCRIPTIONS

3.1   Medications to be dispensed to in-patients who are being discharged
       should be returned to the pharmacy for relabeling.
3.2   The out-patient prescription label should bear the following informa-
       tion.:
       a. Patient's full name
       b. Prescription identification number
       c. Specific directions for use
       d. Date of issue
       e. Name or initials of dispenser
       f. Name of prescribing physician
       g. Where physician requests or hospital policy dictates, identity and
            strength should be on the label
       h. A "Keep out of reach of children" label
       i. Name, address, and telephone number of hospital
3.3   Prescriptions should have noted thereon, at the time dispensed, the
       source and batch identifying number of the medication and the initials
       of the dispenser.
3.4   An identifying check system to insure proper identification of out-
       patients should be established.

SECTION IV

CARE OF DRUGS AND DRUG CABINETS IN NURSING UNITS

4.1   Medication centers should be functional and provide:
       a. Adequate space so that drugs can be placed and arranged in ac-
            cordance with 4.2
       b. Adequate space to allow all container labels to be clearly visible
       c. Adequate lighting so that labels can be clearly read
       d. Adequate ventilation
       e. Adequate work space protected from traffic and noise
       f. Hot and cold running water
       g. Sufficient equipment and supplies in readily usable form
       h. Refrigeration
       i. Inner-lockable narcotic cabinet
       j. Adequate means of security
4.2   Medications should be placed in drug cabinets in accordance with an
       established plan for a particular hospital which provides standardized
       compartments for:
       a. Internal medications
       b. Narcotics, barbiturates, amphetamines
       c. Poisons and external-use drugs
       d. Emergency drugs
       e. Ampuls
       f. Investigational drugs
4.3   Drugs should be arranged alphabetically within the above mentioned
       groups insofar as possible.
4.4   Medication cabinets or rooms and narcotic compartments should be
       kept locked and the keys should be available only to the nurse in charge
       or her alternate.

4.5 Storage of drugs on mobile dressing carriages is discouraged unless properly secured.

4.6 Not more than one hypodermic tablet should be placed in a capsule for the purpose of protection against breakage or to facilitate counting or control.

4.7 Pharmacy should supply exact quantities for preparation of specific amounts of solution, or should preferably supply the finished preparation. Maintenance of bulk chemicals or stock drugs on the nursing units for preparation of solution should be discouraged.

4.8 Separate storage facilities should be provided for:
   a. Test reagents
   b. General disinfectants and antiseptics
   c. Cleansing agents

4.9 Only drugs and the equipment for preparation and administration should be stored in medication cabinets.

4.10 Drug cabinets should be examined weekly or more often by the nurse in charge. Drugs which appear to have deteriorated, exceeded their expiration date, or are not being used should be returned to the pharmacy for proper disposition. Monthly, or more frequent, inspections should be made by the Directors of Pharmacy and Nursing Service or their delegates.

4.11 Controlled drugs in the nursing unit shall be inventoried, recorded, and inspected in accord with an approved system.

4.12 Investigational drugs should be handled as directed in the Statement of Principles Involved in the Use of Investigational Drugs in Hospitals issued by the American Hospital Association and AMERICAN SOCIETY OF HOSPITAL PHARMACISTS.

4.13 Reconstitution of antibiotics and other unstable drugs on the nursing unit should be kept to a minimum. They should be diluted in accordance with directions supplied by the pharmacy.

4.14. Antibiotics and other unstable drugs reconstituted on the nursing unit should carry a nurse prepared label with essentially the following information:
   a. Expiration date
   b. Nurse's name or initials
   c. Dosage or strength per unit volume

4.15 Empty medication containers should be returned to the pharmacy.

4.16 Flammable or explosive liquids such as ether or acetone should be kept in as small supply as possible and in accordance with state and local fire regulations.

SECTION V

MEDICATION ORDERS

5.1 Medications should be given only on the written order of a physician. Exceptions to this policy should be covered by a written policy established by the Medical Board or Medical Staff of the hospital, as for example 5.2 and 5.3.

5.2 Emergency verbal orders may be accepted by a nurse. The physician should check the prepared emergency dose and container before the medication is administered. An order for the medication should be written by the physician at the earliest time possible.

5.3 *Stat* telephone orders may be accepted by a nurse. The order should be recorded in the doctor's order sheet, followed by the name of physician giving the order, the time, and the signature of the nurse receiving it. The nurse should repeat the order to the physician from her written record for confirmation. The physician should countersign this order on his next visit to the station. The nurse accepting a telephone order should be personally responsible for its execution.

5.4   Medication orders should be automatically cancelled under the following conditions:

    a. Patient goes to delivery room or operating room

    b. Transfer of patient to another service

    c. In accordance with written policy of the Medical Board adopted in connection with the Automatic Stop Order statement of the Joint Commission on Accreditation of Hospitals

    d. In accordance with written policy of the Medical Board adopted in connection with Suggested Regulations for Handling Narcotics in Hospitals by the AMERICAN SOCIETY OF HOSPITAL PHARMACISTS and approved by the American Hospital Association

5.5   The physician will specify the time a stat or single order was written. After the nurse administers the medication, she should write, "Given," the time administered, and her signature.

5.6   Medication orders should be legibly written and should include:

    a. Name of medication

    b. Dosage expressed in the metric system, except in instances where dosage is commonly expressed otherwise

    c. Signature of the physician

    d. Route of administration, if other than oral

    e. Date and hour

5.7   The use of abbreviations and chemical symbols in the writing of medication orders is discouraged and, if used, should be limited to those agreed upon and jointly adopted by the nursing, pharmacy, and medical staffs of a particular hospital.

5.8   Any question arising from a medication order, including the interpretation of illegible order, should be referred to the physician writing the order. The nurse should not be expected to attempt to carry out the order until the question is resolved.

SECTION VI

MEDICATION CARDS

6.1   A medication card should be made and used for the preparation and administration of all medications and should carry essentially the following information:

    a. Patient's first and last names

    b. Location of patient and hospital number

    c. Name of drug

    d. Dosage

    e. Route of administration if other than oral

    f. Frequency of administration

    g. Time(s) of administration

    h. Any special precautions or observations

    e. Initials of nurse preparing or verifying the medication order

    j. Expiration date of order

    k. Date card made out

6.2   The medication card should be clearly written in ink or printed and verified by the nurse against the physician's order.

6.3   Cards for "Delayed" or "Omitted" medications should be removed from the regular medication card file and placed in a designated place.

6.4   On assuming charge of a patient unit, the nurse should check the medication cards against the doctor's order to insure the following:

    a. All cards are in their proper place

    b. Cards for "Delayed" or "Omitted" medications have been removed

    c. Cards for medications to be resumed following "Omit" or "Delay" are returned to their proper place in the file

    d. Cards for discontinued order are removed and destroyed

SECTION VII

PREPARATION OF MEDICATIONS FOR ADMINISTRATION

7.1   Ascertain that prescribed dose has not previously been administered.

7.2   Select medication card(s) or drug(s) to be administered.

7.3   Check medication card(s) for expiration time and date and omission.

7.4   Arrange medication cards with medicine cups in the order in which medications are to be administered. Use a separate cup for each medication unless otherwise ordered.

7.5   Expose each medication card singly while preparing the medication.

7.6   Give full attention while preparing medication.

7.7   Select drug and compare it to medication.

7.8   Ascertain that the container is completely and properly labeled, including strength when indicated. Never use unlabeled medications.

7.9   Read the label three (3) times

    a. Before removing from shelf

    b. Before measuring or preparing the dose

    c. Before replacing on shelf

7.10   Medications prepared for administration, but not used, should be discarded.

7.11   The pharmacist should be contacted when there is a question regarding the mixing of medications in the same syringe or container.

7.12   A copy of the hospital formulary, an up-to-date incompatibility chart for possible parenteral medication mixtures, and an antidote chart should be maintained at each nursing station.

7.13   Pharmaceutical calculations required in the administration of medications should be checked by another nurse or, if possible, with the pharmacist.

7.14   The metric system, to the extent possible, should be used in prescribing, administering, and recording medications. Approximate metric and apothecary equivalents and information for computing dosage should be readily available on the nursing unit.

SECTION VIII

ADMINISTRATION OF MEDICATIONS

8.1   Medications should be administered only if information regarding the drug is available in the form approved by the Pharmacy and Therapeutics Committee. The nurse should know and consider:

    a. General use of the drug

      b. Therapeutic action

      c. Usual dosage

      d. Factors modifying the dosage

      e. Factors modifying the effects

      f. Untoward actions, side effects, precautions, and contraindications

      g. Antidote, if known

      h. Medium, route and frequency of administration

      i. Signs of deterioration of drug

8.2   Medications shold be prepared and given as near the specified time as possible.

8.3   The patient for whom the medication is intended should be positively identified by checking the identification band or hospital number, or by other means as specified by hospital policy.

8.4   The person administering the medication should stay with the patient until the medication has been taken. Exceptions to this rule are selected medications which may be left at the patient's bedside on the physician's written order.

8.5   All medications should be administered by the person who has prepared the dose. For exceptions to this rule, see (5.2) (8.8).

8.6   Parenteral medications which are not to be mixed in a syringe should be given in different sites.

8.7   The administration of blood and blood derivatives should be the responsibility of the physician. The physician should be responsible for starting intravenous and subcutaneous infusions, for administering all intravenous medications, and for adding medications to flowing intravenous fluids. Exceptions should be covered by written policy established and endorsed by the Medical Board of the hospital, which policies should be in compliance with existing state nursing, pharmacy, and medical practice acts and regulations, or rulings of the office of the state attorney general.

8.8   In instances when the administration of medications is delegated to another person, the nurse should assume the responsibility for supervision of the procedure.

SECTION IX

RECORDING OF MEDICATIONS

9.1   All administered medications or omitted medications should be recorded on the patient's medical record according to an established procedure.

9.2   Hospital policy determine the responsibility for recording medications administered by the physician.

SECTION X

MEDICATION ERRORS

10.1   Each hospital should set up a clear statement of policy for all medication errors. Such policy should include:

      a. Reporting

      b. Recording

      c. Review

      d. Channel for analysis and necessary action

      e. Written report

10.2   If an error occurs in the administration of medication, the physician and the proper administrative representative should be informed immediately.

10.3   A written report, in accordance with hospital policy, should be prepared and sent to the proper hospital officials within 24 hours.

DRUG INTERACTION SURVEILLANCE

The safe use of medications in hospitals, extended care facilities and nursing homes goes beyond the assurances that the appropriate drug has been dispensed and that the label information is correct. Generally, the introduction of a unit dose system into the operation tends to eliminate many of the errors in medication administration and, at the same time, provides the ultimate in drug control, packaging and dispensing.

To assure the patient and physician or total drug safety, it is essential that the pharmacist maintain a drug interaction surveillance program. Such a program should include a method to check on drug-drug and drug-laboratory test reactions. Because more than one mechanism may be involved, and because each mechanism may be quite complex, the classification of drug interaction mechanisms is very difficult and the practice thereof constitutes a form of specialization in pharmacy. However, the average practitioner of hospital pharmacy can maintain adequate surveillance by instituting a program of working from a direct copy of the physician's original order sheet; preparing a patient drug profile (PDP); and a drug interaction reporting form (DIRF).[10] These combined with the judicious selection and use of the latest textbooks on the subject will assure all concerned that proper drug safety techniques are being practiced.[11,12]

JOINT COMMISSION ON PRESCRIPTION DRUG USE

In November 1976, Senator Edward M. Kennedy announced the formation of the Joint Commission On Prescription Drug Use (JCPDU) with a mandate to (1) define a means by which information on the epidemiology of prescription drug use in the United States could be determined and distributed to interested parties in the United States and (2) describe a post-marketing surveillance (PMS) system that could be used to detect, describe and quantitate the anticipated and unanticipated effects of marketed drugs. The system should be economically feasible and scientifically sound.

The rationale for the creation of the JCPDU is that the regulation of prescription drugs has focused on the pre-marketing phases. Millions of dollars, public and private, are spent to assure that a product is safe and effective for a specific purpose before it is marketed. Once marketed, a physician may use a drug in any dosage, for any purpose— whether or not that purpose has been scientifically evaluated. Thus, the actual use of prescription drugs operates outside the regulatory framework and little is known about how drugs are actually used once marketed.

After 3 years of deliberation, the JCPDU concluded that a Center for Drug Surveillance be created to: (1) obtain and coordinate the information from multiple sources regarding drug use and effects; (2) initiate research that will lead to development of new and necessary methodologies of surveillance and fill voids in the existing body of knowledge about the effects and uses of prescription drugs; (3) report the information so that its medical and social implications can be appropriately understood and acted upon by health care providers, patients, the FDA, the pharmaceutical industry and others responsible for making decisions about drugs; (4) provide training opportunities or a training center for epidemiologists and other scientists and health care providers who will contribute to PMS; and (5) serve as a readily available resource center on drug information to the entire country.

Copies of the JCPDU's report have been distributed to the libraries of all medical and pharmacy schools in the United States as well as to the libraries of professional societies (including the ASHP and A.Ph.A.). Hospital and clinical pharmacists should take an active role in any post-marketing prescription drug surveillance program in order to assure drug use safety. In addition they should become more involved in drug usage review, medical audit and other patient care review procedures.[13,14]

SELECTED READINGS

ASHP Technical Assistance Bulletin on Handling Cytotoxic Drugs in Hospitals. Am. J. Hosp. Pharm., *42*:131–137, 1985.

Avis, K.E. and Levchuk, J.W.: Special Considerations in the Use of Vertical Laminar-flow Workbenches. Am. J. Hosp. Pharm., *41*:81–87, 1984.

REFERENCES

1. ASHP Technical Assistance Bulletin on Hospital Drug Distribution and Control. Am. J. Hosp. Pharm., *37*:1097–1103, (Aug.) 1980.
2. Archambault, George F.: Pharmacy Accidents Can Be Prevented. Hospitals, J.A.H.A., *31*:7:68, 1957.
3. Schlossberg, Eli: Sixteen Safeguards Against Medication Errors. Hospitals, J.A.H.A., *32*:19:62, 1958.
4. Anon: Hospitals, J.A.H.A., Guide Issue (August 1, Part II), *38*:513, 1964.
5. Archambault, George F.: Labels for Nursing Station Medication Containers. Hospitals, J.A.H.A., *32*:18:50, 1958.
6. Wagner, Charles: Planning the Patient Care Unit in the General Hospital, *Public Health Service Publication* No. 930-D-1, U.S. Government Printing Office, Washington, D.C.
7. Anon.: Incident Reporting System. Hospitals, J.A.H.A., *32*:15:46, 1958.
8. Francke, Don E.: Safety Practices and Procedures (An Editorial). Am. J. Hosp. Pharm., *19*:11:553, 1962.

9. Anderson, R. David *et al.*: Guidelines Relative to the Safe Use of Medications in Hospitals. Am. J. Hosp. Pharm., *19*:11:577, 1962.
10. Arnold, Thomas R.: Drug Interaction Reporting in a Small Hospital. Hospital Pharmacy, *7*:3:79, 1972.
11. Hansten, Philip D.: *Drug Interactions,* 5th Ed. Lea & Febiger, Philadelphia, 1985.
12. Hartshorn, Edward A.: *Handbook of Drug Interactions.* Drug Intelligence Publications, Hamilton Press Inc., Hamilton, Illinois, 1973.
13. Stolar, M.H.: Conceptual Framework for Drug Usage Review, Medical Audit and Other Patient Care Review Procedures. Am. J. Hosp. Pharm., *34*:139–145, (Feb.) 1977.
14. Brodie, D.C., Smith, W.E., Jr. and Hlynka, J.N.: Model for Drug Usage Review in a Hospital. Am. J. Hosp. Pharm., *34*:251–254, (Mar.) 1977.

29|

The Small Hospital, Nursing Homes, Hospices and Part-Time Pharmacists

Nearly 2500 hospitals in the United States do not employ either a full-time or a part-time pharmacist to provide pharmaceutical services to their patients and physicians. In these institutions, non-pharmacist personnel handle the drugs which do not require compounding. All others are purchased from local community pharmacies.[1]

It is sometimes overlooked that these same drugs which are daily handled by untrained hospital personnel are required, by law, to be dispensed in the retail pharmacy or the large hospital by duly qualified, licensed pharmacists. By permitting this double standard to exist, trustees, administrators, pharmacists, and pharmacy law enforcement officers are, in effect, denying the small hospital's patient high quality pharmacy service. In addition, the institution's officers and administration are openly inviting both criminal and civil actions should a serious drug accident occur within the hospital.

The American Hospital Association, the American Society of Hospital Pharmacists and the American College of Apothecaries have held that the size of the hospital should not in any way limit or deprive the patient of the pharmacy service to which he is entitled.[2]

Although the ideal goal to ensure adequate pharmaceutical services in all hospitals, irrespective of size, is to place a pharmacist on each staff, we fully realize that this would be a utopian state. Accordingly, a more practical approach must be sought.

Fortunately, a number of far-sighted, economically and safety minded small hospital administrators have explored and developed a number of plans for the provision of adequate pharmaceutical services with their institutions.

This chapter concerns the study of the four principal methods of handling drugs in the hospital without a full-time pharmacist. These same methods may be utilized in the nursing home or extended care facility with minor modification.

MODEL NURSING HOME-PHARMACIST RETAINER AGREEMENT

Whereas, the _____ (hereinafter referred to as "Nursing Home") desires to provide
(name of Nursing Home)
quality pharmaceutical services to its inpatients; and

Whereas, _____ (hereinafter referred to as "Pharmacist") is a pharmacist in good
(name of Pharmacist)
standing licensed to practice his profession under the laws of this state;

Now, therefore, on this _____ day of _____, 196__, in consideration of the mutual agreements and prom-
(date)   (month)
ises hereinafter set forth, the parties hereto agree:

1. The _____ Nursing Home agrees to retain Pharmacist and Pharmacist agrees to provide Nurs-
ing Home with pharmaceutical services. Nursing Home agrees that during the period of this retainer that Pharmacist shall
have the exclusive right to furnish medication and all related medical and health supplies and devices which Pharmacist is
legally and professionally qualified to provide.

2. The retainer of Pharmacist shall commence on the date of this Agreement and shall continue for _____
(months, years) from the date hereof. Subject to this Agreement continuing in full force and effect for said period, Pharmacist shall have the option to continue his retainer hereunder for an additional like period by giving Nursing Home written
notice of his intention so to do not less than _____ days nor more than _____ days prior to the expiration of the initial
term. Upon the exercise of this option by Pharmacist, all of the terms and conditions of this Agreement shall continue in
full force and effect for such additional period, except the option to continue the retainer.

3. During the period of the retainer hereunder, Pharmacist shall serve Nursing Home and shall perform any and all
services in pharmaceutical matters required or requested in connection with the operation of the Nursing Home premises
located at _____, including compliance with all regulatory requirements to meet the conditions or
(street address)
standards of participation in any governmental medical or health assistance programs. Pharmacist will perform such other
services of an advisory or educational nature which are related to pharmaceutical services or for which his education,
training, and experience as a pharmacist are especially suited, without further compensation other than that provided for in
this Agreement.

4A. Pharmacist shall devote such time, energy, and skill as his duties hereunder shall require and shall, at least quarterly, or at any time upon request, submit a report of principal activities performed and to be performed by him for Nursing Home, and shall render such assistance as may be requested by Nursing Home in reviewing the provisions and activities relating to pharmaceutical services in connection with governmental inspections or voluntary accreditation programs.

4B. Pharmacist shall devote not less than _____ hours but not more than _____ hours per _____ (week, month, year)
to the performance of his duties under this retainer which shall include all time expended in preparing reports of activities
performed or to be performed by him for Nursing Home and time expended in reviewing the provisions and activities relating to pharmaceutical services in connection with governmental inspections or voluntary accreditation programs.

5A. Nursing Home shall pay to Pharmacist as fees for his professional services under this retainer an aggregate of
$_____ (_____ dollars) per _____ (month, year), in addition to the actual cost of medication sup-
(number)   (spell out)
plied. Nursing Home shall reimburse pharmacist monthly for the actual cost of medication dispensed to patients upon written
statements of account.

5B. Nursing Home shall pay to Pharmacist his usual and customary fee for each prescription order dispensed to Nursing Home patients which shall not be greater than that Pharmacist charges other noninstitutionalized patients. In addition,
Nursing Home shall pay Pharmacist for his professional consultation and other services performed on Nursing Home premises a retainer in the aggregate sum of $_____, (_____ dollars) per _____ (month, year).
(number)

5C. Nursing Home shall pay to Pharmacist his actual cost of ingredients plus a professional fee of $_____
(number)
(_____ dollars) for each prescription order dispensed to Nursing Home's patients. In addition, Nursing Home shall
pay Pharmacist for his professional consultation and other services performed on Nursing Home premises a retainer in the
aggregate sum of $_____ (_____ dollars) per _____ (month, year).
(number)

6. Nursing Home agrees to provide Pharmacist with office and pharmacy space needed in performing the services of
his retainer and with such secretarial service as may be required. Nursing Home agrees to reimburse Pharmacist for expenditures made on behalf of Nursing Home for reference works, physical equipment, and supplies other than drugs needed
in performing his professional duties upon written statements of account rendered monthly: Provided, however, that any
expenditure in excess of $_____ for any one item shall first require the approval of the Nursing Home.

7. Pharmacist is retained and employed by Nursing Home only for purposes and to the extent set forth in this Agreement, and his relation to Nursing Home shall, during the period that this retainer is in effect, be that of an independent
practitioner, and Pharmacist shall be free to dispose of such portion of his time, energy, and skill not required in the performance of his duties hereunder in such manner as he may choose and to such persons, firms, or corporations as he deems
advisable. Pharmacist shall not be considered under the provisions of this Agreement or otherwise as having an employee
status or as being entitled to participate in any plans, arrangements, or other benefits pertaining to pension, or other em-
ployee-benefit plans.

8. Pharmacist agrees to obtain and maintain a suitable professional liability policy to provide adequate coverage
against mistake or neglect in the performance of his professional services under this retainer.

9. Nursing Home shall make such arrangements as may be necessary to assure Pharmacist of effective and actual control of drugs and related supplies, and the records pertaining thereto, under policies and procedures developed in accordance
with sound pharmaceutical practices.

10. Pharmacist shall arrange to provide the services of another pharmacist to perform the obligations of this retainer
during any absence, vacation or other limited periods when Pharmacist is not personally available.

11. This agreement may be terminated by either party at any time for good and sufficient cause provided the alleged
grounds for termination have been presented in writing at least 30 days prior to the effective date of the termination.

In witness whereof, Nursing Home has caused this agreement to be executed through its duly authorized representative
and Pharmacist has accepted its terms and promises on this _____ day of _____, 196_____.

Name of Nursing Home _____

By: (Signature)   _____

Title: _____

Signature of Pharmacist _____

Fig. 93. Model Nursing Home-Pharmacist Retainer Agreement of the type recommended by
the American Pharmaceutical Association and the American Society of Consultant Pharmacists.

METHODS OF HANDLING DRUGS IN HOSPITALS WITHOUT A FULL-TIME PHARMACIST

The four principal methods of handling drugs in hospitals without a full-time pharmacist are as follows:

1. A community pharmacist contracts to provide a full pharmaceutical service to the hospital and he, or his duly licensed agent, goes to the institution and actively participates in performing the service contracted for (Fig. 93).
2. A community pharmacist contracts to provide drug merchandise only. He does not go to the hospital. In this situation, other hospital personnel, principally nurses, function in the institution as drug dispensers or distributors.
3. Pharmacy service in the small hospital is provided by the department of pharmacy of a nearby large hospital.
4. No pharmacist is involved in the hospital's drug service, which is carried on by nurses, technicians or aides.

SMALL HOSPITAL-COMMUNITY PHARMACIST RELATIONSHIP

It has been reported[2] that to insure that a part-time pharmaceutical program in the small hospital will succeed, the following are essential:

1. "a compact, adequate (but not necessarily large) separate drug room."
2. "a pharmacist on active duty in the hospital on an average of three hours per day."
3. "a direct telephone service between the small hospital's drug room to the independent pharmacy for consultation services."
4. "stand-by delivery service from the independent pharmacy to the hospital."
5. "the availability of an emergency telephone number and service for the use of the hospital at all hours."

Since this initial attempt was made to develop ground rules for the quasi professional-commercial relationship between the small hospital and the community pharmacist, the American Hospital Association and the American Society of Hospital Pharmacists have cooperated in the development of the following *Suggested Principles of Relationship Between Smaller Hospitals and Part-Time Pharmacists.*[3]

PRINCIPLES OF RELATIONSHIP BETWEEN SMALL HOSPITALS AND PART-TIME PHARMACISTS[a]

Preamble

ALL HOSPITALS should be cognizant of the contribution made by a sound and organized pharmaceutical service for improved patient care and treatment. The introduction annually of numerous potent drugs requires that all hospitals have the full or part-time service of a registered pharmacist. In small hospitals which cannot obtain or afford a full-time hospital pharmacist, the services of a pharmacist on a part-time or consultative basis may be obtained.

If the services of a hospital pharmacist of another hospital are not obtainable, the services of a local registered pharmacist should be utilized whenever possible. When pharmaceutical service from a local pharmacy is considered, the part-time pharmacist and the hospital might consider certain guiding principles of affiliation. The Principles of Relationship Between Smaller Hospitals and Part-time Pharmacists are suggested to achieve the objective of better patient care.

Basic Principle

1. *The pharmaceutical service of the hospital shall be organized and maintained primarily for the benefit of hospital patients.*

In any hospital, the individual elements which are maintained and coordinated are all subordinate to the main objective of providing care to the sick and injured. Any function either newly added or strengthened, as in this instance drug or pharmaceutical services (from any source whatever or by any arrangement), must be in agreement with this basic principle.

Organization

1. *The hospital pharmaceutical service should be under the direction of a professionally competent legally qualified pharmacist.*

The hospital must exercise due care in its selection of personnel. The hospital safeguards the patient and its public trust by fixing the responsibility for its varied functions by appointing adequately qualified individuals.

2. *A part-time pharmacist, as a professional member of the hospital staff and as the head of a hospital function or department, must assume the responsibilities involved.*

Recognition as a member of the hospital organization will be in direct proportion to the responsibility which the individual is capable of accepting on a part-time basis.

3. *The part-time pharmacist shall be responsible to the proper administrative authority of the hospital for developing, supervising and coordinating the activities of the pharmaceutical services to hospital patients and departments.*

With hospital affiliation, an attendant responsibility is placed on the part-time pharmacist to preserve the unity and coordination of the hospital's component activities as directed by the administrator in policies laid down in behalf of the public which the hospital governing board represents. Thus the part-time pharmacist subscribing to a hospital connection in terms of relationships

---

[a]Approved by the Board of Trustees of the American Hospital Association and the Executive Committee of the American Society of Hospital Pharmacists February, 1959

is primarily responsible to the hospital administrator for those services provided to hospital patients and departments.

Rules, regulations and procedures regarding drug services to hospital patients and departments should not be counter to or in opposition to the hospital's administrator in behalf of the medical staff, and of the hospital governing board and the public it represents.

4. *The organization of hospital pharmaceutical services, the relationship to the hospital and its elements, and the specific services to be provided should be outlined and reviewed periodically by the hospital administrator and the part-time pharmacist who provides pharmaceutical services to hospital patients and departments.*

To keep abreast of changing developments or staff demands for high standards of service and to obviate misunderstandings, relationships should be outlined initially and reviewed periodically. This appears to be particularly necessary in those situations where certain elements of services are provided on the hospital premises, and others in varying degrees emanate from sources away from the hospital environment arranged by delegation to others who may be unfamiliar with hospital safeguards and policies.

5. *The organization of pharmaceutical services should include the utilization of an organized Pharmacy and Therapeutics Committee responsible for the development of rules and regulations pertaining to professional policies related to pharmaceutical services for hospital patients.*

Following the usual practice in hospitals, the medical and pharmacy staffs acting in an advisory capacity are the most qualified to recommend to the hospital such policies as relate to selection, evaluation and distribution of drugs used in the hospital. The composition and specific objectives of the Pharmacy and Therapeutics Committee as well as its appointment may be developed to best meet the needs of the hospital and its standards.

Functions

1. *The primary functions of the service provided by a part-time pharmacist should be to furnish drugs with sufficient dispatch so that patient care will not be hindered, to provide adequate safeguards for the patient and hospital personnel, and to provide therapeutic agents of respected quality.*

Responsibilities do not begin or end with filling prescriptions or furnishing drugs remotely from the hospital. The well-rounded and minimum responsibility might include such personal services by the part-time pharmacist as staff education related to safeguards in use of drugs on the premises, contribution to educational or research programs where extant, provision of maximum consultation services to nursing and medical staffs, inspection of drug storage and distribution throughout the hospital, attendance at committee and department meetings, preparation of fiscal and professional reports where necessary, maintenance of an approved stock of emergency drugs, provision for 24-hour drug services, elimination of waste, etc.

2. *Records concerned with hospital patient services should be maintained separately, preserved for the period prescribed by legal or hospital requirements, and be readily available.*

Such records as narcotic, barbiturate, alcohol, prescription, and requisition requests differ between hospitals and retail pharmacy practice. Identification with a hospital transaction or treatment may be of prime importance.

3. *The relationship between the hospital and the part-time pharmacist in the function of drug procurement or purchasing for both patient and general*

hospital use should be based on fixed responsibilities and meet the following principles on Business Relationships.

The smaller hospital generally purchases supplies through a modified central channel in the organization. The need for expert evaluation of specifications in the drug field is recognized. Hospitals contributing services to indigent patients enjoy special price privileges, and drugs in this category ethically should not be diverted to other outlets. The complexity in the area of procurement and possibility of abuses by either the hospital or the part-time pharmacist require careful evaluation of the procedure.

a. That basis of financial arrangement between a hospital and part-time local pharmacist should be followed which would best meet the local situation. It is recognized that no one basis would seem applicable or suitable in all instances.

The hospital and the part-time pharmacist must have a thorough appreciation of each other's business systems and controls. This may involve detailed exploration.

b. Arrangements involving services to patients through voluntary insurance, indigent patients, or employees should be established in accordance with accepted hospital relationships and philosophies involving such programs.

Some insurance plans vary between localities, and in some instances the so-called "no-pay or part-pay" patients comprise a sizable number of persons. Special financial arrangements in accord with hospital policy for other services provided may be required.

c. Arrangements for a regular schedule for the personal services of the part-time pharmacist on the hospital premises should be made on a flexible basis related to time spent and services provided.

The hospital schedule and its 24-hour service to patients demands a varying amount or period spent during regular visits or to meet emergency requirements. In general, an average amount of time may be considered initially. Such an arrangement should be included in a plan, even though many services are provided remotely from the hospital premises.

d. Solicitation of patients or rendering services to the medical staff for their private practice through hospital channels by any person connected with the hospital is unethical.

The privilege of hospital affiliation should not be used to gain unfair advantage over other members of the profession. Patients and physicians are attracted to a particular pharmacy because of its known merit and established reputation for satisfactory service. Implied or open solicitation through hospital connections should not be indulged in by part-time pharmacists.

e. Relationships between a part-time pharmacist and the hospital are considered on the merit of reputable, prompt service to patients ar reasonable cost, ability to serve the hospital in all phases of pharmacy service demanded by hospital requirements, and should subscribe to the suggested principles.

In communities where several pharmacies are available, a hospital may hestitate to engage the services of any one pharmacist because of pressures and ill-feeling against the hospital by other pharmacists. Intra-professional rivalry should not place the hospital in a position of not raising its own pharmacy service standards. The hospital as a community institution should be allowed the privilege of judging its future relationships for expanded services on the basis of a part-time pharmacist's ability to provide those services in the spirit in which patient care is provided in that hospital.

Conclusion

These Principles of Relationship Between Smaller Hospitals and Part-time Pharmacists for Hospitals are suggested. These recommended guides for further development and discussion are a beginning for those hospitals and pharmacists who wish to explore possibilities for developing higher standards of pharmaceutical service in institutions without full-time pharmacists.

A combination of such principles and the Minimum Standard for Pharmacies in Hospitals can provide both smaller hospitals and part-time pharmacists a working basis for a higher level of pharmaceutical service.

Under a part-time plan, the community pharmacist contracts to provide the small hospital with prescription orders and other drug merchandise. He does not agree to partake in any of the routine activities normally engaged in by the hospital pharmacist.

An agreement of this type usually provides that the nurse or the physician telephone to the community pharmacist the patient's drug needs. The compounded prescription is then to be delivered to the hospital with a properly identified charge slip. The hospital then bills and collects for the prescription medication along with the routine hospital charges. At the end of a specified billing period, the community pharmacy renders to the hospital a detailed bill of all prescriptions and other drug stocks less a previously agreed upon discount from the total charges. This discount, therefore, provides the community hospital with a small income from its drug service to compensate for its expenses in the billing and collection of the drug charges.

RESPONSIBILITIES OF COMMUNITY OR CONSULTING PHARMACISTS EXTENDED CARE FACILITIES AND SMALL HOSPITALS

Since most extended care facilities and small hospitals do not employ full time pharmacists, many of them contract for such service. Pharmacists who agree to provide such a service are required by the Medicare law to assume certain responsibilities and perform specific functions. These go far beyond the dispensing of prescriptions for patients but include an interdisciplinary approach towards the provision of consulting pharmaceutical service.

DISPENSING PRESCRIPTIONS FOR EXTENDED CARE FACILITIES AND SMALL HOSPITAL PATIENTS

Extended care facilities, nursing homes and small hospitals do not maintain a full service pharmacy on the premises. Thus, the medical staff relies upon community pharmacists to dispense medications from the local pharmacy and have them delivered to the facility. The labels on these prescriptions, in addition to the customary information, should also indicate:

a. Name of Medication
b. Strength
c. Name of Manufacturer
d. Lot and/or control number

The above information is desirable in the event of a drug recall.

CONSULTING PHARMACEUTICAL SERVICE

Generally, the community or consulting pharmacist is expected to work with the organized medical staff, the Director of Nursing and the Administrator for the purpose of establishing written policies and procedures for the control and utilization of medications in the facility.

These policies are normally referred to as the *Policy and Procedural Manual for Pharmacy Services* and should include, among others, the following subject headings:

1. Automatic "Stop Order" policy.
2. Control system for alcohol and spiritous liquors.
3. Control system for all drugs covered by the Controlled Substances Act of 1971. This Act controls the use of narcotics, barbiturates, amphetamines and certain stimulant and depressant medications.
4. Controls for the use of research drugs.
5. Control of physician's drug samples.
6. Policy governing self administration of medications.
7. Emergency drug kits
   a. Contents
   b. Inspection procedure.
8. Reporting of medication errors.
9. Reporting of adverse drug reactions
10. Periodic inspection of nursing station medication cabinets to insure—
    a. That external medications are kept apart from internal use drugs.
    b. That biological refrigerator has a thermometer, that temperature range of refrigerator is 35.5° to 50° F. (Ice cube section used for small pox, yellow fever, measles and polio vaccines, if stocked, and of types requiring below freezing storage.) Biologicals may also be kept in general use refrigerator providing they are stored in a separate box.
    c. That there are no outdated medications (antibiotics, biologicals, etc.).
    d. That medication cabinets are kept locked.

    e. That Metric-English weight and measure conversion charts are at each nursing station medication center.

    f. That working text references on drug uses, side effects and contraindications, such as the American Hospital Formulary Service of the American Society of Hospital Pharmacists are at nursing station medication centers.

11. Policy on medication labeling.
12. Policy and procedure on removal of medications from pharmacy or drug room in absence of pharmacist.
13. Policy and procedure on medications to be taken home by the patient.
14. Pharmacy or store room inventory control system including the dating of stocks on receipt.
15. Macroscopical (light-testing) examination of parenterals.
16. Policy concerning additives to parenterals.
17. The creation and activities of the Pharmacy and Therapeutics Committee including the keeping of written minutes of meetings.
18. The establishment and maintenance of a formulary of drug list.
19. Fire control provisions.
20. Qualification of pharmacists and experience requirements.
21. Policy on record keeping.
22. Policy on Poison Control Center Communications and references.
23. Audit of narcotics and other "controlled" drugs at nursing stations.
24. An "official" (medical staff approved) list of medical abbreviations applicable to drug administration and dispensing.
25. Application of FDA medication lot number recall "alarm" to the facility.
26. Policy and procedures relative to the writing and signing of medication orders.

SMALL HOSPITAL-LARGE HOSPITAL PHARMACY RELATIONSHIP

Many large hospitals often provide assistance to the smaller hospitals by providing pathology and radiology services. In addition, the small hospital often sends to the larger hospital various specimens of human fluids for comprehensive or special laboratory procedures. Since the avenue of cooperation is opened by the above, is there any reason why the large hospital cannot also provide pharmaceutical coverage?

The pharmacy service between the two hospitals can be handled in the same manner that a retail pharmacist would assume full responsibility for the pharmacy service. In this case it is much simpler for telephone service between the two institutions is open around-the-clock, the pharmacist who is on-call at the larger hospital may also cover the small hospital; and finally the inventory of the large hospital is usually more than adequate to provide for emergency items for the small hospital.

This type of arrangement is mutually advantageous to both hospitals in that it provides the smaller hospital with the services of experienced hospital pharmacists and permits the larger hospital with another opportunity to contribute to the over-all improvement of medical care in the community.

PROGRAM FOR SMALL HOSPITAL WITH NO PHARMACY OR PHARMACIST RELATIONSHIP

Hospitals in this category of having no pharmacy or pharmacist relationship usually rely upon other personnel to handle their daily services. Although nurses are primarily engaged in this practice, it is a known fact that the aides and technicians are also utilized.[1]

Drugs used by these institutions are usually stored in a small room, often referred to as the "drug room." Invariably, it is overcrowded, with no semblance of inventory control.

Even under these conditions, the hospital administrator can undertake a simple program to improve his pharmacy service even though he is unable to secure the minimal services of a part-time pharmacist. The proposed program consists of the following steps:

1. The administrator should call a meeting of representatives of his medical and nursing staffs for the purpose of reviewing the present drug inventory and selecting the medications which the hospital should keep and at the same time ascertain those items not in the inventory but which should be procured.
2. Merchandise in the drug room, not on this list, should be discarded or, where possible, exchanged for medications which have been requested to be added to the inventory.
3. A subscription to the American Hospital Formulary Service should be entered because this will make available to the administrator, doctor and nurse a single, concise and authoritative source of information on the drugs carried in the drug room.
4. All of the drugs and related diagnostic agents should then be purchased in the smallest units possible in order that they may be dispensed to the nursing station without repackaging or labeling (both of which are pharmacy acts). Strip packaging is ideally suited for this type of dispensing.
5. If at all possible, place the responsibility for the drug room in the hands of the hospital's most competent nurse or nursing supervisor.
6. Make some arrangement with the local pharmacy for the purchase of prescriptions calling for mixtures of medications for individual patients.
7. The administrator should meet with his medical and nursing staff at least twice a year in order to keep the inventory current and maintain the interest of all concerned in this aspect of patient care.

Because this program requires the purchase of medications in small individual use packages, the cost per dose of the medication will necessarily be higher to both the hospital and to the patient. This, however, should not deter the administrator from undertaking such a program for in exchange for this slightly higher cost per dose of medication he is providing as safe a pharmaceutical service as is possible under the circumstance.

PHARMACY'S ROLE IN NURSING HOMES—EXTENDED CARE FACILITIES

The United States Public Health Service in its Nursing Home Standards Guide defines the term nursing home as—

"a facility or unit which is designated, staffed and equipped for the accommodation of individuals who are not in need of hospital care but who are in need of nursing care and related medical services which are prescribed by or performed under the direction of persons licensed to provide such care or services in accordance with the laws of the state in which the facility is located."

With the advent of Medicare, a great deal of attention has been focused on the nursing home and the role which it must play in the care of our elderly citizens.

The Nursing Homes and Related Facilities Branch, Division of Medical Care Administration, Public Health Service published a report on licensed nursing homes[4] and related facilities which showed that as of June 1965, there were 18,958 facilities with 760,441 beds in the country who were providing either nursing home services, personal care with nursing services, or plain custodial care.

Other statistics that are of interest are that in 1975 there were as many as 25 million people in this country who were 65 years of age or older; that an additional 70,000 nursing home beds were under construction and that the average nursing home had approximately 66 beds with a range of 40- to 100-bed capacity.

Clearly then, these patients require medical, nursing and pharmaceutical services in a volume which is far greater in scope and concentration than we are able to provide due to the personnel shortages within these three professions.

Thus many community pharmacists and hospital pharmacists will have to do double duty in order for the profession of pharmacy to meet its obligation to these patients.

The relationship between the community pharmacist and/or the local hospital pharmacist would be similar to that of servicing a small community hospital. Since these have been presented earlier in the chapter they will not be repeated here.

Public Law 89–97 provides for certain conditions for a pharmaceutical service in the extended care facility. For the convenience of the reader these are hereinafter reproduced and will serve as guidelines for those pharmacists who do respond to the call for pharmaceutical services in the nursing home.

CONDITION OF PARTICIPATION FOR EXTENDED CARE FACILITIES

PHARMACEUTICAL SERVICES

WHETHER DRUGS ARE GENERALLY PROCURED FROM A COMMUNITY PHARMACY OR STOCKED BY THE FACILITIES, THE EXTENDED CARE FACILITY HAS METHODS AND PROCEDURES FOR ITS PHARMACEUTICAL SERVICES THAT ARE IN ACCORD WITH ACCEPTED PROFESSIONAL PRACTICES.

Standard A

Procedures for Administration of Pharmaceutical Services

The extended care facility provides appropriate methods and procedures for the obtaining, dispensing and administering of drugs and biologicals, developed with the advice of a staff pharmacist, a consultant pharmacist, or a *pharmaceutical advisory committee* which includes one or more licensed pharmacists.

FACTOR 1. If the extended care facility has a pharmacy department, a licensed pharmacist is employed to administer the pharmacy department.

FACTOR 2. If the facility does not have a pharmacy department, it has provision for promptly and conveniently obtaining required drugs and biologicals from community pharmacies.

FACTOR 3. If the facility has only a drug room where bulk drugs are stored:
  (i) The consultant pharmacist is responsible for the control of all bulk drugs and maintains records of their receipt and disposition.
  (ii) The consultant pharmacist dispenses drugs from the drug room, properly labels them and makes them available to appropriate licensed nursing personnel. Wherever possible, the pharmacist in dispensing drugs works from the prescriber's original order or a direct copy.
  (iii) Provision is made for emergency withdrawal of medications from the drug room.

FACTOR 4. An emergency medication kit approved by the facility's group of professional personnel is kept readily available.

Standard B

Conformance With Physician's Orders

All medications administered to patients are ordered in writing by the patient's physician. Oral orders are given only to a licensed nurse, immediately reduced to writing, signed by the nurse and countersigned by the physician within 48 hours. Medications not specifically limited as to time or number of doses, when ordered, are automatically stopped in accordance with written policy approved by the physician or physicians responsible for advising the facility on its medical administrative policies.

FACTOR 1. The charge nurse and the prescribing physician together review monthly each patient's medications.

FACTOR 2. The patient's attending physician is notified of stop order policies and contracted promptly for renewal of such orders so that continuity of the patient's therapeutic regimen is not interrupted.

FACTOR 3. Medications are released to patients on discharge only on the written authorization of the physician.

Standard C

Administration of Medications

All medications are administered by licensed medical or nursing personnel in accordance with the Medical and Nurse Practice Acts of each State.
Each dose administered is properly recorded in the clinical record.

FACTOR 1. The nursing station has readily available items necessary for the proper administration of medication.

FACTOR 2. In administering medications, medication cards or other State approved systems are used and checked against the physician's orders.

FACTOR 3. Medications prescribed for one patient are not administered to any other patient.

FACTOR 4. Self-administration of medications by patients is not permitted except for emergency drugs on special order of the patient's physician or in a predischarge program under the supervision of a licensed nurse.

FACTOR 5. Medication errors and drug reactions are immediately reported to the patient's physician and an entry thereof made in the patient's clinical record as well as on an incident report.

FACTOR 6. Up-to-date medication reference texts and sources of information are provided, such as *ASHP Hospital Formulary* and *Physicians Desk Reference*.

Standard D

Labeling and Storing Medications

Patients' medications are properly labeled and stored in a locked cabinet at the nurses' station.

FACTOR 1. The label of each patient's individual medication container clearly indicates the patient's full name, physician's name, prescription number, name and strength of drug, date of issue, expiration date of all time-dated drugs, and name, address and telephone number of pharmacy issuing the drug. It is advisable that the manufacturer's name and the lot or control number of the medication also appear on the label.

FACTOR 2. Medication containers having soiled, damaged, incomplete, illegible, or makeshift labels are returned to the issuing pharmacist or pharmacy for re-labeling or disposal. Containers having no labels are destroyed in accordance with State and Federal laws.

FACTOR 3. The medications of each patient are kept and stored in their originally received containers and transferring between containers is forbidden.

FACTOR 4. Separately locked, securely fastened boxes (or drawers) within the medicine cabinet are provided for storage of narcotics, barbiturates, amphetamines and other dangerous drugs.

FACTOR 5. Cabinets are well lighted and of sufficient size to permit storage without crowding.

FACTOR 6. Medications requiring refrigeration are kept in a separate, locked box within a refrigerator at or near the nursing station.

FACTOR 7. Poisons and medications "for external use only" are kept in a locked cabinet and separate from other medications.

FACTOR 8. Medications no longer in use are disposed of or destroyed in accordance with Federal and State laws and regulations.

FACTOR 9. Medications having an expiration date are removed from usage and properly disposed of after such date.

Standard E

Compliance With Laws Controlling Narcotics, Etc.

The extended care facility complies with all Federal and State laws relating to the procurement, storage, dispensing, administration and disposal of narcotics, hypnotics, amphetamines, certain psychosomatic medications, and other legend drugs.

FACTOR 1. A narcotic record is maintained which lists on separate sheets for each type and strength of narcotic the following information: date, time administered, name of patient, dose, physician's name, signature of person administering dose, and balance.

DRUG SAFETY

The consultant pharmacist serving the nursing home and the extended care facility has the obligation of ensuring safe medication practices in the facility. This goes far beyond the accepted procedures of proper dispensing and labeling of medications and their containers. The horizon for the initiation of control measures is limitless and depends upon the ingenuity of the consultant. However, two tried and true methods are readily available.

First, the consultant pharmacist should maintain a patient drug profile on each and every patient in the unit. Again, these profiles vary with the facility and the pharmacist however. Reference to Figure 94 provides the pharmacist with one type of profile. Some of the items on this profile may appear to be superfluous to some yet they have proven useful on occasion. These are the data on "religion" and SIL (seriously ill list). The religion information has been useful whenever the patient was likely to have blood or blood products prescribed and the use of such products was against his religious beliefs. The data indicating whether or not the patient was considered so ill as to warrant placement on the seriously ill list may be of use to the pharmacist in his discussions

PBBH

I. GENERAL INFORMATION | Frequency |

TPR		Diet: Regular	Activities of Daily Living:	
BP		Special: specify	Bathing:	
Intake			Eating:	
Output		Fluids:	Mobility:	

Date	II.	Medications		III. Diagnostic Tests				
			Date Ord.	X-ray	Date Done	Lab.	Date Done
				EKG			
				Special			

IV.

No. _____ Adm. Date _____ Religion _____ SIL _____

Name _____ Adm. Diagnosis _____

FORM 241

Fig. 94.   Patient profile form in use in one institution.

with the physician and nursing staff. In addition, it helps to emphasize the urgency with which changes in the therapeutic regimen must be made.

Second, the routine inspection of the nursing station is of great importance in that it helps to remove out-dated and deteriorated medications from the medication closet and helps to check to see that products are properly labeled and stored. A sample check list is presented in Figure 95.

HOSPICE PROGRAMS

The National Hospice Organization defines the hospice concept as follows:[5]

A hospice is a centrally administered program of palliative and supportive services which provides physical, psychological, social, and spiritual care for dying persons and their families. Services are provided by a medically supervised interdisciplinary team of professionals and volunteers. Hospice services may be available in either the home or in an institutional setting. Home care can be provided on a parttime, intermittent, regularly scheduled, or around the

PETER BENT BRIGHAM HOSPITAL
Nursing Unit Inspection Guide
Department of Pharmacy

Unit_____
Date_____

Routine_____
Follow-up_____

A. INDIVIDUAL PATIENT DRUGS:
  1. Present arrangement and space allotment for inpatient med-
      dications is satisfactory . . . . Yes___No___
  2. All drugs have been returned to pharmacy for credit fol-
      lowing discontinuation or patient discharge . . . . . . Yes___No___
  3. All labels on medication containers are accurate, are
      not defaced, and necessary accessory labels are present . Yes___No___
  4. Injectable medications are properly labeled as to date
      of reconstitution, concentration, expiration date (in
      addition to patient room-number, name and date). . . . .. Yes___No___
  5. Drugs requiring refrigeration are properly stored . . . . Yes___No___

B. CHARGE FLOOR STOCK DRUGS:
  1. Stock level for each item is adequate . . . . Yes___No___
  2. All items have charge voucher attached . . . . Yes___No___
  3. All items are appropriately labeled and stored . . . . . Yes___No___

C. FREE FLOOR STOCK-DRUGS:
  1. Present arrangement and space allotment for floor stock
      is satisfactory . . . . Yes___No___
  2. All items are properly labeled . . . . Yes___No___
  3. All labels are in satisfactory condition . . . . Yes___No___
  4. Internal drugs are separated from external drugs . . . .. Yes___No___
  5. All items are in adequate supply . . . . Yes___No___

D. EMERGENCY STOCK DRUGS:
  1. Emergency box is in proper place . . . . Yes___No___
  2. Emergency cart is ready for use . . . . Yes___No___
  3. All drugs are in date . . . . Yes___No___

E. REFRIGERATED DRUGS:
  1. All drugs are in the appropriate compartment . . . . Yes___No___
  2. All drugs are properly and completely labeled
      (expiration date, concentration, reconstitution date
      etc.) . . . . Yes___No___

F. NARCOTICS, BARBITURATES AND CONTROLLED SUBSTANCES:
  1. The narcotic drawer is locked . . . . Yes___No___
  2. The key is with the Head Nurse (or nurse in charge) . . . Yes___No___
  3. All drugs are currently being used . . . . Yes___No___

Notes and comments as a result of discussion of inspection form with
Nurse:_____
_____
_____
_____

All Drugs Removed from the Unit have been reviewed with the Nurse.

Signed:
_____Pharmacist_____Nurse

Copy-1 - Pharmacy   Copy-2 - Nursing Unit   Copy-3 - Nursing Unit

Fig. 95. Sample Nursing Unit Inspection Guide.

clock on-call basis. Bereavement services are available to the family. Admission to hospice program of care is on the basis of patient and family needs.

Many home health agencies have developed hospice care programs designed to meet the needs of the terminally ill patient and his or her family. Pharmacist involvement with hospices has been limited and varies with each setting. Some functions performed by consulting pharmacists include but are not limited to the following.[5]

1. Provides skilled evaluation of the use of drugs and biologicals in hospice care with emphasis on drug interactions and symptom control.
2. Conducts a monthly review of the drug protocol of each hospice patient.
3. Serves as a liaison with other community pharmacists and pharmacies to provide 24-hour pharmaceutical service for patients and their families.
4. Conducts in-service training for hospice staff.

SELECTED READINGS

Chappell, N.L. and Barmes, G.E.: The Practicing Pharmacist and the Elderly Client. Contemp. Pharm. Pract., 5:3:170, (Summer) 1982.
Chase, P.A.: Progressive Pharmaceutical Services in a Community Hospital. Am. J. Hosp. Pharm., 41:7:1338, (July) 1984.
Shannon, R.C. and DeMuth, J.E.: Application of Federal Indicators in Nursing-Home Drug-Regimen Review. Am. J. Hosp. Pharm., 41:5:912, (May) 1984.
Sones, S.S.: Compensation for Consultant Pharmacy Services to Long-Term Care Facilities. Contemp. Pharm. Pract., 5:3:161, (Summer) 1982.

REFERENCES

1. Francke, D.E., Latiolais, C.J., Francke, G.N. and Ho, N.F.H.: *Mirror To Hospital Pharmacy,* p. 169. American Society of Hospital Pharmacists, Washington, D.C.
2. Extending Pharmacy Services in Smaller Hospitals. Am. Prof. Pharm., 22:6:540, 1956.
3. Suggested Principles of Relationship Between Smaller Hospitals and Part-Time Pharmacists. Am. J. Hosp. Pharm., 16:3:124, 1959.
4. Conditions and Participation for Extended Care Facilities, U.S. Dept. Health, Education and Welfare, Washington, D.C., Government Printing Office (HIM 3 1966).
5. Whigham, Jr. W.D. and Roberts, K.B.: Considerations When Proposing Consultant Pharmacist Services to Hospice Programs. Contemp. Pharm. Pract., 5:4:239, (Fall) 1982.

30|

Computers in the Hospital Pharmacy

With the improved technology in word processing and computer hardware, the cost of this equipment is within reach of most hospital pharmacies. The literature is replete with innovative programs utilizing computers for automated inventory control,[1] drug interaction computer data base,[2] IV admixture programs,[3] clinical pharmacy services,[4] departmental productivity reporting,[5] drug information filing[6] and unit dose drug distributions.[7]

Prior to commencing work on the acquisition of a computer, the hospital pharmacist should become knowledgeable with the specialized terminology used by computer sales personnel; consult with the institutional data processing manager to determine whether the system to be installed is dependent or independent of the central computer; and finally to ascertain the capability of the equipment and program.

TERMINOLOGY

The following are some of the commonly used words and phrases that the student should master prior to embarking upon a program to acquire a computer.[8]

A *computer* is an apparatus that can perform logical and mathematical operations by mechanical or electrical means, or both, following specific instructions in a controlled sequence.

Hardware means the physical equipment, i.e., the mechanical, magnetic, electrical or electronic devices.

Software means a set of procedures, programs concerned with the operation of the data processing system.

Bytes are characters, either numbers or letters.

Megabytes means 1 million bytes.

32K memory means 32 thousand positions of memory storage.

CPU stands for a central processing unit.

CRT is a cathode-ray tube, a video screen, that is used to display information.

VDT is a video display terminal. Same as CRT.

Mainframe or *HIS (Hospital Information System)* is a hospital-wide system that consists of various departmental modules and can enter or *input* information to and retrieve, or *output,* information from a central source, i.e., the mainframe or computer bank.

"Down" means that period when the system is not operable.

Hard copies are printed records of information that has been entered into the system.

"Stand-alone system" is one that does not depend on the in-house mainframe to operate.

"Floppy" disc is a magnetic recording device, similar to a phonograph record.

Default may be defined as a type of programmed shorthand whereby the system has defined the usual form of data entry for that practice setting.

RAM stands for random access memory.

LANs stands for local area network.

Network is a system of connected computers that permits communication between computers.

PROGRAM CRITERIA

One of the preliminary steps that must be undertaken is to ascertain the capability of the hardware and software to be installed. There are many ways of doing this but the simplest is to interrogate the vendor and the data processing manager. Typical questions are . . . can the proposed system:

1. respond to the need to update patient profiles;
2. readily provide the patient's medication profile;
3. reduce or eliminate the ministerial functions associated with the ordering of patient medications;
4. be supportive of ongoing unit dose dispensing, IV admixture and hyper-alimentation programs;
5. be readily accessed in order to update cost price and charge price. In this same regard, can the system reduce or eliminate the burden or pricing drug order slips for the accounting department;
6. eliminate prescription label typing;
7. provide adequate inventory control;
8. provide better control through effectively monitoring allergies and interactions between two or more drugs, drugs and foods or drugs and laboratory procedures;
9. accommodate the hospital formulary, National Drug Code or the Drug Product Information file of the American Society of Hospital Pharmacists;
10. provide medication labels as a by-product of order entry;
11. accommodate support of an IV admixture program by calculating hand times and drip rates;
12. upon ordering of medications can the system automatically update the medication profile;

13. display all active and discontinued medications plus patient's diagnosis, dietary and allergy precautions;
14. provide a daily "medication administration record" which lists all medications to be administered to a patient during the next 24 hours. This hard copy should be able to be used for the charging function;
15. be used to provide a count of all drugs administered during the patient's entire hospitalization;
16. be used to support a unit dose program by providing daily "fill reports."

Reid[9] reports that computer technology has advanced at such an awesome speed during the last few years that even sophisticated specialists find it difficult to keep up with the latest developments in computer equipment and programs. Thus, he advocates the following "Ten Commandments for Computer Health."

1. Know the vendor's reputation.
2. Know the vendor's experience.
3. Know what features you want and need.
4. Know the true cost.
5. Examine the vendor's proposal.
6. Know and test the system's design quality.
7. Know the system's performance and reliability.
8. Know who's going to install it.
9. Be sure of ongoing support.
10. Is the vendor willing to negotiate?

MANAGING COMPUTER SYSTEM DEVELOPMENT

Once the decision concerning development of a computer system has been made, authorities[10] in the field believe that for the program to succeed consideration should be given to the following:

1. An employee training program should be developed and initiated.
2. A pharmacist should be appointed to coordinate the continued development of the system.
3. Responsibility and methodology for data base accuracy and integrity must be assigned from the start.

The training program may be divided into two parts: a general orientation and a formal training program which should include the following:[11]

1. Computer terminology,
2. Hardware operation demonstration,
3. Description of each function,
5. Delineation of policy and procedures,
6. Manual back-up system description and demonstration of printouts, reports and labels.

Pickett[12] has stated that after recognition of the need to computerize, three general planning or developmental processes need to be completed by the pharmacy manager—operations analysis, financial analysis and administrative analysis. Although these processes represent a common approach to computerization planning for all pharmacy managers, they will vary by degree from one hospital to another.

Operations analysis in computer planning is sometimes called systems audit and serves to quantify and qualify the functions of a department.[12]

The financial analysis must be well developed, with all potential costs and benefits addressed. Examples of costs beyond hardware and software purchases as least costs, include the cost of redundant systems during conversion; additional personnel in training and adaptation; form changes and the purchase of computer paper; professional consultation for problems or changes; additional utility overhead, system maintenance; remodeling and installation requirements; and interface with other automated systems.[12]

Administrative analysis is the consideration of activities and variables that are not part of a financial or operations analysis. For example, reduction in medication error potential or reduction in employee orientation time. The use of the computer may also affect legal or regulatory compliance.[12] System Selection

Because of the widespread use of computers and the lower acquisition cost of hardware and related programs, pharmacists have a choice as to the route to automation. Generally the two routes most considered are the mainframe and the mini-HIS, dedicated standalone.

The mainframe system is the most complex to install yet offers the advantage of being able to serve multiple users and to integrate vast amounts of data, such as patient information, laboratory data, physicians' orders as they are written and daily billing via the patient profile.[13]

The stand-alone system is one that does not have to rely on the in-house mainframe to operate. The advantage of this is that the system remains functional when the mainframe is non-operational. Because this system operates independently of the main system, information present in the main unit has to be entered separately into this system. One way to reduce this duplication of effort is to interface the stand-alone system with the main unit via cable connections and special programming or by having the standalone system produce output in a format that can be interpreted by the main unit through a buffer mechanism which possesses the data.[8]

The disadvantages are that it must serve too many users with varying requirements thus making it difficult to make program changes without compromise, a route that is time consuming and often frustrating.[13] In addition, if the main hospital system is not in operation, the pharmacy module is also non-functional.

The New England Medical Center[14] and The Ohio State University Hospitals[15] have chosen the mainframe system. The success of these installations is purported to be that the control of the system design was vested in pharmacist users and not in system analysts at a distant headquarters.[13]

The pharmacy computer system at the Ohio State University Hospitals was developed to make more efficient use of equipment and professional staff time. Like many other pharmacy systems, this one operates on the mainframe hospital system using computer terminals with light-pen and keyboard access. On-line applications include order entry, patient profiles, pharmacokinetic calculations, and preparation of unit dose cart fill lists. Batch processing functions include drug-use review, drug-drug interactions and financial management reports. It is reported that the system saves considerable staff time in the i.v. admixture and billing areas and relieves pharmacists from performing many clerical and repetitive tasks. The disadvantages of the system include (i) its dependence on another department for patient admission, transfer and discharge information and (ii) delays in obtaining approval for program modification and applications.[15]

The ASHP Technical Assistance Bulletin on Hospital Drug Distribution and Control[16] provides the following data on computerization of the hospital pharmacy.

ASHP TECHNICAL ASSISTANCE BULLETIN ON HOSPITAL DRUG DISTRIBUTION AND CONTROL

Computerization. Many information-handling tasks in the drug control system (e.g., collecting, recording, storing, retrieving, summarizing, transmitting and displaying drug use information) may be done more efficiently by computers than by manual systems. Before the drug control system can be computerized, however, a comprehensive, thorough study of the existing manual system must be conducted. This study should identify the data flow within the system and define the functions to be done and their interrelationships. This information is then used as the basis to design or prospectively evaluate a computer system; any other considerations, such as those of the hospital accounting department, are subordinate.

The computer system must include adequate safeguards to maintain the confidentiality of patient records.

A backup system must be available to continue the computerized functions during equipment failure. All transactions occurring while the computer system is inoperable should be entered into the system as soon as possible.

Data on controlled substances must be readily retrievable in written form from the system.

IMPACT OF THE COMPUTER ON DISPENSING TIME

The effect of computerization on dispensing time in a hospital-affiliated ambulatory care pharmacy was studied.[17]

Based on mean times for each activity, prescription processing time per patient (average of 1.5 prescriptions) was 7.0 minutes for both new and refill prescriptions using manual dispensing, 6.28 minutes for new prescriptions using computer-assisted dispensing, and 4.61 minutes for refill prescriptions using computer-assisted dispensing. Computerization eliminated 78 minutes of time spent on miscellaneous activities each day and added 58.67 minutes of time for computer related activities each day. A net time savings of 196.58 minutes was realized for a prescription volume of 176 prescriptions per day.

MODEL COMPUTER REGULATIONS

The National Association of Boards of Pharmacy has developed a set of Model Computer Regulations[a] which contain important information for use in planning for the computerization of a pharmacy. They are hereinafter reproduced for the convenience of the student and practitioner.

Purpose and Scope

It is the intent of this model regulation to deal with and to define certain procedures that will not only comply with state and federal regulations, but will assist to facilitate the inspection of those pharmacies employing the use of a computer, by the regulatory body charged with compliance. Computerization is a vital component of the pharmacy profession, primarily related to the facet of recordkeeping.

This model regulation will serve as a guideline for all NABP member states wishing to utilize such a composite in developing their own legislation. Jurisdictions may use all or part of this model in promulgating their own regulation or rules to insure compliance with their statutes and/or regulations or rules.

NOTE: Information presented in brackets [   ] represents institutional pharmacy requirements.

---

[a]Available from the NABP copy desk at 1 East Wacker Drive, Suite 2210, Chicago, Ill. 60601

Glossary

AUTOMATED DATA PROCESSING SYSTEM: a system utilizing computer software and hardware for the purposes of recordkeeping

CRT: cathode ray tube used to impose visual information on a screen

COMPUTER: programable electronic device capable of multifunctions including but not limited to storage, retrievel, and processing of information

CONTROLLED (DANGEROUS) SUBSTANCES: those drug items regulated by federal (CSA of 1970) and/or state controlled (dangerous) substances acts

DOWNTIME: that period of time when a computer is not operable

HARDWARE: the fixed component parts of a computer

NABP: National Association of Boards of Pharmacy

PHYSICIAN DRUG ORDER: In institutional practice/settings, this is a drug order written in the patient's chart for a specific patient which is generally sent by the pharmacy to the nursing station for administration. It is not necessarily reduced to writing as a prescription would be.

PRESCRIBER: a practitioner authorized to prescribe and acting within the scope of this authorization

PRESCRIPTION: a written order from a practitioner authorized to prescribe and acting within the scope of this authorization (other terminology: prescription order), or a telephone order reduced to writing by the pharmacist.

PRINTOUT: a hard copy produced by computer that is readable without the aid of any special device

REGULATORY AGENCY: any federal or state agency charged with enforcement of pharmacy or drug laws and regulations

SOFTWARE: programs, procedures and storage of required information data

STOP DATE: In institutional settings, the physician normally indicates on his drug order, the length of time to administer the medication. In absence of such a notation, a committee will have determined by policy, the length of administration of drugs by category.

Regulation

    I. Prescription [or drug order] Requirements

        A.   Prescriptions [or drug orders] shall include, but not be limited to:

            1. date of issuance;

            2. name and address of patient [or patient location if an institution];

            3. name and address of prescriber [if not a staff physician of institution];

            4. DEA number of prescriber in the case of controlled substances;

5. name, strength, dosage form and quantity [or stop date, and route of administration] of drug prescribed;
6. refills authorized;
7. directions of use for patient.

II. Records of Dispensing

  A. Records of dispensing for original and refill prescriptions are to be made and kept by pharmacies for five years and shall include, but not be limited to:

    1. quantity dispensed, if different;
    2. date of dispensing;
    3. serial number [or equivalent if an institution];
    4. the identification of the pharmacist responsible for dispensing;
    5. documentation of satisfaction of state requirements for drug product selection;
    6. records of refills to date.

III. Automated Data Processing Systems

  A. As an alternative to procedures in section I and II, an automated data processing system may be employed for the recordkeeping system if the following conditions have been met:

    1. the system shall have the capability of producing sight-readable documents of all original and refilled prescription information. The term sight-readable means that a regulatory agent or Attorney General shall be able to examine the record and read the information. During the course of an on-site inspection, the record may be read from the cathode ray tube (CRT), microfiche, microfilm, printout or other method acceptable to the Board. In the case of administrative proceedings before the Board, records must be provided in a paper printout form.

    2. such information shall include, but not be limited to the prescription requirements and records of dispensing as indicated in sections I and II of this regulation.

    3. the individual pharmacist responsible for completeness and accuracy of the entries to system must provide documentation of the fact that prescription information entered into the computer is correct. In documenting this information, the pharmacy shall have the option to either:

      a. maintain a bound log book, or separate file, in which each individual pharmacist involved in such dispensing shall sign a statement each day, attesting to the fact that the prescription information entered into the computer that day has been reviewed and is correct as shown. Such a book or file must be maintained at the pharmacy employing such a system for a period of five years after the date of last dispensing; or

      b. provide a printout of each day's prescription information. That printout shall be verified, dated, and signed by the individual pharmacist verifying that the information indicated is correct and then sign this document in the same manner as signing a check or legal document (e.g., J. H. Smith, or John H. Smith). Such printout must be maintained five years from date of last dispensing.

    4. Documentation in No. 3 above, must be provided to the pharmacy within 72 hours of date of dispensing.

    5. An auxiliary recordkeeping system shall be established for the

documentation of refills if the automated data processing system is inoperative for any reason. The auxiliary system shall insure that all refills are authorized by the original prescription and that the maximum number of refills is not exceeded. When this automated data processing system is restored to operation, the information regarding prescriptions filled and refilled during the inoperative period shall be entered into the automated data processing system within 96 hours. However, nothing in this section shall preclude the pharmacist from using his professional judgment for the benefit of a patient's health and safety.

6. Any pharmacy using an automated data processing system must comply with all applicable state and federal laws and regulations.

7. A pharmacy shall make arrangements with the supplier of data processing services or materials to assure that the pharmacy continues to have adequate and complete prescription and dispensing records if the relationship with such supplier terminates for any reason. A pharmacy shall assure continuity in the maintenance of records.

IV. Security
A. To maintain the confidentiality of patients' prescriptions [or drug orders], there must exist adequate safeguards or security of the records.

(Optional Sections)

V. Pharmacies utilizing automated data processing systems must satisfy all information requirements of a manual mode for prescription transferral. Transfer between pharmacies of prescription information for refill purposes:
A. The transfer of original prescription information for the purpose of refill dispensing is permissable between pharmacies subject to the following requirements:
1. The transfer is communicated directly between two licensed pharmacists and the transferring pharmacist records the following information:
a. write the word "VOID" on the face of the invalidated prescription;
b. record on the reverse of the invalidated prescription the name and address of the pharmacy to which it was transferred and the name of the pharmacist receiving the prescription information;
c. record the date of the transfer and the name of the pharmacist transferring the information.
B. The pharmacist receiving the transferred prescription information shall reduce to writing the following:
1. write the word "TRANSFER" on the face of the transferred prescription;
2. provide all information required to be on a prescription pursuant to state and federal laws and regulations and include:
a. date of issuance of original prescription;
b. original number of refills authorized on original prescription;
c. date of original dispensing;

        d.   number of valid refills remaining and date of last refill;

        e.   pharmacy's name, address, and original prescription number from which the prescription information was transferred;

        f.   name of transferor pharmacist.

   C.   Both the original and transferred prescription must be maintained for a period of five years from the date of last refill.

      1.   Pharmacies utilizing automated data processing systems must satisfy all information requirements of a manual mode for prescription transferral.

VI.   Pharmacies utilizing automated data processing systems must satisfy all information requirements of a manual mode for prescription transferral. Transfer between pharmacies of prescription information for Schedules III, IV, and V controlled (dangerous) substances for refill purposes:

   A.   The transfer of original prescription information for a controlled (dangerous) substance listed in Schedules III, IV, or V for the purpose of refill dispensing is premissable between pharmacies on a one time basis subject to the following requirements:

      1.   The transfer is communicated directly between two licensed pharmacists and the transferring pharmacist records the following information:

        a.   write the word "VOID" on the face of the invalidated prescription;

        b.   record on the reverse of the invalidated prescription the name, address, and DEA registration number of the pharmacy to which it was transferred and the name of the pharmacist receiving the prescription information;

        c.   record the date of the transfer and the name of the pharmacist transferring the information.

   B.   The pharmacist receiving the transferred prescription information shall reduce to writing the following:

      1.   Write the word "TRANSFER" on the face of the transferred prescription.

      2.   Provide all information to be on a prescription pursuant to state and federal laws and regulations and include:

        a.   date of issuance of original prescription;

        b.   original number of refills authorized on original prescription;

        c.   date of original dispensing;

        d.   number of valid refills remaining and date of last refill;

        e.   pharmacy's name, address, DEA registration number, and original prescription number from which the prescription information was transferred;

        f.   name of transferor pharmacist.

      3.   Both the original and transferred prescription must be maintained for a period of five years from the date of last refill.

SELECTED READINGS

Knight, J.R.: Computers in Hospital Pharmacy: A Review of the Literature. Topics in Hosp. Pharm. Mgt., *1*:4:1, (Feb.) 1982.

Browning, W.C., Hurd, P.D., Bootman, J.L., Tausik, D.A. nd McGhan, W.F.: Diffusion of

Innovation: Computer Technology in Hospital Pharmacy. Am. J. Hosp. Pharm., *41*:2343–2437, 1984.
Swanson, D.S., Broekemeir, R.L., and Anderson, M.W.: Hospital Pharmacy Computer Systems—1982. Am. J. Hosp. Pharm., *39*:2109–2117, 1982.
Lockwood, Jr. W.A. and Bauman, N.R.: Current and Coming Technology in Hospital Pharmacy Automation. Topics in Hosp. Pharm. Mgt., *4*:1:1, (May) 1984.
Seiker, B.R.: Outpatient Hospital Computer Systems. Topics in Hosp. Pharm. Mgt., *4*:1:26, (May) 1984.

REFERENCES

1. Bradish, R.A.: Changing an Automated Drug Inventory Control System to a Data Base Design. Am. J. Hosp. Pharm., *39*:1502–1505, (Sept.) 1982.
2. Fraser, D.G.: The Development or Purchase of a Drug Interaction Computer Data Base. Topics in Hosp. Pharm. Mgt., *4*:1:52, (May) 1984.
3. Pope, R.A., Slack, M.V., Janousek, J.P., and Mattson, C.J.: A Computer-based IV Admixture System. Topics in Hosp. Pharm. Mgt., *4*:1:43, (May) 1984.
4. Chamberlain, M.A.: Computerized Support of Clinical Pharmacy Services. Topics in Hosp. Pharm. Mgt., *1*:4:37, (Feb.) 1982.
5. Adams, C., Tuck, B.A., and Hung, Jr. M.L.: Departmental Productivity Reporting Through Computerized Systems. Topics in Hosp. Pharm. Mgt., *1*:4:47, (Feb.) 1982.
6. Decker, E.L.: The Drug File: Foundation of the Computerized Pharmacy. Topics in Hosp. Pharm. Mgt., *4*:1:35, (May) 1984.
7. Gouveia, W.A.: Computerized Applications in Unit Dose Drug Distribution Systems. Am. J. Hosp. Pharm., *41*:2092–2093, 1984.
8. Sica-Mancini, J.: Basic Concepts to Consider Before Computerizing a Hospital Pharmacy. Cur. Concepts in Hosp. Pharm. Mgts., *3*:4:14 (Klinter) 1981.
9. Reid, W.: Ten Commandments to Ensure a Healthy Computer System. L. & H. Perspective, *9*:1:19, 1983.
10. Gouveia, W.A. and Nold, E.G.: Computer Systems Planning, Development and Impact Assessment. Am. J. Hosp. Pharm., *30*:2117–2124, 1982.
11. Mildenberger, J. and Gouveia, W.A.: Managing the Implementation of a Pharmacy Computer System. Am. J. Hosp. Pharm., *39*:1692–1701, 1982.
12. Puckert, Jr. W.H.: Developing a Request for Proposal for a Pharmacy Computer System. Topics in Hosp. Pharm. Mgt., *1*:4:19, (Feb.) 1982.
13. Nold, E.G.: Pros and Cons of Main Frame Pharmacy Computer Systems. Am. J. Hosp. Pharm., *41*:1812–1813, 1984.
14. Gouveia, W.A., Mildenberger, J.M., Decker, E.L., and Lynn, V.: The Pharmacy Computer System at the New England Medical Center. Am. J. Hosp. Pharm., *41*:1812–1823, 1984.
15. Moore, T.D., Dzierba, S.H., and Miller, A.: The Pharmacy Computer System at the Ohio State University Hospitals. Am. J. Hosp. Pharm., *41*:2384–2389, 1984.
16. ASHP Technical Assistance Bulletin on Hospital Drug Distribution and Control. Am. J. Hosp. Pharm., *37*:1097–1103, (Aug.) 1980.
17. Moss, R.L. and Pounders, J.N.: Impact of Computerization on Dispensing Time in an Ambulatory-care Pharmacy. Am. J. Hosp. Pharm., *42*:309–312, 1985.

31|

Professional Practices and Relations

The hospital pharmacists of this country can, and in many instances do, carry on a professional and public relations program. The literature is replete with evidence of the need of promoting pharmacy to its kindred professions and to the public.

Hospital pharmacists are in an excellent position to do the profession a great service because of their daily contact with the members of the allied professions and a sizeable segment of the public.

OPPORTUNITIES FOR A PUBLIC RELATIONS PROGRAM

The hospital pharmacy in an average size hospital is the focal point for about 15 to 20 physicians each day in addition to a number of nurses, technicians, and other allied specialists. Therefore, hospital pharmacists can promote pharmacy by instituting and following through with a good professional relations program. Obviously, the execution of such a program will cost very little from a monetary standpoint but will call for an investment of time and effort on the part of those participating. Moreover, despite the tremendous amount of money spent by the drug industry in promoting their products to physicians, there are some doctors who just will not be detailed, will not read their direct mail or journal advertising or who cannot be contacted; but there are relatively few doctors who do not have hospital affiliations and, therefore, they can be contacted by the hospital pharmacist.

Walsh and Hassan[1] have stated that a reasonable program of professional promotion for hospital pharmacy involves the application of the following:

1. Publishing and distributing a pharmacy bulletin.
2. Cooperating in hospital teaching program.
3. Taking an active role in administrative committee work.
4. Taking an active role in pharmaceutical organizations.
5. Cooperating with the medical research staff.
6. Maintaining an adequate reference library.
7. Cooperating with community pharmacists.

8. Accepting speaking engagements.
9. Preparing hospital pharmacy displays.
10. Developing and maintaining the hospital formulary.
11. Maintaining an efficient, professional pharmacy.
12. Being a safety expert.
13. Maintaining a well-controlled manufacturing section.
14. Making special promotional efforts.

PARTICIPATION IN ADMINISTRATIVE COMMITTEE WORK

There seems to be no limit to the number and kind of committees on which the hospital pharmacist may serve. This type of work offers him the opportunity of demonstrating his ability and college training in the medical sciences as well as business administration. Many hospital pharmacists are currently serving on such committees as the Current Practice Committee, Safety Committee, Infection Control Committee, Antibiotics Committee and the Administrative Policy Committee.

The American Society of Hospital Pharmacists has long recognized the important role to be played by the hospital pharmacist as a member of the institution's infection control committee, a view that has now been supported by the American Hospital Association. The following **Statement on the Hospital Pharmacist's Role in Infection Control**[7] is a valuable tool for the institutional practitioner:

ASHP STATEMENT ON THE HOSPITAL PHARMACIST'S ROLE IN INFECTION CONTROL[a]

Hospital-acquired (nosocomial) infections are a significant and complex problem having broad implications for almost every hospital department. In addition, infections acquired in the community and present at the time of hospital admission have nosocomial significance because of the measures required to prevent their spread to other patients and hospital personnel.

Therefore, it is imperative that a hospital have an infection control committee or an equivalent organized method for dealing with the probelm of hospital-associated infections. This "infection control mechanism" should include (at a minimum) representatives from the medical, nursing, pharmaceutical,[b] microbiological and administrative staffs of the hospital. Among its basic responsibilities are the following:

1. Development of written standards for hospital sanitation and asepsis.
2. Development and promulgation of procedures and techniques for meeting these standards and monitoring compliance with them.
3. Development and implementation of a system for eliciting, reporting and

---

[a]Approved by the ASHP Board of Directors, November 14–15, 1977, and by the ASHP House of Delegates, May 15, 1978.

[b]The American Hospital Association has endorsed the recommendation that infection control committees include a pharmacist.

evaluating data concerning infections in the hospitals' patient and personnel populations.
4. Development and implementation of a system for the routine surveillance and review of antimicrobial use within the hospital.

The infection control system operates through, and in cooperation with, the appropriate hospital committees and departments.

Infection Control and the Department of Pharmaceutical Services

The department of pharmaceutical services in a hospital, via its role in controlling and distributing antimicrobial drugs and disinfectants, will obviously play an important part in such infection-control activities as antibiotic use monitoring. However, it also is true that the hospital pharmacy can be the cause, as well as part of the cure, of nosocomial infection problems. Contaminated drug products, prepared and/or distributed by the pharmacy, can and have been the source of hospital-acquired infections. Few hospitalized patients do not receive drugs. Therefore, pharmacists have a clear mandate to take the steps necessary to eliminate, to the extent possible, this source of infection.

The Pharmacist's Role in Infection Control

In light of the foregoing, it is obvious hospital pharmacists have a key role in hospital infection control. In meeting this obligation, they must:

1. Actively participate in the affairs of the infection control committee or its equivalent.
2. Assure the microbiological integrity of all products distributed by the pharmacy, particularly those required to be sterile. Of utmost importance is that the best possible aseptic technique and attendant environmental control be used in the preparation and administration of parenteral admixtures, prefilled syringes, ophthalmics and other sterile products.
3. Advise the hospital on the selection and use of appropriate antimicrobial drugs, disinfectants and sterilants.
4. Establish and operate (in cooperation with the medical staff) an ongoing antibiotic use review program for assessing and improving the quality of antibiotic therapy. In addition to this quality assurance mechanism, quantitative data on antimicrobial drug use should be routinely generated and analyzed.
5. Develop and conduct relevant continuing education programs for hospital staff concerning antimicrobial drug products and their use.
6. Encourage the use of single dose packages of sterile drugs in place of multiple dose containers.
7. Work with the microbiology laboratory to improve microbial sensitivity screening tests and the reporting of their results.

Through these and other activities, pharmacists can help reduce the problems of hospital-associated infections to the lowest possible level.

Those pharmacists who feel that they are too busy to undertake these extra-curricular activities soon find that they are excluded from the professional group within the hospital. This is brought about by the fact that the failure to participate in the problems of the hospital and related professions implies that the pharmacist is either not knowledgeable or is uninterested in the welfare of the institution and, indirectly, the patient.

MEMBERSHIP IN PROFESSIONAL ASSOCIATIONS

There are a number of associations which represent the various segments of American pharmacy. Of these, the *American Pharmaceutical Association* purports to represent the profession as a whole; the *American Society of Hospital Pharmacists* represents the hospital pharmacist; the *American College of Apothecaries* speaks for the professional pharmacist; the *National Association of Retail Druggists* represents the retail store owner plus a number of other associations representing manufacturers, wholesalers, colleges of pharmacy and the various scientific disciplines of pharmacy.

The American College of Clinical Pharmacy (ACCP) was founded on October 8, 1979 and is the profession's first formally established organization devoted entirely to the advancement of clinical pharmacy. The goal of this group is to foster the clinical pharmacy movement and promote the clinical pharmacist as an individual who is competent to participate in the decision-making progress of drug therapy.

With the specialization of the practice of hospital pharmacy, numerous specialty organizations have developed and concentrate on areas of the practice. Examples include but are not limited to the American Society of Consultant Pharmacists, the Academy of Pharmaceutical Management and the Society of Veterinary Hospital Pharmacists which was established in 1980.

Certainly, the minimal membership which the hospital pharmacist should hold should be in the *American Pharmaceutical Association* and the *American Society of Hospital Pharmacists.* It is also desirable for him to belong to his regional and local pharmaceutical associations.

Many hospital administrators advocate personal membership in state and national hospital associations. If the pharmacist finds it possible to become a member of these groups, he will not only enhance his professional stature, but will also give himself an opportunity to learn about and understand the problems of his professional associates, thereby better qualifying him for his own position.

It has been stated[1] that approximately 63% of the practicing physicians of the United States belong to the *American Medical Association,* whereas about 20% of the practicing pharmacists belong to the *American Pharmaceutical Association.*

Clearly then the pharmacists of America, and more particularly the hospital pharmacists, must make every effort to strengthen their professional organizations in order that they may provide all branches of pharmacy with the leadership and services essential to a growing profession.

In addition, the mere joining of our professional associations is not sufficient. It is mandatory that, in order to ensure developmental growth of both the individual and the association, each member must take an active role in the sponsored programs and committee assignments.

COOPERATE WITH MEDICAL RESEARCH STAFF

Clinical research, as it is conducted today, requires the cooperation of all of the allied health services. Pharmacy is no exception. The hospital pharmacist can become an integral part of this research in a number of ways.

1. He can be of invaluable assistance to the busy physician by controlling the inventory and distribution of the investigative material.

2. He can maintain an accurate record on the chemistry, pharmacology, posology, and toxicology of the compounds being studied. This information is oftentimes vital to another physician who is called in an emergency to treat a patient who is taking the research drug when the original investigator cannot be located.

3. By suggesting and preparing better vehicles or physical forms of the new compounds undergoing trial.

4. The astute pharmacist will offer to develop and operate a double or triple blind study for the clinical evaluation of the research drug.

5. Because the pharmacist is usually a member of local social or fraternal groups, he is in an excellent position to assist the physician in the recruiting of normal human subjects for controlled *in vivo* studies of investigational use drugs.

COOPERATE WITH LOCAL PHARMACISTS

This phase of the program requires delicate handling on the part of those concerned. Many times the cry is heard from the community practitioner of pharmacy that the hospital pharmacist is not cooperative and is driving him into bankruptcy because of the low prices quoted in hospitals for many medications. This fighting between the ranks is uncalled for and can be eliminated if both parties will learn to cooperate with and not compete against each other.

Some means of cooperation between retailer and hospital pharmacist are as follows: lending each other products, making available from the hospital pharmacy special formula medications, supplying copies of prescriptions when legal restrictions do not apply, and finally, supporting organizations and legislation sponsored by the community pharmacists.

A step in the right direction was taken when the *American Pharmaceutical Association* and the *American Society of Hospital Pharmacists* joined together to create a *Commission to Study Outpatient Hospital Pharmacy Service.*

Among the elements to be studied by the commission will be (1) the hospital pharmacy in essential patient service, (2) the need for the public to have medications dispensed by pharmacists, (3) professional opportunities in community and hospital pharmacy, (4) the effect of the number of community and hospital pharmacies on professional opportunities, (5) effects of location on status, and (6) legal implications.

COOPERATE WITH NURSING STAFF

ASHP AND ANA GUIDELINES FOR COLLABORATION OF PHARMACISTS AND NURSES IN INSTITUTIONAL CARE SETTINGS[a]

This document describes the benefits and responsibilities of pharmacy and nursing collaboration within the institutional setting. The value of this collaborative effort is reflected in the quality of patient care. The responsibilities of the nurse and the pharmacist are to their respective professions; their accountability is to their patients. As members of the health care team, nurses and pharmacists collaborate with other professionals and members of other disciplines. The complexity of drug therapy requires consultation between nurses and pharmacists on a regular basis.

Pharmacists are well acquainted with the complex problems associated with drug therapy and possess knowledge concerning medications that is useful to nurses in providing patient care. Pharmacists' intensive basic and continuing education in drug therapy, practical application of this knowledge, and presence in institutions make them the appropriate health professional to supply drug information. Since nurses are responsible for direct patient care and are in close contact with the patient, they can provide valuable information regarding beneficial and adverse responses to drug therapy.

In order to promote the exchange of information between nurses and pharmacists, the following guidelines are proposed:

1. Orientation for nurses and student nurses to the institution should include introduction to the pharmacy so that the available services can be discussed and demonstrated.
2. Orientation for pharmacists and pharmacy students should include in-

---

[a]Approved by the ASHP Board of Directors on April 21, 1979, and by the ANA Congress for Nursing Practice on July 12, 1979; developed by the Joint Committee of the American Nurses' Association and the American Society of Hospital Pharmacists.

troduction to a patient-care unit so that its services can be discussed and demonstrated.

3. Collaboration between the nurse and the pharmacist should occur on a regular basis whenever either professional is developing a program to which the other can contribute. Interprofessional collaboration should also occur whenever the perceived roles of the professionals overlap, e.g., in patient education, monitoring adverse drug reactions, cardiopulmonary resuscitation, nurse-pharmacist rounds in critical care areas, and nursing care plans.

Nurses equipped with adequate drug information and knowledge of the patient are able to administer drugs properly and detect the occurrence of desirable or undesirable drug effects.

It is important for the pharmacist to work in collaboration with the nurse when medications are administered. The following are examples of information that should be provided to the nurse by the pharmacist:

> Information on new drugs
> Information on investigational drugs used in the institution
> Drug side effects and therapeutic risks
> Contraindications to particular drug therapy
> Compatibility and stability of drugs, including intravenous admixtures
> Drug computations
> Drug metabolism, excretion, and blood level data (and likelihood of a cumulative effect)
> Drug interactions (including drug/drug, drug/food, and laboratory test modifications)
> Effect of patient age and pathophysiology on drug action

Drug information services should include the following:

1. A pharmacist should be available on site or on call 24 hours a day to provide drug information when needed. It is important that nurses have sufficient information to instruct patients in the use of their medications. Telephone communication should be used only if personal contact in the patient-care area cannot take place.
2. The pharmacist should consult with the nurse, preferably by personal contact, in regard to drugs prescribed for specific patients. The information exchange is best provided in the patient-care area, where the pharmacists can obtain patient data from other professionals, the patient, and the patient's record, as well as from the nurse. The pharmacist should record information that is important to the patient's medication regimen in the patient's record. Specific allergies to drugs should be highlighted on the patient's record.
3. Drug information bulletins and newsletters compiled by pharmacists should be distributed to the nursing staff.
4. Each nursing unit should be provided with reference material on drugs, e.g., *American Hospital Formulary Service,* and the staff should be instructed on the efficient use of these resources. A current formulary, accessible in the patient-care area, should be provided and should contain information about drugs used in the institution.
5. Pharmacists should participate with nurses and physicians in review of patients' medications in relation to patient need, therapeutic duplications, and possible drug interactions. This can be done either by making

rounds or jointly reviewing records, including the drug history. The pharmacist should maintain a drug profile, which can be useful in this review.

6. A program of continuing education on drug therapy should be provided by pharmacists in the institution. New information on drugs and information on new drugs should also be provided.

Pharmacists and nurses can both be involved in providing patient education. A collaborative team effort should be made in the development of programs for patient education. Counseling, teaching, and informing patients on their drug therapy should be a part of the patient education program in all institutions.

Communication among health professionals should begin during their educational years. Pharmacy and nursing organizations should offer periodic joint continuing education programs that provide drug information and programming on patient education and other areas where these two professions can share information. As fellow professionals, nurses and pharmacists should strive toward the common goal of quality patient care.

MAINTAIN AN EFFICIENT PROFESSIONAL PHARMACY

A clean, well-organized pharmacy with alert personnel can do much toward the furtherance of professional and public good will. It makes no difference where the pharmacy is located, how old it is, or how little equipment it has; it can still reflect cleanliness, organization, and alertness of personnel. The effect of a good library and reference files and of committee participation has already been discussed.

ACCEPT SPEAKING ENGAGEMENTS

The hospital pharmacist is usually the unseen but essential member of the hospital health team. Patients expect and get his services; however, they seldom if ever get to know anything about the role played by the hospital pharmacist.

Therefore, the public relations aspect of the recommended program can be greatly benefited if the hospital pharmacists will give a part of his free time to the addressing of civic, fraternal, and church organizations.

Another means of creating good professional relations is to be of service to the pharmaceutical manufacturers by accepting invitations to appear on their sales training programs.

It goes almost without saying that hospital pharmacists should welcome a chance to appear on refresher course programs offered by the colleges of pharmacy or on the programs of local, regional or national hospital and pharmaceutical associations.

HOSPITAL PHARMACY DISPLAYS

The old Chinese proverb of "one picture is worth a thousand words" can be readily applied to this part of the program.

A display in the hospital lobby during *National Pharmacy Week* can do a great deal for both public and professional relations. Displays depicting the role of hospital pharmacy in the hospital picture can be of inestimable value when arranged in conjunction with local nursing and medical meetings or conventions.

PARTICIPATION IN COMPREHENSIVE HEALTH CARE PROGRAMS

The preparation and formulation of a health services delivery system designed to meet the legislative and administrative guidelines developed by the Federal Government have been delegated to the local community. In this setting providers of all facets of health care are expected to interface and work cooperatively with the consumer to develop new systems for the delivery of comprehensive medical care at reasonable cost. As a result thereof, programs such as the Regional Medical Programs (RMP), Model Cities Demonstration Act, Health Maintenance Organizations (HMO's), Home Care Services and neighborhood health centers have developed. In July of 1973, the Federal Government introduced Professional Service Review Organizations (PSRO's) and Certificate of Need (CofN) requirements for the review of medical care and utilization and for the determination of need for new facilities, equipment and services. In addition, a number of new prepaid health insurance plans have come upon the scene. Pharmacists, pharmacy as a profession and colleges of pharmacy must be prepared to participate in the planning, organization and operation of these units if pharmacy is to be included in the reimbursement rate for the so-called "comprehensive health care services."[2]

Of primary importance to the institutional pharmacist is the position taken by the American Hospital Association as is evidenced by the following excerpts from its *Statement* on *Health Care for the Disadvantaged:*

"The fullest possible involvement of hospitals in the delivery of community health services is in the best interests both of the citizens of the community and the hospital. It guarantees an improvement in the total fabric of health care."[3]

From the point of view of having an experienced force participate in the planning of community health needs, the *Statement* provides:

"The hospital is the key community center of high quality health services. The hospital, together with its medical staff, is the health resource that has demonstrated great success in assembling sophisticated equipment and expert personnel. It has also encouraged the introduction of the improvement of elements of community control, and internal quality checks, and administrative and organizational knowledge. These factors qualify it to assume leadership in improving health care for all, rich and poor, urban and rural."[3]

Although it is not possible to provide the student with a detailed discussion of all of the concepts for providing comprehensive health care to all Americans, it is important to touch upon some of the better known and utilized plans. In this connection, the American people have decided that the right to optimal health care is necessary for all people to enjoy their constitutional right to life, liberty, and the pursuit of happiness. To achieve this, a great deal of thought and study went into various methodologies and there merged a general consensus that the ideal health system should achieve the following goals:[4]

   a. Accessibility.
   b. Availability.
   c. Acceptability to the consumer and provider.
   d. Phased implementation, assuring that the system is able to accept the increased demand before money is poured into health care.
   e. Minimal government regulation.
   f. Consumer participation in the cost and in the organization of services.
   g. Quality assurance.
   h. Cost predictability.

HEALTH MAINTENANCE ORGANIZATIONS

On February 18, 1971, President Richard M. Nixon delivered a special message to the Congress titled "Building a National Health Strategy." In it he stated:[5]

"In recent years, a new method for delivering health services has achieved growing respect. This new approach has two essential attributes. It brings together a comprehensive range of medical services in a single organization so that a patient is assured of convenient access to all of them. And it provides needed services for a fixed contract fee which is paid in advance by all subscribers."

"Such an organization can have a variety of forms and names and sponsors. One of the strengths of this new concept, in fact, is its greater flexibility. The general term which has been applied to all of these units is 'HMO'—Health Maintenance Organizations."

The term "Health Maintenance Organization" or "HMO" was coined by Dr. Paul M. Elwood, Jr. in a January 1970 meeting with federal officials considering ways and means to contain the $2 billion cost overrun in Medicare and Medicaid programs.

Thus, it is clear that a Health Maintenance Organization (HMO) is based upon four principles:[5]

   a. "It is an *organized system* of health care which assures the delivery of
   b. "an agreed upon set of *comprehensive health maintenance* and *treatment services* for
   c. "a voluntarily *enrolled group* of persons in a geographic area and
   d. "is reimbursed through a pre-negotiated and fixed periodic payment made by or on behalf of each person or family unit enrolled in the plan."

Each of these principles should be more fully defined and described.

An *organized system* of health care is one that is capable of bringing together directly, or arranging for, the services of physicians and other health professionals with the services of inpatient and outpatient facilities for preventive, acute, and other care, as well as any other health services which a defined population might reasonably require. The system is organized in such a way as to assure for the enrollee the most efficient and effective entry into the health care system. In addition, it arranges for continuity of care for the enrollees through linkages between the components of the system via the utilization of a single medical record.

Comprehensive health maintenance and treatment services means that the HMO is capable of providing or arranging for the provision of the health services that a population of enrollees might require, including primary care, emergency care, acute inpatient hospital care, and inpatient and outpatient care and rehabilitation for chronic and disabling conditions.

An agreed upon set of services means that the consumers and the HMO will agree upon which services will be purchased from the HMO in return for the pre-payment figure. Since some HMO's may have groups of enrollees paid for by Medicare or Medicaid, or by employer-employee arrangements, the benefit schedule for various groups within an HMO may differ.

The *enrolled group* means those individuals or groups of people who voluntarily join the HMO through a contract arrangement in which the enrollee agrees to pay the fixed monthly or other periodic payment (or have it paid on his behalf) to the HMO. The enrollee agrees to use the HMO as his principal source of health care. The contract is for a specified period of time—usually a year.

An HMO can be organized and sponsored by either a medical foundation (usually organized by physicians), by community groups who bring together various interested leaders or organizations, by labor unions, by a governmental unit, by a profit or non-profit group allied with an insurance company (Blue Cross) or some other financing institution. The HMO may be hospital-based, medical school-based, or be a freestanding outpatient facility or group of such facilities.

CONTINUING CARE SERVICE—HOME CARE SERVICE

In addition to being responsible for inpatient care, the hospital must also help to provide a matrix in which seemingly disparate parts of the health care rendered can be linked into an organic whole—a health care network. Thus, hospitals, particularly those in the medical center setting, have developed continuing care and home care services.

The Continuing Care Service is the link between the hospital, nursing home, extended care facility or rehabilitation facility. At times, it can include the patient's home. The service generally plans for the range of continuing care needs of patients after discharge from the hospital.

The Home Care Service provides continuing medical care of the patient when he has been discharged to his home. Such a service coordinates the activities of the patient's physician and the visiting nurse and brings into the home environment the services of the dietitian and social service workers.

DRUG REHABILITATION PROGRAMS

Because of the widespread abuse of drugs, this area of endeavor is quite popular on the community front. Accordingly, participation in these programs by the individual who knows most about drugs—the pharmacist—is mandatory in order to preserve good public and professional relations. In addition to drug abuse educational programs, the pharmacist should encourage these members of the program to study and participate in the following areas:

a. Drug abuse problems treated in the hospital.
b. Legal and ethical issues involved in treating drug abuse.
c. Medical and psychiatric approaches to the treatment of drug abuse.
d. Problems associated with detoxification, especially with concurrent medical or surgical disease.
e. The use of various drugs in detoxification programs.
f. Drug abuse treatment programs in the urban and suburban areas served by the hospital.

DRUG CONSULTATION PROGRAMS

One study on the significance of drug consultation programs conducted by pharmacists to the discharged hospital patient concluded that discharged patients who had such consultation showed less deviation from prescribed drug regimens and had fewer medication problems at home than did patients who had not been accorded this service.[6]

Obviously, drug consultation programs are important from the point of view of patient safety, however, a great deal of good public relations benefit can accrue to the hospital from this professional practice.

In discussing drug therapy with the patient, the following points are recommended for discussion by Cole and Emanuel:[6]

1. "Determination of medication already being taken which may duplicate or interfere with newly prescribed medications.
2. The optimum dosage administration schedule to be followed.
3. Measures to be taken in the management of side effects of the prescribed medications.
4. The importance of administering all doses of the medications as prescribed."

CONTINUING EDUCATION PROGRAMS

It is recognized and accepted that the modern day health care professionals must continually update their basic education in order to provide safe and skillful care to their patients. Continuing education has been mandated by professional organizations and some regulatory bodies for re-licensure. Therefore, the program content of many institutes, conventions and seminars carries continuing education unit credits which the individual must submit to the regulatory agency in order to satisfy the re-licensure requirement. Currently, not all jurisdictions require pharmacists to participate in continuing educational programs as a pre-requisite for re-licensure; nonetheless, most hospital and clinical pharmacists voluntarily participate.

The American Society of Hospital Pharmacists has been a major provider of continuing educational programs for the hospital practitioner. In recognition of its obligation to its membership, the Society has enunciated its commitment to continuing education in the following **ASHP Statement on Continuing Education:**[8]

ASHP STATEMENT ON CONTINUING EDUCATION[a]

Next to integrity, competence is the first and most fundamental moral responsibility of all the health professions. . . . Each of our professions must insist that competence will be reinforced through the years of practice. After the degree is conferred, continuing ed-

[a]Approved by the ASHP Board of Directors, November 14–15, 1977, and by the ASHP House of Delegates, May 15, 1978. Supersedes the Statement dated December 2–3, 1971.

ucation is society's only real guarantee of the optimal quality of
health care.

—Edmund D. Pellegrino

Preamble

In an era of rapidly accelerating change in health care delivery, the roles of
institutional pharmacy practitioners are being constantly redefined. As roles
change, competency requirements change, and as institutional pharmacy practitioners assume the increased responsibilities demanded in these new roles,
they must make a corresponding commitment to improve their professional
competence. Continuing education is the primary means by which practitioners
can gain the knowledge and skills necessary to maintain and improve their
performance.

The purpose of continuing education for health professionals is the improvement of patient care and health maintenance and the enrichment of health
careers. Every institutional pharmacist should set for himself personal educational objectives based upon his needs for performance improvement and
his career goals. He should attempt to achieve these objectives through continuing education experiences judiciously selected from among area, regional
and national resources which most effectively serve his needs. While every
practitioner should assume personal responsibility for maintaining and improving professional competence through life-long, self-directed education, he
may often require assistance in identifying gaps between actual and desired
performance, in setting educational objectives and establishing their relative
priorities, and in selecting learning activities which will contribute most toward
achieving the objectives. It should be the role of the Society to facilitate the
efforts of the institutional pharmacist in his self-directed education.

Objectives

The objectives of the continuing education program of the American Society
of Hospital Pharmacists shall be:

1. To help institutional pharmacists develop a more complete understanding
   of the importance and methods of life-long, self-directed education and
   to encourage and assist them toward this goal;
2. To help institutional practitioners evaluate their professional performance, identify areas where improvement is needed, and set realistic, attainable educational goals;
3. To provide to practitioners information on available area, regional and
   national educational resources which will help achieve their personal
   educational objectives;
4. To assist institutional pharmacists in selecting educational resources
   which fulfill most effectively their individual needs;
5. To provide to pharmacists continuing education resources in a variety of
   formats and media best suited for the subject matter and the needs of the
   greatest number of learners; and
6. To assist pharmacists in evaluating the effectiveness of their continuing
   education experiences.

Implementation

To achieve the foregoing objectives, the Society recognizes the necessity to
develop appropriate procedures which identify the real educational needs of

practitioners, based upon expected or acceptable standards of performance. The Society also recognizes that such standards, expressed in terms of observable and measurable behaviors, do not now exist. Therefore, it will be a long-range goal of the Society to work toward the development of standards of performance for institutional pharmacy practitioner, based upon the competencies expected of them. Concomitantly, the Society will also seek to develop effective methods of assisting practitioners in assessing their personal professional educational needs through self-evaluation.

Authority

The continuing education program of the American Society of Hospital Pharmacists is established by the authority of its Board of Directors under the direction of the Council on Education and Manpower. All matters of policy relating to this program will be considered by the Council on Education and Manpower and will be submitted to the Board of Directors of the Society for approval.

Policies

The following policies will guide the development and conduct of the continuing education programs and activities of the American Society of Hospital Pharmacists, including classroom, self-study and other formats, where applicable:

1. Continuing education programs will be planned and conducted in accordance with the Criteria for Quality of the Continuing Education Provider Approval Program of the American Council on Pharmaceutical Education.
2. Continuing education activities will be cost justified. The Society's overall continuing education program is intended to be self-supporting.
3. The Society may limit or restrict the enrollment for any continuing education program, depending upon the nature and requirements of the particular program.
4. The Society will collaborate, when appropriate, with other professional organizations, agencies, and educational institutions in the planning and conduct of continuing education activities.
5. The Society will maintain close liaison with affiliated chapters and other institutional pharmacy groups in the planning and conduct of continuing education activities.
6. When appropriate, due consideration will be given to the multidisciplinary approach in the planning and conduct of continuing education activities.

SUMMARY

The points and the program that have been discussed are basic signs that can be followed on the road to better professional relations between all branches of the medical profession and the laymen.

Better understanding, however, achieved, always leads to better and mutual respect.

A better program of professional relations will help us as pharmacists to better serve the needs of humanity. Perhaps the great Dr. Albert Schweitzer summed up what should be our real objective when he said:

"I do not know what your destiny will be, but one thing I do know: The only people who will be really happy are those who will have sought and found how to serve."

SELECTED READINGS

McKenzie, M.W.: Communicating With Patients. Tomorrow's Pharmacist, 5:2:4, (Jan.–Feb.) 1984.
Schendt, R.L.: Pharmacy Ethics in the '80s. Curr. Concepts in Hosp. Pharm. Management, 5:1:16, 1983.

REFERENCES

1. Walsh, R.A. and Hassan, W.E.: A 14 Point Program for Promoting Professional and Public Relations by the Hospital Pharmacist. The Bulletin Am. Soc. Hosp. Pharm., 13:4:315, 1956.
2. Emanuel, Sr., D.C. and Barr, Martin: The Role of Wayne State University College of Pharmacy in the Development of an Innovative and Comprehensive Health Care Program. J.D. Ph.A., NS11:10:551, 1971.
3. ———: Statement of Health Care for the Disadvantaged 5-60. American Hospital Association, Chicago, Illinois 60611 (1970).
4. Ainsworth, Thomas H., Jr.: The Significance of the HMO Concept to Hospitals and to the Hospital System, M.H.A. Newsletter Supplement, Vol. XXIII No. 2, February 1972, Massachusetts Hospital Association, Burlington, Massachusetts 01803.
5. ———: Health Maintenance Organizations, The Concept and Structure, U.S. Dept. of Health, Education and Welfare, Health Services and Mental Health Administration, 5600 Fishers Lane, Rockville, Md. 20852.
6. Cole, Philip and Emanuel, Sr.: Drug Consultation: Its Significance to the Discharged Hospital Patient and Its Relevance as a Role for the Pharmacist. Am. J. Hosp. Pharm., 28:12:954, 1971.
7. ASHP Statement on the Hospital Pharmacist's Role in Infection Control. Am. J. Hosp. Pharm., 35:814–815, (Jul.) 1978.
8. ASHP Statement on Continuing Education. Am. J. Hosp. Pharm., 35:815–816, (Jul.) 1978.

INDEX

Page numbers in *italics* indicate figures.

671